High Risk
Pregnancy and Deli

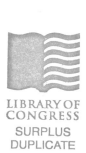

High Risk Pregnancy and Delivery

Second Edition

Editor-in-Chief
Hemant Deshpande MD
Professor and Head
Department of Obstetrics and Gynecology
Dr DY Patil Medical College and Hospital
Dr DY Patil Vidyapeeth (Deemed to be University)
Pune, Maharashtra, India

Associate Editor
Priyanka A Dahiya MD
Assistant Professor
Department of Obstetrics and Gynecology
Kalpana Chawla Government Medical College
Karnal, Haryana, India

Foreword
Sir Sabaratnam Arulkumaran

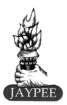

JAYPEE BROTHERS MEDICAL PUBLISHERS
The Health Sciences Publisher
New Delhi | London

Jaypee Brothers Medical Publishers (P) Ltd

Headquarters

Jaypee Brothers Medical Publishers (P) Ltd
EMCA House, 23/23-B
Ansari Road, Daryaganj
New Delhi 110 002, India
Landline: +91-11-23272143, +91-11-23272703
+91-11-23282021, +91-11-23245672
Email: jaypee@jaypeebrothers.com

Corporate Office

Jaypee Brothers Medical Publishers (P) Ltd
4838/24, Ansari Road, Daryaganj
New Delhi 110 002, India
Phone: +91-11-43574357
Fax: +91-11-43574314
Email: jaypee@jaypeebrothers.com

Overseas Office

JP Medical Ltd
83 Victoria Street, London
SW1H 0HW (UK)
Phone: +44 20 3170 8910
Fax: +44 (0)20 3008 6180
Email: info@jpmedpub.com

Website: www.jaypeebrothers.com
Website: www.jaypeedigital.com

Inquiries for bulk sales may be solicited at: jaypee@jaypeebrothers.com

High Risk Pregnancy and Delivery

First Edition: 2011

Second Edition: **2021**

ISBN: 978-93-90020-81-2

Printed at: Samrat Offset Pvt. Ltd.

Contributors

Achanta Vivekanand
Professor and Head
Department of Obstetrics and Gynecology
Prathima Institute of Medical Sciences
Karimnagar, Telangana, India

Ambarisha Bhandiwad
Ex-Professor and Head
Department of Obstetrics and Gynecology
JSS Medical College
Mysuru, Karnataka, India

Amol Agarwal
Senior Consultant and
Interventional Cardiologist
Sterling Hospitals, Ahmedabad
Director
Aditya Heart Clinic
Ahmedabad, Gujarat, India

Amrita Chaurasia
Professor and Head
Department of Obstetrics and Gynecology
Moti Lal Nehru Medical College
Allahabad, Uttar Pradesh, India

Anjali Deshpande
Department of Pathology
Dr DY Patil Medical College
Pune, Maharashtra, India

Ashok Kumar Behera
Ex-Professor and Head
Department of Obstetrics and Gynecology
MKCG Medical College
Berhampur, Odisha, India

Ashok Kumar
Director-Professor
Department of Obstetrics and Gynecology
Dr Ram Manohar Lohia Hospital
New Delhi, India

BS Jodha
Professor
Department of Obstetrics and Gynecology
Sampurnanand (SN) Medical College
Jodhpur, Rajasthan, India

Chandrakant Madkar
Professor
Department of Obstetrics and Gynecology
Dr DY Patil Medical College
Pune, Maharashtra, India

Deepa Lokwani Masand
Professor and Head
Department of Obstetrics and Gynecology
National Institute of Medical Sciences and Research
(NIMS)
Jaipur, Rajasthan, India

Hara P Pattanaik
Joint Director
Health Services, Odisha
Consultant Gynecologist and Laparoscopic Surgeon
Cuttack, Odisha, India

Haresh U Doshi
Professor and Head
Department of Obstetrics and Gynecology
GCS Medical College
Ahmedabad, Gujarat, India

Hemant Deshpande
Professor and Head
Department of Obstetrics and Gynecology
Dr DY Patil Medical College and Hospital
Dr DY Patil Vidyapeeth (Deemed to be University)
Pune, Maharashtra, India

Hemant Talnikar
Professor
Department of Dermatology
Dr DY Patil Medical College
Pune, Maharashtra, India

Hiralal Konar
Professor and Head
Department of Obstetrics and Gynecology
Government Medical College and GB Pant Hospital
Agartala, Tripura, India

Janki Pandya
Assistant Professor
Department of Obstetrics and Gynecology
AMC MET Medical College and Sheth LG Hospital
Ahmedabad, Gujarat, India

Jayanti Reddy
Professor and Head
Department of Obstetrics and Gynecology
SVS Medical College
Mahabubnagar, Telangana, India

JB Sharma
Professor
Department of Obstetrics and Gynecology
All India Institute of Medical Sciences
New Delhi, India

Kishor Rajurkar
Head, Department of Obstetrics and Gynecology
Sanjay Gandhi Memorial Hospital
New Delhi, India

Madhukar Shinde
Associate Professor
Department of Obstetrics and Gynecology
Dr DY Patil Medical College
Pune, Maharashtra, India

Manjula S Patil
Consulting Obstetrician and Gynecologist
Bengaluru, Karnataka, India

Minnu M Panditrao
Professor and Head
Department of Anesthesiology
Adesh Medical College
Bathinda, Punjab, India

Mridul M Panditrao
Professor and Head
Department of Anesthesiology and Critical Care
Aadesh Medical College, Bathinda, Punjab, India

Munjal Pandya
Assistant Professor
Department of Obstetrics and Gynecology
AMC MET Medical College
Sheth Lallubhai Gordhandas Municipal General Hospital
Ahmedabad, Gujarat, India

Niharika Dhiman
Associate Professor
Department of Obstetrics and Gynecology
Maulana Azad Medical College
New Delhi, India

Nilesh Balkawde
Consultant, Obstetrician and Gynecologist
and Laparoscopic Surgeon
Oasis IVF, Pune, Maharashtra, India

Nitin S Kshirsagar
Professor
Department of Obstetrics and Gynecology
Krishna Institute of Medical Sciences
Karad, Maharashtra, India

N Palaniappan
Professor
Department of Obstetrics and Gynecology
Sri Ramchandra Medical College
Tamil Nadu, Chennai, India

Pankaj Desai
Dean (Students) and Associate Professor (VRS)
Department of Obstetrics and Gynecology
Medical College and SSG Hospital
Baroda, Gujarat, India

Prakash Mehta
Consulting High Risk Pregnancy Specialist
Bhagwan Mahaveer Jain Hospital
Bengaluru, Karnataka, India

Pralhad Kushtagi
Professor
Department of Obstetrics and Gynecology
Kasturba Medical College
Mangaluru, Karnataka, India

Priya Ballal
Professor and Head
Department of Obstetrics and Gynecology
Kasturba Medical College
Mangaluru, Karnataka, India

Priyanka A Dahiya
Assistant Professor
Department of Obstetrics and Gynecology
Kalpana Chawla Government Medical College
Karnal, Haryana, India

Rajendra P Shitole
Assistant Professor
Department of Obstetrics and Gynecology
Dr DY Patil Medical College
Pune, Maharashtra, India

Raju V Giraddi
Consultant
Department of Obstetrician and Gynecologist
Raichur, Karnataka, India

Ritu Sharma
Associate Professor
Department of Obstetrics and Gynecology
Government Institute of Medical Science
Greater Noida, Uttar Pradesh, India

RP Rawat
Professor and Head
Department of Obstetrics and Gynecology
Government Medical College
Kota, Rajasthan, India

Sanjana Kumar
Department of Obstetrics and Gynecology
Karnataka Institute of Medical Sciences
Hubli, Karnataka, India

S Habeebullah
Professor
Department of Obstetrics and Gynecology
MGM Medical College, Puducherry, India

Shailaja Mane
Professor (Pediatrics)
Dr DY Patil Medical College
Pune, Maharashtra, India

Shashwat Jani
Assistant Professor
Department of Obstetrics and Gynecology
Smt NHL Municipal Medical College
Ahmedabad, Gujarat, India

Shikha Seth
Professor and Head
Department of Obstetrics and Gynecology
Government Institute of Medical Sciences (GIMS)
Greater Noida, Uttar Pradesh, India

Shilpa Chaudhari
Professor
Department of Obstetrics and Gynecology
Smt. Kashibai Navale Medical College
Pune, Maharashtra, India

Shipra Kunwar
Professor and Head
Department of Obstetrics and Gynecology
ERA Medical College
Agra, Uttar Pradesh, India

Shubharanjan Smantarai
Associate Professor
Department of Obstetrics and Gynecology
Prathima Institute of Medical Sciences
Karimnagar, Telangana, India

S Manikyarao
Professor and Head
Department of Obstetrics and Gynecology
Kurnool Medical College
Kurnool, Andhra Pradesh, India

Sonali Deshpande
Professor
Department of Obstetrics and Gynecology
Government Medical College
Aurangabad, Maharashtra, India

Srinivas Krishna Jois
Associate Professor
Department of Obstetrics and Gynecology
Bangalore Medical College and Research Institute
Bengaluru, Karnataka, India

Sujatha Patnaik
Associate Professor
Department of Obstetrics and Gynecology
Andhra Medical College
Visakhapatnam, Andhra Pradesh, India

Suman Mittal
Professor
Department of Obstetrics and Gynecology
Sawai Man Singh (SMS) Medical College
Jaipur, Rajasthan, India

Sumitra Yadav
Professor
Department of Obstetrics and Gynecology
Mahatma Gandhi Memorial (MGM) Medical College and
MY Group of Hospitals
Indore, Madhya Pradesh, India

Suyajna Joshi D
Head
Department of Obstetrics and Gynecology
District Civil Hospital
Bellary, Karnataka, India

Vandana Kanumury
Professor and Head
Department of Obstetrics and Gynecology
ASRAM Medical College
Eluru, Andhra Pradesh, India

Veena Ranjan
Professor
Department of Obstetrics and Gynecology
Kasturba Medical College
Manipal, Karnataka, India

Virendra Kumar CM
Professor
Department of Obstetrics and Gynecology
Vijayanagar Institute of Medical Sciences
Bellary, Karnataka, India

Vidya Gaikwad
Professor
Department of Obstetrics and Gynecology
Dr DY Patil Medical College
Pune, Maharashtra, India

Vidya Thobbi
Professor and Head
Department of Obstetrics and Gynecology
Al-Ameen Medical College
Bijapur, Karnataka, India

Yukti Wadhawan
Consultant Gynecologist
LaOrigin IVF
New Delhi, India

Foreword

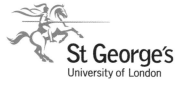

Medicine, Biomedical Sciences, Health and Social Care Science
Cranmer Terrace
London SW17 0RE
e-mail;sarulkum@sgul.ac.uk
Direct
+44 7710470270
www.sgul.ac.uk
Sir Sabaratnam Arulkumaran PhD DSc FRCS FRCOG
Professor Emeritus of Obstetrics & Gynaecology
Room 1.126, First Floor Jenner Wing

I am delighted to provide the foreword for this excellent textbook on *High Risk Pregnancy and Delivery* edited by Professor Hemant Deshpande. He does not need an introduction to the maternity care audience. I had the privilege of lecturing alongside him in conferences and listened to his clear dispensation of the subject with organized thought process. This ability is reflected in the editorial process in producing this textbook. This book with 52 chapters provides a comprehensive cover of all the topics in 'High Risk Pregnancy' that one should know. The book starts with problems of various types of anemia followed by endocrine, medical, obstetric and infective disorders encountered in managing any pregnancy. The final chapters deal with difficult and complex problems of managing a pregnancy after solid organ transplant and oncofertility and pregnancy after malignancy. There are special chapters on Intensive Care and Human Milk Banking. With such an extensive coverage the readers can get the knowledge needed in 'High Risk Pregnancy' from this one dedicated textbook alone.

I must congratulate the well-renowned authors who have tackled each of the subjects well. The designation of authors indicate that almost all of them are senior Professors and Heads of departments. Accordingly the chapter not only reflect the evidence-based practice but also provides suggestions based on their wisdom of experience. The chapters are well-written and comprehensively illustrated with figures, photographs and imaging pictures. There are tables and algorithms and important points given in concise bullet format. This makes it easy for the readers to understand and remember the subject. The chapters have the recent references that provides the readers with the up-to-date knowledge.

This textbook should be in the hands of every health professional who practices obstetrics/maternity care. It is a valuable asset to postgraduates and clinicians at consultant level. Special credit must be given to Professor Hemant Deshpande who has undertaken the great effort in bringing this book for the health care personal to serve our patients better.

Yours sincerely

Sir Sabaratnam Arulkumaran
Past President of the RCOG (07-10), FIGO (12-15) and BMA (14-15)

Acknowledgments

We are especially thankful to Shri Jitendar P Vij (Group Chairman), Mr Ankit Vij (Managing Director), Mr MS Mani (Group President), Ms Chetna Malhotra Vohra (Associate Director—Content Strategy), Ms Pooja Bhandari (Production Head), Dr Rajul Jain (Development Editor) and the publishing staff at Jaypee Brothers Medical Publishers (P) Ltd, New Delhi, India, for their work in completing this book successfully.

Contents

CHAPTER 1

Iron-deficiency Anemia in Pregnancy

Suyajna Joshi D

INTRODUCTION

Anemia is the most common hematological disorder in pregnancy which has significant maternal as well as perinatal morbidity and mortality. Anemia among pregnant women is a serious global health concern. According to the World Health Organization (WHO) report, about million pregnant women suffer from anemia worldwide, of which 0.8 million women are severely anemic. An estimate by the WHO attributes about 591,000 maternal deaths globally to iron-deficiency anemia (IDA), directly or indirectly. Majority of the cases of anemia in pregnancy are due to nutritional deficiency of which >50% cases are attributable to IDA followed by folate and vitamin B_{12} deficiency. Other causes such as hemoglobinopathies, autoimmune hemolytic anemia, aplastic anemia, chronic infections, rheumatoid arthritis, and chronic renal disease, though less commonly found, should arouse suspicion in the clinician based on symptomatology for the better management of the case.

DEFINITION

Anemia is defined as a decrease in the oxygen-carrying capacity of the blood due to a decrease in the hemoglobin concentration or due to a reduced number of red blood cells (RBCs).

CLASSIFICATION OF ANEMIA

Anemia is classified based on etiology (**Box 1**), severity (**Table 1**), and trimester (**Table 2**).

IRON METABOLISM

Iron is an essential component of every cell in the body. Although best known for its critical role in the transport and storage of oxygen (in hemoglobin and myoglobin, respectively), within a large variety of enzymes, iron also acts as a carrier for electrons, a catalyst for oxygenation and hydroxylation, and is necessary for cellular growth and proliferation. Iron supplements are widely administered to treat IDA, particularly in chronic diseases such as kidney disease, heart failure, or inflammatory bowel disease. Without a sufficient supply of iron, hemoglobin cannot be synthesized and the number of erythrocytes in the blood cannot be maintained at an adequate level.

Iron usually exists in the ferrous (Fe^{2+}) or ferric (Fe^{3+}) state, but since Fe^{2+} is readily oxidized to Fe^{3+}, which in

BOX 1: Classification of anemia based on etiology.

- Anemia with nutritional deficiency
  - Iron-deficiency
  - Folic acid deficiency
  - Vitamin B_{12} deficiency
  - Combined deficiency
- Anemia associated with decreased production of RBC
  - Bone marrow disorders
  - Hypothyroidism
  - Chronic renal pathology
  - Bone marrow suppression
- Anemia associated with increased RBCs' destruction
  - Hemolytic anemias
    - Inherited and acquired
    - Sickle cell anemia
    - Thalassemia
  - Hereditary spherocytosis
    - Autoimmune hemolytic anemia
  - Hemolytic uremic syndrome
    - Thrombotic thrombocytopenic purpura
    - Malaria
- Anemia due to blood loss
  - Abnormal uterine bleeding
  - GIT bleeding
  - Obstetric hemorrhage

TABLE 1: Classification of anemia according to severity.

Category of anemia	WHO (Hb in g/dL)	ICMR (Hb in g/d)
Mild	9–10.9	10–11
Moderate	7–8.9	7–10
Severe	4–6.9	4–7
Very severe	<4	<4

(Hb: hemoglobin; ICMR: Indian Council of Medical Research; WHO: World Health Organization)

TABLE 2: Classification of anemia according to trimester.

Pregnancy state	Hemoglobin (g/dL)
First trimester	<11
Second trimester	<10.5
Third trimester	<11

neutral aqueous solutions rapidly hydrolyzes to insoluble iron(III)—hydroxides, iron is transported and stored bound to proteins. Effective binding of iron is essential not only to ensure that it is available where and when required, but also because Fe^{2+} can catalyze the formation of reactive oxygen species, which cause oxidative stress, damaging cellular constituents.

Total body Fe in man is 4–5 g. Daily losses, e.g., in epithelial desquamation from the gastrointestinal tract or skin, are small. Excretion in urine, bile, and sweat is negligible. The normal daily Fe requirement is thus only 1 mg, increasing with physiological need, as in growth, pregnancy, and blood loss. An additional 1,000 mg Fe is required in pregnancy and 0.5 mg Fe/mL in case of blood loss.

Three key proteins regulate the transport and storage of iron **(Fig. 1)**. Transferrin transports iron in the plasma and the extracellular fluid. The transferrin receptor, expressed by cells that require iron and present in their membranes, binds the transferrin di-iron complex and internalizes it into the cell. Ferritin is an iron-storage protein that sequesters iron keeping it in a readily available form. About 60% of iron is found in the erythrocytes within hemoglobin, the oxygen transport protein. The remainder is found in myoglobin in the muscles, in a variety of different enzymes ("heme" and "non-heme"), and in storage form. Most stored iron is in the form of ferritin, found in the liver, bone marrow, spleen, and muscles. Serum iron (i.e., iron bound to transferrin) represents only a very small proportion of the total body iron (<0.2%). Moreover, the relationship between physiological iron compartments is highly dynamic: Erythrocytes are broken down in the liver and the spleen and new red blood cells are produced in the bone marrow. The total serum iron pool is approximately 4 mg, but the normal daily turnover is not >30 mg, such that minor changes in the serum level due to exogenous iron administration are clinically meaningless. In this setting, conventional measurements of serum iron concentration provide no relevant information about the availability of functional iron for physiological processes, and other evaluation strategies must be pursued. A schematic representation of iron metabolism is shown in **Figure 1**.

■ IRON-DEFICIENCY ANEMIA

Iron is essential for normal hemoglobin (Hb) synthesis to maintain oxygen transport as well as necessary for metabolism and synthesis of DNA and enzymatic processes. Iron stores may be measured using several indices, although serum ferritin and transferrin saturation are the most common.

Iron-deficiency anemia is defined as a low Hb concentration in combination with iron-deficiency and is characterized by a defect in Hb synthesis, resulting in abnormally small (microcytic) red blood cells with a decreased Hb content (hypochromic), resulting in reduced capacity of the blood to deliver oxygen. The prevalence of Fe deficiency is much higher. Without adequate Fe supplementation, ferritin falls to subnormal levels toward the end of pregnancy, even in the industrialized nations.

Iron-deficiency anemia evolves through three distinct stages **(Table 3)**. Depletion of storage iron occurs in the first phase (stage I), where total body iron is decreased but red cell indices and hemoglobin (Hb) synthesis remain unchanged. Both these indices change when the supply of

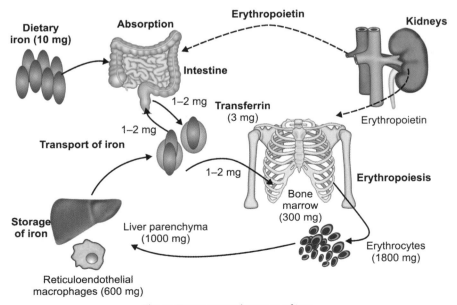

Fig. 1: Transport and storage of iron.

TABLE 3: Stages in the development of iron-deficiency.

Parameters	Normal	Iron depletion	Iron-deficient erythropoiesis	IDA
Hemoglobin	150 g/L (15 g%)	130 g/L (13 g%)	100 g/L (10 g%)	50 g/L (5 gm%)
MCV	N	↓	↓	↓↓
MCHC	N	N	↓	↓↓
Iron stores	Present	Reduced	Absent	Absent
Serum Fe/TIBC (μg/L)	1,000/3,000	75/3,000	500/4,500	250/6,000
Serum ferritin (μg/L)	100	20	10	<10
RBCs	Normal	Normal	Normal	Hypochromic microcytosis

(IDA: iron-deficiency anemia; MCHC: mean corpuscular hemoglobin concentration; MCV: mean corpuscular volume; RBC: red blood cells; TIBC: total iron-binding capacity)

iron to bone marrow is reduced (stage II or iron-deficient erythropoiesis). Stage III, eventually iron-deficiency anemia develops due to insufficient supply of iron to sustain a normal Hb concentration.

Signs and Symptoms of Iron-deficiency Anemia

Although the Hb test is recommended at the first antenatal visit, examination for signs of pallor of the palpebral conjunctiva, tongue, nail beds, and palm should be regularly done. Some iron-deficient patients, with or without clinical signs of anemia, may have alopecia, atrophy of lingual papillae, or dry mouth due to reduced salivation.

The symptoms specific to iron-deficiency anemia include the syndrome of Plummer–Vinson or Paterson–Kelly (dysphagia with esophageal membrane and atrophic glossitis), gastric atrophy, stomatitis due to rapidly turning over of epithelial cells, spoon-shaped nails (koilonychias), and pallor. These changes were caused by the reduction of iron-containing enzymes in epithelial and gastrointestinal (GI) tracts. The restless leg syndrome might be striking neurological squeal prevalent in pregnancy. Pica, the eating disorder in which there is an appealing desire to lick or eat nonfood items such as gypsum, chalk, soil, ice (pagophagia), or paper, is prevalent in pregnant women. Pagophagia (intense desire to eat ice) is quite specific to Iron-deficiency and responds quickly to treatment.

Diagnosis of Iron-deficiency Anemia

There are four groups of tests which are available for detection of IDA:

1. Hb, mean corpuscular volume (MCV), red cell distribution width (RDW), reticulocyte Hb content, % hypochromic cells, red cell size factor, and low Hb density
2. Direct measurements of iron stores through assessment of serum iron, total iron-binding capacity (TIBC), % saturation, serum ferritin, bone marrow biopsy iron
3. Assessment of iron heme form through assessment of free erythrocyte protoporphyrin (EPP)
4. Assessment of iron uptake by measuring the soluble serum transferrin receptor (sTfR), soluble transferrin receptor-log[ferritin] (sTfR-F) index, and zinc protoporphyrin (ZPP)

A primary step in the diagnosis of IDA is to consider the complete blood count, including Hb, MCV, mean corpuscular hemoglobin (MCH), and mean corpuscular hemoglobin concentration (MCHC), which is simple, inexpensive, rapid to perform, and help early prediction of IDA.

Changes in Hb concentration and hematocrit occur only in later stages; both these tests are indicators of Iron-deficiency. Low Hb with a reduced MCV is usually the initial finding on a routine complete blood count (CBC). The severity of anemia is based on the patient's Hb/hematocrit level.

Altitude above sea level and smoking are the known modifiers of Hb. Currently, the Hb cut-off according to trimester has not been defined by the WHO, but it should be recognized that the Hb falls about 0.5 g/dL in the second trimester. Hb concentration is the most common hematological estimation. There is a strong correlation between Hb concentration and serum ferritin levels. The generally recommended methods of Hb estimation are cyanomethemoglobin and HemoCue@ system. RDW has better sensitivity than MCV for diagnosis of IDA. Falling MCV accompanied by a rising RDW should alert the clinician to the presence of possible IDA which is then confirmed by marked RDW increase occurring early after initiation of therapy.

Peripheral smear shows the presence of microcytic hypochromic red cells and typical "photo pencil cells" being indicative of IDA. Other than IDA, the conditions which cause a microcytic blood picture are anemia of chronic disorder, beta-thalassemia, and sideroblastic anemia.

Of all the available indices, the Meltzer index (MCV/RBC) has been shown as the most reliable index with high sensitivity.

A fall in serum ferritin concentration below 15 µg/L indicates iron depletion in all stages of pregnancy. However, treatment needs to be initiated when the concentration falls below 30 µg/L as this indicates early iron depletion.

In order to make definitive diagnosis, bone marrow biopsy should be considered, when the diagnosis remains ambiguous even after the analysis of laboratory results. The "gold standard" for the diagnosis of IDA is absence of stainable iron.

Prophylactic Measures to Prevent Iron-deficiency Anemia in Pregnancy

To combat the high prevalence of IDA, several government programs and state-level schemes were rolled out in various states of India. The National Nutritional Anaemia Prophylaxis Programme (1970), National Anaemia Control Programme (1991), and 12-by-12 Initiative (2007) are some of the nationwide initiatives.

Few state-specific schemes include Madilu Scheme, Thayibhagya Scheme, and Janani Suraksha Yojana. In spite of government's persistent and prolonged efforts, the problem continues to fester as is documented by recent surveys: National Family Health Survey 4 (NFHS-4, 2015–2016) which shows that the prevalence is 23.6–61.4%. The prevalence is higher in urban areas (23.6–61.7%) as compared to rural areas (19.6–58.1%). Diverse religions, cultures, languages, food habits, and traditions influence management practices and present a challenge to the implementation of the health program. Hence, there is a continuing requirement for a country-specific harmonized guideline for the control of IDA in India.

As the prevalence of low iron stores and IDA in women of reproductive age is more in developing countries, iron supplementation is essential in all pregnant women for the following reasons:
- Increase in the demand for absorbed iron
- Increase in the maternal requirement
- Inadequate dietary intake
 The measures to be taken to prevent anemia in general are as follows:
- Dietary intake is increased by advising diet rich in iron such as green leafy vegetables, sprouts, jaggery, meat, and liver
- Cooking in iron vessels and consumption of water boiled in iron containers
- Avoiding of overcooking is advised
- Fortification of the food by iron
- Motivating adolescents and young adults to take iron-rich diet
- Screening for anemia in schools and colleges
- Parasite control measures to prevent hookworm infestations and malaria

■ IRON SUPPLEMENTATION

According to the WHO guidelines:

Iron should be started within the first trimester and provided during antenatal visits.

For developing countries where the prevalence of anaemia is >80%, the WHO recommends daily supplementation of 60 mg elemental iron in the form of ferrous salts along with 400 µg of folic acid for a duration of at least 6 months during pregnancy and 3 months' postpartum.

According to the Ministry of Health (MOH), Government of India, it is recommended to give 100 mg of elemental iron and 500 µg of folic acid for at least 100 days from 14 weeks of gestation for all pregnant women. This is given free of cost by the government of India.

■ TREATMENT

- Food-based strategies—dietary modification, food fortification
- Supplementation—oral iron therapy, parenteral iron therapy

Methods to Treat Iron-deficiency

1. Oral iron preparations
2. Parenteral iron preparations
3. Dietary iron supplementation
4. Blood transfusions
 A comparison of different methods of iron therapy is given in **Table 4**.

Oral Versus Parenteral Iron Therapy

Oral iron therapy: It is very well known that oral iron is less than ideal treatment mainly because of:
- Gastrointestinal adverse effects (particularly when using ferrous iron compounds)
- Lack of adherence to therapy
- Insufficient length of therapy for the degree of iron-deficiency
- Poor duodenal absorption due to concomitant gastrointestinal pathologies [inflammatory bowel

TABLE 4: Comparison of different methods of iron therapy.

	Efficacy	Cost	Side effects
Oral FeSO$_4$	Excellent	Cheap	Abdominal discomfort
Parenteral	Good	Expensive	Fever, rash joint pain shock, death
Dietary iron	Mediocare	Expensive	Weight gain
Blood transfusion	Good	Expensive	TTI—HIV, hepatitis, fever, shock, death

(HIV: human immunodeficiency virus; TTI: transfusion transmitted infection)

disease (IBD) or any other cause of chronic inflammation, malignancy]

- Long course of treatment needed to resolve anemia (1–2 months) and replenish body iron stores (another 3–6 months)

Noncompliance to a prescribed course of oral iron is common and even in compliant patients, poor intestinal absorption fails to compensate for the iron need in the presence of ongoing blood losses or in inflammatory conditions. In addition to that, adequate iron stores are essential to achieve maximum benefit from erythropoiesis-stimulating agents (ESAs). Decreased iron stores or decreased availability of iron are the most common reasons for resistance to the effect of these agents. Thus, oral iron therapy should not be considered for chronic kidney disease (CKD), patients on hemodialysis, and cancer patients receiving ESAs because of the inflammatory state. In this scenario, oral iron is poorly absorbed from the intestinal tract due to upregulation of hepcidin, a peptide hormone that plays a central role in iron homeostasis. In addition to this, in IBD, the possibility that iron may further damage the intestinal mucosa should be a serious indication for the use of IV rather than oral iron therapy.

Recommendations for oral iron therapy:
- It is best taken in an empty stomach early in the morning or 2 hours after food.
- Absorption is impaired with phosphates, phytates, and tanins.
- Iron absorption is increased with vitamin C, orange, or lemon juice.

Factors which inhibit iron salts are:
- Calcium supplements
- Milk and dairy products
- Egg and cereals
- Proton-pump inhibitors
- Antacids
- H_2 receptor antagonists

Oral iron is considered as first-line therapy since it is inexpensive and effective when taken properly.

The recommended oral daily dose for the treatment of IDA in pregnant women is in the range of 120–200 mg/day of elemental iron, depending on the severity of anemia. This may require iron tablets/capsules to be taken two to three times daily.

Ferrous salts are the most appropriate and effective oral iron therapy, and the below preparations are commonly used:
- *Ferrous fumarate:* 300 mg (100 mg elemental iron) per tablet/capsule
- *Ferrous sulfate:* 150 mg/200 mg (45 mg/60 mg elemental iron) per tablet/capsule

- *Ferrous gluconate:* 300 mg (30 mg elemental iron) per tablet/capsule

The tablets supplied by the government of India can be used two times a day. The efficacy of all iron salts mentioned above is similar, and no one preparation is superior to the other. Some enteric-coated, sustained-release preparations such as carbonyl iron, iron polymaltose complex, and ferrous glycine sulfate are also available. These are more expensive but poorly absorbed because they do not release the drug in the duodenum where iron is best absorbed. These preparations are not superior to the ferrous salts mentioned above and are not recommended.

Side effects: Approximately 30% or more of women will have gastrointestinal symptoms as follows:
- Nausea
- Constipation or diarrhea
- Epigastric distress and/or vomiting

Women should be reassured that the side effects will usually subside after 10–14 days of continuous usage.

Parenteral iron therapy
History of parenteral iron therapy:
The ferric hydroxide preparation was the first iron compound for parenteral use introduced early in the 20th century. However, the lack of a carbohydrate shell of this compound resulted in immediate iron release and severe toxic reactions, which led to it being recommended only in extraordinary circumstances. The first high-molecular-weight iron dextran (HMW-ID) for intramuscular and IV use (Imferon) was introduced in 1954. HMW-ID consists of an iron oxyhydroxide core, which is surrounded by a carbohydrate shell made of polymers of dextran.

In 1992 and 1996, two new compounds—Iron Dextran Injection USP (INFeD) containing low-molecular-weight iron dextran (LMW-ID) and Dexferrum with HMW-ID, respectively—were approved by the Food and Drug Administration (FDA) for clinical use in the United States. These formulations can be administered as an IV bolus or total dose infusion (TDI) with doses up to 1,000 mg. Both of them required a test dose and had black box warnings.

In November 2000, iron sucrose (IS) (Venofer) was approved in the United States although it had also been used for a long time in Europe with the greatest experience with this formulation being published in the literature.

With the introduction of ferric carboxymaltose (FCM) as an IV iron formulation which can be used at high doses and allows rapid administration (up to 1,000 mg in a single dose infused in 15 minutes), treatment of IDA is becoming further easier. Because it is free of dextran and its derivatives, FCM does not cross-react with dextran antibodies and never needed the administration of a test dose.

TABLE 5: Administration guidelines for parenteral iron products.

	Iron dextran	*Iron sucrose*	*Ferric gluconate*
Concentration	50 mg/mL (2 mL vial)	20 mg/mL (5 mL vial)	12.5 mg/mL (5 mL ampule)
IV injection (maximum rate)	NTE 50 mg/min	NTE 20 mg/min	NTE 12.5 mg/min
Test dose	Required on the infusion first	Physician discretion	Physician discretion
Test dose	25 mg IV slow push	25 mg IV slow push	25 mg IV slow push or 25 mg in 50 mL of NS IV over 60 minutes
Dosing	100 mg	100 mg	125 mg
IV injection	100 mg over 2–5 minutes	100 mg IV over 5 minutes	125 mg IV over 10 minutes
Maintenance dose	Daily until calculated total amount required has been reached	1–3 times week	1,000 mg over dialysis 8 sessions
Minimum cumulative dose	Based on iron replacement calculations	1,000 mg	1,000 mg
Stability	Not reported	48 hours (concentration of 0.5–2 mg/mL)	Not reported
Diluent	0.9% sodium chloride	0.9% sodium chloride	0.9% sodium chloride
Total dose infusion	Yes	No	No
Infusion	Dilute dose in 250–1,000 mL of 0.9% NS infuse over 1–6 hours	100 mL 0.9% NS IV over 15 minutes	125 mg in 100 mL of NS IV over 1 hour
Routes	IM (INFed) IV infusion	IV injection IV infusion	IV injection IV infusion

Recommendation for parenteral iron therapy **(Table 5)**: India has always been a country with a high prevalence of anemia. Indian obstetricians and nutrition scientists earlier documented that pregnant women were the most vulnerable group for anemia. They reported adverse health consequences of anemia in pregnancy on the mother and the child. Obstetricians then embarked on a series of research studies to combat anemia in pregnancy.

- Daily oral iron folate therapy (100 mg of elemental iron and 500 µg of folic acid) prevented fall in Hb levels seen in pregnancy and resulted in some improvement in birth weight
- Daily administration of two or maximum tolerated doses of oral iron folic acid (100 mg of elemental iron and 500 µg of folic acid) from the time of diagnosis of anemia till delivery succeeded in correction of mild anemia provided the compliance was good.
- Moderate anemia (seen in about 15–20% of pregnant women, majority of whom come to the antenatal clinic after 20 weeks of gestation) did not respond well to oral iron therapy because:
  - One or two tablets a day was insufficient to raise the Hb levels beyond 11 g/dL
  - Attempts to increase the dose resulted in increased side effects and reduced compliance
  - Increased dose also increased gut motility and reduced iron absorption

As a result, oral iron therapy was not found useful for the treatment of moderate anemia.

Indications of parenteral iron therapy:

- Reduced compliance of oral iron owing to poor tolerability and side effects
- Unresponsiveness to oral iron
- The GI adverse effects of oral iron may further exacerbate the pregnancy-associated GI disturbances which include indigestion, constipation, nausea, vomiting, and reflux esophagitis.
- Need for quick recovery from anemia
- In patients who need rapid restoration of iron stores
- Parenteral iron may be used from the second trimester and during the postpartum period.

Prerequisites for parenteral iron therapy:

- Diagnosis of IDA needs to be confirmed before starting parenteral therapy.
- The infusion should be carried out only in a health facility with adequate supervision.
- Availability for the management of anaphylaxis
- Sensitivity test prior to infusion is recommended.

Contraindications to parenteral iron:

- History of anaphylactic reactions to parenteral iron therapy
- First-trimester pregnancy, chronic liver disease, and active infection (acute or chronic). No evidence of use of IV iron in the first trimester of pregnancy is present.
- Oral iron should be stopped at least 24 hours prior to therapy to avoid toxic reaction.

CALCULATION OF TOTAL IRON DOSE

The total iron dose was calculated by a formula, rounded to the nearest multiple of 100.

Total iron dose = Weight (kg) × [Target Hb (g/L) – Actual Hb (g/dL)] × 0.24 + 500 mg

The target Hb was taken as 12 g/dL because of physiological hemodilution during pregnancy. Actual Hb was Hb at the time of inclusion, 0.24 was correction factor, and 500 mg is average stored iron in adults.

PARENTERAL INTRAVENOUS IRON AND FOLIC ACID (PIFA)

In pregnant women, oral iron is often used for prophylaxis of iron-deficiency and is recommended as first-line treatment for pregnant women with IDA. However, oral iron substitution has shown to be insufficient for the treatment of severe IDA and is often associated with gastrointestinal side effects. Therefore, guidelines recommend that physicians consider IV iron administration in pregnant women with severe IDA (Hb < 9.0 g/dL), and in case of intolerability to oral iron as well, insufficient Hb increase after oral iron treatment or if there is a need for rapid Hb reconstitution.

Ferric carboxymaltose (FCM) is an IV iron formulation which can be used at high doses and allows rapid administration (up to 1,000 mg in a single dose infused in 15 minutes). Because it is free of dextran and its derivatives, FCM does not cross-react with dextran antibodies and never needed the administration of a test dose. More recently, the European Medicines Agency (EMA) concluded that no test dose should apply to IV iron products authorized in the European Union yet staff and facilities to evaluate and manage anaphylactic or anaphylactoid reactions should be immediately available. At least four postpartum studies compared the safety and efficacy of FCM versus oral iron. Faster and greater Hb responses were achieved in FCM-treated patients compared to those receiving oral iron and FCM replenished iron stores efficiently. Rather few studies or cases with limited numbers of FCM-treated pregnant women have been reported.

When Christian Brymann started using Inj. Iron Sucrose IV, we had a new hope and there was no looking back. In 1995–1996, we did a randomized controlled trial (RCT) at Vijayanagar Institute of Medical Sciences (VIMS) comparing Inj. Imferon with Inj. Iron Sucrose IV, and the results were more than encouraging. In spite of a satisfactory increase in Hb%, the suboptimal dose, multiple infusions with adverse patient compliance were some of the inhibitory factors of IV Iron Sucrose.

We introduced Inj. FCM in pregnancy in the face of reservations by conventional evidence-based medicine dependent obstetricians. We at Knowledge Skill Transfer Program (KSTP)—Ballari had visualized that parenteral intravenous iron and folic acid (PIFA) by a single dose of 1,000 mg of Inj. FCM is a holistic approach to eradication of pregnancy anemia. In 2012 PIFA with Inj. FCM was started as a community program, now we are seeing the positive results of this program. As an established antenatal prophylaxis for anemia of pregnancy, PIFA with 1,000 mg of Inj. FCM IV is given to all pregnant women after completion of 12 weeks of gestation. PIFA prophylaxis by Suyajna Joshi has become the mainstay in the Eradication of Pregnancy Anemia project.

NEWER INTRAVENOUS IRON FORMULATIONS

In the last 2 years, three new IV iron compounds have been released for clinical use in patients with IDA. Two are currently approved for use in Europe [FCM and iron isomaltoside 1000 (Monofer®)] and one in the United States [Ferumoxytol (FeraHeme®)]. In their preregistration trials, all of these three new compounds potentially had better safety profiles than the more traditional IV preparations, particularly because these products may be given more rapidly and in larger doses than their predecessors with the possibility of complete replacement of iron in 15–60 minutes.

Ferric Carboxymaltose (Fig. 2)

Ferric carboxymaltose is a new parenteral dextran-free iron product and the first of the new agents approved for rapid and high-dose replenishment of depleted iron stores. FCM is an iron complex that consists of a ferric hydroxide core stabilized by a carbohydrate shell. The design of the macromolecular ferric hydroxide carbohydrate complex allows controlled delivery of iron to the cells of the reticuloendothelial system (RES) and subsequent delivery to the iron-binding proteins, ferritin and transferrin, with minimal risk of releasing large amounts of ionic iron into the serum. FCM is a stable complex with the advantage of being non-dextran-containing and with a very low immunogenic potential, and therefore the risk of anaphylactic reactions is low. Its properties permit the administration of large doses

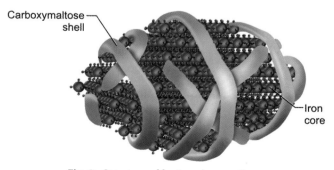

Fig. 2: Structure of ferric carboxymaltose.

(15 mg/kg; maximum of 1,000 mg/infusion) in a single and rapid (15-minute) infusion without the requirement of a test dose.

The therapeutic efficacy of IV FCM has been evaluated in several randomized, open-label, controlled, multicenter trials under different conditions associated with absolute or functional iron-deficiency with or without anemia, including patients with IBD, heavy uterine bleeding, postpartum IDA, chronic heart failure, and CKD patients on hemodialysis or not.

Most of these trials compared FCM with oral iron and found it to have a better efficacy in terms of improving Hb levels and particularly with regard to the body iron replenishment; it was significantly faster and higher than with ferrous sulfate. FCM is approved in Europe, Asia, and Australia, but has not yet been approved by the FDA due to unexplained hypophosphatemia 2 weeks after infusion in patients with CKD and an imbalance in cardiovascular events and deaths in the treatment compared to the placebo arm. However, it should be noted that none of the deaths in the submitted data were considered related to the administration of this IV iron.

The benefit of FCM is the efficacy of IV iron administration without the inconvenience of multiple small-dose injections and long infusion times. For example, if a patient requires 1,000 mg of IV iron to correct the iron-deficiency, then this can be administered 20 times more rapidly with FCM than with iron dextran (0.25 hours vs. 2.7 hours). The administration time for 1,000 mg of FCM in 250 mL of NS is 15 minutes in one visit compared with 161 minutes needed for IS administration. The resulting efficiency ratio is over 10 times better for FCM versus IS. Moreover, FCM effectiveness is associated with real cost-saving benefits for hospitals, healthcare providers, and patients (less frequent and shorter hospital visits).

Ferumoxytol (FeraHeme®)

This formulation was approved by the FDA in 2009 for iron replenishment in CKD patients with IDA. It can be administered as a relatively large dose (maximum 510 mg) in a rapid (<20 seconds) session without test dose requirement. The published safety profile of ferumoxytol is consistent with that of LMW-ID, FG, and IS. However, this product is not currently approved in Europe and the FDA is continuing to evaluate ferumoxytol due to reports of serious cardiac disorders. In addition, ferumoxytol administration may transiently interfere with the diagnostic ability of magnetic resonance imaging which is frequently used for the diagnosis and follow-up of IBD; consequently, this does not seem to be an appropriate IV iron compound for IBD patients. A warning about potentially life-threatening events was added to the instructions for use of ferumoxytol in a recently mandated change.

Iron Isomaltoside 1000 (Monofer®)

The newest IV iron agent, iron isomaltoside 1000 (Monofer®), was introduced in Europe in 2010. This formulation is a nonbranched, nonanaphylactic carbohydrate, structurally different from the branched polysaccharides used in iron dextran (**Fig. 3**). Iron isomaltoside 1000 has a very low immunogenic potential and a very low content of free iron and can therefore be administered as a rapid high-dose infusion of up to 2,000 mg without the application of a test dose, which offers considerable dose flexibility, including the possibility of providing full iron repletion in a single infusion (one-dose iron repletion). Most IV iron agents are colloids with spheroidal iron–carbohydrate nanoparticles. Each particle consists of a carbohydrate shell that stabilizes the iron–oxyhydroxide core (Fe[III]). However, the structure of Monofer® is somehow different, as the linear oligosaccharide isomaltoside 1000 allows the formation of a matrix with interchanging iron and carbohydrate, instead of a classical spheroidal iron–carbohydrate nanoparticle.

The availability of stable parenteral iron compounds allowing for higher dose infusion may greatly facilitate iron replacement therapy in IDA patients. The use of these stable compounds carries benefits for both the patient (less disruption of life, less time away from home/work, reduced injections, few side effects, etc.) and the hospital/health service (reduced visits, reduced physician and nurse time, improved out-patient management, improved cost-effectiveness, etc.). Other benefits of high-dose or TID

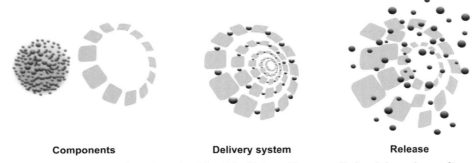

Components   Delivery system   Release

Fig. 3: Matrix structure of iron isomaltoside 1000 which enables controlled and slow release of iron.

(three times daily) infusions are the significant reduction of treatment period and the higher ferritin obtained, which may be important to delay the recurrence of IDA.

MONITORING OF RESPONSE TO TREATMENT

Response to treatment should be monitored using Hb concentration and serum ferritin levels after 3, 6, and 8 weeks, and there should be improvement in those parameters. Other measures were improvement in serum iron level, reticulocyte count, TIBC, and MCV.

Due to iron metabolic pathways, a rise in the reticulocyte count will occur during the second week and thereafter, provided bleeding is not excessive, one can expect a rise in hemoglobin of approximately 1.5 g/week.

Intravenous iron therapy is safe, convenient, and more effective than oral iron therapy in the treatment of IDA and when compliance is the problem and when patients are coming from difficult geographical conditions and approaching the hospital late in pregnancy. There is a decrease in the rate of transfusion use postpartum. Limitations with intravenous iron replacement include the need for medical supervision in the setting of limited healthcare resources.

Parenteral iron therapy helps in achieving target hemoglobin levels in anemic patients and if given in time, parenteral iron therapy will help to reduce the risk of anemia and subsequent maternal and fetal complications as well as risk of blood transfusion during pregnancy and at the time of delivery. Moreover, the compliance of patients with parenteral iron is much better due to reduction of gastrointestinal side effects. So, the current guidelines for the management of IDA should incorporate parenteral iron therapy as effective and safe treatment in pregnant women with IDA.

BLOOD TRANSFUSION

The indications for blood transfusion in pregnancy are as follows:
- Severe anemia at any gestational age
- Moderate anemia beyond 36 weeks' gestational age
- Failure of response to iron therapy
- Obstetric hemorrhage
- Sickle cell anemia and thalassemia in pregnancy

Properly grouped and cross-matched packed cell volume is used for transfusion which is administered slowly over 4–6 hours.

MANAGEMENT DURING LABOR

Apart from the general management protocols of labor monitoring, the following points should be considered as well:

- Fluid overload should be avoided taking care of the adequate nutrition and hydration.
- Vigilant monitoring for signs and symptoms of congestive cardiac failure and pulmonary edema
- Continuous/intermittent oxygen inhalation based on the severity of anemia
- Active management of the third stage of labor should be carried out to prevent the blood loss as even a milder degree of blood loss in anemic patients may jeopardize the maternal health.

POSTPARTUM ANEMIA

Symptoms of anemia in the postpartum period include dyspnea, lethargy, palpitations, and maternal infections, which may influence the ability to care for and bond with a newborn. In addition, there are long-term effects of postpartum hemorrhage related to postpartum anemia, including impaired quality of life, poor cognitive performance, emotional instability, increased risk for postpartum depression, and poor lactation. These occur remote from delivery and constitute a significant health problem in women of reproductive age. Lactation also results in loss of iron via breast milk. Though postpartum anemia is typically seen subsequent to postpartum hemorrhage, it is most commonly associated with antepartum IDA combined with blood loss at delivery. While there currently is no clear classification of postpartum anemia, it is generally described as an Hb concentration < 100 g/L at 24–48 hours after delivery. Approximately 15% of women will have a blood loss > 500 mL at the time of delivery. It is generally recommended that antepartum anemia caused by iron-deficiency and postpartum anemia should be treated. Parenteral iron has been shown to produce a faster and greater increase in Hb concentration than oral supplementation without the risks associated with a blood transfusion. Parenteral iron is emerging as an alternative treatment for significant postpartum anemia.

CONTRACEPTION

It is advisable to enable birth spacing and replenish iron stores. Injectable contraception, combined oral contraceptive pills, or progesterone-only pills are used. Though intrauterine copper T devices are not contraindicated, they are better avoided as they can be a cause for heavy menstrual bleeding.

KEY POINTS
- Provide appropriate dietary advice specially to vegetarians, antihelminthic therapy and iron therapy to ensure satisfactory hemoglobin status before and

during pregnancy, especially in communities where iron deficiency is a common problem.

- Anemia is defined Hb < 11g% in first trimester and Hb <10.5 g% in second and third trimester.

- All pregnant women should be screened for anemia in pregnancy as IDA is associated with low birth weight, preterm birth, perinatal morbidity, maternal morbidity and mortality. Healthcare professionals should be aware of IDA and its associated risks for mother and the fetus.

- Prophylactic iron and folate supplements are necessary for pregnant women to maintain or increase predelivery hemoglobin levels and to prevent the complications due to anemia in pregnancy.

- Those with IDA should be treated with supplemental 100–200 mg elemental iron daily in addition to prenatal vitamins and advised on correct administration to optimize absorption.

- Selective use of oral iron preparations containing ferrous salts with minimal side effects are preferred choice for oral iron therapy with repeat full blood count in 2–3 weeks.

- Parenteral iron therapy after calculating the required dosage is beneficial and effective if oral iron treatment is unsuccessful because of noncompliance, poor follow up or poor absorption.

- During second trimester and late pregnancy, parenteral iron therapy with iron sucrose or Ferric carboxymaltose is more appropriate option than first line oral iron for rapid and effective correction of anemia with additional benefit of vitality and social function.

- In cases of IDA, once the hemoglobin attains the normal range, supplements should be continued for 3 months and at least until 6 weeks postpartum to replenish the iron stores.

- Blood transfusion to be considered in patients with symptomatic severe anemia who are close to delivery, imminent cardiac compromise or symptoms requiring immediate attention.

- Eradication of pregnancy anemia—a concept to be realized is possible by PIFA with Inj. FCM 1000 mg. as developed by Suyajna Joshi.

■ SUGGESTED READING

1. Adamson JW. Iron deficiency and other hypoproliferative anemias. In: Jameson JL, Fauci AS, Kasper DL, Hauser SL, Longo DL, Loscalzo J. Harrison's Principles of Internal Medicine, 20th edition. New York: McGraw Hill.

2. Cançado RD, Muñoz M. Intravenous iron therapy: how far have we come? Rev Bras Hematol Hemoter. 2011;33(6):461-9.

3. FOGSI. (2017). FOGSI general clinical practice recommendations: Iron deficiency anemia in pregnancy. [online] Available from https://www.fogsi.org/wp-content/uploads/2017/07/gcpr-recommendation-ida.pdf [Last accessed September, 2020]

4. Gabbe S, Niebyl J, Galan H, Jauniaux E, Landon M, Simpson J, et al. Obstetrics: Normal and Problem Pregnancies, 6th edition. Gurgaon: Elsevier India; 2016.

5. Geisser P, Burckhardt S. The pharmacokinetics and pharmacodynamics of iron preparations. Pharmaceutics. 2011;3:12-33.

6. Kalaivani K. Use of intravenous iron sucrose for treatment of anaemia in pregnancy. Indian J Med Res. 2013;138:16-7.

7. Mishra R (Ed). Ian Donald's Practical Obstetric Problems, 7th edition. Gurgaon: Wolters Kluwer India; 2014.

8. Nanthini R, Mamatha KR, Shivamurthy G, Kavitha R. A prospective study to assess the efficacy and safety of iron sucrose in pregnant women with iron deficiency anemia in a tertiary care hospital. Int J Basic Clin Pharmacol. 2015;4(6):1271-5.

9. Nash CM, Allen VM. The use of parenteral iron therapy for the treatment of postpartum anemia. J Obstet Gynaecol Can. 2015;37(5):439-42.

10. Perewusnyk G, Huch R, Huch A, Breymann C. Parenteral iron therapy in obstetrics: 8 years experience with iron–sucrose complex. Br J Nutr. 2002;88:3-10.

11. Seshadri L, Arjun G. Essentials of Obstetrics, 1st edition. Gurgaon: Wolters Kluwer India; 2015.

12. Sharma JB, Shankar M. Anemia in pregnancy. JIMSA. 2010;23(4):53-60.

13. Silverstein SB, Rodgers GM. Parenteral iron therapy options. Am J Hematol. 2004;76:74-8.

Megaloblastic Anemia in Pregnancy

Niharika Dhiman, Anjali Deshpande

INTRODUCTION

Anemia in pregnancy is the most commonly affecting medical disorder. According to the National Family Health Survey-4 (NFHS-4) the incidence varies as per the maternity status—58% of breastfeeding women are anemic as compared to 50% of females who are pregnant.[1] Megaloblastic anemia constitutes about 25% of the anemia in pregnancy in developing countries.

Megaloblastic anemia is described as a group of anemia caused by impaired deoxyribonucleic acid (DNA) synthesis. It is characterized by presence of macroovalocytes on peripheral smear and abnormal finding of megaloblastic hyperplasia in the bone marrow sample.[2] Addison in 1849 first characterized it as anemia, general lethargy, and debility.[3] In 1877, Osler and Gardner noted its association with neuropathy, following which in 1887 Lichtheim documented its association with myelopathy. Ehrlich was the first one to demonstrate megaloblasts.

METABOLISM OF FOLIC ACID AND VITAMIN B$_{12}$

Folic acid (pteroylglutamate) functions in its active form tetrahydrofolate. The dietary sources of folic acid include green leafy vegetables, fruits (banana, lemon, oranges, and melons), cereals, nuts, beef, meat, fish, liver, and kidney. It is heat labile and is destroyed by overcooking.

Folic acid absorption occurs in the small intestine. Majority of it is absorbed both actively and passively in the jejunum by binding to reduced-folate transporter-1 and 2 (RFT-1, 2) and folate-binding protein (FBP). A small part of it is absorbed passively in the ileum. Folic acid is absorbed in its monoglutamate form from the enterocytes where it is converted to methyltetrahydrofolate and transported into the systemic and enterohepatic circulation. Intracellularly methyltetrahydrofolate is converted into its active and functional form tetrahydrofolate. Part of the intracellular methyltetrahydrofolate is utilized in the synthesis of thymine which is one of the four pyrimidine bases of DNA. In case of folic acid the above thymine synthesis does not occur and uracil is incorporated in place of thymine thus altering the DNA structure and leading to abnormal nuclear maturation.[4]

TABLE 1: Recommended daily allowance for folic acid and vitamin B$_{12}$.		
Group	Folic acid (µg)	Vitamin B$_{12}$ (µg)
Reproductive age	400	2
Pregnancy	600	2.6
Lactation	500	2.6

The main source of cobalamin or cyanocobalamin is animal food, plant food does not contain cobalamin. Vitamin B$_{12}$ is absorbed from the digestive system in three stages. In stomach it binds to R protein and transported to the duodenum and jejunum. In the alkaline pH of duodenum and jejunum R protein is degraded and cobalamin binds to intrinsic factor (IF). This stable IF-cobalamin complex is taken up by the enterocytes of ileum where IF is degraded and cobalamin binds to transcobalamin II (TCII) binding protein and enters the systemic circulation. Intracellularly cobalamin exists in two active forms—(1) methylcobalamin and (2) adenosylcobalamin. Methylcobalamin acts as a coenzyme in synthesis of tetrahydrofolate and methionine, this is the common pathway for biological action of both cobalamin and folic acid. In case of cobalamin deficiency methyltetrahydrofolate cannot be demethylated for methionine synthesis moreover it cannot be polyglutamized to keep it anchored to the cell as a result it escapes into the circulation without being used. This is also called as *folate trap/Methyltetrahydrofolate trapping.*[5]

Adenosylcobalamin acts as a coenzyme in conversion of methylmalonyl to succinic acid, accumulation of methylmalonyl in a state of cobalamin deficiency has been attributed to the development of neuropathy.[6]

The recommended daily allowance has been shown in **(Table 1)**.

ETIOPATHOGENESIS

Megaloblastic anemia is primarily caused by deficiency of folic acid and vitamin B$_{12}$ which can be due to dietary deficiency or any other factors hampering its absorption **(Table 2)**.

TABLE 2: Etiological factors for megaloblastic anemia.

Causes of folic acid deficiency	Causes of vitamin B_{12} deficiency
Dietary deficiency: Malnutrition, alcohol consumption, goat milk intake	Strict vegetarians
Absorption problems: Celiac disease, Crohn's disease, tropical sprue, Whipple's disease, diabetes mellitus, amyloidosis, small bowel resection	Pernicious anemia, partial gastrectomy, *Helicobacter pylori* infection, gastritis
Drugs: Trimethoprim, pyrimethamine, phenytoin, valproic acid, antiretroviral drugs	
Liver disease, hypothyroidism and chronic hemolytic disease	

Megaloblastic anemia is result of ineffective erythropoiesis which is caused by lack of formation of thymine; it is one of the pyrimidine bases required for DNA synthesis. Uracil is incorporated instead of thymine which alters the structure of pure DNA. As a result the damaged DNA is repaired by p53 cellular apoptosis process. This leads to asynchronous maturation between the nucleus and the cytoplasm leading to release of immature erythropoietic precursors as blasts into the circulation.

Megaloblastic anemia caused by folic acid deficiency usually presents latter half of the pregnancy (20–28 weeks) when the stores are depleted, occurs commonly in multiple pregnancies. It may also present during the puerperium up to 5 months postpartum [oral contraceptive pill (OCP) users/antiepileptic drugs].[7]

Pernicious anemia caused by IF deficiency leading to failure of absorption of vitamin B_{12} is rarely found during pregnancy as most of these women present with infertility.

■ CLINICAL MANIFESTATION

The clinical features of megaloblastic anemia are insidious in onset; the features of vitamin B_{12} deficiency develop over years. It usually presents with features of anemia syndrome, i.e., easy fatigability, weakness, lassitude and breathlessness. Gastrointestinal problems leading to megaloblastic anemia may also present with nausea, vomiting, reflux, gastritis and diarrhea. Cobalamin deficiency leads to specific neurological features which include paresthesia, hypoesthesia, tingling in toes and fingers, gait abnormalities, muscle weakness. These neurological symptoms mostly affect the lower extremities. These neurological symptoms have been attributed to the demyelination and gliosis of the gray column caused by methionine deficiency and accumulation of methylmalonic acid which causes subacute combined degeneration of posterior and lateral gray column of spinal cord. A role of elevated tumor necrosis factor alpha and epidermal growth factor has also contributes to the neurological effects.[8]

On examination the following features are seen in megaloblastic anemia—pallor, change of hair color, glossitis, hyperpigmentation of skin and nails, however features of koilonychia and platynychia are not seen in megaloblastic anemia. Petechial rash over skin can be seen in cases of megaloblastic anemia with thrombocytopenia. Such cases need to be differentiated from aplastic anemia and leukemia. Splenomegaly is found in 10–15% of cases.

On neurological examination signs of vitamin B_{12} deficiency reveal a positive Romberg's and Babinski sign, presence of spasticity, hyporeflexia, and clonus.

■ LABORATORY DIAGNOSIS

The basic workup of megaloblastic anemia includes: complete blood count, flow cytometry, peripheral blood smear, serum folate, and vitamin Cobalamine levels **(Table 3 and 4)**.

Flow cytometry: Macrocytes are found >75% of the cases. Mean corpuscular volume (MCV) > 100 fL (mild: 100–105, moderate: 106–115, and severe >116 fL), mean corpuscular hemoglobin (MCH) > 33 pg, and normal mean corpuscular hemoglobin concentration (MCHC). Red cell distribution width (RDW) is increased.

TABLE 3: Criteria for diagnosis of megaloblastic anemia.[8]

Criteria for diagnosis of megaloblastic anemia (the hemoglobin level should be below 10 g% and at least two out of five should be present):
1. More than 4% of neutrophil polymorphs have five or more lobes.
2. Orthochromatic macrocytes with diameter > 12 mm.
3. Presence of Howell–Jolly bodies
4. Nucleated red blood cells (RBCs)
5. Presence of macropolycytes (giant polymorphs within buffy coat layer)

TABLE 4: Specific diagnostic tests.[7]

Test	Value	Interpretation
Serum folate	<2 ng/mL	Diagnostic
	2–4 ng/mL	Measure methylmalonic acid and homocysteine levels
	>4 ng/mL	Normal
RBC/intraenterocyte folate	<165 µg/mL	Diagnostic
	165–190 µg/mL	Normal
Serum cobalamin	<200 pg/mL	Diagnostic
	200–300 pg/mL	Measure methylmalonic acid and homocysteine levels
	>300 pg/mL	Normal
Methylmalonic acid	70–270 mmol/L	Normal
Homocysteine	5–14 mmol/L	Normal

Peripheral blood smear: Presence of macrocytes, hypersegmented neutrophils (>5% of neutrophils with 5 segments or >1% with 6 segments), anisocytosis (varying size of RBCs), giant polymorphs, and basophilic stippling. Few Howell–Jolly bodies and giant hypersegmented granulocytes can also be seen. There is varying degree of thrombocytopenia, leukopenia, and reticulocytopenia (reticulocyte count <1%). Peripheral smear usually reveals a picture of pancytopenia with suppression of all myeloid lineages. RBCs appear to be thicker and hyperchromic because of increased central pallor **(Figs. 1 and 2)**.[9]

Ineffective erythropoiesis cause intramedullary hemolysis leading to raised serum lactate dehydrogenase (LDH) and elevated indirect bilirubin. Haptoglobin levels can be reduced due to some amount of intravascular hemolysis.[9]

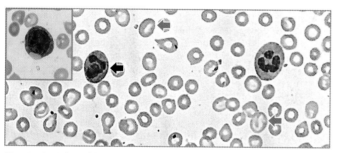

Fig. 1: Peripheral blood smear (40X): Hypersegmented neutrophil (black arrow), macro-ovalocytes (purple arrows); Inset: Megaloblast in a bone marrow aspirate smear.
Courtesy: Dr Harpreet Walia (Senior Consultant and Head), Department of Pathology, SGHS Hospital, Mohali, Punjab.

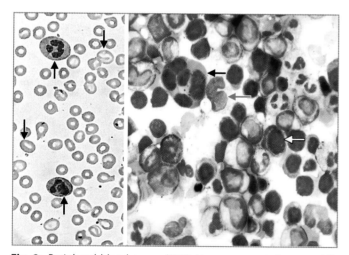

Fig. 2: Peripheral blood smear (40X): Hypersegmented neutrophils (upward arrows), macro-ovalocytes (downward arrows); Bone marrow aspirate smear (100X): Giant metamyelocyte (blue arrow), megaloblast (white arrow), and hypersegmented megakaryocyte (black arrow).
Courtesy: Dr Harpreet Walia (Senior Consultant and Head), Department of Pathology, SGHS Hospital, Mohali, Punjab.

Iron deficiency anemia is masked by folic acid and vitamin B_{12} deficiency as the synthesis of RBCs is reduced leading to raised serum iron, transferrin, and ferritin levels.

Bone marrow aspiration: Bone marrow aspiration (BMA) is routinely not indicated in all cases of megaloblastic anemia except when a diagnosis of refractory anemia, leukemia or myelodysplastic disease is suspected. Bone marrow appears hypercellular, erythroid series—the orthostatic erythroblasts are enlarged with nuclear cytoplasmic asynchrony. In the myeloid series megaloblasts manifest as large band cells.[7,9]

Effect of Folic Acid Deficiency on Pregnancy

As the pregnancy progresses the folate levels reduce to half as compared to the nonpregnant state. This is mainly due to hemodilution, increased renal clearance, and hormonal changes. During the latter half in the pregnancy the increased utilization by the developing fetus and the placenta and rapidly proliferating cells as well as increased catabolism of folic acid results in a negative feedback.

Deficiency of folic acid has been associated with spontaneous abortions, recurrent pregnancy loss, preterm delivery, abruptio placentae, pre-eclampsia, and growth restriction. High homocysteine levels can act as predictor for abruptio placentae and pre-eclampsia. Fewer studies have also linked folate deficiency to HELLP syndrome (hemolysis, elevated liver enzymes and low platelets).[8,10]

Effect of Folic Acid Deficiency Fetus and Neonate

Folic acid is has an essential role in the early embryonic development a deficiency during this period can lead to neural tube defect (NTD), heart defects and orofacial defects. As 50% of the pregnancies are unplanned, only 5–20% of the pregnant women start preconceptional folic acid. Preconceptional folic acid and supplementation during the pregnancy can reduce NTD by 72%. In low risk population who are planning to become pregnant or are not using any contraceptive method should start folic acid supplementation 30 days prior to conception in a dose of 400 µg (0.4 g) daily and continue this through the first trimester. In high risk women (history of NTD in previous pregnancies, partner affected by NTD, first-degree relative affected by NTD, prepregnancy diabetes mellitus, on antiepileptics-valproate and carbamazepine) should be given 4 g of synthetic folic acid.[11]

Fetal growth restriction, prematurity, low birth weight, and very low birth weight babies have been associated with maternal deficiency of folic acid.[10]

■ TREATMENT

Folic acid deficiency is treated by giving 5 mg of synthetic folic acid daily till 4 weeks postpartum. The reticulocyte count increases drastically within 4–7 days of starting treatment. Leukopenia and thrombocytopenia also gets corrected within days. The hemoglobin levels rises over a period of weeks. Iron supplementation should be started as soon as effective erythropoiesis starts. Hypersegmented neutrophils will persist for 10–14 days. Serum LDH levels and indirect bilirubin levels will normalize rapidly, a failure to fall may indicate iron deficiency anemia or error in diagnosis.

Vitamin B_{12} deficiency is mainly treated by parenteral therapy—1,000 µg daily for 1–2 weeks followed by weekly dose till hematocrit normalizes (6 weeks). Oral cobalamin (1,000–2,000 µg) can be given thereafter.[12]

Folic acid supplementation should not be started in megaloblastic anemia if cobalamin deficiency is not ruled out definitively. Treatment with folic acid will only correct the anemia and will worsen the neurological symptoms of cobalamine deficiency. Both folic acid and cobalamin should be given if vitamin B_{12} deficiency has not been ruled out.

In case of severe anemia blood transfusion should be given followed by parenteral therapy.

PREVENTION OF MEGALOBLASTIC ANEMIA

- Consume food rich in folic acid and vitamin B
- Do not overcook as these micronutrients are heat labile
- Use of fortified food, e.g., fortified wheat (folic acid, vitamin B, and iron)
- Folic acid prophylaxis

SUMMARY

Megaloblastic anemia is not an uncommon condition during pregnancy. Most of the cases are diagnosed in the latter half of the pregnancy when the demand of folic acid and vitamin B_{12} increases. High incidence is seen in multipara women and those with short interconceptional period. The most common cause of megaloblastic anemia is dietary deficiency. Folic acid prophylaxis should be started 30 days prior to planned conception; it effectively prevents NTD in the newborn. Megaloblastic anemia can be managed by pharmacotherapy however associated neurological symptoms may require a longer treatment and follow up.

ACKNOWLEDGMENT

My sincere thanks to Dr Harpreet Walia (Senior Consultant and Head), Department of Pathology, SGHS Hospital, Mohali, Punjab for providing elaborate and well-illustrated pictographs of peripheral smear and BMA.

REFERENCES

1. Rchiips. (2009). Key Findings from NFHS-4. [online] Available from http://rchiips.org/NFHS/factsheet_NFHS-4.shtml [Last accessed July, 2020].
2. Allen RH, Stabler SP, Savage DG, Lindenbaum J. Metabolic abnormalities in cobalamin (vitamin B12) and folate deficiency. FASEB J. 1993;7(14):1344-53.
3. Addison T. Anaemia-disease of the suprarenal capsules. Med Gazette. 1849;43:517-8.
4. Bailey LB, Gregory JF 3rd. Folate metabolism and requirements. J Nutr. 1999;129(4):779-82.
5. Watanabe F, Nakano Y. Comparative biochemistry of vitamin B12 (cobalamin) metabolism: biochemical diversity in the systems for intracellular cobalamin transfer and synthesis of the coenzymes. Int J Biochem. 1991;23(12):1353-9.
6. Herbert V, Zalusky R. Interrelations of vitamin B12 and folic acid metabolism: folic acid clearance studies. J Clin Invest. 1962;41(16):1263-76.
7. Carmel R, Green R, Rosenblatt DS, Watkins D. Update on cobalamin, folate, and homocysteine. Hematology Am Soc Hematol Educ Program. 2003:62-81.
8. Letsky E. Blood volume, haematinics, anameia. In: de Swiet M (Ed). Medical Disorders in ObstetricPractice, 3rd edition. Oxford: Blackwell; 1995. pp. 33-60.
9. Rodríguez de Santiago E, Ferre Aracil C, García García de Paredes A, Moreira Vicente VF. Pernicious anemia. From past to present. Rev Clin Esp. 2015;215(5):276-84.
10. Sharma JB. Medical complications in pregnancy. In: Sharma JB (Ed). The Obstetric Protocol, 1st edition. New Delhi: Jaypee Brothers Medical Publishers Pvt Ltd.; 1998. pp. 78-98.
11. Figo Working Group On Best Practice In Maternal-Fetal Medicine; International Federation of Gynecology and Obstetrics. Best practice in maternal-fetal medicine. Int J Gynaecol Obstet. 2015;128(1):80-2.
12. Andrès E, Dali-Youcef N, Vogel T, Serraj K, Zimmer J. Oral cobalamin (vitamin B(12)) treatment. An update. Int J Lab Hematol. 2009;31(1):1-8.

CHAPTER 3

Sickle Cell Disease in Pregnancy

Sumitra Yadav

INTRODUCTION

The most important hemoglobinopathy encountered during pregnancy because of severity of complications associated with this condition. It is an inherited disease, causing chronic anemia due to hemolysis.

Sickle cell disease (SCD) is a cause of extravascular chronic hemolytic anemia. The red blood cells (RBCs) are destroyed in reticuloendothelial system characterized by elevated unconjugated bilirubin, increased urinary urobilinogen and reticulocytosis and elevated lactate dehydrogenase (LDH).

Sickle cell disease included a group of single gene autosomal recessive disorder caused by the "sickle" gene which affects the hemoglobin (Hb) molecule. In India, MP has highest load, with an estimated number of 961,492 sickle heterozygotes and 67,861 sickle homozygotes.[1] The prevalence of HbS varies from 10 to 33%.[1]

TYPES OF SICKLE CELL DISEASE

- It is caused by point mutation in β-globin chain on chromosome 11. This results in substitution of valine by glutamine in position 6 in β-globin chain of Hb molecule. This enhances the polymerization in deoxygenated state and causes increase RBC rigidity and sickling. The

disease is characterized by chronic hemolytic anemia and occurrence of acute, life-threatening vaso-occlusive crisis. This hereditary blood disorder has been classified into various categories **(Table 1)**.[2]

PATHOPHYSIOLOGY

Clinical consequence of SCD is sickle cell crisis which include the following:

- *Vaso-occlusive crisis or painful crisis*: Micro- or macro-infarct leading to organ damage
- *Anemia crisis*: Severe hemolysis, red cell aplasia, splenic sequestration
- *Acute chest syndrome*: Leading cause of maternal mortality
- Neurological events.

Vaso-occlusive Crisis or Painful Crisis[3]

- Most common type of SCD crisis
- Reason for hospital admission
- Most common site for pain is bone due to osteonecrosis of bone marrow especially head of femur and humerus
- Most pain occurs in third trimester and postpartum period

TABLE 1: Categories of SCD.[2]

Sickling syndromes	Name	Genetics	Severity
HbSS	Sickle cell anemia	One sickle cell gene (S) from each parent	Typically the most severe
HbSC	SC disease	Sickle cell gene (S) from one parent and abnormal HbC from other parent	Milder form
A. HbS β0-thalassemia B. HbS β+-thalassemia	Sickle cell β-thalassemia Sickle cell β-thalassemia	Sickle cell gene (S) from one parent and gene for β-thalassemia from other parent Sickle cell gene (S) from one parent and gene for β-thalassemia from other parent	Severe form Milder form
HbSD HbSE HbSO	SD disease SE disease SO Arab disease	Sickle cell gene (S) from one parent and abnormal Hb from other parent	Varies
HbAS	Sickle cell trait	One normal gene (A) from one parent and one sickle cell gene (S) from other parent (If the husband is a carrier, there is 80% chance that the infant will be homozygous for SCD	

(SCD: sickle cell disease)
Note: Sickling occurs in homozygous condition (HbSS) or in compound heterozygous states (e.g., HbSC, HbS β-thalassemia) or sickle cell trait (HbAS).

Flowchart 1: Predisposing factors of sickle cell disease.

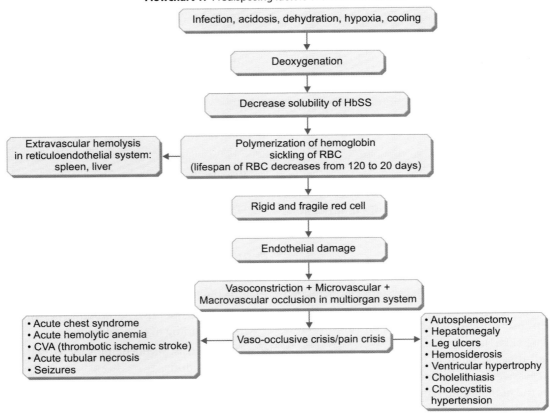

■ Precipitating factor to be ruled out such as toxemia of pregnancy or infection and other causes.

Pain episodes have not been associated with apparent change in the umbilical flow despite increase vascular resistance.

Acute Hemolytic Anemia[4]

■ Rare in SCD
■ Due to acute sequestration of RBC in spleen
■ Acute abdominal pain due to rapid enlargement of spleen.

Acute Chest Syndrome[5]

■ Leading cause of maternal morbidity and mortality in SCD crisis.
■ Acute lung injury caused by *fat embolism* from bone marrow during vaso-occlusion crisis along with RBC sequestration.
■ Characterized by chest pain, respiratory distress with tachypnea, coughing, wheezing, fever, hypoxia, leukocytosis, and abnormal pulmonary function test.
■ *Chest X-ray posterior anterior (PA) view*: Pulmonary infiltrate involving at least one complete lung segment and multilobar involvement is common.

■ *Diagnosis*:[6] Microscopic analysis of sputum or bronchial sampling.
■ *Poor prognosis.*
  Differential diagnosis: Pneumonia.

Neurological Events[7]

Thromboembolic cerebrovascular accident leads to infarction and seizure disorder.

Diagnosis and Management of Sickle Cell Disease

Prenatal: At prenatal visit, following issues to be addressed with couple:

■ Patients and partner's Hb electrophoresis report.
■ Counsel against conception until disease status is optimized.
■ Frequency and management of crisis in prepregnancy period.
■ History of number of previous blood transfusion because of multiple donors, there is risk of RBC isoimmunization.[8]
■ Past obstetrical history and outcomes.
■ Contraception history.
■ *Drugs history*:[9] Ensure folic acid supplements; hydroxyurea (is a disease modifying drug that increases

HbF and decreases sickling crisis) is a teratogenic drug which should be discontinued 3 months prior to conception in both men and women.

- Need of multidisciplinary team approach such as obstetrician, hematologist, anesthetist, neonatologist, and need of ICU care.
- Need of repeated antenatal care (ANC) visits.
- Discussion of maternal and fetal risk in SCD after conception.

Effect of Pregnancy on Sickle Cell Disease

Physiological changes in CVS in pregnancy such as increased cardiac output, due to decreased systemic vascular resistance; increased left ventricular end diastolic volume leads to decompensation of cardiac function.

Also, due to increased tidal volume, minute ventilator volume, total pulmonary resistance, added with reduced functional lung capacity and residual volume lead to cardiopulmonary compromise in women with SCD who are pregnant.

Thus previously asymptomatic women may become symptomatic and symptoms worsen with advancing pregnancy.

Effect of Sickle Cell Disease on Pregnancy

- High miscarriage rate,[10] spontaneous abortions 35–65%, compared to controls.
- Increased risk of *P*lacental abruption, *P*re-eclampsia, *P*reterm labor.
  Preterm labor and eclampsia were higher in patients requiring blood transfusion for SCD. That is to say, any acute or chronic vascular injury in pregnancy increases the risk of obstetric complications in SCD.
- Mode of delivery remains unaltered in SCD.[10]
- Antepartum hemorrhage (APH) and postpartum hemorrhage (PPH) rates are not increased in SCD.
- Retained placenta was more prevalent in a Jamaican study,[11] while postpartum endometritis was higher in another study.[12]
  Integrated multispecialty approach with antenatal supervision, patient education, and regular follow-ups reduce maternal morbidity and mortality in SCD.
  In the last three decades with the improvement in obstetric and neonatology services, perinatal mortality has reduced fivefold from 53% to almost 0–10%.[13]
- In SCD, chronic anemia and vaso-occlusion due to sickling leads to placental damage thus causing intrauterine growth retardation (IUGR) and low birth weight. Doppler flow studies show a positive correlation between reduce uterine flow and birth weight.[14]

Maternal Complications in Pregnancy

Maternal complications in pregnancy complicated by sickle cell syndrome:

Preexisting medical disorder:[11]
- Cardiomyopathy [left ventricular hypertrophy (LVH)]
- Pulmonary hypertension
- Recurrent urinary tract infection (UTI)
- Renal failure
- Cardiac failure.

Pregnancy complications:
- Cerebral vein thrombosis
- Pneumonia
- Pyelonephritis
- Deep vein thrombosis
- Pulmonary embolism
- Sepsis syndrome
- Preterm labor
- Gestational hypertension/preeclampsia
- Eclampsia
- Placental abruption
- Postpartum hemorrhage
- Recurrent pregnancy failure.

Fetal complication:
- Intrauterine growth retardation
- Intrauterine fetal death (IUFD)[15]
- Stillbirth
- Preterm birth
- Prematurity
- Neonatal morbidity and mortality.

Management during pregnancy:
- Early booking appointments with planned schedule of care with multidisciplinary team approach management.
- Provide frequent antenatal care.
- Close supervision during each ANC visit such as TPR to rule out infection, weight and BP, and urine albumin by urostick for screening of preeclampsia.[16]
- Laboratory test such as complete blood count, reticulocyte count, Hb electrophoresis (if not previously done or available), peripheral smear, LDH, renal function test (RFT), liver function test (LFT), urine R/M and urine culture and sensitivity, serum ferritin level and folate level.
- Continue folic acid 4 mg throughout the pregnancy.
- Assessment of fetal well-being by serial ultrasonography and color Doppler examination and timely antenatal fetal surveillance by NST, biophysical profile.
- Labor and delivery close supervision by senior obstetrician is needed.

MANAGEMENT OF SICKLE CELL CRISIS DURING ANTENATAL PERIOD

- *Intravenous hydration*: 1 L of NS 250 mL/h then 125 mL/h with careful input output charting.
- Pain relief by IV morphine, fentanyl by pump using patient-controlled analgesia.
- Partial exchange blood transfusion.
- Intravenous antibiotics covering capsulated organisms.
- *Oxygenation*: As per nasal cannula 3 mL/min.

BLOOD TRANSFUSION

Blood transfusion is main treatment of SCD.

Aim of blood transfusion is to keep HbSS < 50%; hematocrit > 25–30%; and Hb > 10 g.[17]

Indication of Blood Transfusion[18]

- Hemoglobin < 5 g/dL (acute anemia)
- Vaso-occlusive crisis
- Acute chest syndrome
- Neurological symptom.

There are two methods of blood transfusion:
1. *Simple blood transfusion:* Packed cell volume (PCV).
2. Isovolemic partial exchange transfusion.

Protocols for Isovolumetric Partial Exchange Transfusion

Obtain baseline Hb, hematocrit, matching type and crossmatch, to infuse four units, leukocyte poor, and packed red blood cell:

- Infuse 500 mL of normal saline solution (1 hour)
- Remove 500 mL of blood from opposite side (30 minutes)
- Transfuse two units of packed red blood cell warmed under pressure
- Rest patient for 4 hours
- Repeat procedure
- Obtain postprocedure Hb hematocrit and Hb electrophoresis.

Complications of frequent blood transfusion:

- Red blood cell (RBC) isoimmunization
- Delayed blood transfusion reaction
- Iron overloading
- Hemochromatosis
- Transmission of infection such as hepatitis A, B, C, and HIV.

MANAGEMENT DURING LABOR

- Keep the patient warm
- Maintain proper hydration and avoiding volume overloading
- Avoid any factors that increase risk of sickle cell anemia (SCA) crisis

- Epidural analgesia for pain relief
- Maternal vital monitoring such as TPR charting, BP, strict input and output charting
- Continuous electronic fetal monitoring
- Avoid prolonged labor
- Operative delivery for obstetric indications
- Blood transfusion if Hb < 7 g.

Postpartum Care

- Patients should maintain adequate hydration
- Vitals such as blood pressure, pulse, temperature, and respiratory rate should be monitored.

Postpartum Thromboprophylaxis

It is indicated in:
- Patients who have experienced sickle cell crisis in pregnancy
- Women who have lesser degrees of mobility
- On the basis of high-risk assessment.

Neonatal Care and Management

Infants having SCA, the Hb components are HbF + small amount of HbS (no HbA).

Early diagnosis reduces mortality and morbidity in infants by prevention of pneumococcal sepsis.

Cord blood or heel-prick sample can be taken but both are subject to small error rate primarily involving carrier phenotypes. Cord blood samples are less conclusive.

Isoelectric focusing and liquid chromatographic techniques are used for screening:
- Neonatal screening and follow-up with pediatrician
- Babies should get antipneumococcal vaccination at 2 months of age
- Long-term prophylaxis with penicillin treatment and regular evaluation should be done
- Exclusive breastfeeding should be done.

CONTRACEPTIVES

- *Oral contraceptive pill (OCP)*: Theoretical risk of thromboembolism, but low-dose OCP are not contraindicated.
- *Progesterone-based contraceptives*: Depot medroxyprogesterone acetate (DMPA, Depo-Provera, ANTARA) is the drug of choice. It has the additional benefit of stabilizing the erythrocyte membrane thereby decreasing sickling.
- *Intrauterine contraceptive devices (IUCDs)*: Relative contraindication due to pelvic infection.
- *LNG devices*: Lower risk of pelvic infection can be used where other methods are contraindicated.
- *Barrier methods*: High failure rate.
- *Permanent methods*: On completion of family.

FUTURE TREATMENT

- *Hydroxyurea* is used because it is relatively nontoxic and its myelosuppressive effects are readily reversible. Myelosuppression caused by hydroxyurea induces F-cell formation in bone marrow leading to rapid erythroid regeneration.
- *Erythropoietin* can be used with hydroxyurea to stimulate production of fetal Hb.
  Hydroxyurea is a proven teratogen in animals and hence it is contraindicated in pregnancy.
- 5-azacytidine—it was the first drug to be used which stimulates by globin gene activation.
  Cytotoxic drugs that act at molecular level increasing the percentage of HbF and HbA form the mainstay of treatment.

> ### KEY POINTS
>
> - The most important hemoglobinopathy encountered during pregnancy.
> - Autosomal recessive disorder caused by point mutation in globin chain on chromosome.[11] This results in substitution of valine by glutamine in position 6 in globin chain of Hb molecule.

REFERENCES

1. Colah RB, Mukherjee MB, Martin S, Ghosh K. Sickle cell disease in tribal populations in India. Indian J Med Res. 2015;141(5):509-15.
2. Nelson-Piercy C. Handbook of Obstetric Medicine, 4th edition. New York: Informa Healthcare; 2010.
3. Gregory J, Foster K, Tyler H, Wiseman M. The Dietary and Nutritional Survey of British Adults. London: Her Majesty's Stationery Office; 1990.
4. RCOG (2007). Blood Transfusions in Obstetrics (Green-top Guideline No. 47). [online] Available from: https://www.rcog.org.uk/en/guidelines-research-services/guidelines/gtg47/ [Last accessed July, 2020].
5. Van Wyck DB, Martens MG, Seid MH, Baker JB, Mangione A. Intravenous ferric carboxymaltose compared with oral iron in the treatment of postpartum anemia: a randomized controlled trial. Obstet Gynecol. 2007;110:267-78.
6. Perewusnyk G, Huch R, Huch A, Breymann C. Parenteral iron therapy in obstetrics: 8 years experience with iron-sucrose complex. Br J Nutr. 2002;88:3-10.
7. Bayoumeu F, Subiran-Buisset C, Baka NE, Legagneur H, Monnier-Barbarino P, Laxenaire MC. Iron therapy in iron deficiency anemia in pregnancy: intravenous route versus oral route. Eur J Obstet Gynecol Reprod Biol. 2005;123:S15-S19.
8. RCOG (2011). Sickle Cell Disease in Pregnancy, Management of (Green-top Guideline No. 61). [online] Available from: https://www.rcog.org.uk/en/guidelines-research-services/guidelines/gtg61/ [Last accessed July, 2020].
9. Hendrickse JP, Watson-Williams EJ, Luzzato L, Ajabor LN. Pregnancy in homozygous sickle-cell anaemia. J Obstet Gynaecol Br Commonw. 1972;79:396-409.
10. Hassel K. Pregnancy and sickle cell disease. Hematol Oncol Clin North Am. 2005;19(5):903-16, vii-viii.
11. Serjeant GR, Loy LL, Crowther M, Hambleton IR, Thame M. Outcome of pregnancy in homozygous sickle cell disease. Obstet Gynecol. 2004;103(6):1278-85.
12. Seoud MA, Cantwell C, Nobles G, Levy DL. Outcome of pregnancies complicated by sickle cell and sickle-C hemoglobinopathies. Am J Perinatol. 1994;11(3):187-91.
13. Rust OA, Perry KG Jr. Pregnancy complicated by sickle hemoglobinopathy. Clin Obstet Gynecol. 1995;38(3):472-84.
14. Billett HH, Langer O, Regan OT, Merkatz I, Anyaegbunam A. Doppler velocimetry in pregnant patients with sickle cell anemia. Am J Hematol. 1993;42(3):305-8.
15. Larrabee KD, Monga M. Women with sickle cell trait are at increased risk for preeclampsia. Am J Obstet Gynaecol. 1997;177(2):425-8.
16. Mahomed K. Prophylactic versus selective blood transfusion in sickle cell anaemia during pregnancy. Cochrane Database Syst Rev. 2002;(2):CD000040.
17. Xu K, Shi ZM, Veeck LL, Hughes MR, Rosenwaks Z. First unaffected pregnancy using preimplantation genetic diagnosis for sickle cell anemia. JAMA. 1999;281(18):1701-6.
18. Eissa AA, Tuck SM. Sickle cell disease and β-thalassaemia major in pregnancy. Obstet Gynaecol. 2013;15:71-8.

CHAPTER 4

Thalassemia in Pregnancy

Hara P Pattanaik

■ INTRODUCTION

Thalassemia is a group of hereditary hemolytic diseases caused by faulty hemoglobin synthesis, widespread in Mediterranean, African, and Asian countries. The defective red blood cells (RBCs) with inadequate hemoglobin content leads to extravascular hemolysis with release of erythroid precursors into peripheral circulation and result in anemia. About 70,000 babies are born with thalassemia every year and about 100 million individuals are asymptomatic carriers.

There are two types of thalassemia, (1) alfa and (2) beta, depending upon which protein chain of the hemoglobin molecule is missing in RBC. Thalassemia is also categorized into three groups depending on its severity. Thalassemia major (homozygous β-thalassemia) result from inheritance of a defective β-globin gene from each parent resulting in a severe transfusion-dependent anemia, the heterozygous state β-thalassemia trait (thalassemia minor) causes mild to moderate microcytic anemia with no significant detrimental effect on overall health. Thalassemia intermedia is defined as a group of patients with variation of disease severity. Many patients may be diagnosed accidentally with mild anemia and splenomegaly

On the other end, patients are usually within 2–6 years of age group with impairment of growth and development though regular blood transfusion may not be required.

Multiple transfusions cause iron overload resulting in hepatic, cardiac, and endocrine dysfunction. The anterior pituitary is very sensitive to iron overload resulting in delayed puberty, low bone mass, and subfertility due to hypogonadotropic hypogonadism.[1] Women with thalassemia who require repeated blood transfusions often have a higher rate of infertility.[2,3] However some women with the disease are able to become pregnant.[4,5] For them screening, counseling, and prenatal diagnosis are important components of prenatal care. The improved blood transfusion technique and effective chelation protocol have improved quality of life and survival of these patients.[6,7]

■ PRECONCEPTION CARE

Thalassemia is associated with an increased risk to both mother and the fetus, in particular due to complication of cardiomyopathy in the mother due to iron overload and increased risk of fetal growth retardation. In addition new endocrinopathies such as diabetes mellitus, hypothyroidism, and hypoparathyroidism develop due to increased iron burden. So the women with thalassemia are best evaluated preconceptionally regarding transfusion requirements, compliance with chelation therapy and assessment of body iron burden including optimization of management and screening for end-organ damage.

Thyroid

Hypothyroidism is frequently found associated with patients of thalassemia. Longitudinal studies show that patients who have been chelated optimally are less likely to suffer from endocrinopathies or cardiac problem.[8] Women should be euthyroid in prepregnancy state to decrease maternal morbidity as well as perinatal mortality and morbidity.

Pancreas

Diabetes mellitus is common in adults with thalassemia. The cause is multifactorial due to insulin resistance, iron-induced islet cell insufficiency, genetic factor, and autoimmunity.[8] Good glycemic control is essential in prepregnancy. Women with established diabetes mellitus should have ideally HbA1c level of < 43 mmol/mol at least 3 months prior to conception in order to reduce the risk of congenital anomaly. Serum fructosamine level is preferred nowadays as HbA1c is diluted by repeated blood transfusion resulting in underestimation.

Heart

The cardiac status of the woman to support a pregnancy as well as the severity of iron-related cardiomyopathy should be evaluated by a cardiologist. Electrocardiogram, echocardiogram, and T2 cardiac magnetic resonance imaging (MRI) should be done.

Liver

Ultrasonogram of liver, gallbladder and spleen if present should be done to detect cholelithiasis, liver cirrhosis due to iron overload or transfusion-related viral hepatitis. Iron concentration of liver should be assessed by using liver

FerriScan or T2 MRI. If it exceeds the target range, intensive chelation is required preconceptionally.

Bone

Osteoporosis is a common finding in thalassemia along with vitamin D deficiency which should be treated before pregnancy.[9]

Red Cell Antibodies

Alloimmunity occurs in 16.5% of individuals with thalassemia. Red cell antibodies may indicate a risk of hemolytic disease of the fetus and newborn. If antibodies present there may be a challenge in obtaining suitable blood for transfusion.

Genetic Screening

If a partner is a carrier of a hemoglobinopathy that may adversely interact with the woman's genotype. So genetic counseling should be offered to a couple preconceptionally. In vitro fertilization/intracytoplasmic sperm injection (IVF/ICSI) with a preimplantation genetic diagnosis (PGD) should be considered in the presence of hemoglobinopathy in both partners so that a homozygous or compound heterozygous pregnancy can be avoided.

Immunization

Women requiring blood transfusion regularly or intermittently are at a risk of transfusion transmitted infections. Therefore all HbsAg negative women who are on transfusion should be vaccinated. Hepatitis C status should be ascertained and in a positive case, RNA titer should be found out and referred to a hepatologist. All splenectomized patients should be vaccinated for pneumococcus and *Haemophilus influenzae*, penicillin prophylaxis should be given, and folic acid 5 mg daily should be given 3 months prior to conception.

■ ANTENATAL CARE

Women with thalassemia are best cared for in a multidisciplinary team setting including an obstetrician with expertise in managing high-risk pregnancy, a hematologist, diabetologist, and a cardiologist.

Antenatal checkup should be done every month until 28 weeks of gestation and thereafter fortnightly. Thyroid function should be monitored periodically and dose of thyroxin should be altered. Cardiac assessment is essential to determine cardiac function, further iron chelation as well as planning of labor. Monthly assessment of serum fructosamine concentration should be reviewed by a diabetologist. Chelation with Desferrioxamine is safe during ovulation induction in these patients. Aggressive chelation in preconception stage can reduce and optimize a body iron burden reducing end-organ damage, but due to lack

of safety data all chelation therapy in first trimester should be regarded as potentially teratogenic. Desferrioxamine is the only agent can be used in second and third trimester. It has short half life.

Role of Ultrasound

Early scan at 7–9 weeks of gestation should be done to know the viability of the fetus as β-thalassemia and diabetes mellitus both have a higher risk of early pregnancy loss. Also fertility treatment with ovulation induction leads to multiple pregnancy. In addition to routine first trimester scan (11–14 weeks) and a detailed anomaly scan at 18–20 weeks gestation, serial fetal biometry is done every 4 weeks from 24 weeks onward because maternal anemia results in fetal growth retardation.

Transfusion Regimen

Decision of blood transfusion depends upon woman's symptoms and fetal growth. If there is worsening of maternal anemia or evidence of fetal growth retardation, regular transfusion is required to maintain hemoglobin level at 10 mg/100 mL. It should be monitored every month and a two unit of transfusion given if the level falls below it. In every woman hemoglobin falls at different rate after transfusion. So, close surveillance is necessary. Thalassemia intermedia patients, who are asymptomatic with normal fetal growth may require blood transfusion in late pregnancy. Generally in nontransfused patients if hemoglobin is above 8 g% at 36 weeks gestation, transfusion can be avoided prior to delivery, postnatal transfusion can be given. Otherwise a top-up transfusion of two units can be recommended.

Role of Thromboprophylaxis

Woman with thalassemia major and intermedia have a prothrombotic tendency due to presence of abnormal cell fragments especially if they have undergone splenectomy. This leads to increased risk of venous thromboembolism. Risk is highest in woman with thalassemia intermedia, not receiving transfusion since a good transfusion suppresses end-organ erythropoiesis. Women with splenectomy or platelet count > 600 × 10⁹/L should continue low-dose aspirin of 75 g/day. Those not using prophylaxis should be advised to use on hospitalization.

Management of Iron Chelation

This should be managed by a hematologist with experience in iron chelation therapy particularly in pregnancy. Those women with high risk, cardiac decompensation present as increasing breathlessness, paroxysmal nocturnal dyspnea (PND), orthopnea, syncope, palpitation, and edema. Cardiac MRI is safe in pregnancy for risk evaluation. Those at higher risk should start low-dose subcutaneous desferrioxamine 20 mg/kg/day for a minimum of 4–5 days in a week. Women with severe hepatic iron loading can be carefully reviewed and considered for iron chelation after 20 weeks.

INTRAPARTUM CARE

Thalassemia in itself is not an indication for cesarean section. Timing and mode of delivery should be based on national guidelines dependent on any issue identified in pregnancy [diabetes and intrauterine growth retardation (IUGR)]. Depending on the hemoglobin level of the woman, cross-matched blood should be kept ready. In woman with thalassemia major, IV desferrioxamine 2 g over 24 hours should be administered throughout labor. Continuous electronic fetal monitoring should be done to diagnose early fetal hypoxia. Third stage of labor should be managed actively to reduce blood loss.

POSTPARTUM CARE

Women with thalassemia are at a great risk of venous thromboembolism and should receive low molecular weight heparin prophylaxis while in hospital and seven days postpartum following normal vaginal delivery and 6 months following cesarean.

Breast feeding is safe and should be encouraged. Desferrioxamine is secreted in breast milk, but is not orally absorbed and not harmful to children. Hence, safe in postpartum period.

CONTRACEPTION

No contraindication for hormonal methods of contraception such as combined oral contraceptive (OC) pills, progesterone only pills or MIRENA (IUCD).

CONCLUSION

With development of newer techniques[10,11] such as chorionic villus sampling at 11–14 weeks gestation, amniocentesis (15–18 weeks), and fetal cord blood sampling (18–21 weeks), the genetic defect of the baby born to the thalassemic mother can be diagnosed at an earlier stage and decision regarding continuation of pregnancy taken easily. If both the spouses are at risk of having a baby with thalassemia major, they can choose to conceive using PGD technique in an infertility clinic. Preconception screening and counseling with advanced pregnancy management brings a better prognosis for the thalassemic mother.

KEY POINTS

- Thalassemia major patients are generally infertile.
- Thalassemia is the only anemia where iron therapy is contraindicated.
- Diagnosis of thalassemia is made by hemoglobin electrophoresis

- Endocrinopathies such as diabetes mellitus, hypothyroidism, and hypoparathyroidism develop in these patients due to increased iron burden.
- Optimization of iron burden from repeated transfusions should be balanced by chelation therapy to avoid complications related to iron overload particularly, cardiomyopathy and diabetes.
- Iron chelators like deferasirox and deferiprone should be withheld 3 months prior to conception and women switched over to desferrioxamine iron chelation.
- Serum fructosamine level is preferred over HbA1c nowadays for monitoring glycemic control as the later is diluted by repeated blood transfusion resulting in under estimation.
- Genetic screening is of paramount importance in these patients. If the male partner is a carrier of hemoglobinopathy, then genetic screening has to be offered as it may interact with woman's genotype. PGD should be considered in IVF/ICSI in presence of hemoglobinopathies in both the partners, so that a homozygous or compound heterozygous pregnancy is avoided.
- IVF involving egg or sperm donation should always be screened for hemoglobionpathies.
- Indore had first exclusive blood bank giving blood for thalassemia children (pediatric thalassemia unit)

REFERENCES

1. Chatterjee R, Katz M, Cox TF, Porter JB. Prospective study of the hypothalamic-pituitary axis in thalassaemic patients who developed secondary amenorrhoea. Clin Endocrinol (Oxf). 1993;39:287-96.
2. De Sanctis V, Vullo C, Katz M, Wonke B, Hoffbrand AV, Bagni B. Hypothalamic-pituitary-gonadal axis in thalassemic patients with secondary amenorrhea. Obstet Gynecol. 1988;72:643-7.
3. Modell B, Khan M, Darlison M. Survival in beta-thalassaemia major in the UK: data from the UK Thalassaemia Register. Lancet. 2000;355(9220):2051-2.
4. Protonotariou AA, Tolis GJ. Reproductive health in female patients with β-thalassemia major. Ann NY Acad Sci. 2000;900:119-24.
5. Skordis N, Christou S, Koliou M, Pavlides N, Angastiniotis M. Fertility in female patients with thalassemia. J Pediatr Endocrinol Metab. 1998;11(Suppl 3):935-43.
6. Ryan K, Bain BJ, Worthington D, James J, Plews D, Mason A, et al. Significant haemoglobinopathies: guidelines for screening and diagnosis. Br J Haematol. 2010;149:35-49.
7. Shinar E, Rachmilewitz EA. Oxidative denaturation of red blood cells in thalassemia. Semin Hematol. 1990;27:70-82.
8. Weatherall DJ. Pathophysiology of thalassaemia. Baillieres Clin Haematol. 1998;11:127-46.
9. Toumba M, Skordis N. Osteoporosis syndrome in thalassaemia major: an overview. J Osteoporos. 2010;2010:537673.
10. Weatherall DJ. Thalassemia in the next millennium. Keynote address. Ann NY Acad Sci. 1998;850:1-9.
11. Weatherall DJ. The definition and epidemiology of non-transfusion-dependent thalassemia. Blood Rev. 2012;26(Suppl 1):S3-6.

CHAPTER 5

Cardiac Diseases in Pregnancy

Haresh U Doshi, Amol Agarwal

■ INTRODUCTION

Incidence of cardiac disease in pregnancy varies from 0.3 to 3.5%.[1] Different types of heart diseases in pregnancy are:

- Rheumatic heart disease
- Peripartum cardiomyopathy (PPCM)
- Congenital heart disease
- Pregnant women with prosthetic valves
- Cardiac arrhythmias
- Coronary artery disease.

■ SYMPTOMS AND SIGNS

Normal physiological changes in pregnancy include increase in blood volume and cardiac output (40–45%), increase in heart rate (85–90 beats/min), decrease in blood pressure (8–15 mm Hg) and upward and left shifting of heart. These changes produce some of the symptoms and signs that mimic heart disease. Symptoms of dyspnea, fatigue, edema, chest pain, and palpitation can be present in normal pregnancy while severe dyspnea [ortho, paroxysmal nocturnal dyspnea (PND)], nocturnal cough, hemoptysis, severe chest pain, and syncope suggest definite heart disease. In signs neck veins pulsation, systolic murmur < Grade III, displaced apex beat, third heart sound, and sinus tachycardia can be present in normal pregnancy while neck veins distension, systolic murmur > Grade III, diastolic murmur, definite cardiomegaly, loud P2, wide split S2, fourth heart sound, persistent arrhythmia, cyanosis and clubbing suggest definite heart disease.

■ RHEUMATIC HEART DISEASE

The ratio of rheumatic to congenital heart disease has decreased from 9:1 in past to 3:1 now due to better control of rheumatic fever in childhood and more patients of congenital heart disease are reaching child bearing age with better treatment.

In rheumatic heart disease mitral valve is most commonly involved, i.e., 85% of cases followed by aortic valve in 10% of cases and both in 5% of cases.

Mitral Stenosis

Normal mitral valve surface area is 4–6 cm². Symptoms appear when it is reduced to <2.5 cm². Less than 1 cm² is called critical mitral stenosis (MST).

Due to stenosis there is obstruction to blood flow from left atrium to left ventricle, so left atrial pressure is elevated and this leads to increased pulmonary venous and capillary pressure and pulmonary hypertension. The increase in left atrial volume (atrial dilatation) makes it vulnerable to arrhythmias and atrial fibrillation. With stagnation of blood and fibrillation, thrombus formation may occur with embolic complications.

Pregnancy alterations of increased cardiac output, tachycardia, and fluid retention predispose patients to pulmonary edema and heart failure.

Management

Prepregnancy counseling: Patients with heart disease should be counseled before pregnancy regarding: (1) risk of maternal death, (2) prolonged hospitalization, (3) risk of congenital heart disease to baby, (4) risk of intrauterine growth retardation (IUGR) and prematurity, and (5) medications and their side effects.

Antepartum management: The patient should be managed in high-risk pregnancy clinic. Patient is classified according to New York Heart Association (NYHA) functional classification **(Box 1)**[2] of heart disease.

Complete cardiology workup, e.g., cardiologist consultation, X-ray chest with shielding, ECG and echocardiography is done and drugs are started as per

---

BOX 1: New York Heart Association (NYHA) functional classification.

Class I: No limitation of physical activity. Ordinary physical activity does not cause symptoms

Class II: Slight limitation of physical activity. Ordinary physical activity results in fatigue, palpitation, dyspnea (shortness of breath)

Class III: Marked limitation of physical activity. Comfortable at rest. Less than ordinary activity causes fatigue, palpitation, or dyspnea

Class IV: Unable to carry on any physical activity without discomfort. Symptoms of heart failure at rest

cardiologist's advice. Frequent antenatal visits, i.e., every 2 weeks up to 28 weeks then every weekly up to delivery.

New York Heart Association class I and II patients are admitted 2 weeks before EDD or if they develop any cardiac symptom during pregnancy. Class IV patient is continuously hospitalized while class III can take breaks from hospitalization if stable.

Adequate rest is ensured. Excessive weight gain is avoided. Prevention, early detection, and treatment of anemia, infection, and hypertension should be done.

Continue prophylaxis against recurrence of rheumatic fever, i.e., injection Penidure 2.4 mega units I/M even 3 weeks. Ensure endocarditis prophylaxis during any minor surgical procedure.

Patients having high risk for mortality should be advised medical termination of pregnancy (MTP). These include: (1) Eisenmenger syndrome, (2) Primary pulmonary hypertension, (3) Coarctation of aorta complicated, and (4) Marfan's syndrome with aortic involvement. Relative indications include: (a) Class III and IV diseases if family is completed, (b) Severe aortic stenosis (AST), (c) Cyanotic congenital heart disease, and (d) History of congestive cardiac failure (CCF) in previous pregnancy or in between pregnancy.

In patients continuing pregnancy and worsening of disease valvotomy is now performed by *percutaneous balloon mitral valvotomy*.

Indications:
- Critical MST
- Progressive pulmonary hypertension
- Profuse and uncontrollable hemoptysis
- Pulmonary edema
- History of CCF in previous pregnancy
- Failure to respond to medical Rx.

Intrapartum management: Vaginal delivery is preferred in spite of the physical efforts required in labor as it has less morbidity and mortality. Cesarean section (CS) is reserved for obstetric indications only. However in present times with better anesthetic facilities, newer cardiac drugs, and multipara monitors available CS is liberally done. Induction of labor is avoided unless absolutely necessary.

First stage: Supine position is avoided. Propped up semirecumbent position is the best.

Adequate sedation—tramadol 100 mg I/M as pethidine is not freely available. Continuous epidural analgesia is the method of choice for pain relief. Epidural narcotics, i.e., fentanyl + bupivacaine are now used. It is avoided in cyanotic heart disease, severe AST, and in patients who are on anticoagulant therapy.

Oxygen therapy is given as required. Pulse oximetry should be done. Central venous pressure (CVP) monitoring

is advisable. Nutrition is maintained by oral drinks. I/V fluid should be restricted to <60 mL/hour. Pulse, BP, respiration monitoring, and chest examination should be done every 30 minutes or more frequently if needed. Continuous ECG monitoring is advised and in cases of pulmonary hypertension Swan–Ganz catheter to measure pulmonary capillary wedge pressure is advocated.

Antibiotics prophylaxis against infective endocarditis is given by ampicillin or cephalosporins with gentamycin. As per American College of Obstetricians and Gynecologists (ACOG) guidelines this is not indicated for uncomplicated delivery. However in our patients we should continue to give it as strict asepsis cannot be ensured.

Second stage: Lithotomy position should be avoided. Pulse and respiration are measured every 10 minutes. Outlet forceps (preferred) or vacuum should be used to shorten the second stage.

Third stage: Active management of third stage is *not* done. If there is atonic PPH concentrated oxytocin 20 units in IV drip or prostaglandin I/M injection (carboprost) 250 μg is administered. Ergometrine is better avoided.

Postpartum management: Careful observation is must as heart failure can occur immediate postpartum (sudden additional blood load from the uterus) or later (mobilization of extravascular fluid in the vascular system).

Adequate bed rest with gentle leg exercises and breathing exercises is advocated to prevent thromboembolic and chest complications. Breast feeding is allowed except in patient with heart failure.

Contraception:
Permanent: Vasectomy is preferred to female sterilization. However, it is recognized that women with severe disease have a shortened life span and the male may wish to preserve his fertility to have a family in future. In female minilap tubal ligation (TL) under local anesthesia after at least 1 week of delivery or interval laparoscopic tubal ligation (Lap TL) using less gas and less head low position can be the option.

Temporary: Oral pills are avoided due to risk of thromboembolism. Progesterone only contraceptives can be used. Intrauterine contraceptive device (IUCD) is avoided due to risk of infection. Barrier method is the method of choice but high failure rate is a problem.

Other Valvular Lesions
Aortic Stenosis

It is either congenital or rheumatic in origin. Pregnancy is poorly tolerated in such cases with high maternal mortality of 15%. Strict limitation of physical activity is must. Hypovolemia and hypotension must be avoided. Balloon valvotomy or aortic valve surgery may be indicated during pregnancy.

Mitral Incompetence (MI) Mitral Regurgitation (MR) Aortic Incompetence (AI) Aortic Regurgitation (AR)

These are tolerated during pregnancy because the decrease in systemic vascular resistance will increase forward flow. Associated MST usually decides the prognosis.

Pulmonary and Tricuspid Valve Diseases

These are rare and they are usually well tolerated.

■ PERIPARTUM CARDIOMYOPATHY

Diagnostic criteria suggested by Demakis and Rahimtoola[3] include:

- Heart failure in last month of pregnancy or 5 months postpartum
- Absence of prior heart disease
- No identifiable cause of heart failure
- Echocardiography shows left ventricular dysfunction. Echo changes suggested by Hibbard et al.[4] include: (i) ejection fraction < 45%, (ii) fractional shortening < 30%, and (iii) left ventricle end diastolic dimension > 2.7 cm/m^2.

Typical clinical features include fatigue, dyspnea on exertion, orthopnea, nonspecific chest pain, peripheral edema, and abdominal discomfort. Although rare, it carries high risk of mortality, i.e., 25–50%. It is found more in patients with hypertension, multiple pregnancy, and increased maternal age and parity. The exact cause of PPCM is unknown. Treatment of heart failure is on usual lines. Medical therapy for PPCM may be initiated during pregnancy and continued postpartum. Digoxin, diuretics, and hydralazine may be used safely during pregnancy and while breast feeding. Beta blockers may improve left ventricular function in patients with cardiomyopathy. When conventional medical therapy is unsuccessful, women with PPCM may require intensive intravenous therapy, mechanical assist devices, or even cardiac transplantation.

More than half of women with PPCM completely recover normal heart size and function within 6 months of delivery. Because of high risk of recurrence, future pregnancy is contraindicated.

■ CONGENITAL HEART DISEASES

- *Left-to-right shunts*: Atrial septal defect (ASD), ventricular septal defect (VSD), and patent ductus arteriosus (PDA) are reasonably well tolerated during pregnancy. Size of the defect is the main determinant factor of degree of disability.
- *Coarctation of aorta*: It is rare in woman and is frequently associated with bicuspid aortic valve and cerebral artery aneurysms. Pregnancy increases the risk of aortic dissection, infective endocarditis and cerebral hemorrhage.
- Cesarean section is recommended only for obstetric indications.
- *Tetralogy of Fallot*: It consists of (1) pulmonary stenosis, (2) right ventricular hypertrophy, (3) large VSD, and (4) overriding of aorta.
- In patients who have not had surgical repair, pregnancy is poorly tolerated, so MTP is advised.
- *Marfan's syndrome*: It has an autosomal dominant inheritance. There is myxomatous degeneration of heart valves and cystic medial necrosis of the aorta resulting in aneurysms. Pregnancy is dangerous in such case because of aortic dissection and rupture.
- *Pulmonary stenosis*: Usually well-tolerated during pregnancy. In severe stenosis congestive heart failure can occur.
- *Eisenmenger's syndrome*: It is characterized by pulmonary hypertension secondary to right-to-left or bidirectional shunt. Because of high maternal and perinatal mortality (severe maternal hypoxemia and polycythemia) MTP is advised.
- *Idiopathic hypertrophic subaortic stenosis (IHSS)*: There is marked hypertrophy of ventricular septum leading to outflow obstruction. Hypovolemia should be avoided as in AST.

■ PREGNANT WOMAN WITH PROSTHETIC VALVES

Bioprosthetic valve do not require anticoagulation during pregnancy. But due to short life of such valves mechanical prosthetic valves are now used, which require lifelong anticoagulation.

Anticoagulants

Warfarin: Warfarin freely crosses the placental barrier and can harm the fetus, but it is safe during breastfeeding. The incidence of *warfarin embryopathy* (abnormalities of fetal bone and cartilage formation) is about 4–10%; the risk is highest when warfarin is administered during 6–12 weeks of gestation. The risk of warfarin embryopathy is low in patients who take 5 mg or less per day.

Unfractionated heparin: Unfractionated heparin (UFH) does not cross the placenta so it is safe for the fetus. Its use however, has been associated with maternal osteoporosis, hemorrhage, thrombocytopenia or thrombosis [heparin-induced thrombocytopenia and thrombosis (HITT) syndrome], and a high incidence of thromboembolic events UFH is used subcutaneously with starting does is 15,000–20,000 U twice daily. The appropriate dose adjustment is based on an activated partial thromboplastin time (aPTT) of 2–3 times the control level. High doses of UFH are often required to achieve the goal aPTT, because of the hypercoagulable state of pregnancy. Heparin is stopped as soon as the labor pains start or 6 hours before elective cesarean sections and is again started at 6–12 hours of completion of labor. UFH can be reversed with *protamine sulfate*. 1 mg of drug neutralizes 100 units of heparin. It is given I/V slowly.

Low-molecular-weight heparin: Low-molecular-weight heparin (LMWH) produces a more predictable anticoagulant response than UFH and is less likely to cause HITT. Its effect on maternal bone mineral density appears to be minimal. LMWH can be administered subcutaneously and dosed to achieve an antifactor Xa level of 1.0–1.2 U/mL 4–6 hours after injection.

It is advisable to stop warfarin when the pregnancy is discovered and to use UFH or LMWH, at least until after the 12th week. Heparin restarted at approximately 36 weeks in anticipation of delivery.

Pregnancy and Cardiac Surgery

Open heart surgery including valve replacement surgery has the same risks as in nonpregnant patient but it is associated with very high fetal loss.

◼ CARDIAC ARRHYTHMIAS

Significant cardiac arrhythmias are rare during pregnancy. Management of arrhythmias is similar to that in the nonpregnant state. Drug treatment is indicated when women are symptomatic and commonly used antiarrhythmic medications are safe during pregnancy. Exceptions are amiodarone which can cause neonatal hypothyroidism and sotalol which can cause fetal IUGR. Electrocardioversion is usually safe during pregnancy and can be used when indicated.

◼ CORONARY ARTERY DISEASE

Acute myocardial infarction (AMI) during pregnancy is rare, occurring in 1 in 35,000 pregnancies. Angiotensin-converting enzyme (ACE) inhibitors and statins are contraindicated during pregnancy. Clopidogrel and glycoprotein IIb/IIIa receptor inhibitors have been used safely in individual pregnant patients. Percutaneous coronary intervention using both balloon angioplasty and stenting has been successfully performed in pregnant patients with AMI, with the use of lead shielding to protect the fetus.

Different scoring systems for predicting adverse outcome during pregnancy or are CARPREG I and II scoring and ZAHARA prediction score.

Siu and Colman[5] suggested four risk factors to estimate the risk of cardiac complications during pregnancy (CARPREG score) **(Table 1)**.

Risk estimation of cardiovascular maternal complications is 5% if there is 0 point. It is 27% if there is 1 risk factor and it increases to 75% if there is > 1 risk factor.

CARPREG II score[6] is now suggested which include 10 risk factors whichare shown in **Table 2**.

Risk of cardiac event is 5% if score is 1, 10% if score is 2, 15% if score is 3, 22% if score is 4, and 41% if score is >4.

Zahara Prediction score[7] has been described in **Table 3**.

TABLE 1: Risk factors to estimate the risk of cardiac complications during pregnancy (CARPREG score).

	Cardiac risk factor	Point
1	Prior heart failure, TI attacks, arrhythmia, stroke	1
2	NYHA > II, cyanosis	1
3	Ejection fraction < 40%	1
4	Left-sided heart obstruction, i.e., mitral < 2 cm², aortic valve < 1.5 cm² or peak left ventricular outflow tract gradient > 30 mm on echo	1

(NYHA: New York Heart Association; TI: transient ischemic)

TABLE 2: CARPREG II score.

	Predictor	Points
1	Prior cardiac event or arrhythmias	3
2	Baseline NYHA >2 or cyanosis	3
3	Mechanical valve	3
4	Systemic ventricular dysfunction LVEF < 55%	2
5	High-risk valve disease or left ventricular outflow tract obstruction (aortic valve area < 1.5 cm², subaortic gradient > 30, or moderate-to-severe aortic regurgitation, mitral stenosis < 2.0 cm²	2
6	Pulmonary hypertension RVSP > 49 mm Hg	2
7	High-risk aortopathy	2
8	Coronary artery disease	2
9	No prior cardiac intervention	1
10	Late pregnancy assessment	1

(LVEF: left ventricular ejection fraction; NYHA: New York Heart Association; RSVP: right ventricular systolic pressure)

TABLE 3: Zahara prediction score.

Predictors	Points	Total points	Risk
Prior arrhythmias	1.5	0	2.9%
NYHA class ≥ 2	0.75	0.5–1.5	17.5%
Left heart obstruction (PG > 50 mm Hg or AVA < 1 cm²)	2.5	1.51–2.50	43%
Cardiac medication before pregnancy	1.5	2.51–3.50	43.1%
Systemic AV valve regurgitation	0.75	>3.51	70%
Pulmonary AV valve regurgitation	0.75		

(AV: atrioventricular; AVA: aortic valve area; NYHA: New York Heart Association)

TABLE 4: World Health Organization classification.

Class	Risk of pregnancy	Condition
I	No detectable increased risk of maternal mortality, No/mild increased risk of morbidity	Uncomplicated, small or mild PST, PDA, mitral valve prolapsed Successfully repaired ASD, VSD or PDA Isolated ventricular or atrial ectopic beats
II	Small increased risk of maternal mortality or moderate increased risk of morbidity	Unoperated ASD or VSD Repaired tetralogy of Fallot Most arrhythmias Class II or III (depending on individual) Mild left ventricular impairment Hypertrophic cardiomyopathy Native or tissue valvular disease not considered WHO class I or IV Marfan syndrome with aortic dilatation Repaired coarctation
III	Significantly increased risk of maternal morbidity or mortality	Mechanical valve Systemic right ventricle Fontan circulation Cyanotic heart disease Other complex congenital heart disease Aortic dilatation 40–45 mm in Marfan syndrome
IV	Extremely high-risk of maternal mortality or severe morbidity; pregnancy is contraindicated	Pulmonary artery hypertension of any cause Previous peripartum cardiomyopathy with residual impairment Severe systemic ventricular dysfunction (LVEF < 30%, NYHA III or IV) Marfan syndrome with dilated aorta > 45 mm Native severe coarctation K

(ASD: atrial septal defect; LVEF: left ventricular ejection fraction; NYHA: New York Heart Association; PDA: patent ductus arteriosus; VSD: ventricular septal defect)

Modified World Health Organization (WHO) classification[8] integrates all known maternal cardiovascular risk factors. The patients are classified in four classes as shown in **Table 4**.

KEY POINTS

- Etiology for congenital heart lesion is multifactorial and include genetic, diabetes, systemic lupus erythematosus (SLE), infections, e.g., rubella and alcohol ingestion.
- Heart disease is temporarily worsened by one grade NYHA, there is no long-term deleterious effect of pregnancy on heart disease.
- Risk of transmission to fetus in case of congenital heart diseases varies from 2 to 20% for different lesions. In fetuses with increased nuchal translucence of > 95th centile 2% will have major cardiac defect.

◼ REFERENCES

1. Konar H, Chaudhuri S. Pregnancy Complicated by Maternal Heart Disease: A Review of 281 Women. J Obstet Gynaecol India. 2012;62(3):301-6.
2. The Criteria Committee of the New York Heart Association. Nomenclature and Criteria for Diagnosis of Diseases of the Heart and Great Vessels, 9th edition. Boston: Little, Brown and Co.; 1994. 253-6.
3. Demakis JG, Rahimtoola SH. Peripartum cardiomyopathy. Circulation. 1971;4:964-8.
4. Hibbard JU, Lindheimer M, Lang RM. A modified definition for peripartum cardiomyopathy and prognosis based on echocardiography. Obstet Gynecol. 1999;94(2):311-6.
5. Siu SC, Sermer M, Colman JM, Alvarez AN, Mercier LA, Morton BC, et al. Prospective multicenter study of pregnancy outcomes in women with heart disease. Circulation. 2001;104(5):515-21.
6. Slversides CK, Grewal J, Mason J, Sermer M, Kiess M, Rychel V, et al. Pregnancy Outcomes in Women with Heart Disease. The CARPREG II study. J Am Coll Cardiol. 2018;71(21):2419-30.
7. Drenthen W, Boersma E, Balci A, Moons P, Roos-Hesselink JW, Mulder BJ, et al. Predictors of pregnancy complications in women with congenital heart disease. Eur Heart J. 2010;31(17):2124-32.
8. European Society of Gynecology (ESG); Association for European Paediatric Cardiology (AEPC); German Society for Gender Medicine (DGesGM), Regitz-Zagrosek V, Blomstrom Lundqvist C, Borghi C, et al. ESC guidelines on the management of cardiovascular diseases during pregnancy: the Task Force on the Management of Cardiovascular Diseases during Pregnancy of the European Society of Cardiology (ESC). Eur Heart J. 2011;32(24):3147-97.

CHAPTER 6

Hypertensive Disorders in Pregnancy

Suyajna Joshi D, Raju V Giraddi

■ INTRODUCTION

Hypertension is the most common medical problem encountered during pregnancy, complicating 2–8% of pregnancies. 16% is the maternal death attribution to hypertensive disorders. The terminology and classification recommended by the National Institute of Health [National High Blood Pressure Education Program (NHEBP) Working Group] is preferred over the older but widely used term pregnancy-induced hypertension (PIH) because it is more precise. Preeclampsia occurs in approximately 5% of all pregnancies, 10% of first pregnancies, and 20–25% of women with a history of chronic hypertension. Hypertensive disorders in pregnancy may cause maternal and fetal morbidity and remain a leading source of maternal mortality.

Earlier, the diagnosis of PIH was classically described as a triad of hypertension, proteinuria, and edema. However, the triad is no longer necessary and ideally the use of the term PIH should be abandoned as its meaning in clinical practice is unclear and often confusing.

In 2013, the American College of Obstetricians and Gynecologists removed proteinuria as an essential criterion for diagnosis of preeclampsia (hypertension plus signs of significant end-organ dysfunction are sufficient for diagnosis). They also removed massive proteinuria (5 g/24 hours) and fetal growth restriction (FGR) as possible features of severe disease because massive proteinuria has a poor correlation with outcome, and FGR is managed similarly whether or not preeclampsia is diagnosed. Oliguria was also removed as a characteristic of severe disease.

■ DIAGNOSIS AND CLASSIFICATION

Hypertension in pregnancy is defined as a sustained systolic blood pressure (SBP) of 140 mm Hg or more and/or a diastolic blood pressure (DBP) of 90 mm Hg or more. This is best confirmed on two occasions at least 6 hours apart but within 7 days of using the same arm.

Severe hypertension should be defined as a SBP of 160 mm Hg or a DBP of 110 mm Hg. For severe hypertension, a repeat measurement should be taken for confirmation after 15 minutes. A DBP of 90 mm Hg identifies a level above which perinatal morbidity is increased in nonproteinuric hypertension, and DBP is a better predictor of adverse pregnancy outcomes than SBP.

A classification recommended by the National Institute of Health (NHEBP Working Group 2000) divides hypertension in pregnancy into four types:
1. Chronic hypertension.
2. Preeclampsia–eclampsia.
3. Preeclampsia superimposed on chronic hypertension.
4. Gestational hypertension (transient hypertension of pregnancy or chronic hypertension is identified in the latter half of pregnancy).

The changes proposed in this classification are elimination of edema and using relative increase in BP (i.e., >30 mm Hg in SBP and 15 mm Hg in DBP from the basal BP) for diagnostic criteria. The Korotkoff V sound was adopted to determine the DBP. BP should be measured with the woman in the sitting position with the arm at the level of the heart. An appropriately sized cuff (i.e., length of 1.5 times the circumference of the arm) should be used. In particular, Korotkoff phase V should be used for designation of DBP, as it is more reliable.

This recommendation replaces the previous recommendation to use both phase IV and phase V. Phase IV (muffling) should be used for DBP only if Korotkoff sounds are audible as the level approaches 0 mm Hg. A cuff that is too small overestimates SBP by 7–13 mm Hg and DBP by 5–10 mm Hg. A cuff should never be placed over clothing. Supine positioning has the potential to cause hypotension, and left lateral positioning has the potential to give the lowest BP value, because the right arm is frequently elevated above the level of the heart during BP measurement. Most errors in office BP measurements are operator dependent and correctable.

■ NORMAL MATERNAL CHANGES FOR FETAL GROWTH

Maternal changes during pregnancy provide for nutritional needs for the fetus to grow and mature. The blood flow to the placenta is impaired in hypertensive women when compared to normotensive women. Uterine blood flow is preferentially distributed to the placental bed, leading to increased placental blood perfusion. The local prostanoid production, extra renal renin–angiotensin activity, and placental progesterone production affect the hemodynamic changes within the uterine vasculature. To support increased perfusion of the uterus, there is a need for increased blood volume, together with uterine arterial vasodilatation. While the prostacyclin (PGI2):thromboxane ratio shifts more toward a vasodilatory profile, it also creates a state of partially compensated relative hypovolemia, resulting in the activation of volume receptors. This causes a stimulation of antidiuretic hormone (ADH) and renin production. The increased angiotensin II produced is, however, diverted toward aldosterone production away from its activity as a vasoconstrictor. This seems necessary to counteract the natriuretic effect of progesterone on the distal tubule. The vasoconstrictor effect of angiotensin is blunted by the endothelial production of vasodilators such as PGI2 and nitric oxide (NO). In other words, there is vascular refractoriness to the effect of angiotensin II. Thus, there is fluid and electrolyte retention by kidneys; the resulting increase in blood volume helps to fill the expanded vascular system.

■ CHANGES IN HYPERTENSION

Placenta as a Triggering Factor

Many of the adaptive changes seen in normal pregnancy are absent in preeclampsia. The invasion of the myometrial segment of spiral arteriole which normally occurs between 12 and 20 weeks was found to be specifically affected during the second phase of placentation. Tunica media in such patients is responsive to vasoactive agents. It is believed that placental ischemia results in the release of a substance "Factor X." Therefore, the maternal systemic changes seen in preeclampsia may be in response to factors released secondarily to placental ischemia. Similar placental findings are seen in intrauterine growth restriction (IUGR). Other factors mentioned below are required to turn placental insufficiency into the systemic pathology of preeclampsia. Preeclampsia is characterized by inadequate trophoblastic invasion with loss of vascular refractoriness (**Figs. 1 to 3**).

Vasospasm

While failure of trophoblastic invasion of the spiral vessels seems to be the fundamental defect, the altered PGI2/thromboxane A2 (TXA2) ratio favoring TXA2 seems to be a major player in causing preeclampsia. Vasoconstrictor

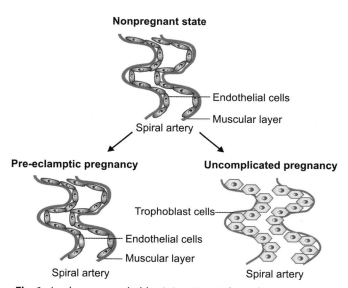

Fig. 1: Inadequate trophoblastic invasion with resultant responsive muscular layer and endothelial dysfunction is seen in preeclampsia.

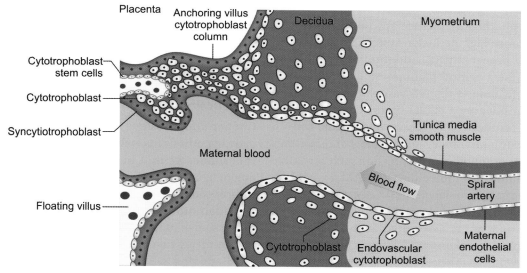

Fig. 2: Normal trophoblastic invasion with increased blood flow.

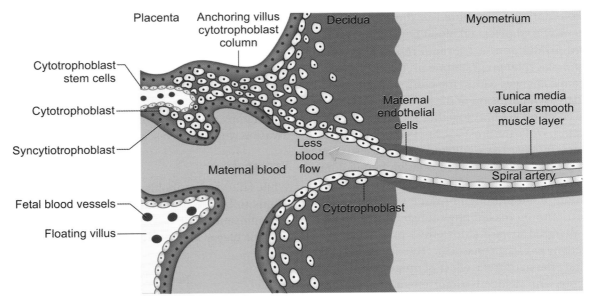

Fig. 3: Abnormal trophoblastic invasion with less placental blood flow.

prostanoid profile and the lack of nonprostanoid vasodilators play a major role in generalized vascular constrictor activity resulting in a failure of necessary expansion of the blood volume. As a result, there is poor perfusion of peripheral organs and tissues including the placenta. The renin–angiotensin system now functions as in a nonpregnant individual leading to worsening vasoconstriction, hypertension, and fluid retention. Gant and coworkers (1973)[1] demonstrated that increased vascular sensitivity to angiotensin II clearly preceded the onset of hypertension.

Endothelial Dysfunction

Nitric oxide or endothelial-derived relaxing factor (EDRF) is a potent vasodilator. Like PGI2, it too decreases the affinity for platelet aggregation. NO converts uteroplacental circulation from a high-resistance low perfusion system to a low-resistance high perfusion system. Its production is deficient in preeclampsia. Endothelial dysfunction is accepted to be a central pathophysiological event in preeclampsia leading to altered vascular reactivity and loss of vascular integrity. Cellular fibronectin, an isoform of fibronectin synthesized locally by endothelial cells in response to tissue injury, is elevated in preeclampsia. Other cellular markers of endothelial dysfunction such as soluble intercellular adhesion molecule 1 (sICAM 1), soluble vascular cell adhesion molecule 1 (sVCAM 1), E selectin, and plasma fibronectin are also elevated in patients with preeclampsia and/or are associated with an increased risk of developing preeclampsia. Evidence of endothelial dysfunction in women with preeclampsia is associated with an increased risk of small for gestational age (SGA) babies

and preterm babies. In contrast, women with preeclampsia but without hyperuricemia and elevated cellular fibronectin did not show evidence of increased risk for preterm birth and SGA babies.

Immunological Factors

The immunological reactions could result in the abnormalities of implantation and invasion. The risk of hypertension in pregnancy is appreciably enhanced in circumstances where the formation of blocking antibodies to the antigenic site on the placenta might be impaired. This may arise where the number of antigenic sites provided by the placenta is unusually great compared with the amount of antibody as with multiple fetuses. The immunization concept is supported by the observation that preeclampsia develops more frequently in multiparous women impregnated by a new consort.

Hoff and associates found a maternal–fetal human leukocyte antigen (HLA)–antigen D related (DR) relation with preeclampsia.

Genetic Predisposition

Cooper and Chesley (1986)[2] concluded that the single gene hypothesis fits well in the etiology, but multifactorial inheritance cannot be excluded. Women carrying the angiotensinogen gene variant T235 had a higher incidence of preeclampsia. Some found high incidence of factor V Leiden mutation in preeclamptic women. The high expression of tumor necrosis factor (TNF) alpha gene may have a major role in mediating endothelial disturbances predisposing women for hypertension. The role of endothelial NO synthetase (*eNOS*) gene in the development

Flowchart 1: Genesis of preeclampsia as a two-stage disorder (Roberts and Taylor).

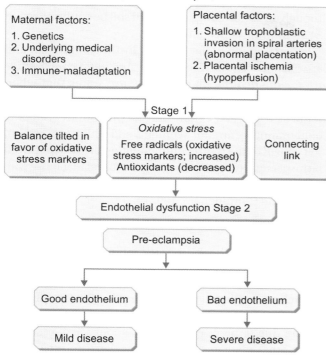

of familial preeclampsia was evaluated by analysis among affected sister pairs. Chromosome 7q36 encoding the *eNOS* gene has been localized.

▪ PREECLAMPSIA

Preeclampsia is a multisystem, pregnancy-specific disorder of unknown etiology with onset after 20 weeks of gestation **(Flowchart 1)**. It is classified as mild and severe. Hypertension is the most important sign of preeclampsia. Hence, care should be exercised in measuring the BP.
Women are at a high risk of preeclampsia if they have:

▪ *One of the following high-risk factors:*
  – A history of hypertensive disease during a previous pregnancy
  – Chronic kidney disease
  – Autoimmune disease, such as systemic lupus erythematosus (SLE) or antiphospholipid syndrome
  – Type 1 or type 2 diabetes
  – Chronic hypertension:
    - Thrombophilia
▪ *Two or more of the following moderate-risk factors:*
  – First pregnancy
  – Aged 40 years or older
  – Pregnancy interval of >10 years
  – Body mass index (BMI) of 35 kg/m² or greater at the first visit

  – Family history of preeclampsia
  – Multiple pregnancy.

Management

Management of preeclampsia poses a stiff challenge as it is an unpredictable disorder whose only definitive cure is termination of pregnancy. Hence, management is directed toward early detection and amelioration of its progression, the objective being to continue the pregnancy to achieve fetal maturity and prevent maternal complications, especially in mild hypertension. In order to prolong the pregnancy, day-to-day assessment of maternal and fetal condition is of vital importance.

Diagnostic Criteria for Preeclampsia

▪ *Blood pressure:*
  – SBP of 140 mm Hg or more or DBP of 90 mm Hg or more on two occasions at least 4 hours apart after 20 weeks of gestation in a woman with a previously normal BP
  – SBP of 160 mm Hg or more or DBP of 110 mm Hg or more [Severe hypertension can be confirmed within a short interval (minutes) to facilitate timely antihypertensive therapy].
▪ *Proteinuria:*
  – 300 mg or more per 24-hour urine collection (or this amount extrapolated from a timed collection) or
  – Protein/creatinine ratio of 0.3 mg/dL or more or dipstick reading of 2+ (used only if other quantitative methods are not available)
  – In the absence of proteinuria, new-onset hypertension with the new onset of any of the following:
    - *Thrombocytopenia:* Platelet count <100,000 * 10⁹/L
    - *Renal insufficiency:* Serum creatinine concentrations > 1.1 mg/dL or a doubling of the serum creatinine concentration in the absence of other renal diseases
    - *Impaired liver function:* Elevated blood concentrations of liver transaminases to twice normal concentration
    - *Pulmonary edema:* New-onset headache unresponsive to medication and not accounted for by alternative diagnoses or visual symptoms.

The presence of frontal or occipital headache which does not respond to simple analgesics indicates a worsening condition. Controlling the hypertension may relieve the headache as it is of vascular origin. **Box 1** shows the list of criteria which indicate the severity of preeclampsia.

BOX 1: Diagnostic criteria for severe preeclampsia (ACOG Practice Bulletin 2002).

- Blood pressure > 160–180 mm Hg systolic or >110 mm Hg diastolic
- Proteinuria > 5 g/24 hours
- Oliguria defined as <500 mL/24 hours
- Upper abdominal pain
- Cerebral or visual disturbances
- Pulmonary edema
- Epigastric or right upper quadrant pain
- Impaired liver function of unclear etiology
- Thrombocytopenia
- Fetal intrauterine growth retardation or oligohydramnios
- Elevated serum creatinine
- Grand mal seizures (eclampsia)

(ACOG: American College of Obstetricians and Gynecologists)

Laboratory Findings

The tests are usually normal in case of mild preeclampsia. The laboratory tests reflect the effect of disease on the various systems.

Urine examination is one of the oldest and frequently performed tests in clinical practice. Proteinuria is a sign of preeclampsia which is defined as ≥300 mg of protein in a 24-hour urine collection. The diagnosis is questionable in its absence. It usually correlates with 30 mg/dL or a 1+ reading in dipstick in a random urine specimen. Proteinuria is also valuable as a sign of severity, and a value ≥ 5 g in 24 hours is one of the criteria to classify as severe. The 24-hour urine collection for protein is the gold standard in the diagnosis of preeclampsia. However, a quicker method such as dipstick has a good although not perfect correlation with the protein in the urine. A 1+ dipstick has a 92% positive predictive value to predict 30 mg/dL of protein in the urine. However, a negative or trace dipstick result does not rule out proteinuria and up to 66% of these women have >30 mg/dL of protein in the urine. The proteinuria in preeclampsia is nonselective containing mixture of several proteins of different molecular weights. The urinary sediment is usually unrevealing and in most cases shows abundance of fine and coarse granular casts. The presence of a nephritic (red cell casts) or nephrotic (birefringent lipid, wax casts) must alert the clinician to the possibility of an underlying renal pathology. It is very sensitive and reliable in predicting the severity of the disease. Trace levels to +1 proteinuria are acceptable, but levels of +2 or greater are abnormal. The concentration of protein in urine is dependent on several factors including the volume excreted, posture, contamination with vaginal discharge, and urinary tract infection (UTI). Hence, for screening, a clean midstream sample must be collected. If the urine is positive for bacterial culture in a woman with hypertension, the tests for urine proteins must be repeated after treatment with appropriate antibiotics. Recently, spot urine specimens for protein:creatinine ratios have been validated as screening tools for abnormal proteinuria during pregnancy. They appear to be more accurate than urinalysis, although an abnormal result should still be confirmed with a 24-hour urine collection.

Expert opinion in the National Institute for Health and Care Excellence (NICE) guideline *Antenatal care, routine care for the healthy pregnant woman* states that when BP is measured at each antenatal check, a urine sample should be tested at the same time for proteinuria (National Collaborating Centre for Women's and Children's Health, 2008). NICE based this recommendation on evidence from a retrospective study of 53 women that found that those with proteinuria > 500 mg/day had a high risk of preeclampsia (Stettler and Cunningham, 1992).[3]

Complete Blood Count

Hemoglobin levels > 13 g/dL suggest the presence of hemoconcentration. Low levels may be due to microangiopathic hemolysis or iron deficiency. In cases in which an incidental platelet count is <150,000/μL, 75% are secondary to dilution thrombocytopenia of pregnancy, 24% are due to preeclampsia, and about 1% of cases are due to other platelet disorders not related to pregnancy. Counts < 100,000/μL suggest preeclampsia or idiopathic thrombocytopenic purpura (ITP). This may occur in 7% of the mild disease and 50% of the severe patients. Thrombocytopenia is characteristic of preeclampsia since it does not occur in essential hypertension. Examination of the peripheral blood smear for evidence of microangiopathic hemolysis and thrombocytopenia may reveal the presence of red blood cell (RBC) fragments. In this setting, the diagnoses of hemolytic-uremic syndrome (HUS), thrombotic thrombocytopenic purpura (TTP), and HELLP syndrome (*H*emolytic anemia, *E*levated *L*iver enzymes and *L*ow *P*latelet count) are a form of severe preeclampsia.

Liver Function Tests

Preeclampsia can be associated with hepatic dysfunction indicated by elevated levels of gamma glutamase, serum glutamic-oxaloacetic transaminase [SGOT; aspartate aminotransaminase (AST)], serum glutamic pyruvic transaminase [SGPT; alanine aminotransferase (ALT)], lactate dehydrogenase (LDH), and alkaline phosphatase. It should be noted that even placenta contributes to the concentration of alkaline phosphatase. Elevated hepatic transaminases may occur in the absence of epigastric/right upper quadrant (RUQ) pain.

Renal Function Tests

Decreased clearance of uric acid usually precedes the changes of glomerular filtration rate (GFR). Tubular dysfunction occurs earlier to glomerular dysfunction.

A serum uric acid level of >5 mg/dL is abnormal and is a sensitive, but nonspecific, marker of tubular dysfunction in preeclampsia. A rising level of serum uric acid in preeclampsia during the last trimester may indicate poor fetal prognosis. However, it is a poor predictor of the disease as it rises along with the clinical appearance of the disease. Blood urea and serum creatinine are lower in pregnant women than in a nonpregnant state due to increased GFR and the rise in plasma volume. Serum creatinine of >0.8 mg/dL during pregnancy suggests intravascular volume contraction or renal involvement in preeclampsia.

Coagulation Studies

Prothrombin time (PT) and/or international normalized ratio (INR) and/or activated partial prothrombin time (aPTT) results may be abnormal in consumptive coagulopathy and disseminated intravascular coagulopathy (DIC) complicating severe preeclampsia. Checking the PT/INR/aPTT is not necessary in the absence of abnormal liver transaminases or thrombocytopenia.

Serum Electrolytes

Serum sodium and potassium levels are low during normal pregnancy due to hemodilution. Persistent low levels of potassium in a hypertensive woman may indicate accelerated hypertension or an underlying mineralocorticoid-producing tumor of the adrenal gland (Conn syndrome).

Mild Preeclampsia

Primarily, the management is determined by the gestational age and the severity of the disease. In cases of mild hypertension, the pregnancy is continued up to 37 weeks if possible with close maternal and fetal surveillance to ensure adequate growth and maturity of the child. In such cases, the pregnancy outcome is similar to that found in normotensive pregnancy. Maternal evaluation includes measurements of BP, weight, urine protein, and questioning about symptoms of headache, upper abdominal pain, and visual disturbances. The frequency of these tests may be modified based on clinical findings and patient symptoms. Following the initial documentation of proteinuria and the establishment of the diagnosis of preeclampsia, additional quantifications of proteinuria are no longer necessary. Although the amount of proteinuria is expected to increase over time with expectant management, this change is not predictive of perinatal outcome and should not influence the management of preeclampsia. The BP should be checked every 15 minutes until the woman is stabilized and every 30 minutes in the initial phase of assessment. BP should be checked every 4th hourly if the patient is stable and asymptomatic.

NICE concluded that advice on rest, exercise, and work for women at risk of hypertensive disorders of pregnancy should be the same as the advice given to healthy pregnant women in their guideline *Antenatal care, routine care for the healthy pregnant woman* (National Collaborating Centre for Women's and Children's Health, 2008).

In the HYPITAT (Hypertension and Preeclampsia Intervention Trial at Term) trial, women with gestational hypertension and preeclampsia without severe features after 36 weeks of gestation were allocated to expectant management or induction of labor. The latter option was associated with a significant reduction in a composite of adverse maternal outcome including new-onset severe preeclampsia, HELLP syndrome, eclampsia, pulmonary edema, or placental abruption. In addition, no differences in rates of neonatal complications or cesarean delivery were reported by the authors.[4]

Fetal evaluation includes ultrasonography (USG), daily fetal movement count, and nonstress testing (NST). In the acute setting, an initial assessment with cardiotocography should be undertaken. This gives information about fetal well-being at that time but does not give any predictive information. Women in labor with severe preeclampsia should have continuous electronic fetal monitoring. If conservative management is planned, then further assessment of the fetus with ultrasound measurements of fetal size, umbilical artery Doppler, and liquor volume should be undertaken. Serial assessment will allow the timing of delivery to be optimized. The value of Doppler in other fetal vessels has yet to be clarified.

The main pathology affecting the fetus, apart from prematurity, is placental insufficiency leading to IUGR. IUGR occurs in around 30% of preeclamptic pregnancies. Ultrasound assessment of fetal size, at the time of the initial presentation with hypertension, is a valuable one-off measurement to assess fetal growth. Growth restriction is usually asymmetrical, so measurement of the abdominal circumference is the best method of assessment. Reduced liquor volume is also associated with placental insufficiency and FGR. Serial estimations of liquor volume can detect fetal compromise. Randomized trials have shown that investigation with umbilical artery Doppler assessment, using absent or reversed-end diastolic flow, improves neonatal outcome and serial investigations of this and other fetal vessels can be used to follow pregnancies under treatment and optimize delivery (**Box 2**).

BOX 2: Criteria for delivery in mild preeclampsia.

- Abnormal biophysical profile
- Criteria for severe preeclampsia met

Severe Preeclampsia

It is mandatory to admit a woman with a diagnosis of severe preeclampsia. The management of severe preeclampsia is based on careful assessment, stabilization, continued monitoring, and delivery at the optimal time for the mother and her baby. This means controlling BP and, if necessary, prevent the convulsions. Senior obstetric and anesthetic staff and experienced midwives should be involved. There is a general consensus that severe hypertension should be considered as urgent and treated in pregnancy to decrease maternal morbidity and mortality even in the absence of symptoms.

Treatment of hypertension is the cornerstone of preeclampsia management. In our study of 164 eclampsia patients (1997–99), maternal mortality was 11.4% when the mean arterial pressure (MAP) was >110 mm Hg and it was 4.5% when the MAP was <110 mm Hg. This stresses the need for adequate treatment of hypertension in eclampsia. Unfortunately, in most of the Indian centers once eclampsia develops, anticonvulsive management is practiced without concurrent adequate antihypertensive management. Maternal outcome can be improved by simultaneous and effective application of all the principles of eclampsia management.

Antihypertensive treatment should be started in women with a SBP > 160 mm Hg or a DBP > 110 mm Hg. In women with other markers of a potentially severe disease, treatment can be considered at lower degrees of hypertension. Labetalol, given orally or intravenously; nifedipine, given orally; or hydralazine, given intravenously, can be used for the acute management of severe hypertension. Atenolol, angiotensin-converting enzyme (ACE) inhibitors, angiotensin receptor-blocking (ARB) drugs, and diuretics should be avoided. Nifedipine should be given orally, not sublingually. Doctors should use the drug with which they are familiar.

There is a continuing debate concerning women with a BP between 100 mm Hg systolic and 110 mm Hg diastolic. Maternal treatment is associated with a reduction of severe hypertensive crises and a reduction in the need for further antihypertensive therapy; however, there appears to be a small reduction in infant birth weight. With treatment, prolongation of pregnancy of an average of 15 days is possible as long as there is no other reason to deliver **(Table 1)**.

Hypertensive Emergency and Urgency

Depending on the severity of elevations of BP and presence of end-organ damage, severe hypertension is defined as either hypertensive emergency or hypertensive urgency. A hypertensive emergency is associated with acute end-organ damage and should be treated with an immediate titratable short-acting IV antihypertensive agent. Severe hypertension without end-organ damage is referred to as hypertensive urgency and is usually treated with oral antihypertensive agents.

Altered autoregulation occurs in patients with hypertensive emergency, and since end-organ damage is present already, rapid and excessive correction of the BP can further reduce perfusion and propagate further injury. Therefore, patients with a hypertensive emergency are best managed with a continuous infusion of a short-acting, titratable antihypertensive agent. Due to unpredictable

TABLE 1: Antihypertensive agents in acute hypertension (Clarke).			
Drug	*Mechanism of action*	*Dosage*	*Comment*
Hydralazine hydrochloride	Arterial vasodilator	5 mg IV, then 5–10 mg IV/20 min	Must wait 20 min for response between IV doses; possible maternal hypotension
Labetalol	Selective alpha- and nonselective beta-antagonist	20 mg IV, then 40–80 mg IV/10 min to 300 mg total dose; IV infusion 1–2 mg/min, titrated	Less reflex tachycardia and hypotension than with hydralazine
Nifedipine	Calcium channel blocker	10 mg by mouth, may repeat after 30 min	Oral route only; possible exaggerated effect if used with $MgSO_4$
Nitroglycerin	Relaxation of venous (and arterial) vascular smooth muscle	5 µg/min infusion, double every 5 min	Requires arterial line for continuous BP monitoring; potential methemoglobinemia
Sodium nitroprusside	Vasodilator	0.25 µg/kg/min infusion; increase 0.25 µg/kg/min/5 min	Requires arterial line for continuous BP monitoring; potential cyanide toxicity
Diazoxide	Peripheral arteriolar vasodilator	30–60 mg IV/5 min; IV infusion 10 mg/min, titrated	Possible rapid hypotension, hyperglycemia, decreased uterine contractility
Captopril enalapril	Angiotensin-converting enzyme inhibitor	Oral route only	Contraindicated during pregnancy due to potential fetal side effects (anuria or renal failure)
Methyldopa	Dopa decarboxylase inhibitor	1 g loading dose; then 250–500 mg IV/6 hours	Slow onset of action (4–6 hours) after IV injection; not ideal for hypertensive crises

pharmacodynamics, the sublingual and intramuscular (IM) routes should be avoided. Patients with a hypertensive emergency should be managed in an intensive care unit (ICU)/high dependency unit (HDU) with close monitoring. The immediate goal is to reduce DBP by 10–15% or to approximately 110 mm Hg over a period of 30–60 minutes. In our hospital, we use IV labetalol to control acute severe hypertension. In VIMS protocol (Vijayanagar Institute of Medical Sciences, Bellary), we use 15 mg of IV labetalol every 15 minutes until the desired BP is achieved up to a maximum of 225 mg.

Doses of the most commonly used agents used for the treatment of a BP of 140–159/90–*105 mm Hg:*

- Methyldopa 250–500 mg po bid-qid (max 2 g/d). There is no evidence to support a loading dose of methyldopa.
- Labetalol 100–400 mg po bid-tid (max 1,200 mg/d).
Some experts recommend a starting dose of 200 mg po bid:
- Nifedipine PA tablets (10–20 mg po bid-tid, maximum 180 mg/d) or XL preparation (20–60 mg po OD, maximum 120 mg/d). Caution should be exercised in ensuring that the correct form of nifedipine has been prescribed.

Drug Treatment of Preeclampsia

NICE reviewed the available evidence and concluded that (National Collaborating Centre for Women's and Children's Health, 2010): There is limited good-quality evidence about treatment of preeclampsia. There is no evidence that lowering BP in women with mild or moderate preeclampsia improves pregnancy outcomes compared with starting treatment once the woman has developed severe hypertension. However, there is insufficient evidence to know whether antihypertensive treatment prevents rarer outcomes such as a stroke or placental abruption. There is some evidence about appropriate target BP. There seems to be an increased risk of severe hypertension with less tight control (diastolic values above 90 mm Hg or 100 mm Hg). There is some evidence from a randomized controlled trial that labetalol reduces the risk of progression to severe hypertension. There is little evidence on the use of calcium-channel blockers.

NICE considered that the association of beta- blockers with reduced fetal growth was a result of excessive lowering of BP. Expert opinion from NICE is that labetalol seems to be as effective and safe as other drugs used for hypertension for managing preeclampsia and it is licensed for use in pregnancy. Labetalol should be used as first-line treatment. Alternative treatment includes methyldopa and nifedipine, and these should be offered after considering adverse effect profiles for the woman, fetus, and newborn baby.

For the first 2 weeks after the birth: Continue the antihypertensive treatment used during pregnancy, unless the woman is taking methyldopa. If she is taking methyldopa, this should be stopped 2 days after the birth, as it may increase the risk of depression.

Prophylactic Anticonvulsant Therapy

Magnesium sulfate ($MgSO_4$) should be considered for women with preeclampsia for whom there is concern about the risk of eclampsia. This is usually in the context of severe preeclampsia once a delivery decision has been made and in the immediate postpartum period. In women with less severe disease, the decision is less clear and will depend on individual case assessment.

The Magpie (MAGnesium sulphate for Prevention of Eclampsia) study has demonstrated that administration of $MgSO_4$ to women with preeclampsia reduces the risk of an eclamptic seizure. Women allocated $MgSO_4$ had a 58% lower risk of an eclamptic seizure [95% confidence interval (CI) 40–71%]. The relative risk reduction was similar regardless of the severity of preeclampsia.

Fluid Management

Fluid management in severe PIH consists of crystalloid infusions of normal saline or lactated Ringer's solution, at a rate of 80–100 mL/h or 1–2 mL/kg/h. Additional fluid volumes, in the order of 1,000 mL, may be required prior to the use of epidural anesthesia or vasodilator therapy to prevent maternal hypotension and fetal distress. Fluid restriction is advisable to reduce the risk of fluid overload in the intrapartum and postpartum periods. IV fluids are known to cause a decrease in colloid oncotic pressure (COP) in laboring patients. In addition, baseline COP is decreased in patients with preeclampsia and may decrease further in the postpartum period as a result of mobilization of interstitial fluids. This may be clinically relevant with respect to the development of pulmonary edema in patients who are receiving betamimetic. Therefore, close monitoring of fluid intake and output, hemodynamic parameters, and clinical signs must be undertaken to prevent an imbalance of hydrostatic and oncotic forces that potentiate the occurrence of pulmonary edema. Over the last 20 years, pulmonary edema has been a significant cause of maternal death. Fluid administration should not be routinely administered to treat oliguria (<15 mL/h). For persistent oliguria, neither dopamine nor furosemide is recommended. Central venous access is not routinely recommended, and if a central venous catheter is inserted, it should be used to monitor trends and not absolute values. The regime of fluid restriction should be maintained until there is a postpartum diuresis, as oliguria is common with severe pre-eclampsia. If there is associated maternal hemorrhage, fluid balance is more difficult and fluid restriction is inappropriate.

Delivery

The presence of preeclampsia does not guarantee accelerated lung maturation, and a high incidence of neonatal respiratory complications has been associated with premature delivery for preeclampsia. Antenatal corticosteroid therapy (i.e., Dexamethasone 6 mg IM every 12 hours for four doses) should be considered for all women who present with preeclampsia before 34 weeks' gestation as it accelerates fetal pulmonary maturity and decreases neonatal mortality and morbidity; a high incidence of neonatal respiratory complications has been associated with premature delivery for preeclampsia.

For women with any hypertension in pregnancy, vaginal delivery should be considered unless a caesarean section is required for the usual obstetric indications. If vaginal delivery is planned and the cervix is unfavorable, then cervical ripening agents should be used to increase the chance of a successful vaginal delivery. The delivery should be well planned, done on the best day, performed in the best place, by the best route, and with the best support team. A few hours' delay in delivery may be helpful if it allows the neonatal unit to be more organized or allows the transfer of the mother to a place where a cot is available. This assumes that the mother is stable before delivery and prior to transfer.

If the gestation is >34 weeks, delivery after stabilization is recommended. If <34 weeks and the pregnancy can be prolonged in excess of 24 hours, steroids help to reduce fetal respiratory mortality. There is a probable benefit from steroid therapy even if delivery is <24 hours after administration. Conservative management at very early gestations may improve the perinatal outcome but must be carefully balanced with maternal well-being. Vaginal delivery is generally preferable but, if gestation is below 32 weeks, caesarean section is more likely as the success of induction is reduced. After 34 weeks with a cephalic presentation, vaginal delivery should be considered. The consultant obstetrician should discuss the mode of delivery with the mother. Vaginal prostaglandins will increase the chance of success. Antihypertensive treatment should be continued throughout assessment and labor. Continuous fetal monitoring is performed as these fetuses are most often growth restricted with oligoamnios and are vulnerable to fetal distress. Adequate pain relief is necessary to decrease the hypertensive response to labor pain. Epidural analgesia is highly effective and helps to easily control BP and improves the perinatal and maternal outcomes. Regional analgesia and/or anesthesia are appropriate in a woman with a platelet count > 75,000/μL unless

there is coagulopathy, falling platelet concentration, or co-administration of an antiplatelet agent [e.g., acetylsalicylic acid (ASA)] or anticoagulant (e.g., heparin).

The third stage should be managed with five units of IM Syntocinon or five units IV Syntocinon, given slowly. Ergometrine or Syntometrine should not be given for prevention of postpartum hemorrhage, as this can further increase the BP.

Clinicians should be aware of the risk of late seizures and ensure that women have a careful review before discharge from the hospital. Antihypertensive medication should be continued after delivery as dictated by the BP. It may be necessary to maintain treatment for up to 3 months, although most women can have treatment stopped before this. Clinicians should be aware that up to 44% of eclampsia occur postpartum, especially at term, so women with signs or symptoms compatible with preeclampsia should be carefully assessed.

A summary of the management of severe preeclampsia is shown in **Flowchart 2**.

Complications of Severe Preeclampsia

HELLP syndrome: HELLP syndrome is a variant of severe preeclampsia, affecting up to 12% of patients with preeclampsia–eclampsia. As mentioned earlier, HELLP

Flowchart 2: Summary of the management of severe preeclampsia.

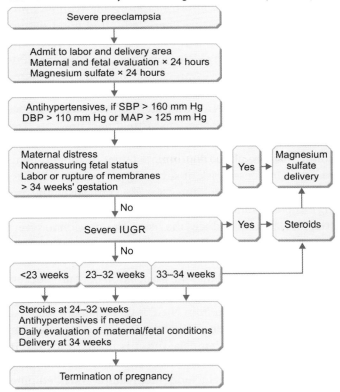

(DBP: diastolic blood pressure; IUGR: intrauterine growth restriction; SBP: systolic blood pressure)

> **BOX 3:** Recommended criteria for HELLP syndrome.
>
> - Hemolysis (at least two of the following):
>   - Peripheral
>   - Smear (schistocytes, burr cells)
>   - Serum bilirubin (>1.2 mg/dL)
>   - Low serum haptoglobin
>   - Severe anemia unrelated to blood loss
> - Elevated liver enzymes:
>   - ALT or AST ≥ twice upper level of normal
>   - LDH ≥ twice upper level of normal
> - Low platelets < 100,000/mm³
>
> (ALT: alanine aminotransferase; AST: aspartate aminotransferase; LDH: lactate dehydrogenase)

> **BOX 4:** Medical and surgical disorders confused with the HELLP syndrome.
>
> - Acute fatty liver of pregnancy
> - Appendicitis
> - Diabetes mellitus
> - Gallbladder disease
> - Gastroenteritis
> - Glomerulonephritis
> - Hemolytic-uremic syndrome
> - Hepatic encephalopathy
> - Hyperemesis gravidarum
> - Idiopathic thrombocytopenia
> - Kidney stones
> - Peptic ulcer
> - Pyelonephritis
> - Systemic lupus erythematosus
> - Thrombotic thrombocytopenic purpura
> - Viral hepatitis

syndrome is characterized by *h*emolysis, *e*levated *l*iver enzymes, and *l*ow *p*latelets (Weinstein, 1982). The acronym, HELLP syndrome, was coined by Weinstein in 1982, but the hematological changes were described by Pritchard et al. in 1954. Pritchard et al. credited association of thrombocytopenia with severe preeclampsia to Stahnke in 1922 and hepatic changes to Sheehan in 1950. Unlike most forms of preeclampsia, HELLP syndrome is not primarily a disease of primigravidas. Several studies have found that nearly half of HELLP syndrome patients were multigravidas, the incidence being almost twice that seen in primigravid patients **(Box 3)**.

Mississippi classification:

- *HELLP Class I:*
  - Platelet < 50,000/ mm³
  - AST or ALT > 70 IU/L
  - LDH > 600 U/L
- *HELLP Class II:*
  - Platelet 50,000–1,00,000/mm³
  - AST or ALT > 70 IU/L
  - LDH > 600 U/L
- *HELLP Class III:*
  - Platelet < 1,000,000/mm³
  - AST or ALT > 70 IU/L
  - LDH > 600 U/L.

The clinical signs and symptoms of patients with HELLP syndrome are classically related to the impact of vasospasm on the maternal liver. Thus, the majority of patients present with signs or symptoms of liver compromise. These include malaise, nausea (with or without vomiting), and epigastric pain. In most series, hepatic or RUQ tenderness to palpation is seen consistently in HELLP syndrome patients.

Clinically, many HELLP syndrome patients do not meet the standard BP criteria for severe preeclampsia. In one series of 112 women with severe preeclampsia–eclampsia complicated by HELLP syndrome, admission DBP was <110 mm Hg in 31% of cases and <90 mm Hg in 15% (Sibai, 1986).[5] In some patients, preeclampsia may first seem to be

a cause of jaundice, gastrointestinal bleeding, hematuria, or abdominal pain. They may be misdiagnosed as having other diseases **(Box 4)**. Numerous misdiagnoses are associated with this syndrome, and a delay in diagnosis may be life-threatening. A pregnant woman with thrombocytopenia, elevated serum transaminase levels, or epigastric pain should be considered to have HELLP syndrome until proven otherwise. A rare but interesting complication of HELLP syndrome is transient nephrogenic diabetes insipidus.

The presence of HELLP syndrome is associated with an increased risk of maternal death (0–24%) and an increased rate of maternal morbidities such as pulmonary edema (8%), acute renal failure (ARF; 3%), DIC (15%), abruptio placentae (9%), acute respiratory distress syndrome, sepsis, and stroke. There is also an increased rate of wound hematoma and increased need for blood and blood products. Development of HELLP syndrome in the postpartum period increases the chance of ARF and pulmonary edema. The chance of placental abruption in HELLP syndrome patients is 20 times higher than that seen in the general obstetric population. The reported perinatal death is 7–20%.

As with other severe preeclampsia variants, delivery is ultimately the treatment of choice. The timing of delivery, however, remains controversial. Several investigators recommend immediate delivery, while others reasonably suggest that under certain conditions with marked fetal immaturity, delivery may safely be delayed for a short time. Clark and associates have demonstrated transient improvement in patients with HELLP syndrome following bed rest and/or corticosteroid administration. Following an initial improvement, however, each patient's clinical condition worsened. Thus in a mother with a very premature fetus and borderline disturbances in platelet count or serum transaminase values, and in the absence of other absolute indications for delivery, careful hospital observation may at times be appropriate. Certainly, uncontrollable BP, significantly rising liver enzymes, or a serum creatinine would mandate immediate delivery irrespective of the gestational age.

The mode of delivery should depend on the state of the cervix and other obstetric indications for cesarean birth. HELLP syndrome, by itself, is not an indication for cesarean delivery. A high percentage of patients with HELLP syndrome, however, will undergo operative delivery. A commonly encountered situation involves a mother with a premature fetus, an unfavorable cervix, and a platelet count < 100,000/μL. In such patients, cesarean delivery is often preferred to avoid the necessity of later operative delivery for failed induction in the face of more significant thrombocytopenia. Maintain platelet counts > 20,000/μL for vaginal delivery and >40,000/μL for cesarean delivery. 6–10 units of platelet transfusion may be necessary before cesarean section in cases <40,000/μL. Laboratory abnormalities usually return to normal within a short time after delivery; it is not unusual, however, to see transient worsening of both thrombocytopenia and hepatic function in the first 24–48 hours' postpartum. An upward trend in platelet count and a downward trend in LDH concentration should occur in patients without complications by the fourth postpartum day. The treatment of patients with postpartum HELLP syndrome is the same as that of the antepartum period including the use of $MgSO_4$.

In a study of postpartum HELLP syndrome (Martin et al. 1997),[6] dexamethasone 10 mg intravenously at 12-hour intervals was given until disease remission was noted in treated patients, at which time up to two additional 5 mg intravenous doses were given at 12-hour intervals. Most impressive was a clinically significant reduction of indicated transfusion and respiratory therapy, invasive hemodynamic monitoring, infectious or bleeding-related morbidity, and length of the postpartum hospital course. Cochrane database review (2004) concludes that there is insufficient evidence to determine whether adjunctive steroid use in HELLP syndrome decreases maternal and perinatal mortality and major maternal and perinatal morbidity. However, in this review, patients treated with dexamethasone had faster resolution of laboratory parameters.

■ ECLAMPSIA

Eclampsia is the inevitable consequence of the disease progression in preeclampsia characterized by grand mal tonic-clonic seizures occurring in a patient with preeclampsia with other neurological and medical disorders being ruled out.

Physicians of ancient civilizations of Egypt, Greece, India, and China possibly knew of the syndrome. Mention about eclampsia can be found in records of 2200 BC Kahun Papyrus which states "to prevent women from biting her tongue, avite means a small wooden stick pound upon her jaws." The term "eclampsia" (to flash out suddenly, to come on suddenly, flash of lightning, to shine forth) was coined by Verandeus in 1668. Mauriceaus recognized that the disease could be treated by prompt delivery.

The incidence of eclampsia varies from 1 in 100 to 1 in 1,700 in developing countries and 1 in 2,000 in developed countries. The incidence in India varies from 1 in 30 to 1 in 500. In 80–85% cases, it is preceded by a stage of imminent eclampsia characterized by warning signs and symptoms that include headache, giddiness, and visual disturbances (flashes of light, dimmed vision, photophobia, and complete blindness). It arises without any obvious symptoms in 15–20% of the cases. Eclampsia unheralded by hypertension and proteinuria occurred in 38% of cases reported in the United Kingdom (Douglas, 1994).[7] Douglass and Redman concluded, "the term pre-eclampsia is misleading because eclampsia can precede preeclampsia." Eclamptic seizures occur prior to the delivery in roughly 80% of patients. In the remainder, convulsions occur postpartum usually within 48 hours and they have been reported up to 23 days following delivery. An awareness of the diverse presentations is important to allow prompt and adequate treatment. The differential diagnosis includes epilepsy, coincidental cerebrovascular accident, space-occupying lesions, infections (meningitis, encephalitis), metabolic disturbances, and hysteria.

The precise cause of seizures in preeclampsia remains unknown. Hypertensive encephalopathy, vasospasm, hemorrhage, ischemia, and edema of the cerebral hemispheres have been proposed as etiologic factors. Thrombotic and hemorrhagic lesions have been identified on autopsy of preeclamptic women.

The actual convulsive attack consists of four stages:

1. *Stage 1 (premonitory stage):* This stage lasts for a few seconds to half a minute; patient becomes unconscious, pupils dilate, eyes roll from side-to-side, turned to one side and fix, twitching of the face and the hands.

2. *Stage 2 (tonic stage):* This stage lasts for a few seconds; the body becomes rigid with distorted features, hands are clenched, and arms flexed.

3. *Stage 3 (clonic stage):* This stage lasts for half a minute to 2 minutes; alternative contraction and relaxation of the muscles, clenching of the jaw, tongue bites, twitching in the face starting around the angle of the mouth extending to the arm and leg of one side of the body. The face becomes cyanosed, tongue protrudes

out with frothing in the mouth, and breathing becomes steratorius.

4. *Stage 4 (stage of coma):* In this stage, the movements cease, the patient lies quiet, coma supervenes, and respiration gradually quietens down. The patient wakes up after a short time with amnesia of the events; sometimes, the patient may go into deep coma from which he/she may not recover. Fits may occur in quick succession leading to a condition called "status eclampticus." During convulsions, the temperature rises (rise of >39° is a grave sign suggestive of cerebral hemorrhage) as well as the pulse rate and BP. The first convulsions are usually the forerunner for others with the number of convulsions varying from 1 or 2 in mild cases to even 100 or more in untreated severe cases. As a rule, death does not occur until after frequent repetitive convulsions occur. During convulsions, the placental blood flow decreases and this combined with maternal hypoxemia and lactic acidosis cause fetal bradycardia. However, this usually recovers in 3–5 minutes; persistence of bradycardia for >10 minutes needs other causes, such as placental abruption, to be ruled out. It is at times difficult to distinguish between postpartum eclampsia and postpartum cerebral vein thrombosis.

The basic approach revolves around the following principles:

- General management
- Anticonvulsant management
- Antihypertensive management
- Obstetric management.

General Management

Patients with eclampsia require nursing in specialized ICUs with all necessary equipment. All external provoking stimuli are reduced to the minimum. They are nursed on railed cots in quiet dark rooms with minimum handling and examinations. Anticonvulsants are given as per the hospital protocol; suction apparatus is used to keep the throat clear. The head end may be lowered to facilitate postural drainage. Sometimes, a left lateral position may be needed. Oxygen is given by mask at 8–10 L/min to correct maternal and fetal hypoxia. During a convulsion a soft, firm mouth gag is used to prevent injury to the tongue. If asphyxia sets in, patients are intubated and positive-pressure ventilation is given; tracheostomy may be needed. One of the most important aspects of management is the maintenance of fluid balance. Fluid replacement should be with Ringer's lactate/normal saline at the rate of 60 mL/h up to a maximum of 125 mL/h. Once the patient is little stable and not restless, she is catheterized with an indwelling Foley catheter and vaginal

examination is performed to assess the cervical status. Care is taken to prevent bedsores/pneumonia.

Anticonvulsant Management

Parenteral $MgSO_4$ has emerged as the drug of choice for treating and preventing eclampsia with its major advantages of efficacy and relative safety to the mother/baby. The Eclampsia Collaborative Trial Group concluded, "there is now compelling evidence in favor of $MgSO_4$ for the treatment of eclampsia." In 2002, the results of the "Magpie trial," another large multicentric trial, were published which showed beyond any reasonable doubt the efficacy of $MgSO_4$ in reducing the risk of eclampsia. Pritchard gets the credit for popularizing $MgSO_4$ for preeclampsia and eclampsia in modern obstetrics by his famous Parkland Hospital regimen, popularly known as the "Pritchard's regimen." Others who made significant contribution to establish $MgSO_4$ as the first-line anticonvulsant in eclampsia were Zuspan, Sibai, Duley, Flowers, Chesley and Pepper, Eastman, and Cruik Shant.

Mechanism of Action

The precise mechanism of action of $MgSO_4$ in eclampsia is not clear with a great deal of controversies still existing. The postulated mechanisms include the following:

- *Central action*—blockade of N-methyl-D-aspartate (NMDA) subtype of glutamate channel receptor in a voltage-dependent manner. Preferential uptake by the hippocampus and cerebral cortex rich in NMDA receptors with potent cerebral vasodilatation is demonstrated by Doppler studies. Increased $MgSO_4$ concentration was demonstrated in cerebrospinal fluid after infusion.

- *Peripheral action*—at the neuromuscular junction causing blockage of calcium entering the cell and blocking calcium at the intracellular sites/membranes, reducing the presynaptic acetylcholine release at the endplate, and reducing the motor end plate sensitivity to acetylcholine (reducing neuromuscular irritability). Direct action of a neuromuscular block, though suggested, seems unlikely, as the serum concentration for its anticonvulsive action is well below that needed for neuromuscular block.

Magnesium sulphate is also known as the Epsom salt. It is $MgSO_4 \cdot 7 H_2O \cdot USP$. It has a molecular weight of 246, and 1 g of the salt contains 98 mg of elemental magnesium. The normal serum levels vary from 1.6 to 1.1 mEq/L **(Table 2)**. Magnesium is not absorbed orally; it attracts water in the colon (basis for its use as a laxative). By about 90 minutes, 50% of the infused magnesium move intracellular and by 4 hours about 50% are excreted in urine. Tubular reabsorption of magnesium depends on the parathyroid

TABLE 2: Serum levels of magnesium toxicity.	
Normal therapeutic level	4–6 mEq/L
Loss of patellar reflex	8–12 mEq/L
Feelings of warmth, flushing	9–12 mEq/L
Somnolence	10–12 mEq/L
Slurred speech	10–12 mEq/L
Muscular paralysis	15–17 mEq/L
Respiratory difficulty	15–17 mEq/L
Cardiac arrest	30–35 mEq/L

TABLE 3: Pritchard's protocol.

Loading dose	Maintenance dose
4 g (20 mL of 20%) IV over not <3 minutes immediately to be followed by 10 g (20 mL of 50%) IM, 5 g in each buttock. If convulsions persist after 15 minutes 2 g (10 mL of 20%) is given over 2 minutes. If the woman is large, 4 g is given	5 g (10 mL of 50%) is given every 4 hours at alternate sites after assuring presence of knee reflex respiratory rate > 14/min urine output > 100 mL

TABLE 4: Baha M Sibai regimen.

Loading dose	Maintenance dose
6 g IV (30 mL of 20%) in 100 mL of 5% dextrose over 10–15 minutes	(20 g of 50%) added to 1,000 mL of 5% dextrose given as IV infusion at 100 mL/h (2 g/h). Adjust to get a serum magnesium level of 4.8–9.6 g/dL.

hormone level. Magnesium administered parenterally promptly crosses the placenta and achieves equilibrium in the fetal serum and less in the amniotic fluid. The kidneys excrete magnesium. Calcium is the physiological antidote for magnesium.

Magnesium sulfate is commercially available as 25% or 50% w/v, with 1 g of $MgSO_4$ containing 98 mg of elemental ion. Sibai (1984)[8] found no therapeutic advantages of intravenous over intramuscular administration except for avoidance of muscle pain.

Intravenous dose is always diluted because bolus may cause cardiac arrhythmia/arrest.

Magnesium sulfate is not an innocuous drug, so strict monitoring of patients on $MgSO_4$ is needed to prevent serious side effects to the mother/fetus.

Fetal effects may include:

- Neurological and neuromuscular depression
- Protective effect against cerebral palsy
- Hyporeflexia
- Reduced FHR variability.

Management of $MgSO_4$ toxicity is by calcium. Calcium is the logical antidote for magnesium. Intravenous calcium as 10 mL of 10% calcium gluconate infusion is given slowly over 3 minutes. It increases the acetylcholine liberated at the neuromuscular junction by the action potential.

If respiratory arrest ensues, prompt endotracheal intubation and ventilation are life-saving.

Different MgSO₄ Regimens

There are many $MgSO_4$ regimens which are widely used in different parts of the world. The very fact that there is no single standardized protocol in the world gives scope for tailoring the regimen according to the local needs. This becomes all the more relevant in resource-poor settings.

Suyajna Joshi's Classification of MgSO₄ Regimens (1998)

- High-dose regimens, loading dose > 10 g, e.g., Pritchard regimen

- Low-dose regimen, loading dose < 10 g, e.g., Zuspan, Suman Sardesai regimen, Dhaka regimen
- Single-dose regimen, e.g., Joshi's regimen (VIMS regimen).

Pritchard's protocol and Baha M Sibai regimen are given in **Tables 3** and **4**, respectively.

■ MODIFICATIONS OF STANDARD REGIMENS

In the last decade, researchers in the developing countries have been constantly striving to steadily decrease the dosage of both loading and maintenance doses of $MgSO_4$ regimens to suit the local conditions. Disciplined use of standard Western regimens is hard to achieve in developing countries. There is definitely a transnational difference in response to $MgSO_4$ in the third world with racial characteristics being important in determining the response; there is danger in applying the results of the trials as such in different countries. As discussed in the Magpie trial report (2002), the most important question would be "what is the minimal effective dose?" If a woman is known to be or appear to be small, the dose should probably be limited (Pritchard). In recent years, Andrea Witlin in her review article on eclampsia comments, "One may also speculate that magnesium sulphate dosing should vary according to the patient's weights or body mass index. However, this has never adequately been evaluated."

Sardesai Suman et al., considering the small weight of Indian women, tried low-dose $MgSO_4$ therapy in eclamptic women for control of convulsion and in imminent eclampsia as seizure prophylaxis. In a study of 570 eclamptic women, they gave 4 g of $MgSO_4$ as loading dose intravenously and subsequently 2 g of $MgSO_4$ was given every 3rd hourly IV/IM with a recurrence rate of 7.89%. Begum et al. used low-dose "Dhaka regimen" comprising 10 g of loading dose; following this, 2.5 g was given intramuscularly 4th hourly in 65 patients. Only 1 (1.53%) developed recurrence. She concluded that half of the standard dose appeared to be sufficient to control convulsions. Mahajan et al. in a study of 95 women used 6 g loading dose and 4 g maintenance dose and reported a recurrence rate of 1.05%. In Chowdhury et al. study of 630 women, 480 women received IM $MgSO_4$ as maintenance dose according to the Pritchard regimen and 150 women were subjected to a low-dose IV regimen of $MgSO_4$ (0.6 g/h). There was no significant difference in the recurrence of convulsion (3.3% in the IM and 2% in the IV group).

The results of the Magpie trial suggest that a shorter course of treatment may be adequate. In this study, most of the women probably received only the loading-dose injection before being referred on to the recruiting hospital. For these women, there was no difference in the outcome between those given further $MgSO_4$ or placebo (relative risk 1.24, 95% CI 0.49–3.11). The argument for a short course is further supported by the trial data, which suggest that the drug may continue to be beneficial long after the treatment has been given. Since, eclamptic fits can occur at any time up to 7 days after delivery, for most of the time at which the women were at risk, they would have had subtherapeutic serum concentrations of $MgSO_4$. Despite this situation, prophylaxis seems to have been successful. To make $MgSO_4$ available to women at risk from eclampsia, a short regimen is suitable for use in underdeveloped countries; ideally, this would include a single $MgSO_4$ injection (Andrew D Weeks, Lancet 2002).[9]

■ NEWER INITIATIVE IN SAFE MOTHERHOOD

It should be noted that most of these regimens are used at medical colleges and many eclampsia cases occur in rural places where immediate treatment to arrest the seizures is not readily available. Despite the compelling evidence in favor of $MgSO_4$, health personnel at the primary care level do not administer $MgSO_4$. Most of these women either receive no immediate treatment or receive some anticonvulsants such as diazepam and sent to tertiary care centers for further management. Transportation of these highly irritable eclamptic women is far from ideal in most of the third-world countries including India.

Eclampsia is one of the important direct causes of maternal mortality. Eclampsia-related mortality can be reduced by early referral and effective institution of anticonvulsant therapy. $MgSO_4$ is the drug of choice for eclampsia. There is delay in starting the $MgSO_4$ therapy. Most often, eclamptic women are referred to tertiary care hospitals in a moribund state with consequent poor

fetomaternal outcome. Such a catastrophe can be avoided if $MgSO_4$ therapy is started at the earliest.

The eclampsia mortality rate is relatively more in the resource-poor settings of developing countries. In the Sibai study, the excellent maternal outcome is attributed to the experience of the physicians and use of a standardized protocol. In contrast, Lopez-Llera reported 13.9% maternal deaths while Adetoro reported 14.4% of maternal mortality. However, many of these patients were admitted in a moribund state with multiple complications. This finding emphasizes the importance of early and proper referral of such patients. The anticonvulsant regimen alone cannot change the maternal and fetal outcomes. The other principles of eclampsia management should be simultaneously and effectively instituted. Sibai recommends that the patient should be stabilized regarding BP and control of convulsion before transport and the patient should be sent in an ambulance with medical personnel in attendance.

The need of the hour is to arrest seizures at the earliest, especially in primary healthcare (PHC) settings, so that convulsion to treatment interval is brought to minimum. This strategy will help in improving the maternal and fetal outcome. 10% of these patients may convulse again after receiving loading dose. This recurrence may be acceptable considering the potential benefits of seizure control during transportation to higher centers. Most of these women will become seizure-free after an additional dose 2 g $MgSO_4$.

Suyajna Joshi et al. studied the effect of single-dose $MgSO_4$ "Suyajna Joshi's regimen" (VIMS Regimen) (4 g diluted intravenously plus 4 g intramuscularly) on 513 patients with a recurrence rate of 9.1 and 3.3% maternal mortality.

Administration of a traditional $MgSO_4$ regimen requires regular supervision by trained staff; hence, it would seem particularly important to assess the minimum effect dose and duration of treatment. As endorsed by the Magpie trial, Andrew D Weeks, and based on the encouraging results, we rationalize that the shorter $MgSO_4$ therapy should be readily available for immediate use at primary care levels. Doctors and trained paramedical staff should be extensively made aware about the shorter versions of $MgSO_4$ therapy.

Considering the constraints of women health care in resource-poor settings of developing countries, *the single-dose regimen can be safely used outside the established obstetric centers (at the PHC level itself where maximum cases of eclampsia occur)* and transferred to a tertiary care center for definitive, disciplined management of these cases.

Thus, crucial time is not wasted and almost seizure-free transportation can be ensured. Convulsion to medication interval is brought to minimum. Thus, many more lives of mothers can be saved.

Seizures refractory to standard $MgSO_4$ regimens may be treated with a slow 100 mg IV dose of thiopental sodium (Pentothal) or 1–10 mg of diazepam. Alternatively, sodium amobarbital (up to 250 mg) may be administered IV. Alternatively as advocated by Lucas, 1,000 mg of phenytoin is infused over a period of 1 hour and 500 mg of oral dose is given 10 hours later.

■ THREE-STAGE MANAGEMENT PROTOCOL OF ECLAMPSIA OF SUYAJNA JOSHI

Despite the compelling evidence in favor of $MgSO_4$, health personnel at the primary care level do not administer it. Most of the eclamptic women receive either no immediate treatment or some cocktail of anticonvulsants such as diazepam Inj. Phenergan; they are sent to tertiary care centers for further management. Transportation of these highly irritable eclamptic women is far from ideal in most of the third-world countries including India. The need of the hour is to arrest seizures at the earliest, especially in PHC settings, so that convulsion to treatment interval is brought to minimum.

Joshi Suyajna D started single-dose $MgSO_4$ in the year 1998. Joshi et al. studied the effect of single-dose $MgSO_4$ "Joshi's regimen" (4 g diluted intravenously plus 4 g intramuscularly). The results of the study are comparable to other standard regimens. Now this single-dose regimen is initiated at the site of convulsion to reduce the convulsion-treatment interval. After stabilizing the patient with $MgSO_4$ and nifedipine, the patient is transported to a higher center for definitive treatment. With this, the recurrence rate has come down to 3% and case fatality rate to <1%. Hardly 5% of the eclamptic patients reach the tertiary care center in a moribund sate.

■ CONVULSION TREATMENT INTERVAL

In our resource-restricted settings, the patient must be given $MgSO_4$ and antihypertensive at the site of convulsions with maximum importance to keep the airway patent. After stabilizing, the patient has to be transferred to a tertiary care center for definitive, disciplined management of these cases. Thus, crucial time is not wasted and almost seizure-free transportation can be ensured. Convulsion to medication interval is brought to minimum with optimum fetomaternal outcome.

Three-Stage Management Protocol of Eclampsia—Suyajna Joshi:

1. Initial management as early as possible with single-dose $MgSO_4$—4 + 4 g. Oral nifedipine if needed.
2. Convulsion-free transportation of the stabilized patient in a well-equipped ambulance for a repeat dose $MgSO_4$ 2 g if needed.
3. Tertiary care center to manage the patient in HDU.

Continuing the administration of $MgSO_4$ for 24 hours after the last fit in patients with eclampsia is at best empirical.

The anticonvulsant regimen alone cannot change the maternal and fetal outcome. The other principles of eclampsia management should be simultaneously and effectively instituted. BM Sibai[5] recommends that the patient should be stabilized regarding BP and control of convulsion before transport and the patient should be sent in an ambulance with medical personnel in attendance. In tertiary care centers, other causes of maternal mortality such as hypertensive crises, left ventricular diastolic dysfunction, ARF, and coagulatory disorders can be closely monitored and treated to reduce maternal mortality and morbidity.

■ ANTIHYPERTENSIVE MANAGEMENT

$MgSO_4$ alone cannot improve maternal outcome. The other principles of eclampsia management should be effectively instituted. Persistent and severe elevations of BP must be treated to prevent cerebrovascular accidents, pulmonary edema, and ARF. The management has already been discussed in Severe Preeclampsia section.

■ OBSTETRIC MANAGEMENT

Eclamptic patients require delivery without respect to gestational age. Cesarean delivery should be reserved for obstetric indications or for deteriorating maternal condition. The gestational age, cervical status, and fetal condition and position need to be considered before determining the most appropriate route of delivery. Cervical ripening agents can be used for induction of labor. However, prolonged induction should be avoided.

Maternal mortality rates are increased in patients with eclampsia, but the rates have declined dramatically in recent years. Contemporary maternal mortality rates range from 0 to 16%. Mortality rates are more in developing countries as most of these women are admitted to tertiary hospitals in a moribund state. Mortality depends on the early referral, immediate anticonvulsant treatment, experience of the physicians, and associated adverse pregnancy conditions. Pulmonary edema and intracerebral hemorrhage are the leading causes of death in eclampsia. Eclampsia still remains an important cause of maternal mortality in India. Along with sepsis and hemorrhage, the other leading causes, it is called a "lethal triad" of maternal mortality. Overall, the contemporary perinatal mortality rate among eclamptics ranges from 7 to 30% and is most commonly secondary to placental abruption, prematurity, and perinatal asphyxia. Antenatal deaths account for a significant proportion of the overall perinatal mortality. Depending on the gestational age and the clinical circumstances, it is advisable to have a neonatologist available at delivery.

PULMONARY EDEMA

Sibai and colleagues reported a 2.9% incidence of pulmonary edema in severe preeclampsia–eclampsia. 70% of these cases developed postpartum. A higher incidence of pulmonary edemas was noted in older patients, multigravidas, and patients with underlying chronic hypertension. The etiology of pulmonary edema in preeclamptic patients appears to be multifactorial. Nonhydrostatic factors (pulmonary capillary leak and decreased COP) may cause or contribute to pulmonary edema in patients with preeclampsia. In other patients, highly elevated systemic vascular resistance may lead to decreased CO and left ventricular stroke work index (LVSWI), and secondary cardiopulmonary edema may have been seen with normal left ventricular function following iatrogenic fluid overload.

The diagnosis of pulmonary edema is made on clinical grounds. Symptoms of dyspnea and chest discomfort are usually elicited. Tachypnea, tachycardia, and pulmonary rates are noted on examination. Chest X-ray and arterial blood gases confirm the diagnosis. Other life-threatening conditions, such as thromboembolism, should be considered and ruled out as quickly as possible.

Initial management of pulmonary edema includes oxygen administration and fluid restriction. A pulse oxymeter should be placed so that oxygen saturation may be monitored continuously. A pulmonary artery catheter may be considered for severe preeclamptic patients who develop pulmonary edema antepartum, in order to distinguish between fluid overload, left ventricular dysfunction, and nonhydrostatic pulmonary edema, each of which may require different approaches to therapy **(Fig. 4)**.

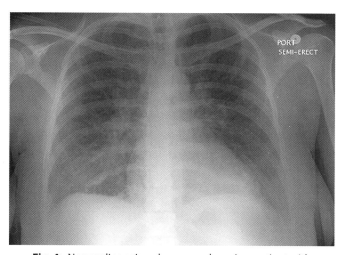

Fig. 4: Noncardiogenic pulmonary edema in a patient with preeclampsia.

Furosemide (Lasix) administered in a 10–40 mg dose IV over 1–2 minutes represents the first line of conventional therapy for patients with pulmonary edema associated with fluid overload. If adequate diuresis does not commence within 1 hour, an 80 mg dose may be slowly administered to achieve diuresis. In severe cases of pulmonary edema, a diuresis of 2–3 L needs to be achieved. Prior to diuresis appropriate fluid management for these hemodynamically complex patients may be clarified by complete hemodynamic evaluation, using parameters derived by a pulmonary artery catheter. An alternative approach in patients without evidence of fluid overload, but with congestive failure secondary to intense peripheral vasospasm (Strauss, 1980), involves the administration of IV nitroprusside. When hypoxemia persists despite initial treatment, mechanical ventilation may be required for respiratory support, pending correction of the underlying problem. In all cases, close monitoring of the patient's respiratory status with frequent arterial blood gases should be performed. Fluid balance is maintained by careful monitoring of intake and output.

RENAL COMPLICATIONS OF PREECLAMPSIA

Renal plasma flow and GFR are diminished significantly in preeclamptic patients. Renal biopsy of preeclamptic patients often demonstrates a distinctive glomerular capillary endothelial cell change, termed *glomerular endotheliosis*. ARF in preeclamptic pregnancies is uncommon. Maternal and perinatal complications were extremely high, although subsequent pregnancy outcome and long-term prognosis were usually favorable in the absence of preexisting chronic hypertension. ARF secondary to PIH is usually the result of acute tubular necrosis but may be secondary to bilateral cortical necrosis. Precipitating factors include abruption, coagulopathy, hemorrhage, and severe hypotension. Renal cortical necrosis associated with preeclampsia may be secondary to other underlying medical disorders, especially in an older, multiparous patient. If ARF occurs, hemodialysis or peritoneal dialysis may be required.

Liver Rupture

Hepatic infarction may lead to intrahepatic hemorrhage and development of a subcapsular hematoma, which may rupture into the peritoneal space and result in shock and death. The diagnosis of a liver hematoma may be aided by use of USG, radionuclide scanning, computed tomography (CT), and selective angiography. The maternal and fetal prognoses of liver rupture are poor. When the diagnosis of liver hematoma is suspected in severe preeclampsia prior to delivery of the fetus, immediate exploratory laparotomy and cesarean section should be considered in order to prevent rupture of the hematoma secondary to increased abdominal pressure in the second stage of labor, in vomiting, or during eclamptic convulsions. Prompt delivery is also mandatory. When the diagnosis of liver hematoma is made in the postpartum period, conservative management with blood transfusion and serial USG may be reasonable. Liver rupture with intraperitoneal hemorrhage, when suspected, requires laparotomy. Hemostasis may be achieved by compression, simple suture, topical coagulant agents, arterial embolization, omental pedicles, ligation of the hepatic artery, or lobectomy, depending on the extent of the hepatic damage.

Cerebral Edema

Cerebral hemorrhage and cerebral edema are two major causes of maternal mortality in preeclampsia. The three most important etiologic factors include increased intravascular pressure, damage to vascular endothelium, and reduced plasma COP. In preeclampsia, cerebral edema is thought to occur secondary to anoxia associated with eclamptic seizures or secondary to loss of cerebral autoregulation as a result of severe hypertension. General therapeutic principles in the treatment of cerebral edema include correction of hypoxemia and hypercarbia, avoidance of volatile anesthetic agents, control of body temperature, and control of BP. Assisted hyperventilation reduces intracranial hypertension and the formation of cerebral edema. The administration of hypertonic solutions such as mannitol increases serum osmolality and draws water from the brain into the vascular compartment, thus reducing brain tissue water and volume. A 20% solution of mannitol is given as a 0.5–1.0 g/kg dose over 10 minutes or as a continuous infusion of 5 g/h. Steroid therapy (dexamethasone, betamethasone, methylprednisolone) is thought to be most effective in the treatment of focal chronic cerebral edema, which may occur in association with a tumor or abscess. Steroid therapy is less beneficial in cases of diffuse or acute cerebral edema.

Temporary Blindness (Amaurosis)

Temporary blindness may complicate 1–3% of cases of preeclampsia–eclampsia. The injury is usually the result of severe damage to the retinal vasculature or occipital lobe ischemia. Cunningham and colleagues evaluated over a 14-year period the clinical courses of 15 women with severe preeclampsia or eclampsia who developed cortical blindness (Cunningham, 1995).[10] Blindness persisted from 4 hours to 8 days but resolved completely in all cases. Based on data from CT imaging and MRI, cortical blindness results from petechial hemorrhage and focal edema in the occipital cortex. Transient blindness usually resolves spontaneously

after delivery of the fetus. Focal neurological deficits such as this require ophthalmologic and neurological consultation and CT or MRI of the brain. Paralysis of the sixth cranial nerve has been reported as a complication of eclampsia.

Cardiovascular Complications

Women with a history of preeclampsia continue to have an elevated risk of cardiovascular disease in subsequent years. Several systematic reviews and meta-analyses have linked preeclampsia with an increased risk of cardiovascular disease (hypertension, myocardial infarction, congestive heart failure), cerebrovascular events (stroke), peripheral arterial disease, and cardiovascular mortality later in life, with an estimated doubling of odds compared with women unaffected by preeclampsia.

Gestational Hypertension

Hypertension without proteinuria developing after 20 weeks of gestation, during labor, or the puerperium in previously normotensive nonproteinuric women is gestational hypertension. It is the most frequent form of hypertensive conditions of pregnancy with a prevalence of 6–15%. 46% of gestational hypertension patients may become preeclamptic. The condition is more frequent in obese women, multiple pregnancy, diabetes, chronic hypertension and in women with a history of preeclampsia. The pregnancy outcomes are worse than in mild preeclampsia. Patients with gestational hypertension have an increased incidence of preterm delivery and SGA babies. They also have an increased incidence of abruptio placentae. 33% of gestational hypertension women will present with a severe form. The management of these patients is as outlined in Preeclampsia section.

Chronic Hypertension in Pregnancy

To diagnose chronic hypertension in pregnancy, it is necessary to diagnose hypertension before pregnancy or prior to 20 weeks of gestation. Some women without chronic hypertension have repeated pregnancies in which *transient hypertension* appears only late in pregnancy and regresses postpartum. This hypertension is evidence of a latent hypertensive vascular disease and is analogous to gestational diabetes.

In most women with hypertension antedating pregnancy, increased BP is the only demonstrable finding. Some have complications that increase the risks during pregnancy and may shorten life expectancy, including hypertensive or ischemic cardiac disease, renal insufficiency, or a prior cerebrovascular event. Such a hypertensive vascular disease in pregnancy is encountered more frequently in older women. Obesity is an important factor predisposing to chronic hypertension. Specifically, chronic hypertension may be increased as much as 10-fold in obese women, and these women are more likely to develop superimposed preeclampsia. Diabetes mellitus is also prevalent in chronically hypertensive women, and its interplay with obesity is overwhelming. Heredity plays an important role, and indeed, a number of genes inherited as mendelian traits have been described to cause hypertension.

Preconceptional Therapy

Women with chronic hypertension should ideally be counseled prior to pregnancy. It is important to establish the basic data of the patient. Medication should be changed to that is acceptable during pregnancy. Diuretics should be gradually diminished and preferably eliminated prior to conception. ACE inhibitors and ARBs are associated with renal anomalies and irreversible renal failure. Hence, they are contraindicated. BP self-monitoring is encouraged. Personal health behavioral modifications include maintaining normal body weight, BMI 18.5–24.9 kg/m^2, consume a diet rich in fruits, vegetables, and low-fat dairy products with a reduced content of saturated and total fat [dietary approaches to stop hypertension (DASH)]; reduce dietary sodium intake to no >100 mmol/day: 2.4 g sodium or 6 g sodium chloride; moderation of alcohol consumption; and avoidance of smoking.

Evaluation

If the practitioner has not had sufficient experience with hypertension in pregnancy, he/she must take advice from a specialist in maternal fetal medicine. Renal, hepatic, and cardiac function should be assessed. Ophthalmologic evaluation is important for women with long-standing chronic hypertension. Echocardiography is indicated in women with any prior adverse outcome or in those with long-term hypertension. Other tests to consider are based on clinical presentation. Suspect SLE in patients with disproportionate proteinuria to the degree of hypertension and one should check antinuclear antibody and double-stranded DNA antibodies.

Maternal and Fetal Effects

In most women with chronic hypertension, BP falls in the second trimester and then rises during the third trimester to early pregnancy levels. Adverse outcomes in these women are dependent largely on whether superimposed preeclampsia develops. Prior adverse events such as a cerebrovascular accident or myocardial infarction, as well as cardiac or renal dysfunction, are especially pertinent. Women with these are at a markedly increased risk for a recurrence or worsening during pregnancy. Those who require multiple medications for hypertension control, or those who are poorly controlled, are also at an increased risk for adverse pregnancy outcomes. Most clinicians believe that pregnancy is relatively contraindicated in women who maintain persistent diastolic pressures of >110 mm Hg despite therapy, require multiple antihypertensives, or have a serum creatinine level of >2 mg/dL. Even stronger contraindications are prior cerebrovascular thrombosis/hemorrhage, myocardial infarction, or cardiac failure.

Most women taking monotherapy and whose hypertension is well-controlled prior to pregnancy do well. Even these women, however, are at an increased risk for superimposed preeclampsia and placental abruption. Pregnancy-aggravated hypertension manifests as a sudden increase in BP.

Systolic pressures > 200 mm Hg or diastolic pressures of 130 mm Hg or more may rapidly result in renal or cardiopulmonary dysfunction. When there is superimposed severe preeclampsia or eclampsia, the outlook for the mother is serious unless the pregnancy is terminated. Placental abruption is another common and serious complication. Indicated preterm delivery, FGR, perinatal mortality, and other adverse outcomes are all increased in these women.

Superimposed Preeclampsia

The features of superimposed preeclampsia are given in **Table 5**.

August and Lindheimer (1999) found that superimposed preeclampsia occurred in 4–40% of these women. The incidence is higher in women with severe hypertension in early pregnancy. Uterine artery Doppler velocimetry showed increased impedance at 16–20 weeks and was predictive of superimposed preeclampsia at 28–32 weeks in women with chronic hypertension. Worsening proteinuria or new-onset proteinuria and new-onset thrombocytopenia help to diagnose superimposed preeclampsia.

Management during Pregnancy

The goal for pregnancy complicated by chronic hypertension is to reduce adverse maternal or perinatal outcomes. Home BP monitoring is advocated and encouraged. The machines must be correctly calibrated. This approach reduces the need for antihypertensive dose and hospitalization. Bed rest is advised. Uterine blood flow is increased in left lateral recumbent position. Antihypertensive therapy has not been shown to improve fetal condition or prevent preeclampsia. However, it controls the acceleration of hypertension and helps to prevent maternal stroke. Methyldopa, labetalol, nifedipines and hydralazine are safely used in pregnancy.

TABLE 5: Features of superimposed preeclampsia.

	Preeclampsia	Chronic hypertension
Age	Extremes of age	More often older
Parity	Nulliparous usually	Often multiparous
Onset	Rare before 20 weeks	BP increase before 20 weeks
History	Negative	Positive, often with hypertension in previous pregnancy
Fundus	Retinal edema, arteriolar spasm	Chronic changes of arteriosclerosis may be present
Cardiac status	Usually normal	Ventricular hypertrophy may be present
Deep tendon reflexes	Hyperactive	Normal
Hemoglobin/hematocrit	Increased values suggest hemoconcentration and support diagnosis	Unchanged
Blood smear	Schistocytes	Unchanged
Platelet count	Significantly decreasing levels or absolute count <50,000/mm³	Unchanged
Serum creatinine	Abnormal or rising levels, especially when associated with oliguria, suggest severe PE	May be elevated in long-standing disease
Proteinuria	Increased	Absent or minimal in essential hypertension
Uric acid	Increased	Normal
Liver function	RUQ pain/tenderness may be present, increased serum transaminases and/or lactate dehydrogenase in severe PE	Normal

(PE: preeclampsia; RUQ: right upper quadrant)

Diuretics should be used as adjuvant therapy and only reserved for patients with excessive fluid retention and for fluid overload. Diuretics are not recommended for leg edema of pregnancy. Avoid using two antihypertensives of the same class when the patient needs more than one drug for control of hypertension (e.g., methyldopa and labetalol) instead use vasodilator as the second agent (e.g., nifedipine).

Most pregnant patients with mild chronic hypertension remain stable. The patient should not be allowed to go beyond term and often delivery before 38th week is necessary. The risk of abruption is 0.7–1.4% in mild cases and 5–10% for those with severe hypertension. Delivery is considered when one of the following exists:

- Superimposed preeclampsia of any severity at term
- Severe preeclampsia at any gestational age
- Fetal compromise, low biophysical profile (BPP), persistent nonreactive NST
- Documented lung maturity
- Moderate or severe hypertension at or beyond 37–38 weeks' gestation.

Prediction of Preeclampsia

Prediction is important because the risk for recurrent preeclampsia can be as high as 65% (Barton & Sibai, 2008).[11] Preeclampsia is associated with substantial maternal and perinatal complications. The ideal screening test must be simple, noninvasive, rapid, inexpensive, easy to be performed early in pregnancy, and must have high sensitivity and predictive value. Unfortunately, currently there is no clinically useful screening test to predict preeclampsia [World Health Organization (WHO), 2004].

However, numerous clinical, biochemical, and biophysical tests have been proposed to predict preeclampsia. These tests take into consideration preconception risk factors, pregnancy-related risk factors, and markers to predict preeclampsia.

Preconception Risk Factors

The first step in the management of a woman with a history of preeclampsia is to conduct a detailed evaluation of potential risk factors **(Table 6)**[11].

Pregnancy-related Factors

Prediction depends on pregnancy risk factors and markers which can be either biophysical or biochemical. Pregnancy risk factors are as follows:

- Hydrops/hydropic degeneration of the placenta
- Multifetal gestation
- Unexplained FGR
- Gestational hypertension
- UTI
- Periodontal infection
- Gestational diabetes.

TABLE 6: Risk for preeclampsia based on previous history and underlying disease.

Risk factors	Risk (%)
Chronic hypertension/renal disease	15–40
Pregestational diabetes mellitus	10–35
Connective tissue disease (lupus, rheumatoid arthritis)	10–20
Thrombophilia (acquired or congenital)	10–40
Obesity/insulin resistance	10–15
Age older than 40 years	10–20
Limited sperm exposure	10–35
Family history of preeclampsia/cardiovascular disease	10–15
Woman born as SFGA	1.5-fold
IUGR, abruptio placentae, IUFD in previous pregnancy	2–3-fold

(IUFD: intrauterine fetal death; IUGR: intrauterine growth restriction; SGFA: small for gestational age)

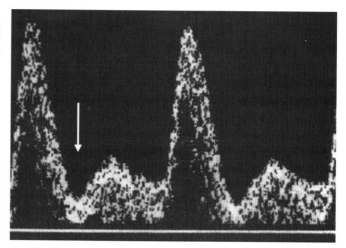

Fig. 5: Presence of diastolic notch in uterine artery Doppler.

SCREENING TESTS FOR PREECLAMPSIA (WHO, 2004)

I. *Placental perfusion and vascular resistance dysfunction:*
   – Mean arterial blood pressure
   – Rollover test
   – Doppler ultrasound
   – Isometric exercise test
   – Intravenous infusion of angiotensin II
   – Platelet angiotensin II binding
   – Platelet calcium response to arginine vasopressin
   – Renin
   – 24-hour ambulatory blood pressure monitoring.

II. *Fetoplacental unit dysfunction:*
   – Human chorionic gonadotropin
   – Alpha fetoprotein
   – Estriol
   – Inhibin A
   – Pregnancy-associated plasma protein A—decreased.

III. *Renal dysfunction:*
   – Serum uric acid—elevated Microalbuminuria—increased
   – Urinary calcium excretion—decreased
   – Urinary kallikrein
   – Microtransferrinuria—elevated.

IV. *Endothelial and oxidant stress dysfunction:*
   – Platelet activation and endothelial cell adhesion molecules—elevated
   – Cytokines—elevated
   – Placenta growth factor—decreased
   – Fibronectin—elevated
   – Endothelin—elevated
   – Thromboxane—elevated
   – Homocysteine—elevated.

Comment

The very fact that so many tests are proposed for prediction explains the futility of the search for a screening test. MAP is a better predictor of preeclampsia than SBP and DBP alone (+ve LR 3.5 and –ve LR 0.46). The rollover test (Gant) and isometric exercise are not of value in predicting preeclampsia because of poor sensitivity and reproducibility. Angiotensin II challenge test is expensive, time consuming, and unreliable. Uterine artery Doppler ultrasound showing a high pulsatility index and/or persistent diastolic notch in the first and second trimesters is a poor predictor of preeclampsia. Uterine artery Doppler plus biochemical markers are showing promising results in the prediction **(Fig. 5)**; however, current data do not support this combination for routine screening for preeclampsia[11]. Serum fibronectin levels are elevated in preeclampsia which confirms the role of vascular endothelial injury. However, the timing of elevation coincides with the onset of clinical disease.

BP remains the cornerstone of early diagnosis. The reliability of these tests is inconsistent. Many suffer from poor specificity and predictive values. None provided a cutoff value that could be clinically useful for the prediction of preeclampsia. Thus, currently there is no clinically useful screening test to predict preeclampsia (WHO, 2004).

RECENT RESEARCH

Researchers in the United Kingdom reported (Renal Week 2010: American Society of Nephrology 43rd Annual Meeting) that an analysis of urine samples obtained before 20 weeks of gestation from 145 pregnant women who either did or did not develop preeclampsia allowed them to identify five protein peaks that predicted preeclampsia with 92% accuracy. The clinical signs of preeclampsia typically do not appear until later in pregnancy, but the researchers theorized that because abnormal placentation or placental insufficiency is central to the pathogenesis of preeclampsia, and placentation is complete by 18 weeks of gestation, changes in the urinary protein profile early in pregnancy might predict the development of the disease.

■ PREVENTION

There is a considerable literature devoted to the prevention of preeclampsia. However, there is some controversy over whether or not prevention of preeclampsia per se is a worthy goal rather than the prevention of the complications of preeclampsia. The prevention has three types: Primary prevention means avoiding the disease, secondary prevention means breaking off the disease process before emergence of an obvious clinical disease, and tertiary prevention implies prevention of complications of the disease.

Primary Prevention

Primary prevention, though best, is possible only when the exact etiology is known. Primary prevention is possible to some extent by modification of some of the risk factors. As the disease process is more common in nulliparous women or in multiparous women with change of partners, it is recommended to have pregnancies with low-risk men, to stay with the same partner, and to have children at an age when the endothelium is still able to cope with the inflammatory stress associated with the pregnancy state. Prevention and/or effective control of obesity could significantly result in the frequency of preeclampsia. Similarly, women with diabetes, chronic hypertension, renal, and other medical disorders should have their primary condition under control before attempting conception. However, it applies only to minority of patients.

Secondary Prevention

The basic requirements for secondary prevention are (1) knowledge of pathophysiological mechanisms, (2) availability of screening methods, and (3) means of intervention and modification of the pathophysiology. None of the three criteria are available for effective secondary prevention. Many screening tests suffer from poor sensitivity and specificity.

Nonpharmacological Interventions

- Bed rest
- Lifestyle changes
- Regular physical activity.

Nutritional Interventions

- Dietary sodium restriction
- Dietary protein and energy intake
- Control of obesity
- Change in dietary habits
- Fish oil—some studies have shown beneficial effects of omega-3 fatty acids in the prevention of preeclampsia. The large European multicentric Fish Oil supplementation Trial in Pregnancy (FOTIP) concluded that fish oils are unlikely to be beneficial in prevention of preeclampsia
- Alcohol intake
- Arginine supplementation—found to be beneficial but it was an isolated study
- Japanese Herbal medicine Toki-shakuyaku-san (TS) may be beneficial in the treatment and prevention of preeclampsia (Takei et al.).[12]

Pharmacological Interventions

- Antihypertensive drugs
- Diuretics
- Zinc supplementation
- Magnesium
- Folic acid and other B vitamins—there is no scientific data that any of B vitamins are beneficial in the prevention of preeclampsia.

Low-dose aspirin: Low-dose aspirin 50–150 mg/day therapy during pregnancy selectively inhibits platelet TXA2 biosynthesis with minimal effects on PGI2 production, thus altering the balance in favor of PGI2. There is alteration in TXA2:PGI2 ratio. This inhibits platelet aggregation. Unfortunately, the initial encouraging results of aspirin to prevent preeclampsia could not be confirmed by a larger multicentric trial. The largest trial to date is the CLASP (collaborative low-dose aspirin) study. Overall, the use of low-dose aspirin was associated with 12% reduction in the incidence of preeclampsia (nonsignificant) and it reduced the incidence of preterm delivery (19.7% vs. 22.3% in the placebo group). Aspirin-treated women had slightly higher risk of abruptio placentae (statistically not significant). A meta-analysis (Duley) of antiplatelet agents for the prevention of preeclampsia did not find difference between treatment and control groups.

The recommendations to use aspirin are based on expert advice from NICE (National Collaborating Centre for Women's and Children's Health, 2010). NICE reviewed evidence from a Cochrane systematic review and a large meta-analysis of individual patient data and concluded that:

- The use of low-dose aspirin was consistent with a small risk reduction for preeclampsia, and there is a clear benefit in their defined high-risk groups.

- Moderate risk has been poorly defined in studies. However, the presence of two moderate risk factors would confer a greater risk than any risk factor considered individually.

- Data on the safety of aspirin in the doses used for the prevention of preeclampsia is sufficient.

The recommendation to start aspirin at 12 weeks' gestation is based on expert advice from NICE, as this is the earliest gestational age for which there is available evidence concerning the use of aspirin for the prevention of preeclampsia (National Collaborating Centre for Women's and Children's Health, 2010). Expert reviewers warned against prescribing aspirin to women with uncontrolled BP. Clinical Knowledge Summaries (CKS) recommends that in such women, it is best to seek specialist advice about whether or not to prescribe aspirin:

- Heparin and low-dose aspirin—only for women with antiphospholipids antibody syndrome and not for routine recommendation.

- *Calcium supplementation:* There is an inverse relation between calcium intake and the frequency of preeclampsia. The largest trial conducted (2 g/day ca supplementation) by Levine in US did not find any benefit. However, Cochrane review (Atallah) observed a modest reduction in preeclampsia and the effect was greatest in high-risk women with low calcium intake. Currently, WHO is conducting a study with 1.5 g/day supplementation in seven locations worldwide.

NICE concluded that there is high quality evidence from a Cochrane systematic review that calcium supplementation reduces the risk of preeclampsia in women who have a low dietary intake of calcium (which does not generally apply to women in the UK). The benefits of calcium supplementation are greatest in women who are at a high risk of pre-eclampsia. If calcium intake is known to be adequate, then there is no statistically significant benefit. Therefore, NICE decided that routine calcium supplementation in the UK could not be justified.

- *NO donors:* NO synthesis is impaired in preeclampsia. The data on the effects of NO donors in prevention of PE are limited and conflicting. A large multicentric double-blind randomized controlled trial is currently underway in India by the Indian Council of Medical Research (ICMR).

- *Antioxidants:* Various antioxidants such as vitamins C and E, lycopene, selenium, N-acetylcysteine, and garlic are used in many studies with encouraging results. However, the Cochrane review 2008 found that antioxidant supplementation may not affect the risk of preeclampsia or clinical outcomes (level 2 evidence).

Long-term Effects

The preeclamptic group had a higher incidence of preeclampsia in their *second pregnancies* (46.8% vs. 7.6%) and in subsequent pregnancies (20.7% vs. 7.7%) when compared with the normotensive group.

According to Chesley, the recurrence of preeclampsia depends on the following:

- *Time required to become normotensive in the postpartum period:* The longer the time required, the higher the chance of recurrence. If hypertension is still present on day 10 after delivery, the probability of recurrence is 59% compared to 21% in those in whom BP is normal.

- *BMI:* The larger the BMI, the higher the chance of recurrence in subsequent pregnancies.

- Weight in pounds divided by height in inches, the value exceeds.

- *Time of onset of eclampsia:* There is an inverse relation between the gestational age and the chance of recurrence in subsequent pregnancy; the later the onset, the lesser the incidence in the next pregnancy.

- *Average SBP during pregnancy:* The higher the BP, the higher the chance of recurrence.

Multiparous women with eclampsia will have a higher incidence of chronic hypertension than do normal control groups or nulliparous eclamptic women. The overall incidence of chronic hypertension was *significantly higher* in the preeclamptic–eclamptic group (14.8% vs. 5.6% Sibai). Patients remaining normotensive in subsequent pregnancies had the lowest incidence of chronic hypertension Mann et al. report a greater incidence of myocardial infarction in women with a history of preeclampsia (three-fold). According to the Royal College of General Practitioners, women who were recruited for an oral contraception study showed that those with a history of hypertension in pregnancy had a significantly increased risk of hypertension, myocardial infarction, and ischemic heart disease later in life. The prevalence of remote hypertension is increased in multiparas who develop preeclampsia and in women with severe early onset disease of any parity (Working Group Report on High Blood Pressure in Pregnancy 2001). Preeclampsia doubles the risk for premature maternal death.

KEY POINTS

- Hypertension is the most common medical problem encountered during pregnancy, complicating 2–3% of pregnancies.
- The use of the term PIH should be abandoned as its meaning in clinical practice is unclear and often confusing.

- Preeclampsia is characterized by inadequate trophoblastic invasion with resultant placental ischemia and predominance of vasoconstrictor profile.
- Proteinuria is characteristic of preeclampsia.
- Primarily, the management of preeclampsia is determined by the gestational age and the severity of the disease.
- NICE considered that the association of beta- blockers with reduced fetal growth was a result of excessive lowering of blood pressure. Expert opinion from NICE is that labetalol seems to be as effective and safe as other drugs used for hypertension for managing preeclampsia and it is licensed for use in pregnancy. Labetalol should be used as first-line treatment. Alternative treatment includes methyldopa and nifedipine.
- Fluid restriction is advisable to reduce the risk of fluid overload in the intrapartum and postpartum periods.
- The presence of preeclampsia does not guarantee accelerated lung maturation, and antenatal corticosteroid therapy should be considered for all women who present with preeclampsia before 34 weeks' gestation.
- The clinical signs and symptoms of patients with HELLP syndrome are classically related to the impact of vasospasm on the maternal liver.
- The Eclampsia Collaborative Trial Group concluded, "there is now compelling evidence in favor of $MgSO_4$ for the treatment of eclampsia."
- $MgSO_4$ acts both centrally and peripherally.
- Magnesium toxicity is treated by 10% calcium gluconate.
- There are several modifications of standard $MgSO_4$ regimens in the developing countries. Joshi's single-dose $MgSO_4$ (VIMS regimen) can be administered by health personnel at first referral unit (FRU) levels and then the patient is transferred to tertiary centers for definitive management. This would ensure almost seizure-free transport.
- Eclamptic patients require delivery without respect to gestational age. Cesarean delivery should be reserved for obstetric indications or deteriorating maternal condition.
- Nonhydrostatic factors (pulmonary capillary leak and deceased COP) may cause or contribute to pulmonary edema in patients with preeclampsia.
- Acute renal failure in preeclamptic pregnancies is uncommon.
- Cerebral hemorrhage and cerebral edema are two major causes of maternal mortality in preeclampsia.
- Temporary blindness may complicate 1–3% of cases of preeclampsia–eclampsia due to occipital lobe ischemia.

- Women with chronic hypertension should ideally be counseled prior to pregnancy.
- The patients with gestational hypertension have an increased incidence of preterm delivery and SGA babies.
- New-onset proteinuria and thrombocytopenia are diagnostic of superimposed preeclampsia in chronic hypertension patients.
- Unfortunately, currently there is no clinically useful screening test to predict preeclampsia (WHO, 2004).
- NICE concluded that there is high quality evidence from a Cochrane systematic review that calcium supplementation reduces the risk of preeclampsia in women who have a low dietary intake of calcium.
- The only group where low-dose aspirin may be justified is in women who are at risk of developing early onset preeclampsia.
- Prevalence of remote hypertension is increased in multiparas who develop preeclampsia and in women with severe early onset disease of any parity (Working Group Report on High Blood Pressure in Pregnancy 2001).

■ REFERENCE

1. Gant NF, Daley GL, Chand S, Whalley PJ, MacDonald PC. A study of angiotensin II pressor response throughout primigravid pregnancy. J Clin Invest. 1973;52:2682-9.
2. Chesley LC, Cooper DW. Genetics of hypertension in pregnancy: possible single gene control of preeclampsia and eclampsia. Am J Obstet Gynecol. 1986;53:851-63.
3. Stettler RW, Cunningham FG Natural history of chronic proteinuria complicating pregnancy Am J Obstet Gynecol. 1992;167:1219- 24.
4. Koopmans CM, Bijlenga D, Groen H, Mc Vijgen S, Aarnoudse J, Bekedam DJ, et al. Induction of labour versus expectant monitoring for gestational hypertension or mild pre-eclampsia after 36 weeks' gestation (HYPITAT): a multicentre, open-label randomised controlled trial. Lancet. 2009;374(9694):979-88.
5. Sibai BM, Taslimi MM, el-Nazer A, Amon E, Mabie BC, Ryan GM. Maternal-perinatal outcome associated with the syndrome of hemolysis, elevated liver enzymes, and low platelets in severe preeclampsia-eclampsia. Am J Obstet Gynecol. 1986;155(3): 501-9.
6. Martin JN Jr, Perry KG Jr, Blake PG, May WA, Moore A, Robinette L. Better maternal outcomes are achieved with dexamethasone therapy for postpartum HELLP (hemolysis, elevated liver enzymes, and thrombocytopenia) syndrome. Am J Obstet Gynecol. 1997;177(5):1011-7.
7. Douglas KA, Redman CWG. Eclampsia in United Kingdom. BMJ. 1994;309:1395-400.
8. Sibai BM, Graham JM, McCubbin JH. A comparison of intravenous and intramuscular magnesium sulfate regimens in preeclampsia. Am J Obstet Gynecol. 1984;150(6):728-33.
9. The Magpie Trial Group. Do women with pre-eclampsia and eclampsia, and their babies, benefit from magnesium sulphate? The Magpie Trial: a randomized, placebo-controlled trial. Lancet. 2002;359:1877-90.

10. Cunningham FG, Fernandez CO, Hernandez C. Blindness associated with preeclampsia and eclampsia. Am J Obstet Gynecol. 1995;172(4 Pt 1):1291-8.

11. Barton, John & Sibai, Baha. Pediction and Prevention of Recurrent Preeclampsia. Obstetrics and gynecology. 2008;112:359-72.

12. Takei H, Nakai Y, Hattori N, Yamamoto M, Kurauchi K, Sasaki H, Aburada M. The herbal medicine Toki-shakuyaku-san improves the hypertension and intrauterine growth retardation in preeclampsia rats induced by Nomega-nitro-L-arginine methyl ester. Phytomedicine. 2004;11(1):43-50.

■ SUGGESTED READING

1. ACOG Practice Bulletin No. 202: Gestational hypertension and preeclampsia. Obstet Gynecol. 2019;133(1):e1.

2. Clarke SL, Phelan JP, Saade GR, Dildy GA, Belfort MA, Hankins GDV. Critical Care Obstetrics. New York: Wiley; 2003.

3. Gabbe SG, Niebyl JR, Simpson JL, Landon MB, Galan HL, Jauniaux ERM, et al. Obstetrics: Normal and Problem Pregnancies. 2016(7).

4. Gary Cunningham F, Leveno KJ, Bloom SL, Dashe JS, Hoffman BL, Casey BM. Williams Obstetrics, 25th edition. New York: McGraw Hill; 2018.

5. Misra R (Ed). Ian Donald's Practical Obstetrics Problems, 7th edition. Boca Raton, FL: CRC Press; 2012.

6. National Institute of Health and Care Excellence (2019). Hypertension in pregnancy: diagnosis and management. [online] Available from: https://www.nice.org.uk/guidance/ng133. [Last accessed September, 2020]

7. Queenan JT, Spong CY, Lockwood CJ (Eds). Queenan's Management of High Risk Pregnancy: An Evidence-based Approach, 6th edition. New York: Wiley Blackwell; 2012.

8. Royal College of Obstetricians & Gynecologists (2006). Severe pre-eclampsia/eclampsia, management (Green-top Guideline No. 10A). [online] Available from: https://www.rcog.org.uk/en/guidelines-research-services/guidelines/gtg10a/. [Last accessed September, 2020]

9. Seneviratne HR, Wijeyaratne CN (Eds). Pregnancy-induced Hypertension. Chennai: Orient Longman; 1998.

10. Studd J, Tan SL, Chervenak FA (Eds). Progress in Obstetrics and Gynecology, 17th edition. Philadephia: Elsevier; 2006.

Gestational Diabetes

Pralhad Kushtagi

INTRODUCTION

Occurrence of hyperglycemia during pregnancy because of pregnancy is more often transitory and resolves itself postpartum. In the past, any hyperglycemia initially detected during pregnancy was considered gestational diabetes mellitus (GDM), regardless of whether the condition actually existed before the pregnancy or not. Although women developing hyperglycemia in pregnancy are at a higher risk of progressing to type 2 diabetes, labeling the condition as gestational diabetes may add to the anxiety that they will have to be on lifelong treatment. It may be wise to refer to them as with *gestational hyperglycemia*. In this chapter, hyperglycemia developing in pregnancy and due to pregnancy will be referred to and discussed as gestational diabetes mellitus (GDM) since the terminology is familiar. It may be remembered that some management principles are common to pre-existing diabetes (type 1 and type 2 diabetes diagnosed prior to pregnancy) and gestational diabetes.

CLASSIFICATION OF HYPERGLYCEMIA IN PREGNANCY

There are several classifications of hyperglycemia or diabetes in pregnancy floated by different authors and specialty bodies. One groups the condition into types 1a and 1b depending on whether insulin is required or not at the onset/first diagnosis during pregnancy. The classification that appears to be comprehensive is given in **Box 1**.

DEFINITION

Gestational diabetes is defined as glucose intolerance resulting in hyperglycemia of variable severity detected after the first trimester of pregnancy that is clearly not overt diabetes.[1]

It does not exclude the possibility of glucose intolerance unrelated to pregnancy that may have begun concomitantly with the pregnancy.

The criteria for glucose intolerance vary depending on the test used and the guideline followed **(Table 1)**.

Overt diabetes mellitus is considered present, if any of these are present:

- In first trimester:
  - Fasting glucose   126 mg/ dL
  - Random glucose/OGCT*   200 mg/dL
  - Glycated hemoglobin (HbA1C)   6.5%
- Later when OGTT** is done after the first trimester, commonly at/after 23 weeks' pregnancy:
  - Fasting glucose   126 mg/dL
  - 2-hour glucose   200 mg/dL (following a 75 g oral glucose load)

*OGCT Oral Glucose Challenge Test; **OGTT Oral Glucose Tolerance Test

PREVALENCE

The prevalence of GDM is increasing worldwide. The global prevalence of hyperglycemia during pregnancy has been estimated at 16.9% (21.4 million live births in 2013) using the World Health Organization (WHO) criteria.[8] Determination of the exact prevalence of GDM is difficult due to wide variations in reporting, the population being studied, and the lack of universal diagnostic criteria. It is considered that for a given population and ethnicity, GDM corresponds to the prevalence of impaired glucose tolerance (IGT; in a nonpregnant adult) within that given population.[9] The pooled prevalence of GDM in Asia has been reported as 11.5%,[10] higher than European countries (5.4%) but lower than African countries (14.0%).[11] The reported prevalence of GDM in India has varied from 3.8 to 21% in different parts of the country. In the United States of America, the prevalence of GDM has shown an increase from 8.1% in 2007 to 8.5% in 2010[12] and the overall prevalence was 9.2%. In India, it is estimated that about 4 million women are affected by GDM at any given time point,[13] and the prevalence has been reported to vary widely from 3.8% to as high as 41%.[14]

BOX 1: Composite classification of hyperglycemia in pregnancy.

- Gestational diabetes mellitus
- Pregestational diabetes mellitus (type 1 or 2):
  - Diagnosed prior to pregnancy:
    - Impaired glucose tolerance test
    - Overt diabetes—types 1 and 2
    - Monogenic diabetes
  - Diagnosed during incumbent pregnancy—hyperglycemia that is likely to have preceded pregnancy:
    - Elevated first-trimester fasting glucose
    - Overt diabetes diagnosed following screening/diagnostic test

TABLE 1: Diagnosis of gestational diabetes—different threshold criteria for glucose intolerance.

Criterion	Gestation at testing (weeks)	Glucose load (g)	Glucose threshold(mg/dL)*				Inference
			Fasting	1 hour	2 hours	3 hours	
Carpenter- Coustan, 1982[2]	24–28	100	95	180	155	140	2 values ≥ cutoff
ADA, 2004[3]	14–18 high and 24–28 for medium risk	100	105	190	165	145	2 values ≥ cutoff
IADPSG, 2010;[4] WHO, 2013;[5] ADA, 2016[1]	24–28	75	92	180	153	–	1 or more values ≥ cutoff
NICE, 2015[6]	As early as possible; high risk	75	100	–	140	–	1 or more values ≥ cutoff
DIPSI, 2010[7]	24–28; universal	75	–	–	140	–	Value ≥ cutoff

(ADA: American Diabetes Association; DIPSI: Diabetes in Pregnancy Study group of India; IADPSC: International Association of the Diabetes and Pregnancy Study Groups; NICE: National Institute for Health and Care Excellence; OGCT: oral glucose challenge test; OGTT: oral glucose tolerance test; WHO: World Health Organization)
Notes: Plasma glucose values in mg/dL: F: Fasting; 1 hour, 2 hours, or 3 hours: Hours after glucose load.
*For values in mmol/L, multiply with 18.

■ RISK FACTORS

A pregnancy with the presence of any of the characteristics given in **Table 2** appears to be at an increased risk of developing GDM, and the presence of multiple risk factors will have an additive effect on the risk.

■ PATHOPHYSIOLOGY

During a healthy pregnancy, due to the addition to various physiological adaptations that the mother's body undergoes, insulin sensitivity shifts depending on the requirements. In early pregnancy, insulin sensitivity increases, promoting the glucose uptake into adipose stores in preparation for the energy demands of later pregnancy.[15] As the pregnancy progresses, a state of insulin resistance (IR) develops due to elaboration of local and placental hormones, the latter including estrogen, progesterone, leptin, cortisol, placental lactogen, and placental growth hormone.[16] This results in slight elevation of blood glucose for transportation across the placenta. This mild state of IR also promotes endogenous glucose production and the breakdown of fat stores, resulting in a further increase in blood glucose and free fatty acid (FFA) concentrations.[17] These changes revert to prepregnancy levels within a few days of delivery.[18] Pregnancies where the normal metabolic adaptations fail to occur adequately result in GDM. It is usually the result of β-cell dysfunction on a background of chronic IR during pregnancy.

β-Cell Dysfunction

β-cell dysfunction may be a result of prolonged, excessive insulin production in response to chronic fuel excess. It may be noted that the majority of susceptibility genes that are associated with GDM are related to β-cell function, including potassium voltage-gated channel KQT-like 1 (*Kcnq1*) and glucokinase (*Gck*). Even a minor deficiency in

TABLE 2: Risk factors for development of gestational diabetes mellitus in the present pregnancy.

Characteristics	Variables
Personal characteristics	• Ethnic group with high prevalence for type 2 diabetes—Hispanic American, African-American, Native American, South or East Asian, Pacific Islander • Maternal age > 25 years • Body mass index > 30 kg/m²
Medical disorders	Metabolic syndrome, polycystic ovary syndrome, hypertension
Family history/genetic factors	Diabetes in first-degree relatives
Past-pregnancy factors	• Gestational diabetes mellitus Unexplained perinatal loss; poor obstetric performance • Birth of a malformed infant • Birth of macrosomic baby (≥4 kg)
Present-pregnancy factors	• Glycosuria at the first antenatal visit in the first trimester • Excessive weight gain in the first 24 weeks • Multiple gestation • Repeated urinary tract infection; vaginal candidiasis
Epigenetic factors	• Overeating, unhealthy dietary pattern, and lack of regular exercise • High-density lipoprotein < 35 mg/dL, triglyceride > 250 mg/dL

the β-cell machinery may get exposed in times of metabolic stress of pregnancy.[19]

Insulin Resistance

The development of IR in women who develop GDM could be due to the following factors:

■ *Diet:* A woman whose diet is not balanced and is rich in fat and/or proteins at the expense of carbohydrates even though the caloric value is appropriate is likely to develop GDM because of IR. According to the glucose-fatty acid cycle of Randle, preferential oxidation of free fatty acids over glucose plays a major role in insulin sensitivity by activating serine kinase cascade leading to defects in insulin signaling. They also inhibit insulin-stimulated glucose uptake to muscle. Although a high intake of dietary proteins has positive effects on energy homeostasis, it has detrimental effects on glucose homeostasis by promoting IR and increasing gluconeogenesis.

- *Failure of insulin signaling:* The rate of insulin-stimulated glucose uptake is reduced in GDM. Insulin signaling occurs by reduced tyrosine or increased serine/threonine phosphorylation. Insulin receptor abundance is usually unaffected. Several risk factors seem to exert their effects by interfering within insulin signaling.

- *Neurohormonal dysfunction:* Facilitation of amino acid transport across the placenta is brought about by increased placental leptin production and interference in insulin signaling by adiponectin expressed from syncytiotrophoblast regulated by cytokines. Adipose tissue elaborates adipokines and cytokines (tumor necrosis factor alpha, interleukin-6, and interleukin-1alpha) actively in to circulation. These may impair insulin signaling and inhibit insulin release from beta cells.

- *Gluconeogenesis:* Upregulated hepatic glucose production may not significantly contribute to IR, but increased protein intake and muscle breakdown may stimulate the process.

- *Changes in gut microbiome:* Diet that decreases the population of *Fermicutes* (e.g., red meat, animal protein) can reduce the metabolism of dietary plant polysaccharides. Mucin degrading *Pervotellaceae* may contribute to gut permeability which may in turn by facilitating movement of cytokines into circulation promote IR.

- *Oxidative stress:* Reactive oxygen species through inhibition of insulin-stimulated glucose uptake and also slowing down of glycogen synthesis in liver and muscle.

- *Placenta:* It contributes to IR through its secretions of glucogenic hormones and cytokines. Placenta in addition to anti-insulin action through placental lactogen, cortisol estrogen, and progesterone also produces insulinase that increases insulin destruction. Placental lactogen has growth hormone-like action, causing increased lipolysis with liberation of free fatty acids.

Pregnancy is therefore considered as a diabetogenic state, and since it induces the mother to utilize fatty acids for her caloric need sparing glucose for the fetus, it is aptly described as a condition of accelerated starvation.

■ EFFECT OF GESTATIONAL DIABETES

Untreated or uncontrolled GDM is associated with an increased risk of complications for both the mother and the child.

Mother

Candida proliferates when the homeostasis of the vaginal microenvironment is disturbed, including changes in mucosal acidity and hormone levels. It is generally believed that pregnant women with GDM are predisposed to *Candida* colonization of the vagina. Elevated glycemia in the vaginal tissue increases fungus adhesion and growth, predisposing the vaginal epithelial cells to binding to *Candida albicans* cells. In addition, hyperglycemia may interfere with host defense mechanism making diabetic patients more sensitive to vulvovaginal candidiasis. The possible mechanisms are: (i) decrease in nonpurposeful migration of neutrophils; (ii) weakening of chemotactic and phagocytic functions of leukocytes.[20] It is for similar reasons that *urinary tract infection* (UTI) can be thought to be more prevalent in GDM. Studies have not shown increased frequency of UTI, upper or lower, in GDM.

Gestational diabetes mellitus is associated with an increased risk of *preeclampsia*, since both conditions share the same risk factors, although it is unclear whether these two conditions share a common pathophysiological pathway.

Spontaneous and indicated *preterm labor delivery* is hypothesized to be associated with poor glycemic control. The possible mechanism could be direct induction of endothelial dysfunction and increased oxidative stress leading to blunted nitric oxide–dependent vasodilatation with hyperglycemia. Decreased synthesis of nitric oxide in the uterus is associated with initiation of labor in animals, and moreover nitric oxide has been shown to be a uterine relaxant.

Increased propensity for vaginal infection and altered local defense along with population of inflammatory cytokines and possibility of *prelabor rupture of membranes* (PROM) are common. Intrauterine pressure due to polyhydramnios may contribute to it. *Chorioamnionitis* and later *subinvolution of uterus* are associated with GDM.

Polyhydramnios is attributed to fetal polyuria in response to hyperglycemia, and macrosomia may result in overdistension of the uterus to result in *hypotonic uterine action in labor.*

Delivery of a macrosomic baby puts a woman with GDM at a higher risk of morbidity due to *traumatic complications* of *vaginal delivery* and higher rates of *cesarean delivery* with associated operative morbidity.

Women with GDM are at a higher risk of developing *type 2 diabetes*; approximately 60% of them develop type 2 diabetes later in life. Each additional pregnancy is reported to confer a threefold increase to the risk and a yearly risk of 2–3% conversion to type 2 diabetes.

The alteration in vasculature of women with GDM is permanent, and this predisposes them to *cardiovascular disease* (CVD). An increased risk of CVD as high as in two-third of the past GDMs could partly, but not fully, be explained by the higher BMI.

Fetus-Neonate

Gestational diabetes mellitus is also associated with a significant risk for the fetus, including stillbirth, macrosomia, shoulder dystocia, and congenital malformations. Neonatal complications are also more frequent and include neonatal hypoglycemia, neonatal hyperbilirubinemia, hypocalcemia, erythrocytosis, and poor feeding.

For *macrosomia*, it is hypothesized by Pederson that maternal hyperglycemia results in fetal hyperglycemia and hyperinsulinemia, which in turn cause excessive fetal growth. Abnormalities in maternal lipid levels may also be an important factor. Placental factors can also affect the supply of nutrients to the fetus and can contribute to fetal overgrowth. Macrosomia has been variously defined as birthweight > 4,000–4,500 g, as well as large for gestational age, in which birthweight is above the 90th percentile for population- and sex-specific growth curves. It may complicate as many as 40–50% of pregnancies in women with GDM.

Preterm birth due to early induction of labor before 39 weeks of gestation and/or prelabor rupture of membranes is one of the complications. Spontaneous onset of preterm labor is also higher in patients with hyperglycemia in pregnancy.

Shoulder dystocia is one of the most serious complications of vaginal delivery in macrosomic babies. It is associated with *birth trauma*, and the risk of brachial plexus injury is approximately 20 times higher when the birth weight is above 4,500 g.

Hypoglycemia, a common occurrence after birth, is due to the hyperinsulinemia of the fetus. Hypoglycemia can lead to more serious complications such as severe central nervous system and cardiopulmonary disturbances. Major long-term sequelae include neurologic damage resulting in mental retardation, recurrent seizure activity, developmental delay, and personality disorders.

Respiratory distress syndrome (RDS) is thought be due to the fact that pulmonary surfactant biosynthesis gets affected by hyperglycemia and hyperinsulinemia. Insulin excess may interfere with the normal timing of glucocorticoid-induced pulmonary maturation in the fetus by blocking cortisol action in fibroblasts reducing the production of fibroblast-pneumocyte factor. Transient tachypnea of the newborn (TTN) occurs two to three times more commonly than in normal infants. The mechanism may be related to reduced fluid clearance in the diabetic fetal lung. Cesarean delivery, which is more frequently performed, may be a contributing factor.

Hyperbilirubinemia may be because of prematurity, impaired hepatic conjugation of bilirubin, and increased enterohepatic circulation of bilirubin resulting from poor feeding. In macrosomia, neonates have a high oxygen demand causing increased erythropoiesis and, ultimately, polycythemia.

Hypocalcemia is seen in infants of gestational diabetic mothers (IDM) and is related to failure from increasing parathyroid hormone (PTH) synthesis following birth. Reduction in PTH secretion and PTH responsiveness is brought about by *hypomagnesemia*. For this reason, in some neonates with hypocalcemia and hypomagnesemia, the hypocalcemia may not respond to treatment until the hypomagnesemia is corrected. It has been proposed that low neonatal levels are due to maternal hypomagnesemia caused by increased urinary loss secondary to hyperglycemia.

Congenital anomalies are seen in babies born of mothers with diabetes. Heart defects and neural tube defects, such as spina bifida, are the most common types of birth defects. Usually, no attributable birth defects result because of gestational diabetes. The high blood sugar level of women with GDM can damage the developing organs of the fetus, leading to congenital anomalies. Hyperketonemia, hypoglycemia, somatomedin inhibitor excess, and excess free oxygen radicals have also been suggested.

Later Complications

Childhood Obesity

There has been evidence of fetal programming of later adiposity amongst offspring exposed to existing diabetes in utero. Exposure to maternal GDM is reported to be associated with a higher BMI, a greater waist circumference, more visceral and subcutaneous adipose tissue, and a more centralized fat distribution pattern. The long-term effects of in utero GDM exposure are not always evident in early childhood, but rather manifest during puberty. An offspring of diabetic mothers is also susceptible to the onset of *metabolic syndromes* such as increased blood pressure, hyperglycemia, obesity, and abnormal cholesterol levels that occur together and increase the risk of heart disease, stroke, and diabetes.

■ SCREENING AND DIAGNOSIS

The exercise helps in early screening for overt diabetes and detecting GDM.

Early Screening for Pregestational Diabetes

Testing early in the first trimester for blood sugars (fasting and postprandial, or random) may help to pick up pregestational diabetes. Glycosylated hemoglobin (HbA1c) percentage estimation can also be used (please vide the section *Definition*, given in the preceding text, for threshold values).

Detecting Gestational Diabetes

A consensus is still elusive regarding an optimal approach to screening for GDM as to whether it should be a two- or a one-step approach.

A *two-step approach* begins with screening using 50 g oral glucose challenge test (OGCT) followed by diagnostic 100 g oral glucose tolerance test (OGTT):

- *Step 1: Oral glucose challenge test:* The woman is administered 50 g glucose without regard to the time of the day or the last meal, and blood is tested for plasma glucose value 1 hour after the glucose ingestion. The test is interpreted as positive if the blood sugar estimate is above 140 mg/dL. This test also helps in identifying cases with diabetes when the result value is 200 mg/dL or more.

- *Step 2: Oral glucose tolerance test:* Women with positive OGCT are subjected to diagnostic OGTT. After overnight fasting of 8 hours following the usual diet, 100 g of glucose in 200–250 mL of water is administered by mouth. Blood samples are obtained in a fasting state before glucose ingestion and three more samples after the ingestion at hourly intervals. Until all blood samples are taken, the woman remains in a fasting state.

  [Interpretation of the test result follows either the Carpenter-Coustan[2] or American Diabetes Association (ADA)[3] threshold values to infer an abnormal test if any two values meet or exceed.]

A *one-step approach* proceeds directly with OGTT and follows 75 g glucose ingestion:

- *WHO:*[5] It involves obtaining a blood sample after 8 hours of overnight fasting following a usual meal, ingestion of 75 g glucose in 200–250 mL water, and taking two additional hourly blood samples for glucose assessments.

  The test is considered as abnormal if any one value meets or exceeds the threshold.

- *Diabetes in Pregnancy Study group of India (DIPSI):*[7] One-step approach is different in that there is no requirement of overnight fasting and only one blood sample is obtained for estimation 2 hours after glucose ingestion.

  The test is interpreted as positive for GDM if the blood sugar estimate is >140 mg/dL.

In the two-step approach, a woman has to return after 50 g OGCT for possible 100 g OGTT which therefore increases the dropout rate. It has two different sets of glucose thresholds to interpret the results. The one-step approach proceeds directly with 75 g OGTT curtailing two visits for the purpose. It would likely increase the number of women with a GDM diagnosis because only one abnormal value is needed for diagnosis. Both the diagnostic tests require the woman to follow overnight fasting and give repeated blood samples.

The single-step approach of DIPSI overcomes the inconvenience of reporting in a fasting state by making repeated visits. The rationale behind choosing the test in the nonfasting state is that glucose concentrations are affected little by the time since the last meal in a normal glucose-tolerant woman, whereas it will affect glucose concentrations in a woman with GDM who has impaired insulin secretion. The reason behind obtaining only a single blood sample 2 hours after the glucose challenge is that the primary outcomes of birth weight, neonatal adiposity, and cord C peptide level > 90th percentile tend to occur as the 2-hour postglucose values increase beyond 140 mg/dL, although there is a continuous relationship between maternal glycemia and neonatal outcomes.

Clinicians and institutions should select one criterion to use consistently, with local rates of diabetes and availability of resources for managing GDM being factored into that decision.

The protocol suggested by the government of India[21] at Indian facilities for Indian women is:

- To follow universal screening.

- Single-step test using 75 g oral glucose and measuring blood sugar 2 hours after the glucose ingestion.

- 75 g glucose is to be given orally after dissolving in approximately 300 mL water irrespective of whether the pregnant woman comes in a fasting or a nonfasting state and of the last meal. The intake of the solution has to be completed within 5–10 minutes.

- A plasma standardized glucometer should be used to evaluate blood sugar 2 hours after the oral glucose load.

- If vomiting occurs within 30 minutes of oral glucose intake, the test has to be repeated the next day, and if vomiting occurs after 30 minutes, the test continues.

- A threshold blood sugar level of ≥140 mg/dL is taken as the cutoff for the diagnosis of GDM.

TABLE 3: Investigations required in workup of a woman with gestational diabetes.

Investigation	When and frequency	Reason

Glycemic status:
Blood sugars
	Fasting with postprandial sugar profile:
	• 10–14 days after medical nutrition therapy
	• 24–48 hours after initiating change in insulin/metformin requirement
	• If requirement is:
	  – Stabilized—every 2 weeks
	  – Not stabilized—individualized
	Random sugar estimation:
	• In labor, every 2–4 hours in those who required insulin
		Glycemic levels are dynamic with fluctuations in a day and across the periods of pregnancy and labor

Complication profile:
• Kidney function tests—(blood) urea, creatinine, uric acid
• Urinalysis:
  – Proteinuria
  – Ketonuria
  – Culture
• Fundus oculi examination
• Obstetric ultrasound
	At diagnosis
	Repeat fortnightly, if glycemic control is poor
	
	If hypertension is present
	If the glycemic control is poor; when in labor, whenever random blood sugar is >160–180 mg/dL
	Every 4 weeks; symptom directed
	At admission; every week if uncontrolled sugars, and monthly if controlled on hypoglycemics
	An interval growth scan at 32–34 weeks or earlier when discrepancy between uterine height and period of pregnancy is detected; biophysical profile at 34 weeks and at 2 weekly intervals in women on hypoglycemics
		As an indicator of hypertensive effect on kidneys since there is a vicious association between hyperglycemia and hypertension
		
		Indicate the severity of maternal effect.
		To monitor (i) fetal growth—macrosomia, growth restriction; (ii) liquor volume abnormalities—polyhydramnios; (iii) fetal well-being

■ MANAGEMENT

The objectives of the management will be to ensure optimal glycemic control during pregnancy and labor, prevent maternal–fetal–neonatal effects, and treat when they occur.

Investigations after diagnosis can be categorized as those to monitor the blood sugars, baseline investigations for complications that may arise, and those for maternal and fetal well-being **(Table 3)**.

Treatment

The objectives of the treatment will be (1) to maintain glycemia under control, (2) to carry pregnancy to term while monitoring for fetal and maternal well-being, (3) prevention/early identification of the complications, (4) timely intervention, and (5) treatment of complications:

■ *Glycemic control:* Management of hyperglycemia involves medical nutrition therapy and treatment with hypoglycemic agents. Trial of changes in diet and exercise are offered to women with GDM when there is no fasting hyperglycemia at the time of diagnosis:
  – *Medical nutrition therapy (MNT):* The objective, in addition to maintaining a normoglycemic state, will be to provide a balanced diet so that adequate nutritional requirements of both the mother and the fetus are addressed **(Box 2)**.

Diet manipulation is the first line of management of GDM in women whose fasting blood sugar (FBS) is <105

BOX 2: Goals of Medical Nutritional Therapy.

• Achieve normoglycemia
• Prevent ketosis
• Provide adequate gestational weight gain based on maternal body mass index
• Contribute to fetal well-being

mg/dL and none of the postprandial values is >200 mg/dL.

For working out a diet, the energy requirement for the woman should be calculated individually based on BMI **(Table 4)**. Women should consume a minimum of 1,800 calories a day to prevent ketosis.

The yield of the energy should be harvested from the main proximate principles. "Diet" does not mean that it is carbohydrate restriction **(Table 5)**. The proportion of carbohydrate in the diet is manipulated to blunt postprandial hyperglycemia. It should be remembered that reducing the carbohydrates to decrease postprandial glucose levels may lead to higher consumption of fat, which may have adverse effects on maternal IR and fetal body composition.

A food chart should be prepared in consultation with the dietician to suit the tastes and likes of the woman. The meal plan for the day could be split such that there will be three major meals and at least two minor meals. It should be seen that during the waking time, there is

TABLE 4: Calorie requirement in gestational diabetes based on the body mass index (BMI).

Body mass index		Energy required (kcal/kg)*
Category	BMI (kg/m²)	
Low	<18.5	Up to 40
Normal	18.5–22.9	30
Overweight	23–28.9	22–25
Obese	>28.9	Up to <15

*Calorie requirement is calculated for the ideal body weight.

TABLE 5: Food composition and proportion of energy in diet.

Proximate principal source	Energy sourced (%)
Carbohydrate	45
Protein	30
Fats	25*

*Saturated fat intake should be <7% of the total calories.

not more than 4 hours' stretch of no food. This will help in preventing breakdown of body fat and protein for energy requirements minimizing the occurrence of IR, and avoids undue peak in plasma glucose levels after ingestion of the total quantity of food at one time. The schedule of food intake can be: 6.30 AM early morning juice/milk, 9 AM breakfast, 11 AM snacks, 1.30–2 PM lunch, 4.30–5 PM snacks with juice/tea/ coffee, 8.30–9 PM dinner, and 10.30–11 PM bedtime juice/milk. After one goes to sleep, the basal metabolic rate will be low and nearly 8 hours of no food is not going to be a significant factor since energy requirement will also be less:

- *Exercise:* The use of exercise as part of the continuum of treatment in women with GDM is accepted and widely encouraged. There are no GDM-specific exercise prescription guidelines published; research has been conducted in general pregnancy and exercise. It is recommended that women with GDM should do both aerobic and resistance exercise at a moderate intensity, a minimum of three times a week for 30–60 minutes each time. Transient improvement of insulin action and passive glucose uptake are seen after exercise for up to 48 hours. Exercise induces increase in skeletal muscle glucose uptake that results from a coordinated increase in rates of glucose delivery, surface membrane glucose transport, and intracellular substrate flux through glycolysis.

Blood sugars are assessed after at least 10 days to 2 weeks post initiation of maternal nutrition therapy and encouragement to exercise. If the glucose values remain higher than the threshold values, induction of hypoglycemic agents is to be made.

- *Hypoglycemic agents:* Pharmacotherapy is considered for management of GDM not controlled on MNT. The drug treatment is initiated at any of the following thresholds:
  - Fasting glucose   > 95 mg/dL
  - 1-hour postprandial glucose   > 140 mg/dL
  - 2-hour postprandial glucose   > 120 mg/dL

Insulin is the first drug of choice and metformin can be considered for optimizing the blood sugar levels:

- *Insulin:* It has been the mainstay of pharmacotherapy for GDM. Insulin is started immediately if FBS is >120 mg/dL while MNT is begun simultaneously. Women are taught self-monitoring of plasma glucose and self-injection. Blood sugars are estimated while fasting and 1.5 hours after each meal.

The dose required varies in different individuals depending on the degree of hyperglycemia. The total requirement of insulin reported is 0.7–2 units/kg/day (of the present pregnancy weight). Requirement increases with increasing gestational age, obesity, and other factors affecting glycemic control. Commonly, the mixed and split dose regimen is used. The glycemia management is carried out in consultation with an internist-endocrinologist.

Insulin management is initiated with lowest calibrable dose of 2–6 units of subcutaneous injection of short acting insulin before meal. The dose is titrated against the blood sugar response (fasting and postprandials) the next day. Dose adjustment is done in increment or decrease of 2–4 units. There is no guideline to guide the adjustment of insulin dose. It can be an individual hospital protocol. It should be remembered that each individual will be different when it comes to insulin sensitivity or resistance. Once the total daily dose requirement is arrived at, it can be split to twice-a-day dosing schedule where two-third of it is administered in the morning and the remaining one-third at night. A mixture of intermediate-acting NPH and short-acting insulin is advised with two-third NPH and one-third short-acting insulin in the morning, and pre-dinner dose being equally divided between NPH and short-acting insulin. The onset of action with short-acting insulin is 30 minutes and lasts for 6–8 hours whereas with NPH it is 1 hour and its action lasts for 10–14 hours.

With this regimen, if the patient continues to have fasting hyperglycemia, the intermediate-acting insulin has to be given at bedtime instead of before dinner.

It is ideal to use human insulin as they are least immunogenic. Insulin of animal source produces antibodies which can cross the placenta and cause insulin-induced macrosomia. Insulin analogs such as lispro insulin and aspart insulin have been approved for use in pregnancy.

Hypoglycemia, pain at the site of injection, and lipodystrophy remain the concerns.

- *Biguanides: Metformin* appears safe in the treatment of GDM, but one-third of the women would require insulin supplementation to achieve glycemic targets. Its advantages are comparable to the use of insulin for GDM. In addition, it is considered to reduce occurrence of pregnancy-related hypertension and gestational weight gain. Metformin is given as 500 mg tablet a day and frequency is adjusted to control the blood sugar. The most common disadvantage is gastrointestinal side effects including the metallic taste in the mouth, nausea, anorexia, abdominal discomfort, and diarrhea. These symptoms are usually mild, transient, and reversible after the dose reduction or discontinuation.

  Its continued use in women with polycystic ovarian disease has shown that metformin may prevent GDM.

- *Sulfonylureas: Glyburide* is considered safe in pregnancy and the clinically important pregnancy outcomes are reported to be similar to those with Metformin. Glyburide can be considered for women with GDM in whom blood glucose targets are not achieved with metformin but who decline insulin therapy or cannot tolerate metformin. The dose of glyburide is 5–10 mg, twice a day. Maternal hypoglycemia is the most common side effect.

  Although metformin and glyburide have not been associated with an increased risk of anatomic birth defects, when either drug is prescribed, patients should be made aware that information regarding the long-term effects of transplacental passage of these drugs is not known, and thus caution is warranted. The fetal drug levels were found to be high with glyburide (70% of maternal level) and for metformin, they were even higher (200% of maternal level). The theoretical risk that fetal exposure to an insulin-sensitizing agent has long-term effects on offspring should be kept in mind.

- *Acarbose:* It is an oral alpha-glucosidase inhibitor oligosaccharide obtained from the fermentation processes of a microorganism, actin. There is only one small randomized trial looking at the use of acarbose in women with GDM. There was no difference in maternal/fetal outcomes compared to insulin although gastrointestinal side effects were increased. The dose can be given as 25 mg, three times a day. The dosage needs to be individualized.

■ While efforts are made to control blood sugars, further management of pregnancy will be guided by the ability to maintain normoglycemia and the results of fetal well-being tests:

- *Good glycemic control:* Pregnancy is monitored and carried to full term. Our practice is to decide in favor of termination of pregnancy if labor has not set in spontaneously by the expected date of delivery.

- *Poor glycemic control:* The objective will be to carry pregnancy at least to late preterm, i.e., beyond 34 weeks. Once that is reached provided there is no fetal compromise, the plan would be to enter early term and decide for termination of pregnancy. Although in GDM sudden fetal death is less common than in overt diabetics, maternal glycemia would exert a similar influence on the fetus.

- *Fetal compromise:* Any evidence of a nonreassuring fetal status should warrant the decision for termination of pregnancy any time after 30–32 weeks of pregnancy in consultation with the patient and her companion, and neonatologist-pediatrician.

■ *Labor and delivery care:* The decision for cesarean delivery, whenever taken, will be because of obstetric indications and not because of GDM. Cesarean delivery will be planned in cases with macrosomia and if the expected baby weight is >4 kg, and the primary indication will be fetopelvic disproportion:

- *Preterm labor:* For inhibition of preterm labor when sets in before 34 weeks of pregnancy, beta-mimetics should be avoided for tocolysis. Corticosteroids are not contraindicated and should be given.

- *Labor or termination of pregnancy up to 37 weeks:* To augment fetal lung maturity, glucocorticoids should be administered. Lung surfactants, especially entry of phosphatidyl glycerol, are delayed even beyond 34 weeks of pregnancy in fetuses because of hyperinsulinemia. Therefore, infants of hyperglycemic mothers will be prone to respiratory distress syndrome. Corticosteroids can initiate acute maternal hyperglycemia and ketoacidosis can manifest. Hence, insulin dosage in these women needs to be increased as guided by sugar estimates. An algorithm that can help to implement increased insulin dosage after corticosteroids can thus be simplified as:

- *Day 1:* Increase the next dose of insulin by 25–30%.
- *Day 2–3:* All insulin doses are increased by 40–50%.
- *Day 4:* All insulin doses are increased by 20–30%.
- *Day 5:* All insulin doses are increased by 10–20%.
- *Days 6 and 7:* The insulin dose is gradually reduced to presteroid levels.

– *Induction of labor:* Labor would be induced electively in the early morning and the morning dose of insulin should be omitted and woman started on dextrose with neutralizing dose of insulin (500 mL of dextrose or dextrose-saline with 15 units of insulin). Capillary blood sugars are monitored every 1–2 hours. Threshold of control will be 126 mg/dL and additional insulin requirement is titrated as dictated by sugar levels **(Table 6)**.

The woman is simultaneously started on 10% dextrose infusion for nutrition during labor at the rate of 125 mL/h.

Presence of ketosis obtunds the action of insulin and render it ineffective. Therefore, the rate of delivery of insulin should be raised whenever ketosis develops. The optimal rate of glucose decline should be 100 mg/dL/h. Do not allow the blood glucose level to fall below 200 mg/dL during the first 4–5 hours of treatment. Hypoglycemia may develop rapidly with correction of ketoacidosis due to improved insulin sensitivity.

– *Cesarean delivery:* When posted for cesarean delivery electively, she will preferably be first on the list of surgeries for the day. As in care during labor, the woman will be skipping the dose of insulin that morning and will be shifted to the surgery area with infusion of glucose with neutralizing dose of insulin. That morning, fasting sugar estimation and report of the electrolytes should accompany the woman.

TABLE 6: Rate of insulin infusion according to the blood sugar level.	
Blood sugar (mg/dL)	Rate of insulin (units/h)
Up to 126	1
126.1–180	2
180.1–240	3
>240	4

POSTPARTUM CARE

After the delivery of placenta, the glucose levels begin to decline and the insulin requirement reduces drastically. It will be wise to halve the insulin requirement for the day if the woman has been on insulin and get estimates of fasting and postprandial sugar values after 48 hours of delivery to decide the need and dose of hypoglycemic agents.

A woman with GDM should be encouraged to breastfeed immediately after delivery and for at least 4 months' postpartum.

There is a long-term maternal risk of dysglycemia. The evidence of impairment of insulin secretion and its action may persist postpartum. At 3–6 months, the postpartum risk of dysglycemia is about 20%.[22] Hence, every woman with GDM who did not require hypoglycemic agents or in whom insulin was stopped after delivery is advised OGTT after the puerperium.

The importance of using effective methods of contraception until the woman is normoglycemic and ready to conceive should be stressed. It will help to minimize the risks of congenital anomalies. Intrauterine devices can be considered the first choice of long-acting reversible contraception. Combined estrogen progesterone preparations can be used. Progesterone-only methods are acceptable alternatives.

STUDIES OF IMPORTANCE

Hyperglycemia and Adverse Pregnancy Outcome[23]

Hyperglycemia and adverse pregnancy outcome (HAPO) was an international multicenter study of a cohort of 25,505 pregnant women in 15 centers tested with a 2-hour 75 g OGTT and followed through pregnancy, generating an expectation of universal convergence for the adoption of a 75 g OGTT for the diagnosis of gestational diabetes as well as for the formulation of diagnostic criteria for GDM. It was designed to study the risks of adverse outcomes associated with degrees of maternal glucose intolerance not meeting the criteria for gestational diabetes. It showed a dose–response gradient across maternal glucose levels for the various adverse pregnancy outcomes.

Australian Carbohydrate Intolerance Study[24]

Australian Carbohydrate Intolerance Study (ACHOIS) was carried out on 1,000 women to determine whether the treatment of GDM reduced the risks of perinatal outcomes. It showed significant reduction in serious perinatal morbidity (1% vs. 4%) and improved the woman's health-related quality-of-life in the treated group.

ACKNOWLEDGMENT

Contribution of Professor Lalit Kapadia, the author of the chapter for the first edition that provided the structure to this chapter revision, is acknowledged.

- Metformin or Glyburide can be used for maintaining euglycemia, but should be switched over to regular insulin as labor approaches or termination of pregnancy is planned.

KEY POINTS

- GDM is defined as glucose intolerance of variable severity detected after first-trimester that is not overt diabetes, not excluding the possibility of concomitant development of glucose intolerance unrelated to pregnancy.
- Prevalence is increasing worldwide and there are wide variations
- There are multitude of risk factors that may increase the risk for developing GDM
- Diagnosis is based on 2-step of 50 g glucose challenge followed by 100g-3h tolerance test or single step procedure using 75 g glucose ingestion.
- Failure of metabolic adaptations of pregnancy to balance increased secretion of placental glucogenic hormones, beta cell dysfunction and mild insulin resistance results in GDM.
- Maternal effect of uncontrolled GDM include increased risk for vulvovaginal candidiasis, UTI, preeclampsia, preterm labor, PROM, chorioamnionitis, subinvolution of uterus, and if there is macrosomia and/or polyhydramnios hypotonic uterine action, traumatic vaginal delivery, and increased incidence of cesarean delivery. Long term effects include predisposition to development of type 2 diabetes and cardiovascular disease.
- Fetal effects are stillbirth, macrosomia, shoulder dystocia, and congenital malformations.
- The frequent neonatal complications are hypoglycemia, respiratory distress, hyperbilirubinemia, hypocalcemia, erythrocytosis, and poor feeding. Childhood obesity and susceptibility for metabolic syndrome are the late effects.
- A blood sugar estimation at first trimester visit and challenge test after 50g glucose intake or the 75 g challenge-cum-tolerance test after at 23–26 weeks of pregnancy are the screening strategies followed by the most.
- Medical nutrition therapy is the first intervention if FBS is <105 and none of postprandial values are >200 mg/dL.
- When pharmacotherapy is required, Insulin is the time-honoured choice. It is started with short-acting regular insulin in low dose 2–6 units before meal, and the requirement titrated against blood sugar response.

REFERENCES

1. American Diabetes Association (ADA). Classification and Diagnosis of Diabetes. Diabetes Care. 2016;39(Suppl 1):S13-S22.
2. Carpenter MW, Coustan DR. Criteria for screening tests for gestational diabetes. Am J Obstet Gynecol. 1982;144:768-73.
3. American Diabetes Association. Diagnosis and Classification of Diabetes Mellitus. Diabetes Care. 2004;27(Suppl 1):s5-s10.
4. International Association of Diabetes and Pregnancy Study Groups Consensus Panel. International Association of Diabetes and Pregnancy Study Groups Recommendations on the Diagnosis and Classification of Hyperglycemia in Pregnancy. Diabetes Care. 2010;33(3):676-82.
5. WHO/NMH/MND/13.2. Diagnostic criteria and classification of hyperglycaemia first detected in pregnancy: World Health Organization Guideline. Diabetes Res Clin Pract. 2014;103:341-63.
6. National Institute for Health and Care Excellence (2015). Diabetes in pregnancy: management of diabetes and its complications from preconception to the postnatal period. [online] Available from: www.nice.org.uk/guidance/ng3 [Last accessed September, 2020]
7. Seshiah V. Fifth National Conference of Diabetes in Pregnancy Study Group. India J Assoc Physic India. 2010;58:329-30.
8. Guariguata L, Linnenkamp U, Beagley J, Whiting DR, Cho NH. Global estimates of the prevalence of hyperglycaemia in pregnancy. Diabetes Res Clin Pract. 2014;103:176-85.
9. Yogev Y, Ben-Haroush A, Hod M. Pathogenesis of gestational diabetes mellitus; In: Hod M, Jovanovic L, Di Renzo GC, de Leiva A, Langer O (Eds). Textbook of Diabetes and Pregnancy, 1st edition. London: Martin Dunitz, Taylor & Francis Group; 2003. p. 46
10. Lee KW, Ching SW, Ramachandran V, Yee A, Hoo FK, Chia YC, et al. Prevalence and risk factors of gestational diabetes mellitus in Asia: a systematic review and meta-analysis. BMC Pregnancy Childbirth. 2018;18:494.
11. Mwanri AW, Kinabo J, Ramaiya K, Feskens EJ. Gestational diabetes mellitus in sub-Saharan Africa: systematic review and meta regression on prevalence and risk factors. Tropical Med Int Health. 2015;20(8):983-1002.
12. DeSisto CL, Kim SY, Sharma AJ. Prevalence estimates of gestational diabetes mellitus in the United States, Pregnancy Risk Assessment Monitoring System (PRAMS), 2007-2010. Prev Chronic Dis. 2014;11:E104.
13. Kayal A, Anjana RM, Mohan V. Gestational diabetes: an update from India. Diabetes Voice. 2013;58:30-4.
14. Mithal A, Bansal B, Kalra S. Gestational diabetes in India: science and society. Indian J Endocrinol Metab. 2015;19(6):701-4.
15. Di Cianni G, Miccoli R, Volpe L, Lencioni C, Del Prato S. Intermediate metabolism in normal pregnancy and in gestational diabetes. Diabetes Metab Res Rev. 2003;19:259-70.
16. Catalano PM, Tyzbir ED, Roman NM, Amini SB, Sims EA. Longitudinal changes in insulin release and insulin resistance in nonobese pregnant women. Am J Obstet Gynecol. 1991;165:1667-72.
17. Phelps RL, Metzger BE, Freinkel N. Carbohydrate metabolism in pregnancy: XVII. Diurnal profiles of plasma glucose, insulin, free fatty acids, triglycerides, cholesterol, and individual amino acids in late normal pregnancy. Am J Obstet Gynecol. 1981;140:730-6.

18. Ryan EA, O'Sullivan MJ, Skyler JS. Insulin action during pregnancy: studies with the euglycemic clamp technique. Diabetes. 1985;34:380-9.

19. Prentki M, Nolan CJ. Islet beta cell failure in type 2 diabetes. J Clin Investig. 2006;116:1802-12.

20. National Health Mission (2014). Diagnosis and management of Gestational Diabetes Mellitus: Technical and Operational Guidelines. [online] Available from: https://nhm.gov.in/New_Updates...Guidelines/Gestational-Diabetes-Mellitus.pdf [Last accessed September, 2020]

21. Nowakowska D, Kurnatowska A, Stray-Pedersen B, Wilczynski J. Activity of hydrolytic enzymes in fungi isolated from diabetic pregnant women: is there any relationship between fungal alkaline and acid phosphatase activity and glycemic control? APMIS. 2004;112:374-83.

22. Kim C, Newton KM, Knopp RH. Gestational diabetes and the incidence of type 2 diabetes: a systematic review. Diabetes Care. 2002;25:1862-8.

23. The HAPO Study Cooperative Research Group. Hyperglycemia and adverse pregnancy outcomes. N Engl J Med. 2008;358:1991-2002.

24. Crowther CA, Hiller JE, Moss JR, McPhee AJ, Jeffries WS, Robinson JS. Effect of treatment of gestational diabetes mellitus on pregnancy outcomes. N Engl J Med. 2005;352:2477-86.

Thyroid Disorders in Pregnancy

Srinivas Krishna Jois

HISTORY

Thyroid was first identified in 1656 by the anatomist Thomas Wharton and he named the gland the thyroid.[1] In 1909, Theodor Kocher from Switzerland won the Nobel Prize in Medicine "for his work on the physiology, pathology and surgery of the thyroid gland."[2]

Sushruta Samhita of Ayurvedic medicine written in about 1500 BC mentions the disease goiter as "Galaganda" along with its treatment. In 1600 BC, the Chinese were using burnt sponge and seaweed for the treatment of goiters.[3]

In 1884, thyroidectomies were successfully performed for the treatment of toxic goiter.[4] Hashimoto's disease was described in 1912.[4]

Case reports of postpartum thyroiditis (PPT) with hypothyroidism or thyrotoxicosis were made by the mid-1970s.[4]

Thyroid dysfunction is not uncommon. The diagnosis of many of these conditions is relatively simple, and the prognosis is excellent if managed in a timely manner. Neonatal screening programs for hypothyroidism are now the standard of care and have shown an incidence of 1 in 3,500-4,500 births.[5]

PHYSIOLOGY[6]

There is an increase in hormone secretion by 40-100% during pregnancy, and a slight increase in the size of the gland (from 12 to 15 mL) is seen. The gland increases by 10% in size during pregnancy in iodine-replete areas and by 20–40% in areas of iodine deficiency.[7]

During the first trimester, because of human chorionic gonadotropin (hCG; intrinsic thyrotropic activity due to similarity in alpha chains), thyroid-stimulating hormone (TSH) decreases.

Estrogen also contributes to an increase in total triiodothyronine (T3) and thyroxine (T4) by increasing thyroxine-binding globulin (TBG).

Thus, subclinical hyperthyroidism occurs in the first trimester which settles later.

But free T3 (FT3) and free T4 (FT4) are normal (T4 may be slightly increased).

The fetus starts secreting T4 by 12 weeks but significant dependence by the fetus is seen on maternal T4. TSH does not cross the placenta but T4 does.[8]

The World Health Organization recommends an iodine intake of 200 µg/day during pregnancy to maintain adequate thyroid hormone production.

It has been reported that the upper 95% confidence interval (CI) for plasma TSH in the first trimester is 2.5 mU/L.[9] It is known that the TSH level descends 60–80% by week 10 and recovers slowly thereafter, but it may not reach the preconception normal range until gestation ends.[10]

The hormone range for pregnancy is about 1.5 times the nonpregnant range **(Table 1)**.

If trimester-specific reference ranges for TSH are not available in the laboratory, then the reference ranges given in **Table 2** are recommended.[11]

IMMUNOMODULATION IN PREGNANCY

This information is relevant while studying thyroid disorders in pregnancy as immunological mechanisms are responsible for most of the cases of thyroid disorders:

TABLE 1: Normal range of thyroid hormones.[6]

Hormones	First trimester	Second trimester	Third trimester	Nonpregnant
TSH (µIU/mL)	0.6–3.4	0.37–3.6	0.38–4.04	0.34–4.35
Total T3 (ng/dL)	97–149	117–169	123–162	77–135
Total T4 (µg/dL)	6.5–10.1	7.5–10.3	6.3–9.7	5.4–11.7
Free T3 (pg/mL)	4.1–4.4	4.0–4.2	–	2.4–4.2
Free T4 (ng/dL)	0.8–1.2	0.6–1.0	0.5–0.8	0.8–1.7

(triiodothyronine; thyroxine; thyroid-stimulating hormone)

TABLE 2: Trimester-wise TSH level.

Trimester	TSH range in mU/L
First trimester	0.1–2.5
Second trimester	0.2–3.0
Third trimester	0.3–3.0

(TSH: thyroid-stimulating hormone)

BOX 1: Level A recommendation by the American College of Obstetricians and Gynecologists (ACOG) 2015-Practice bulletin no 148.

- Universal screening is not recommended.
- Universal screening for thyroid autoantibodies in pregnancy is not recommended
- TSH is the first-line screening test to assess thyroid status in pregnancy.
- TSH and FT4 should be measured to diagnose thyroid disease in pregnancy.
- Treat overt hypothyroid disease in pregnancy with adequate thyroid hormone to minimize risk of adverse outcomes.
- TSH should be monitored in pregnant women who have overt hypothyroidism and the dosage of thyroid replacement adjusted accordingly.
- Pregnant women with overt hyperthyroidism should be treated with thioamide to minimize risk of adverse outcomes.
- FT4 should be monitored in pregnant women with hyperthyroidism and thioamide dose adjusted accordingly

- There is a shift from Th1 to Th2
- Interleukin (IL) 3, 4, 5, 6, 10, and 13 increase.
- NK activity decreases.
- Masking antibodies in the mother block fetal antigens making them nonimmunogenic.
- Free exchange of fetal and maternal antigens and immune tolerance in the maternal compartment leads to the fetal cells/antigens getting lodged in maternal cells including maternal thyroid.
- Post delivery when the immune tolerance is reversed, from Th2 to Th1, autoimmune thyroiditis may occur/exacerbate.

INCIDENCE

The prevalence of hypothyroidism in pregnancy is around 2.5% according to the Western literature.[11] The prevalence of Graves' disease is around 0.1–0.4% and that of thyroid autoimmunity (TAI) is around 5–10%.[12]

A report from Chennai revealed a prevalence of 2.8% of subclinical hypothyroidism (SCH) among women without a known thyroid disease. The thyroid peroxidase antibody (TPOAb) positivity was 57.1% in antenatal women with SCH and 7% in euthyroid.[13] A report from Mumbai found a 4.8% prevalence of hypothyroidism and 6.4% thyroid antibody positivity.[14] Researchers in Delhi found a higher prevalence of 4.58% of overt hypothyroidism (OH).[15]

Thyroid disorders are the most common endocrine conditions affecting women of reproductive age.[16]

SCREENING

What Parameters to Screen, When, and Their Frequency

The best method of screening to identify and subsequently manage thyroid dysfunction pre-pregnancy and during pregnancy is unknown (Cochrane).

While universal screening versus case-finding for thyroid dysfunction increased diagnosis and subsequent treatment, no clear differences for the primary outcomes (preeclampsia or preterm birth) or for the secondary outcomes, including miscarriage and fetal or neonatal death, and neurosensory disability for the infant as a child (IQ < 85 at 3 years), were documented.[17]

The publication of a large randomized trial showed no difference in cognitive function in 3-year-old children of mothers randomized to screening and treatment versus no treatment for subclinical hypothyroid disease, thus giving the first affirmation that universal screening is not recommended.

The second affirmation is that routine measurements of thyroid function in women with hyperemesis gravidarum are still *not* recommended.[18,19]

Level A recommendations by the American College of Obstetricians and Gynecologists (ACOG) are given in **Box 1**.

Because of insufficient evidence to support universal TSH screening in the first trimester, most professional societies, including the American Thyroid Association (ATA), Endocrine Society, and ACOG, recommend targeted case-finding rather than universal screening.[7]

Only high-risk women belonging to the following categories are recommended to be screened:[20]

- Women with a history of hyperthyroid or hypothyroid disease, postpartum thyroiditis (PPT), or thyroid lobectomy
- Women with a family history of thyroid disease
- Women with a goiter
- Women with thyroid antibodies (when known)
- Women with symptoms or clinical signs suggestive of thyroid underfunction or overfunction, including anemia, elevated cholesterol, and hyponatremia
- Women with type I diabetes
- Women with other autoimmune disorders
- Women with infertility who should include screening with TSH as part of their infertility work-up
- Women with previous therapeutic head or neck irradiation
- Women with a history of miscarriage or preterm delivery

This long list of situations where case-finding is recommended includes many women because the symptoms of thyroid deficiency and excess are very nonspecific. The advice against a universal screening program to detect thyroid dysfunction in all fertile women is, therefore, superseded by the clinical situation.

■ THYROID DISORDERS

Any thyroid disorder either presents as a hypothyroid or a hyperthyroid state.

Very rarely thyroid swellings and nodules can present in a euthyroid state, but the diagnosis is very obvious with the patient presenting with a neck mass. Thyroid swellings may show any of the following symptoms which help us to classify them, make specific diagnosis, and be aware of their effects on pregnancy and newborn.

The signs and symptoms and their effect on pregnancy are presented in **Tables 3 and 4**.

Hyperthyroidism

Hyperthyroidism shows an incidence of 0.1-0.4% in pregnancy. This condition is rarely encountered because of low fertility in them, high risk of abortions, and improvement in autoimmune conditions during pregnancy. Hyperthyroidism can occur due to the following reasons:

- *Graves' disease:* 85-90%
- Initial stages of Hashimoto's thyroiditis
- Overtreatment of hypothyroidism
- Subclinical hyperthyroidism
- Toxic nodule
- *Gestational transient hyperthyroidism:* 2–3% of all pregnancies
- Gestational trophoblastic disease (GTD)
- *T3 toxicosis:* Abnormally high levels of T3

Symptoms of hyperthyroidism may mimic those of normal pregnancy, such as an increased heart rate, sensitivity to hot temperatures, and fatigue. Other symptoms have been given in **Table 3**.

- Initial stages of Hashimoto's thyroiditis can show thyrotoxic features as the gland is undergoing destruction.
- If not monitored properly, hypothyroid patients on treatment may go to a state of hyperthyroidism with undetectable TSH.
- Toxic nodules are usually associated with goiter and hyperthyroid features which can be confirmed by neck scan. Rarely surgery may become necessary during pregnancy.
- GTD could be associated with thyrotoxicosis in 25-65% cases.

Graves' Disease

Graves' disease is the most common cause of hyperthyroidism in pregnancy. The features of hyperthyroidism are as follows:

TABLE 3: Signs and symptoms of thyroid disorders.

Symptoms/Signs	Hyperthyroidism	Hypothyroidism
CNS	Anxiety, tremors, nervousness, lid lag, muscle weakness, exophthalmos	Lethargy, insomnia, prolonged DTR, carpal tunnel syndrome
CVS	Palpitations, fatigue perspiration, failure, dyspnea, arrhythmias, cardiomyopathy, pulmonary hypertension	Edema—nonpitting
Metabolism	Heat intolerance, weight loss, hot skin	Cold intolerance, weight gain, cold skin
GIT	Increased appetite, loose motions, nausea, vomiting	Decreased appetite, constipation
Menstrual	Irregularity/oligomenorrhea	Menorrhagia/amenorrhea
Others	Infertility, abortions, onycholysis four times increased risk of ICU admissions	Galactorrhea, infertility, abortion, dry skin, hyperlipidemia, two times increased risk of ICU admissions

(CNS: central nervous system; CVS: cardiovascular system; DTR: deep tendon reflexes; GIT: gastrointestinal tract; ICU: intensive care unit)

TABLE 4: Effects of thyroid disorders on pregnancy and the fetus.[16,28]

Effects	Hyperthyroidism	Hypothyroidism
First trimester	Abortions, anomalies if on medication,* fetal hypothyroidism/hyperthyroidism-antibody mediated	Abortion (20%), RPL (1%), depression
Second trimester	Drug-related issues such as toxicities,† nonimmune hydrops	Abortion, anemia
Third trimester	PTL, PE, IUGR, stillbirth, baby with hearing loss (12 times)	Myopathy, PE, abruption, PTL (10–15%)
Postnatal	Exacerbation, neonatal hyperthyroidism	Psychosis, lactation issues, cretin, impaired neuropsychointellectual development of baby
General	CCF, arrhythmias, hyperemesis	Anemia, goiter, increased drug requirement

(CCF: congestive cardiac failure; IUGR: intra-uterine growth restriction; PE: preeclampsia; PTL: preterm labor; RPL: recurrent pregnancy loss)
*Methimazole is associated with esophageal or choanal atresia, tracheoesophageal fistula, and aplasia cutis.
† Propylthiouracil (PTU) is rarely associated with severe hepatotoxicity in the second trimester.

- Organ-specific autoimmune disorder with TSH-receptor antibodies (TRAb)
- Improves during pregnancy except during the first trimester
- Exacerbates in the postpartum period

- In spite of prepregnancy treatment, the presence of antibodies may cause fetal hyperthyroidism (1%).
- Treatment during pregnancy can cause fetal hypothyroidism as the drugs cross the placenta.
- Pharmacotherapy is the treatment of choice in pregnancy.
- Subtotal thyroidectomy is not usually done in pregnancy.
- Radiofrequency ablation is contraindicated in pregnancy. If treated with radioiodine pregnancy to be avoided for atleast 6 months post-treatment.

TABLE 5: Antithyroid drugs and dosage.

Drug	Dose	Frequency
Propylthiouracil	100–150 mg	tid
Methimazole	5–10 mg	tid

Thyroid storm—managed by
ICU admission, initial thionamide administration (PTU 1,000 mg oral), oral potassium iodide or IV sodium iodide (500–1,000 mg IV tid), if sensitive, lithium carbonate 300 mg 6th hourly. Beta-blockers such as propranolol (10–40 mg oral)/labetalol. Manage anemia, preeclampsia, infection before delivery. Steroids may be necessary as well as management of hyperpyrexia.[6]

Gestational Transient Thyrotoxicosis (GTT)

- Occurs because of excessive hCG in pregnancy
- Multiple pregnancy, molar pregnancy, and hyperemesis gravidarum can be seen in association
- Resolves by 20 weeks and needs no treatment.
- When TSH is very low, a trend in the serum T4 and T3 levels, eye disease, family history, goiter, weight loss, and arrhythmias may help in differentiating transient GTT from a truly thyrotoxic state/Graves' disease.[21]
- Differentiation of Graves' disease from gestational thyrotoxicosis is supported by the presence of clinical evidence of autoimmunity and presence of TRAb. (TPOAb may be present in either case.)[7]

Subclinical Hyperthyroidism

A new section has been included in subclinical hyperthyroidism, which is defined as an abnormally suppressed TSH accompanied by a normal FT4 level. Subclinical hyperthyroidism is present in approximately 1.5% of pregnant women. No adverse outcomes have been associated with this finding, and so, this is one more reason not to check thyroid function tests routinely.[17] It can cause osteoporosis and thyroid failure in the long run.

Pharmacotherapy

- Mild hyperthyroidism (slightly elevated thyroid hormone levels, minimal symptoms) is often monitored closely without therapy as long as both the mother and the baby are doing well.
- When hyperthyroidism is severe enough to require therapy, antithyroid medications are the treatment of choice, with PTU being the historical drug of choice.
- The goal of therapy is to keep the mother's FT4 and FT3 levels in the high-normal range on the lowest dose of antithyroid medication. Targeting this range of free

hormone levels will minimize the risk to the baby of developing hypothyroidism or goiter.

- Maternal hypothyroidism should be avoided. Therapy should be closely monitored during pregnancy. This is typically done by following thyroid function tests (TSH and thyroid hormone levels) monthly.[10]
- Beta-blockers can be used during pregnancy to help treat significant palpitations and tremor due to hyperthyroidism. They should be used sparingly due to reports of impaired fetal growth associated with long-term use of these medications.
- As Graves' disease typically worsens in the postpartum period, usually in the first 3 months after delivery, higher doses of antithyroid medications are frequently required during this time.[10]
- PTU, if available, is recommended as the first-line drug for treatment of hyperthyroidism during the first trimester of pregnancy because of the possible association of methimazole (MMI) with specific congenital abnormalities that occur during first-trimester organogenesis. MMI may also be prescribed if PTU is not available or if a patient cannot tolerate or has an adverse response to PTU. Dosage and frequency of administration is shown in **Table 5**.
- MMI 10 mg is considered to be approximately equal to 100–150 mg of PTU. Recent analyses reported by the U.S. Food and Drug Administration (FDA) indicate that PTU may rarely be associated with severe liver toxicity.
- For this reason, it is recommended that clinicians should change treatment of patients from PTU to MMI after the completion of the first trimester.
- Available data indicate that MMI and PTU are equally efficacious in the treatment of pregnant women.
- If switching from PTU to MMI, thyroid function should be assessed after 2 weeks and then at 2- to 4-week intervals.[7]

Subtotal thyroidectomy may be indicated during pregnancy as therapy for maternal Graves' disease if:

- A patient has a severe adverse reaction to antithyroid drug (ATD) therapy
- Persistently high doses of ATD are required (over 30 mg/d of MMI or 450 mg/d of PTU)
- A patient is nonadherent to ATD therapy and has uncontrolled hyperthyroidism. The optimal timing of surgery is in the second trimester.[10]

Neck ultrasound

Although scintigraphy scans are contraindicated during pregnancy and rarely needed these days anyway, routine ultrasound may be considered when a goiter or nodular disease is suggested by clinical history and examination. This procedure is useful both to characterize thyroid size and degree of thyroiditis present and to delineate all nodules, allowing an evaluation of their growth characteristics on repeated measurements. In addition, sonography can help make the clinical diagnosis of Graves' disease (by excluding nodules) or Hashimoto's thyroiditis (by the typical heterogeneous patterning).

Hypothyroidism

The most common causes of hypothyroidism in women of reproductive age are as follows:

- Iodine deficiency
- Autoimmune thyroid disease
- A history of past total or subtotal thyroidectomy
- Radioiodine ablation
- Transient thyroiditis
- Congenital hypothyroidism
- Lymphocytic hypophysitis (rarely)
- Sheehan syndrome
- Hypophysectomy
- Amiodarone induced

Myxedema coma[22]

A high mortality rate, even with appropriate treatment, ICU admission, passive rewarming, broad-spectrum antibiotic coverage, and corticosteroids may also be needed. The definitive treatment is thyroid hormone replacement administered as IV T4, 200–500 µg as a bolus followed by 50–100 µg daily.

In suspected cases, the algorithm to work up the case is shown in **Flowchart 1**.

Newly Diagnosed Cases

Follow the algorithm shown in **Flowchart 1**.

When maternal TSH is elevated, measurement of serum FT4 concentration is necessary to classify the patient's status as either sub clinical hypothyroidism (SCH) or overt hypothyroidism (OH).

This is dependent upon whether FT4 is within or below the trimester-specific FT4 reference range.

Thyroid autoantibodies were detected in ~50% of pregnant women with SCH and in >80% with OH.

Avoid OH.

Flowchart 1: Algorithm in suspected cases.

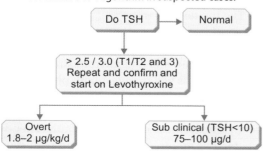

TABLE 6: Levothyroxine dosage guideline.			
Thyroid-stimulating hormone level (mU/L)	5–10	10–20	>20
Levothyroxine dose (µg)	25–50	50–75	75–100

Treat both TPOAb positive and negative subclinical hypothyroid cases.[7]

The drug of choice is Levothyroxine (LT4) **(Table 6)**.

- Repeat TSH once in 4 weeks and adjust the dose till TSH is between 0.5 and 2.5 mU/L.
- Thyroid function tests should be re-measured within 30–40 days and then every 4–6 weeks.[7]
- Iron supplements, calcium, vitamins, or omeprazole may reduce LT4 absorption. In those cases, it is best to advise a 4-hour gap between the medications and LT4.[7]
- Postpartum—probably prepregnancy dose should suffice.

Prevention is primarily done by maintaining an iodine intake of 200-250 µg/day.

Levothyroxine

- *Pregnancy:* Category A
- *Breastfeeding:* Safe.
  Not contraindicated. Levothyroxine is excreted into breastmilk in small quantities.
- *Drug interactions:*
  Interfere with absorption:
  Iron salts, antacids, calcium salts, omeprazole
- *Separate ingestion by >4 hours.*
  Liver microsomal inducers such as rifampicin, phenobarbitone, carbamazepine, and phenytoin can reduce the efficacy of levothyroxine.

Prediagnosed Cases

If the preconception TSH value is <1.6 mU/L, no increment in the thyroxine dosage is required in the first trimester.

A hypothyroid pregnant woman who is already on LT4 replacement therapy will require a dose increase from 25 to 50% on average to maintain desirable TSH concentrations because they have inadequate thyroid reserve.[25] Most hypothyroid pregnant women need a dose increase during the first trimester. In the second trimester, there is generally a plateau in LT4 requirements, but 25–40% of women may need a further dose increase during the third trimester.[26,27]

■ NEONATAL ISSUES

Neonates of women with definitively treated Graves' disease (status post thyroidectomy or treatment with ^{131}I before pregnancy) have a higher risk of neonatal Graves' disease compared with women with Graves' disease who were on thioamide treatment during pregnancy. This is because the definitively treated women still have thyroid-stimulating antibodies that cross the placenta and could affect the fetus but they have no concurrent thioamide treatment, a drug that also crosses the placenta.[18,28]

The infants could become hypothyroid also because of the treatment of Graves' disease with PTU which can affect the thyroid of the fetus.

[131]I should not be given to a woman who is or may be pregnant. If inadvertently treated, the patient should be promptly informed of the radiation danger to the fetus, including thyroid destruction if treated after the 12th week of gestation.

All newborns of mothers with Graves' disease (except those with negative TRAb and not requiring ATD) should be evaluated by a medical care provider for thyroid dysfunction and treated if necessary.[27]

Uncontrolled maternal hyperthyroidism has been associated with fetal tachycardia, small for gestational age babies, prematurity, stillbirths, and possibly congenital malformations. This is another reason why it is important to treat hyperthyroidism in the mother.[10]

■ MEDICAL TERMINATION OF PREGNANCY[29]

The Indian Thyroid Society guidelines do not mention that maternal hypothyroidism is in itself an indication for medical termination of pregnancy (MTP). The thyroid hormone is necessary for fetal brain development and the fact that the early fetus is dependent on maternal sources for its supply is beyond doubt. Untreated or inadequately treated hypothyroidism in mothers has been shown to lead to birth of children with significantly lower IQs. The incidence of learning disabilities is much higher in children born to women with untreated OH **(Table 7)**.

> **Thyroid Autoantibodies**
> These (thyroid peroxidase and thyroglobulin) can be found with normal or increased TSH. They could be responsible for early pregnancy loss. Treatment with levothyroxine has been found to be beneficial by some studies.[23,24]

TABLE 7: Medical termination of pregnancy in thyroid disorders.

Thyroid disorder	<20 weeks	>20 weeks
Overt hypothyroidism	Levothyroxine Assess the severity and other issues*	Levothyroxine MTP cannot be considered in India
Subclinical hypothyroidism	Levothyroxine No need for MTP	Levothyroxine MTP cannot be considered in India
Hyperthyroidism	Antithyroid drugs, Preferably PTU. If MMI has been used, assess at TIFFA scan and decide	Antithyroid drugs

(MMI: methimazole; MTP: medical termination of pregnancy; PTU: propylthiouracil; TIFFA: targeted imaging for fetal anomalies)
*The ease of conception, past babies born with low IQ, family history of low IQ relatives, radioiodine exposure in the past 6 months, parity, age, duration of gestation, and severity of the disease need to be considered if the patient requests for an MTP, but cannot be recommended.

■ THYROID NODULES/CANCER

Fine-needle aspiration (FNA) cytology should be performed for predominantly solid thyroid nodules larger than 1 cm. Nodules of 5 mm to 1 cm in size should be considered for FNA if the pregnant women have a high-risk history or suspicious findings on ultrasound. During the last weeks of pregnancy, FNA can reasonably be delayed until after delivery. Ultrasound-guided FNA is likely to have an advantage for maximizing adequate sampling.[10]

Women found to have cytology indicative of papillary cancer or follicular neoplasm without evidence of advanced disease and who prefer to wait until the postpartum period for definitive surgery may be reassured that delaying surgical treatment until soon after delivery is unlikely to change disease-specific survival.

Radioactive iodine (RAI) with ^{131}I should not be given to women who are breastfeeding or for at least 4 weeks after nursing has ceased.

Furthermore, pregnancy should be avoided for 6 months to 1 year in women with thyroid cancer who receive therapeutic RAI doses to ensure stability of thyroid function and confirm remission of thyroid cancer.[10]

■ POSTPARTUM THYROIDITIS (PPT)[10]

Thyroiditis can cause both thyrotoxicosis and hypothyroidism. In PPT, thyrotoxicosis occurs first followed by hypothyroidism.

Women who are at risk for PPT are those with:

- Autoimmune disorders (such as type 1, or juvenile onset, diabetes mellitus)
- Positive antithyroid antibodies (risk correlates with antibody levels)
- History of previous thyroid dysfunction
- History of previous PPT (20% of women will have recurrence)
- Family history of thyroid dysfunction

The exact cause is not known, but it is believed to be an autoimmune disease very similar to Hashimoto's thyroiditis. In fact, these two disorders cannot be distinguished from one another on pathology specimens.

As in Hashimoto's thyroiditis, PPT is associated with the development of antithyroid (antithyroid peroxidase, antithyroglobulin) antibodies

In the US, PPT occurs in approximately 5–10% of women. The incidence can be greater in certain high-risk populations.

Not all women demonstrate evidence of going through both phases of hyper- and hypothyroidism (approximately one-third of patients will manifest both phases while one-third of patients will have only a thyrotoxic or a hypothyroid phase).

The thyrotoxic phase occurs 1–4 months after delivery and lasts for 1–3 months. It is associated with symptoms including anxiety, insomnia, palpitations, etc. Since these symptoms are often attributed to being postpartum and the stress of having a new baby, the thyrotoxic phase is often missed.

Most women present in the hypothyroid phase, which occurs 4–8 months after delivery and may last up to 9–12 months. Symptoms include fatigue, weight gain, constipation, dry skin, etc.

Most women will have return of their thyroid function to normal within 12–18 months of the onset of symptoms. Around 20% of those who go into a hypothyroid phase will remain hypothyroid.

Treatment depends on the phase of thyroiditis and the degree of symptoms. Women presenting with thyrotoxicosis may be treated with beta-blockers to decrease palpitations and reduce tremors.

As symptoms improve, the medication is tapered off since this phase is transient.

Antithyroid medications are not used for the thyrotoxic phase since the thyroid is not overactive.

The hypothyroid phase is treated with thyroid hormone replacement. If the hypothyroidism is mild, with a few symptoms, no therapy may be necessary. In other situations after the T4 therapy is started, monitor and try to take her off the medication after 12–18 months as 80% would recover from this condition and would not require any treatment by a year or two.

■ OBSTETRIC MANAGEMENT

Antenatal

- Routine antenatal care
- No universal screening recommended
- Look for risk factors and screen
- Newly diagnosed problems—immediate initiation of treatment, being aware of toxic profile
- Escalate the dose in prediagnosed cases of hypothyroidism
- Keep a watch on weight gain, blood pressure, and anemia
- Thyroid scan, FNAC, surgical intervention if necessary (for nodules)
- Cardiac evaluation and beta-blockers in rhythm disturbances
- Admission in cases of cardiac failure/thyroid storm/ myxedema coma or other obstetric complications
- Fetal surveillance for anomalies, thyromegaly, hydrops, cardiac rhythm disturbances, distress, and the frequency to be individualized. More applicable in autoimmune conditions, Graves' disease, and women on medications for hyperthyroidism
- Optimize TSH and FT4/total T4
- Steroid prophylaxis in threatened/established preterm labor

Intranatal

There are three varieties of presentation of cases:

1. *Prediagnosed conditions:* Well controlled, offer routine care
2. *Diagnosed but uncontrolled:* Adequately control and brace up to manage complications
3. *Diagnosed in labor/with complications:* All emergency measures should be available such as IV T4, IV beta-blockers, cardiologist, and ICU care as basically it is a team approach management.
   a. Except for hypertensive disorders of pregnancy, abruption, and intrauterine fetal death, there is no indication for induction of labor.
   b. Augmentation of labor—routine practice is applicable.
   c. For second and third-stage routine care except in cardiac complications, prophylactic forceps may be required.
   d. Careful monitoring of pulse, temperature, blood pressure, urine output (UOP), and conscious level needs to be done and look for thyroid storm, myxedema coma, cardiac failure, acute pulmonary edema, etc.
   e. Lower segment caesarean section (LSCS) for obstetric indications only

Anesthetic Considerations[22]

Hyperthyroidism

The problems that one need to keep in mind are: (1) hyperdynamic circulation leading to high output cardiac failure, (2) cardiac dysrhythmias, (3) difficult airway associated with huge goiter, and (4) thyroid storm.

Regional anesthesia can be preferred for cesarean section. It is easier and safer in such patients. It also avoids manipulation of a potential difficult airway and cardiovascular problems due to inadequate depth. Surgery can be safely performed using a single-shot spinal anesthesia with bupivacaine and hypno-sedation.

Hypothyroidism

Severe hypothyroidism should be managed with IV T3/T4 but, if they are not available, oral T3 is the mode of choice. Hypothermia should be prevented in the operation room as well as in the postoperative period. During surgical stress, hydrocortisone should be given. Regional anesthesia should be favored over general anesthesia. Presence of normal coagulation should be confirmed before regional anesthesia.

Contraception

No restriction for any type of contraceptive use in both hyperthyroidism, hypothyroidism and in simple thyroid swellings. Combined oral contraceptives, any progesterone methods (Injectable, oral, LNG-IUS, implants, emergency contraception), IUCD, sterilization surgery and centchroman can be used in thyroid abnormalities. Hyperthyroidism with cardiac complications estrogen containing contraceptives are avoided till adequately controlled.[30]

KEY POINTS

- Commonest endocrine problem encountered in pregnancy

- Both hypothyroidism and hyperthyroidism can adversely affect the pregnancy outcome
- Screening for thyroid disorders may be incorporated in the investigations done during first trimester (routine screening not recommended by Government of India)
- The cut off values for TSH and thyroid hormones differ in pregnancy
- Early initiation of treatment in both deficiency and excess helps to optimize the outcome
- Propylthiouracil is the preferred drug in hyperthyroidism in pregnancy though methimazole may be used in 2nd and 3rd trimester to avoid serious hepatotoxicity of PPU
- Radioiodine treatment is contraindicated in pregnancy
- Surgery may be considered in indicated cases
- Antenatal, intranatal and postnatal care is routine except when associated with cardiac, hypertensive or neurological complications wherein the management has to be individualized.
- Barrier methods, progesterone only methods, IUCD, centchroman, tubectomy can be safely used for contraception, but estrogen containing contraception is better avoided in hyperthyroidism with cardiac complications but safe in well controlled cases

■ REFERENCES

1. Whonamedit? Thomas Wharton. [online] Available from https://www.whonamedit.com/doctor.cfm/2046.html [Last accessed September, 2020]
2. The Nobel Prize. The Nobel Prize in Physiology or Medicine 1909. [online] Available from https://www.nobelprize.org/prizes/medicine/1909/summary/ [Last accessed September, 2020].
3. V. Leoutsakos, A short history of the thyroid gland, HORMONES 2004;3(4):268-71.
4. Hamdy RC. The thyroid gland: A brief historical perspective. South Med J. 2002;95(5): 471-3
5. Fisher DA. Hypothyroidism. Pediatr Rev. 1994;15:227.
6. Gary Cunningham F, Leveno KJ, Bloom SL, Spong CY, Dashe JS, Hoffman BL. Williams Obstetrics, 24th edition. New York: McGraw Hill; 2014.
7. The American Thyroid Association Taskforce on Thyroid Disease During Pregnancy and Postpartum, Stagnaro-Green A, Abalovich M, Alexander E, Azizi F, Mestman J, et al. Guidelines of the American Thyroid Association for the diagnosis and management of thyroid disease during pregnancy and postpartum. Thyroid. 2011;21(10):1081-125.
8. Dashe JS, Casey BM, Wells CE, McIntire DD, William Byrd E, Leveno KJ, et al. Thyroid-stimulating hormone in singleton and twin pregnancy: Importance of gestational age-specific reference ranges. Obstet Gynecol. 2005;106:753-7.
9. Glinoer D, Lemone M, Bourdoux P, De Nayer P, DeLange F, Kinthaert J, et al. Partial reversibility during late postpartum of thyroid abnormalities associated with pregnancy. J Clin Endocrinol Metab. 1992;74:453-7.
10. American Thyroid Association. Thyroid Disease and Pregnancy. [online] Available at https://www.thyroid.org/thyroid-disease-pregnancy/ [Last accessed September, 2020]
11. LeBeau SO, Mandel SJ. Thyroid disorders during pregnancy. Endocrinol Metab Clin North Am. 2006;35(1):117-36.
12. Hollowell JG, Staehling NW, Flanders WD, Hannon WH, Gunter EW, Spencer CA, et al. Serum TSH, T4, and thyroid antibodies in the United States population (1988 to 1994): National Health and Nutrition Examination Survey (NHANES III). J Clin Endocrinol Metab. 2002;87(2):489-99.
13. Gayathri R, Lavanya S, Raghvan K. Subclinical hypothyroidism and auto immune thyroiditis in pregnancy: A study in South Indian subjects. J Assoc Physicians India. 2009;57:691-3.
14. Nambiar V, Jagtap VS, Sarathi V, Lila AR, Kamalanathan S, Bandgar TR, et al. Prevalence and impact of thyroid disorders on maternal outcome in Asian-Indian pregnant women. J Thyroid Res. 2011;2011:429097.
15. Sahu MT, Das V, Mittal S, Agarwal A, Sahu M. Over and subclinical thyroid dysfunction among Indian pregnant women and its effect on maternal and fetal outcome. Arch Ggynecol Obstet. 2010;281:215-20.]
16. Jefferys A, Vanderpump M, Yasmin E. Thyroid dysfunction and reproductive health. Obstet Gynaecol. 2015;17:39-45.
17. Spencer L, Bubner T, Bain E, Middleton P. Cochrane Database of Systematic Reviews. (2015). Screening and subsequent management for thyroid dysfunction pre-pregnancy and during pregnancy for improving maternal and infant health. [online] https://doi.org/10.1002/14651858.CD011263.pub2 [Last accessed September, 2020]
18. American College of Obstetricians and Gynecologists. Practice Bulletin No. 148: Thyroid disease in pregnancy. Obstet Gynecol. 2015;125(4):996-1005.
19. Marcos Abalovich, De Groot L, Alexander EK, Amino N, Barbour L, Cobin RH, et al. Management of thyroid dysfunction during pregnancy and postpartum: An Endocrine Society Clinical Practice Guideline. J Clin Endocrinol Metab. 2012;92(8):S1-47.
20. Galofre JC, Davies TF. Autoimmune thyroid disease in pregnancy: A review. J Womens Health (Larchmt). 2009;18(11):1847-56.
21. Surks MI. Subclinical thyroid dysfunction: A joint statement on management from the American Association of Clinical Endocrinologists, the American Thyroid Association, and The Endocrine Society. J Clin Endocrinol Metab. 2005;90:586-7.
22. Sannaboraiah SK, Ramaswamy AH, Shaikh S. Thyroid disorders during pregnancy and anesthetic consideration. Anaesth Pain Intensive Care. 2014;18(3):302-7.
23. Stagnaro-Green A, Roman SH, Cobin RH, el-Harazy E, Alvarez-Marfany M, Davies TF. Detection of at-risk pregnancy by means of highly sensitive assays for thyroid autoantibodies. JAMA. 1990;264:1422-5.
24. Negro R, Mangieri T, Coppola L, Presicce G, Casavola EC, Gismondi R, et al. Levothyroxine treatment in thyroid peroxidase antibody-positive women undergoing assisted reproduction technologies: A prospective study. Hum Reprod. 2005;20:1529-33.
25. Alexander EK, Marqusee E, Lawrence J, Jarolim P, Fischer GA, Larsen PR. Timing and magnitude of increases in levothyroxine requirements during pregnancy in women with hypothyroidism. N Engl J Med. 2004;351:241-9.
26. Toft A. Increased levothyroxine requirements in pregnancy—Why, when, and how much? N Engl J Med. 2004;351:292-4.
27. De Groot L, Abalovich M, Alexander EK, Amino N, Barbour L, Cobin RH, et al. Management of thyroid dysfunction during pregnancy and postpartum: An endocrine society clinical practice guideline. J Clin Endocrinol Metab. 2012; 97(8):2543-65.
28. American College of Obstetricians and Gynecologists. Practice Bulletin No. 37: Thyroid disease in pregnancy. Obstet Gynecol. 2002;100:387-96.
29. Kalra S, Ganie MA, Unnikrishnan AG. Overt hypothyroidism in pregnancy: Can we consider medical termination of pregnancy? Indian J Endocr Metab. 2013;17:197-9.
30. UK medical eligibility criteria, FSRH, for contraceptive use | UKMEC 2016.

Renal Disease in Pregnancy

Hiralal Konar

INTRODUCTION

Pregnancy results in significant alteration in renal function due to pregnancy-associated physiologic changes involving the structure and the function of the urinary system. Any alteration beyond the physiological limit may affect the maternal and neonatal outcomes in an adverse way. There are three scenarios: first, renal disease may antedate pregnancy and may be aggravated due to physiologic changes; second, there are specific renal conditions that develop de novo during pregnancy; and third, acute kidney injury in early or late pregnancy.

PHYSIOLOGICAL CHANGES IN THE URINARY SYSTEM DURING PREGNANCY[1-3]

Physiological adaptations during pregnancy which are clinically important include the following:

- The size of the kidneys is increased by 1–1.5 cm and the calyces, renal pelvis, and ureters dilate due to smooth muscle relaxation by progesterone and compression from gravid uterus.
- Increase in glomerular filtration rate (GFR): 50% rise occurs at the end of the first trimester and 55% in the mid-trimester and then plateaus. Renal blood flow reaches a peak rise of 70–80% in the mid-trimester and then falls to 45% above nonpregnant value at term.
- Rise in GFR leads to a fall of serum urea and creatinine levels by 20%. Therefore, in contrast to a nonpregnant state, a serum creatinine level of 0.8 mg/dL is considered abnormal.
- There is a fall of serum albumin by 5–10 g/L.
- Proteinuria up to 200 mg in 24 hours and glycosuria may occur.
- Asymptomatic bacteriuria is common due to dilatation and stasis of the collecting system and vesicoureteral reflex resulting in high incidences of urinary tract infection (UTI).

CHRONIC KIDNEY DISEASE[4-8]

Chronic kidney disease (CKD) is now classified into five stages according to the level of renal function (**Table 1**).

Stages 1 and 2 (normal or mild renal impairment with persistent albuminuria) affect up to 3% of women of childbearing age. Stages 3–5 (glomerular filtration rate < 60 mL/min) affect around 1 in 150 women of childbearing age, but because of reduced fertility and an increased rate of early miscarriage, pregnancy in these women is less common. Studies of CKD in pregnancy have mostly classified women on the basis of serum creatinine values (**Table 2**).

Chronic kidney disease may be detected for the first time during pregnancy. Around 20% of women who develop early pre-eclampsia (≤30 weeks' gestation), especially those with heavy proteinuria, have previously unrecognized CKD.

Effects of Renal Disease on Pregnancy

The fetomaternal outcome depends on the type of renal disease and the underlying pathology, degree of renal dysfunction, degree of hypertension and proteinuria, and presence of infection and anemia.

Some specific renal diseases such as renal scleroderma and polyarteritis nodosa deteriorate grossly during pregnancy, and pregnancy is contraindicated. In

TABLE 1: Stages of chronic kidney disease on the basis of GFR.

Stage	Description	Estimated GFR (mL/min/1.73 m²)
1	Kidney damage with normal or raised GFR	≥90
2	Kidney damage with mildly low GFR	60–89
3	Moderately low GFR	30–59
4	Severely low GFR	15–29
5	Kidney failure	<15 or dialysis

(GFR: glomerular filtration rate)
Source: NKF-KDOQI CKD classification guideline 2002, with permissions.

TABLE 2: Chronic kidney disease on the basis of creatinine level.

Type	Serum creatinine
Mild dysfunction	1.5 mg% or less
Moderate dysfunction	>1.5–2.4 mg %
Severe dysfunction	>2.5 mg%

systemic lupus erythematosus and mesangiocapillary glomerulonephritis, there is a possibility of deterioration.

In mild dysfunction, there is a low risk of worsening during pregnancy and the incidence of superimposed pre-eclampsia is 10%. Although the incidence of preterm and small for gestational age (SGA) is increased, the overall fetal prognosis is good.

In moderate dysfunction, 40% women deteriorate during pregnancy and there is persistence of the damage during the postpartum period. The risk of superimposed pre-eclampsia is 40% and that of preterm labor and SGA is also high.

In severe dysfunction, 80% women develop pre-eclampsia, 70–80% deliver preterm, and the incidence of SGA is 40–50%. There is progression to end-stage renal disease in 30–45% of cases.

Prepregnancy Counseling[5,6]

Women with chronic renal disease need prepregnancy counseling. A baseline assessment of blood pressure (BP), proteinuria, renal function test, and complete blood count is required before planning a pregnancy. Women with serum creatinine > 1.4/dL and certainly those with > 2 mg/dL should be advised to refrain from pregnancy. BP should be controlled and anemia should be treated before pregnancy. The possibility of deterioration of renal function and the onset of superimposed pre-eclampsia with all possible adverse effects on the fetus and mother should be explained before becoming pregnant.

Folic acid 400 µg daily should be given as usual before conception until 12 weeks' gestation. Fetotoxic drugs—such as angiotensin-converting enzyme (ACE) inhibitors and angiotensin II receptor blockers—should be stopped before pregnancy if equally effective drugs are available or as soon as pregnancy is confirmed.

Antepartum Management[4-7]

Antenatal care in women with renal disease need to be under multidisciplinary supervision with an aim to detect a) renal deterioration b) development of superimposed preeclampsia and c) detect fetal growth restriction.

Maternal Surveillance

The frequency of maternal visit is suggested to be every fortnight (once in 2 weeks) up to 28 weeks and weekly thereafter; BP and urine dipstick for proteinuria need to be checked in every visit. If there is proteinuria of +1 or more by dipstick, quantification of proteinuria by 24-hour urine protein and protein/creatinine ratio (PCR) should be done. Renal disease is suspected if there is persistent proteinuria above 500 mg/day before 20 weeks of gestation and it mandates a referral to a nephrologist.

Investigations related to renal function (blood urea and serum creatinine) should be done at the first visit and 4–6 weekly throughout pregnancy. Urine for routine and microscopy (for hematuria and cast, indicating an active parenchymal disease) and urine culture should be done at 4–6-week interval.

Liver function tests [serum glutamic pyruvic transaminase (SGPT), serum glutamic-oxaloacetic transaminase (SGOT), lactate dehydrogenase (LDH)], coagulation profile [prothrombin time (PT), activated partial thromboplastin time (ApTT)], platelet count, and 24-hour urinary protein may be done if superimposed pre-eclampsia is suspected.

Fetal Surveillance

Uterine artery Doppler at 20–24 weeks may be done to predict pre-eclampsia and fetal growth restriction (FGR). Fetal growth is monitored from 26 weeks onward through fetal biometry by ultrasound, and liquor volume is also assessed. If FGR is suspected, umbilical artery Doppler is indicated to know the degree of fetal compromise.

Specific Treatment[6]

Multidisciplinary involvement of nephrologists, physicians, and hematologists is essential.

The folic acid, iron, and calcium supplementation should be given as per the routine protocol.

Low-dose aspirin (50–75 mg) is recommended on confirmation of pregnancy to prevent superimposed pre-eclampsia.

Blood pressure needs to be controlled with labetalol, alpha methyldopa, or nifedipine. The target is to keep BP between 120/80 and 140/90 mm Hg throughout pregnancy. Diuretics are better avoided as they are likely to cause FGR.

Angiotensin-converting enzyme inhibitors and angiotensin receptor renal blockers are contraindicated in pregnancy and need to replaced on the diagnosis of pregnancy.

Women with proteinuria > 1 g/24 hours are at an increased risk of venous thrombosis, and thromboprophylaxis with low-molecular-weight heparin is recommended in them antenatally till 6 weeks' postpartum.

Asymptomatic bacteriuria and UTI need to be aggressively treated. Antibiotic prophylaxis should be given to women with recurrent bacteriuria/UTI.

Subcutaneous recombinant erythropoietin is indicated in women with anemia. Hemodialysis is initiated if serum creatinine is >5 mg/dL and/or blood urea is >120 mg/dL.

Obstetric Management

Many of the cases with chronic renal disease go into preterm labor. There is no contraindication to the standard steroid protocol for fetal lung maturity. Close intrapartum monitoring of mother and fetus is indicated in the event of preterm labor.

In the absence of significant fetomaternal complication/ deterioration, delivery should be planned at or near-term. Early delivery is necessary for severe hypertension and superimposed pre-eclampsia and/or deteriorating maternal renal function and fetal compromise. There is no contraindication to induction of labor. Prostaglandin and oxytocin are both safe for cervical ripening and labor induction. Cesarean delivery is indicated for obstetric reasons.

Postnatal Care

Renal function tests and urine microscopy and culture are to be done in the early postpartum period.

Advise for postpartum contraception should be given.

Women with early onset pre-eclampsia (before 32 weeks) need to be evaluated in the postpartum period for an underlying renal disease.

■ ACUTE RENAL DYSFUNCTION DURING PREGNANCY[8]

Acute renal failure (ARF) or acute kidney injury is characterized by two cardinal features: Oliguria (<400 mL/24 hours) and rise in serum creatinine (>1.2 mg/ dL). Renal failure can be classified as prerenal, renal, and postrenal according to the cause. Prerenal occurs due to hypovolemia and hypoperfusion as in hemorrhage, renal is due to intrinsic renal or renovascular diseases, as in severe pre-eclampsia, and postrenal is due to obstruction of the urinary tract.

There are pregnancy-specific conditions which may cause acute renal dysfunction in women without preexisting renal pathology.

In early gestation, hyperemesis gravidarum may cause prerenal azotemia. Volume depletion due to severe bleeding in early gestation (abortion or ectopic gestation) may lead to acute tubular necrosis. Postabortal sepsis may also lead to acute renal dysfunction.

In late pregnancy and puerperium, the important causes of acute renal dysfunction are pre-eclampsia, antepartum and postpartum hemorrhage, acute fatty liver of pregnancy, and hemolytic uremic syndrome. Sepsis due to chorioamnionitis and puerperal sepsis, disseminated intravascular coagulation following amniotic fluid embolism, or abruption of placenta are also important causes of ARF.

Pyelonephritis, obstructive uropathy, lupus flare, mismatched blood transfusion, and nephrotoxic drugs can cause acute deterioration of renal function during any trimester.

The specific pathology in some of the important causes of acute kidney injury and its specific management are given in **Table 3**.

TABLE 3: Specific pathology and its management in some of the important causes of acute kidney injury.

Condition	Pathology/pathophysiology	Management plan
Pre-eclampsia	Characteristic pathological feature is glomerular capillary endotheliosis resulting in glomerular dysfunction	Termination of pregnancy and supportive care
Acute fatty liver of pregnancy	Rapidly progressing liver failure in late pregnancy associates acute renal dysfunction	Termination of pregnancy and supportive care
Hemolytic uremic syndrome	Characterized by microangiopathic hemolytic anemia, thrombocytopenia, and acute renal failure as a part of multiorgan dysfunction	Serious condition with high maternal mortality, multidisciplinary involvement, and supportive care is required. Plasmapheresis is the treatment of choice
Lupus nephritis	Exacerbation of SLE (flare) can occur in puerperium and in the third trimester. It mimics pre-eclampsia with proteinuria, thrombocytopenia, and elevated liver enzymes	To be treated through a multidisciplinary approach with high dose of intravenous steroids
Acute pyelonephritis	1% of pregnancies are complicated by this serious infection of kidney through ascending infection following asymptomatic bacteriuria. *Escherichia coli* is the most common pathogen. Impaired renal function, thrombocytopenia, hemolysis, and ARDS are the complications	IV broad-spectrum antibiotic initially and to be modified according to urine culture/sensitivity report, adequate hydration, and supportive care
Renal calculi and obstructive uropathy	Presents with renal colic or refractory infection or worsening renal function	Treatment is conservative with hydration, antibiotic, and pain relief. Ureteral stenting/percutaneous nephrostomy/ laser lithotripsy is indicated in single kidney, persistent infection, intractable pain, or worsening of renal function

(ARDS: acute respiratory distress syndrome; SLE: systemic lupus erythematosus)

Management of Acute Renal Failure

The differentiation of prerenal, renal, and postrenal cause of ARF is important. Clinical history is important.

The management is done in consultation with the nephrologist and urologist. In prerenal ARF, fluid challenge is usually done. The amount of transfusion depends on central venous pressure, hourly urine output, and obligatory losses. Low-dose dopamine infusion may help in increasing renal perfusion. In renal cause, fluid restriction is the rule along with supportive care. In postrenal cases, depending on the site of obstruction, ureteral stenting or percutaneous nephrostomy is done by the urologists.

Each renal unit has specific protocols for initiation of dialysis. Common indications are severe metabolic acidosis, electrolyte imbalance, especially hyperkalemia, refractory pulmonary edema, or congestive cardiac failure due to volume overload. The frequency of dialysis depends on subsequent clinical parameters and renal function and serum electrolytes.

Supportive care preferably in a high-dependency unit (HDU) with renal diet, fluid restriction (300 mL + previous day output), antibiotics, and packed cell transfusion are essential during and after dialysis.

■ SOME SPECIAL CONDITIONS

Diabetic Nephropathy

Pregnancy in women with insulin-dependent diabetes does not lead to an increased risk of nephropathy and women with diabetic nephropathy with preserved renal function do not deteriorate as a result of pregnancy. However, women of diabetic nephropathy with moderate-to-severe renal dysfunction have a considerable risk of fetomaternal morbidity. An increased risk of pre-eclampsia and preterm delivery is associated with this condition. There is also an increased risk of congenital malformations of the fetus in women with diabetic nephropathy.

Women on Dialysis[9]

Although a decline in fertility in women with advanced renal disease on dialysis is expected, if pregnancy still occurs, it poses a significant clinical challenge.

The important complications in these women are hypertension (50–70%), pre-eclampsia (18–67%), polyhydramnios (40%), FGR (17–77%), and prematurity and low birth weight (50–100%).[8]

Increased dialysis intensity improves the fetal outcome with a live birth rate of 70–90%.

Different studies comparing peritoneal dialysis and hemodialysis in pregnancy showed no significant difference in the fetomaternal outcome. However, peritoneal dialysis in some cases failed to achieve the desired level of blood urea nitrogen and a switchover to hemodialysis was warranted. In a recent study, continuous ambulatory peritoneal dialysis (CAPD) was found more effective than hemodialysis in improving fetal outcome.

Along with dialysis, supportive care in the form of BP control, maintaining a hemoglobin level around 9–10 g/dL, and keeping the electrolytes in the normal range is essential for good prognosis.

Women with Renal Transplant[10]

More than 7,000 pregnancies have been reported globally in women after renal transplant. The improvement in endocrine and renal function leads to improvement in the fertility of these women.

Women with renal transplant are counseled to conceive when they fulfil the following criteria: (1) At least 2 years following a transplant, (2) optimum health condition with table renal function (serum creatinine < 2 mg/dL and proteinuria < 500 mg/day), (3) good control of BP, and (4) minimal maintenance dose of immunosuppressant with no recent rejection episode.

Among the drugs used for immunosuppression, prednisolone at a dose of 20 mg/day and azathioprine are found to be relatively safe as a very small amount of prednisolone crosses the placenta and azathioprine, although crosses the placenta, cannot be converted to its active metabolite by the fetal liver. Cyclosporin is more likely to cause FGR without significant teratogenic effect.

Overall, the common problems in post-transplant patients are pre-eclampsia, preterm labor, premature rupture of membrane, FGR, low birth weight, infection, and rejection episodes.

There is no contraindication to vaginal delivery. During intrapartum and postpartum periods, prophylactic antibiotic should be given to prevent infection as they are on immunosuppressants.

KEY POINTS

- Due to physiological changes during pregnancy, diagnosis of renal disease becomes difficult. Renal disease also mimics pre-eclampsia. Early onset pre-eclampsia and proteinuria > 500 mg/24 hours before 20 weeks are some clues for diagnosing renal dysfunction during pregnancy.
- The fetomaternal adverse outcome is related to the baseline renal function at the onset of pregnancy. CKD with preserved renal function is likely to have good prognosis.
- Superimposed pre-eclampsia is to be prevented by low-dose aspirin.

- Close maternal and fetal monitoring during pregnancy and multidisciplinary care with collaboration with the nephrologist are an essential part of management.
- There are pregnancy-related causes of ARF which need to be predicted, identified promptly, and treated properly to prevent ARF.
- ARF has a high risk of maternal mortality and morbidity and needs aggressive management with HDU care and hemodialysis, if indicated.

■ REFERENCES

1. Williams DL. Renal disease in pregnancy. Obstet Gynaecol Reprod Med. 2007;17(5):147-53.
2. Sanders CL, Lucas MJ. Renal disease in pregnancy. Obstet Gynaecol Clin N Am. 2001;28(3):593-600.
3. Odutayo A, Hladunewich M. Obstetric nephrology: Renal hemodynamic and metabolic physiology in normal pregnancy. CJASN. 2012;7:2073-80.
4. Williams DL. The implication of pre-existing renal disease in pregnancy. Curr Obstet and Gynaecol. 1999;9:75-81.
5. Fitzpatrick A, Mohammadi F, Jesudason S. Managing pregnancy in chronic kidney disease: Improving outcomes for mother and baby. Int J Women's Health. 2016;8:273-85.
6. Davidson JM, Nelson PC, Kehoe S, Baker P. Renal disease in pregnancy: Consensus views arising from 54th study group. Chapter 20. London: RCOG Press; 2008. pp. 249-51. www.rcog.org.uk
7. Imbasciati E, Gregorinin G, Cabiddu G, Gammaro L, Ambroso G, Del Giudice A, et al. Pregnancy in CKD stages 3 to 5: Fetal and maternal outcomes. Am J Kidney Dis. 2007;49:753-62.
8. Davison J, Baylis C. Renal disease. In: De Swiet M (Ed). Medical Disorders in Obstetric Practice, 3rd edition. Oxford: Blackwell Science; 1995. pp. 226-305.
9. Chou CY, Ting IW, Lin TH, Lee CN. Pregnancy in patients on chronic dialysis. A single centre experience and combined analysis of reported results. Eur J Obstet Gynaecol Reprod Biol. 2008;136(2):165-70.
10. Basaran O, Emirolu R, Secme S, Moray G, Haberal M. Pregnancy and renal transplantation. Transplant Proc. 2004;36(1):122-4.

■ SUGGESTED READING

1. Achour A, Ben Dhia N, Frih A, Ben Dhia R, Mahjoub S, el May M. [Pregnancy with delivery at term in hemodialyzed women]. Rev Fr Gynecol Obstet. 1992;87(1):21-5.
2. Attini R, Montersino B, Leone F, Minelli F, Fassio F, Rossetti MM. Dialysis or a plant-based diet in advanced CKD in pregnancy? A case report and critical appraisal of the literature. J Clin Med. 2019;8(1):123.
3. Cao Y, Zhang Y, Wang X, Zhang Y. Successful pregnancy and delivery in uremic patients with maintenance hemodialysis: A case report. Medicine. 2018;97(50):e13614.
4. Glinoer D, Abalovich M. Unresolved questions in managing hypothyroidism during pregnancy. BMJ. 2007; 335(7614):300-2.
5. Kaul A, Bhadauria DS, Pradhan M, Sharma RK, Prasad N, Gupta A. Pregnancy check point for diagnosis of CKD in developing countries. J Obstet Gynaecol India. 2018;68(6):440-6.
6. Leanos-Moranda A, Campos-Galicia I, Ramirez-Valenzuela KL, Berumen-Lechuga MG, Isordia-Salas I, Molina-Perez CJ. Urinary IgM excretion: a reliable marker for adverse pregnancy outcomes in women with chronic kidney disease. J Nephrol. 2018;32(2):241-50.
7. Nelson DB. Minimal change glomerulopathy in pregnancy. Nephrol Nurs J. 2003;30(1):45-50, 55-6, 122.
8. Piccoli GB, Zakhariva E, Attini R, Hernandez MI, Guillien AO, Alrukhaimi M, et al. Pregnancy in chronic kidney disease: Need for higher awareness. A pragmatic review focused on what could be improved in the different CKD stages and phases. J Clin Med. 2018;7(11):415.
9. Weatherhead S, Robson SC, Reynolds RJ. Eczema in pregnancy. BMJ. 2007. [online] Available from https://doi.org/10.1136/bmj.39227.671227.AE [Last accessed September, 2020]
10. Williams D, Davison J. Chronic kidney disease in pregnancy. BMJ. 2008;336(7637)211-5.

Epilepsy in Pregnancy

Suman Mittal

INTRODUCTION

"Epilepsy" is a Greek word meaning "to seize upon." The Greek physician Hippocrates wrote the first book on epilepsy, "On the Sacred Disease", refuting the idea that epilepsy was a curse or a prophetic power. Hippocrates proved the truth that it is a brain disorder. It is the oldest known and the second most common neurological disorder after migraine. There are many myths and fears associated with epilepsy in India, thus making the patient's life more difficult. Unbelievable as it appears, epilepsy was considered as a valid ground for divorce under *Hindu Marriage Act, 1955*, and *Special Marriage Act, 1954*, till *1995*.

An estimated 0.2–0.7% of pregnant females suffer from epilepsy, the most common major neurological complication occurring during the pregnancy. While approximately over 1.5 million (40% of epileptics) women with epilepsy (WWE) in India are of child-bearing age, to meet their needs, managing maternal epilepsy and monitoring the health of the developing fetus remain two of the most perplexing and engaging issues for all healthcare professionals.

Epilepsy is a disorder of the central nervous system (CNS) characterized either by mild episodic loss of attention or sleepiness (*petit mal*) or by severe convulsions with loss of consciousness (*grand mal*).

Majority of women suffering from epilepsy have normal pregnancy with favorable outcomes. They, however, have higher maternal and fetal risks compared with the general population. Careful planning and management of any pregnancy in a woman who has epilepsy are essential to minimize these risks. The modern management of epilepsy combines the use of improved anticonvulsants with a more sympathetic attitude toward an epileptic patient.

DEFINITIONS

In 1870, Hughlings Jackson, a British neurologist, defined epilepsy as "an intermittent derangement of nervous system due to an excessive and disorderly discharge of cerebral nervous tissue on muscle".

- *Seizure:* Seizure is a paroxysmal event due to abnormal excessive hypersynchronous discharges from an aggregate of CNS neurons.
- *Epilepsy:* This describes a condition in which a person has recurrent seizures due to chronic underlying processes.
- *Status epileptics:* This is defined as 30 minutes of continual seizure activity or a cluster of seizures without recovery.

REPRODUCTIVE ISSUES

Catamenial Epilepsy

A two-fold increase in seizure frequency at a specific period of the menstrual cycle is considered as a catamenial exacerbation. Changes in hormone concentrations, with estrogen being proconvulsant, have been considered as contributory factors. An increase in seizures has also been reported during the follicular phase, when estrogen concentrations are high, and a decrease has been noted in the midluteal phase, at which time progesterone levels are high. Premenstrual tension and fluid retention have also been proposed as contributory factors to catamenial exacerbation of seizures. There have been various approaches to the treatment of catamenial seizures. Trials of administered progesterone and norethisterone have been open and add-on has shown only equivocal benefit.

Fertility

The fertility of men and WWE has been estimated to be 85 and 80% of the expected levels, respectively. Menstrual disorders are common in WWE, particularly polycystic ovarian syndrome and hypogonadotropic hypogonadism.

OBSTETRIC PERSPECTIVE OF EPILEPSY

A majority of WWE will have normal pregnancy and delivery—an unchanged seizure frequency, and over 90% deliver a normal baby. The seizure-free duration is the most important factor in assessing the risk of seizure deterioration. However, many women still present late in pregnancy and are on combinations of anticonvulsant drugs, which significantly increase the risk of birth defects.

PRECONCEPTIONAL COUNSELING

In developing countries where access to an obstetrician and a neurologist may not be possible, counseling with subsequent assessment and care can be provided by general practitioners if they are aware of the impact of different antiepileptic drugs (AEDs). Since 50% of the pregnancies are unplanned, reproductive issues should be raised and discussed by the healthcare provider once the WWE becomes sexually active to allow informed and well-considered choices. Healthcare professionals must be sensitive to a patient's anxieties and be prepared to manage both their seizures and emotional concerns. The woman should be reassured that majority of pregnancies ends in safe confinement and healthy babies. All too often, WWE are referred for review of their treatment when they are 10–14 weeks' pregnant, by which time the most critical period with regard to malformations has probably passed.

The objective is to keep the pregnant woman with epilepsy seizure free while minimizing adverse effects on the pregnancy and the fetus, including possible teratogenic effects. Parents will need counseling to make several changes in their lives to provide a safe environment for the baby.

The recommendations to be discussed with WWE and their partners can be summarized as follows [as per the Royal College of Obstetricians and Gynaecologists (RCOG)]:

- Optimize treatment before conception.
- All WWE should be advised to take 5 mg/day of folic acid prior to conception and to continue the intake until at least the end of the first trimester to reduce the incidence of major congenital malformation.
- Counsel the patient and her partner about the fetal abnormalities that may be detected and those that may be missed by prenatal testing.
- If AED is needed, use monotherapy.
- Choose the most effective AED for seizure and syndrome.
- Use the lowest effective dose.
- Avoid high peak levels of drug used by using multiple doses or extended-release formulations.
- The withdrawal of AEDs should be considered and discussed with the patient if she has been seizure free for more than 2–3 years.
- Counsel about the importance of regular medication.
- Avoid alcohol, smoking, driving, climbing heights, swimming, and other drugs.
- Ensure good nutrition throughout pregnancy.
- Reproductive decision-making in people with epilepsy can be influenced by an overestimation of the risk of inheritance in their offspring.[1] If there are known risk factors for inheritance of epilepsy, or if there is a fear of inheritance, genetic counseling should be offered.[2]

THERAPEUTIC TERMINATION OF PREGNANCY

- Any congenital malformation which is not compatible with survival is a clear-cut indication for termination of pregnancy.
- Uncontrolled seizure after AED therapy
- Unplanned pregnancy which is already exposed to multiple and potential teratogenic drugs and X-rays
- Patient who is mentally not prepared for pregnancy and even after intense counseling, she is still not prepared to continue with the pregnancy.

EFFECT OF PREGNANCY ON EPILEPSY

The effect of pregnancy on seizure frequency is variable and unpredictable among patients. The majority of women (67%) do not experience a seizure in pregnancy.[3] The seizure-free duration is the most important factor in assessing the risk of seizure deterioration.[4]

In women who were seizure free for at least 9 months to 1 year prior to pregnancy, 74–92% continued to be seizure free in pregnancy as well.[4-6] Pregnant women who have experienced seizures in the year prior to conception require close monitoring for their epilepsy.

The data from the EURAP (International Registry of Antiepileptic Drugs and Pregnancy) study showed that pregnant women with idiopathic generalized epilepsies were more likely to remain seizure free (74%) than those with focal epilepsies (60%).[3] There is insufficient evidence to assess whether the rates of status epilepticus are increased in pregnant WWE compared with nonpregnant WWE. Currently, there are no tests to predict the risk of seizure deterioration in pregnancy.

Pregnancy is associated with physiological and metabolic changes that can alter seizure frequency. Physiological and metabolic changes during pregnancy which have their implications on drug disposition are summarized in **Table 1**.

TABLE 1: Physiological and metabolic changes during pregnancy: Effects on drug disposition.

Parameter	Consequences
<ul><li>Total body water, extracellular fluid</li><li>Fat stores</li><li>Cardiac output</li><li>Renal blood flow and glomerular flow rate</li><li>Altered cytochrome P-450 activity elimination</li><li>Maternal albumin of drug for hepatic extraction</li></ul>	<ul><li>Altered drug distribution</li><li>Elimination of lipid-soluble drugs</li><li>Hepatic blood flow leading to elimination</li><li>Renal clearance of unchanged drug</li><li>Altered systemic absorption and hepatic</li><li>Altered free fraction, increased availability</li></ul>

The metabolism of nearly every epileptic drug increases, resulting in lower blood levels, in case the adjustments are not made. The maternal plasma concentration of levetiracetam during the third trimester is about 40% of the baseline concentration without pregnancy, which suggests that therapeutic monitoring can be of value.[7]

Other factors during pregnancy which have their implications on drug disposition include:

- Poor compliance
- Vomiting
- Inappropriate reduction of AED
- Sleep deprivation
- Multiparity
- Hormonal variations of pregnancy: Increased estrogen levels
- Reduction of functional residual capacity with hypercapnia and reduction of cerebral flow
- Hyperventilation causing compensation acidosis
- Retention of sodium and water
- Nitrogen-sparing effect of pregnancy resulting in changes in amino acid concentrations

Sleep deprivation or noncompliance plays a clear role in up to 70% of women who have had an increase in seizures during pregnancy, so it is important to inquire about sleep patterns and compliance in pregnant patients who have epilepsy. Sleep deprivation can result from physical discomforts, movements of the fetus, and nocturia. Marital and financial stress and personal doubts and concerns can contribute to sleep deprivation or cause a more direct increase in the likelihood of seizure occurrence.

Noncompliance with medications is common during pregnancy and is in large part the result of the strong message that any drugs during pregnancy are harmful to the fetus. The teratogenic effects of AEDs are well described, but risks to the fetus are often exaggerated or misrepresented. Proper education about the risks of AEDs versus the risks for seizures can be helpful in assuring compliance during pregnancy.

■ EFFECTS OF EPILEPSY ON PREGNANCY

The effects of epilepsy on pregnancy are varied and include:

- Effects of epilepsy itself
- Effects of seizures
- Effects of AEDs

Effects of Epilepsy Itself

Ninety percent of WWE have uneventful pregnancies, but the incidence of obstetrics complications is higher. Spontaneous abortion is also a common event and may complicate up to 20% of pregnancies in WWE, although the data regarding the risk of abortion in WWE is extremely limited and conflicting.[8] Several complications of pregnancy have been reported to occur more frequently in WWE than in the general population. These include vaginal hemorrhage, placental abruption, pregnancy-induced hypertension, and intrauterine growth retardation.[9] Studies comparing stillbirth rates found higher rates in infants of mothers with epilepsy (1.3–14%) than in infants of mothers without epilepsy. Studies have demonstrated increased rates of neonatal and perinatal deaths.[10]

Effects of Seizures

Seizures can harm in two ways:

1. Decreased uteroplacental circulation leading to impaired oxygenation
2. Trauma to mother and growing fetus

An increased rate of spontaneous abortions as well as an increased risk of fetal malformations is associated with seizures during the first trimester. This risk is probably related to transient fetal hypoxia and acidosis secondary to decreased uteroplacental circulation.

Generalized tonic-clonic seizures (GTCSs) can cause maternal and fetal hypoxia and acidosis. After a single GTCS, fetal intracranial hemorrhages, miscarriages, and stillbirths are reported. A single brief tonic-clonic seizure has been shown to cause depression of fetal heart rate for more than 20 minutes, and longer or repetitive tonic-clonic seizures are incrementally more hazardous to the fetus and the mother. During the seizures, trauma to the mother and the fetus, abruptio placentae, prelabor rupture of membranes, and fetal death may occur. The ultimate concern of seizure during pregnancy is usually not the seizure itself but the potential for blunt abdominal trauma as a result of the patient falling down.

Effects of Antiepileptic Drugs

Each AED crosses the placenta. At term, maternal blood and cord blood levels are approximately equal. Most of the AEDs belong to pregnancy category C or D, and the risk of medication to the fetus must be considered against the risk of maternal seizures.

Teratogenic Risks for Antiepileptic Drugs (Table 2)

Fetal anticonvulsant syndrome: The term "fetal anticonvulsant syndrome" is used to include various combinations of congenital anomalies which have been described with virtually all the AEDs.

Women should be informed that the risk of congenital abnormalities in the fetus is dependent on the type, number, and dose of AEDs.

In WWE who not exposed to AEDs, the incidence of major congenital malformations is similar to the background risk for the general population.[11]

TABLE 2: Teratogenic risks from antiepileptic drug.

	General population	Infants of women who have epilepsy
Congenital heart defects	0.5%	1.5–2%
Cleft lip/palate	0.15%	1.4%
Neural tube defect	0.06%	1–3.8% (VPA), 0.5–1% (CBZ)
Urogenital defects	0.07%	1.7%

(CBZ: carbamazepine; VPA: valproate)

In WWE who are taking AEDs, the risk of major congenital malformation to the fetus is dependent on the type, number, and dose of AED. Among AEDs, lamotrigine and carbamazepine monotherapy at lower doses have the least risk of congenital malformations in the offspring.[12] Data from the EURAP study group[12] suggest that the lowest rates of malformation were observed in women exposed to <300 mg/day of lamotrigine [2 per 100, 95% confidence interval (CI) 1.19–3.24] and to <400 mg/day of carbamazepine (3.4 per 100, 95% CI 1.11–7.71). The rates of major congenital malformation in the UK and Ireland registers[13] were also lower in the levetiracetam monotherapy group (0.7 per 100; 95% CI 0.19–2.51) than the polytherapy group (5.6 per 100, 95% CI 3.54–8.56).[13]

The most common major congenital malformations associated with AEDs are neural tube defects, congenital heart disorders, urinary tract and skeletal abnormalities, and cleft palate.[12,14,15] Sodium valproate is associated with neural tube defects, facial cleft, and hypospadias; phenobarbital and phenytoin with cardiac malformations; and phenytoin and carbamazepine with cleft palate in the fetus. A systemic review and meta-analysis of 59 studies provided estimates of the incidence of congenital malformation in fetuses born to women taking various AEDs.[15] The risk was highest for women taking sodium valproate (10.7 per 100, 95% CI 8.16–13.29) or AED polytherapy (16.8 per 100, 95% CI 0.51–33.05) compared with 2.3 per 100 (95% CI 1.46–3.1) observed in mothers without epilepsy.[15] The risk of recurrence for major congenital malformation was increased (16.8 per 100) in WWE with a previous child with major congenital malformation.[16] There was no significant association between epilepsy type and tonic-clonic seizures in the first trimester and major congenital malformations.

■ POTENTIAL MECHANISM OF ANTICONVULSANT EMBRYOPATHY

The cause of the anticonvulsant embryopathy is likely multifactorial. Anticonvulsant drugs are the most significant offending factor, more so than the actual traits carried by mothers who have epilepsy, environmental factors, or possibly seizures during pregnancy.

The mechanism whereby AEDs are teratogenic have not been definitely established. Possibilities include the formation of epoxide and arene oxide metabolites and cytotoxic free radicals.

Teratogenicity by AEDs is likely to be mediated by several mechanisms including antifolate effects; some are associated with folate deficiency and some drugs such as valproate and lamotrigine interfere with folate metabolism.

Long-term Neurodevelopmental Outcomes of Exposure to AEDs and Maternal Seizure in Infants Born to WWE

Based on limited evidence, in utero exposure to carbamazepine and lamotrigine does not appear to adversely affect the neurodevelopment of the offspring. There is very little evidence for levetiracetam and phenytoin. Children exposed to sodium valproate in utero had a significantly lower developmental quotient when compared with those born to WWE who were not taking AEDs and with those born to women without epilepsy.[17]

High doses of sodium valproate were negatively associated with verbal ability, IQ, nonverbal ability, memory, and executive function and this was not observed with other AEDs.[18] In utero exposure to sodium valproate is associated with increased rates of childhood autism (adjusted hazard ratio 2.9, 95% CI 1.4–6.0).[19,20]

■ ANTIEPILEPTIC DRUGS

Management of AEDs during pregnancy can be complex. Clearance of virtually all of the AEDs increases during pregnancy, resulting in a decrease in serum concentrations. Clearance of most of the AEDs normalizes gradually during the first 2–3 postpartum months. The commonly used AEDs and their doses and side effects are given in **Tables 3 and 4**, respectively.

Antiepileptic drug treatment should be reviewed before conception. For most women with active epilepsy, the appropriate course is to establish them on the minimally effective dose of the single AED that gives the best control of their seizures.

Carbamazepine is the drug of choice: Carbamazepine has enjoyed a reputation as the AED associated with the least teratogenic risk.

■ ANTENATAL CARE

The recommendations as per the RCOG for antenatal care are given in the following text:

First Trimester

- Antenatal care should be started as early as possible.
- Some drugs (carbamazepine) can cause a false-negative

TABLE 3: Commonly used drugs, their doses, and side effects.

Drug	Dose	Maternal effects	Fetal effects
Phenytoin	300–500 mg/day in 1–3 doses	Megaloblastic anemia, gingival hyperplasia, hirsutism	Fetal hydantoin syndrome, cleft lip, palate, flat nasal bridge, etc.
Phenobarbital	90–180 mg/day 2–3 divided doses	Drowsiness, ataxia	CHD, VSD, ASD, cleft lip with/without cleft palate
Primidone	750–1,500 mg/day in 3 divided doses	Nausea, ataxia, drowsiness	Severe embryopathy
Valproic acid	550–2,000 mg/day in 3–4 divided doses	Ataxia, drowsiness	NTD, CV defects, urogenital malformations
Carbamazepine	600–1,200 mg/day in 3–4 divided doses	Drowsiness, leukopenia, ataxia, mild hepatomegaly	Least teratogenic, NTD
Ethosuximide	750–1,250 mg/d (20–40 mg/kg) qid-bid	Nausea, hepatotoxicity, leukopenia, thrombocytopenia	Possible teratogenesis
Trimethadione			Growth delays, cardiac and ocular defects, microcephaly, hypospadias, low-set ears, palatal abnormalities, abnormalities incompatible with pregnancy, two-thirds have major congenital defects

(ASD: atrial septal defect; CHD: congenital heart disease; NTD: neural tube defect; VSD: ventricular septal defect; CV: cardiovascular)

pregnancy test. Confirmation should be done by serum β human chorionic gonadotropin (β-hCG).

■ The multidisciplinary setting should involve an obstetrician, a neurologist, and epilepsy specialist nurses.

  – In women with an unplanned pregnancy, an individualized management plan should be agreed upon between the woman with epilepsy and the neurologist. This may include a change in the dose or type of AED aimed at minimizing the risk to the fetus. AEDs should not be abruptly stopped or changed without appropriate discussion. Even high-risk drugs such as sodium valproate are still the drugs of choice for certain epilepsies, and a discussion of risks and benefits is mandatory.

  – Establish accurate gestational age by clinical data and ultrasonography.

  – Control nausea and vomiting promptly as they interfere with AED absorption and metabolism.

  – Folic acid supplementation should be continued.

  – Preferably monotherapy should be given. Carbamazepine is the drug of choice.

  – Biochemical screening with maternal serum alpha fetoprotein when combined with ultrasonography increases the detection rate for neural tube defects to 94–100%,[21] thereby offering the opportunity to detect these abnormalities in early gestation for WWE.

Second and Third Trimesters

■ Pregnant WWE should have access to regular planned antenatal care with a designated epilepsy care team.

TABLE 4: Newer antiepileptic agents.

Medication	Usual dose (mg/day)	Doses/day	Special notes
Gabapentin	1,200/3,600	3	Not enzyme-inducer antacids interface
Lamotrigine	300–500	1 or 2	Rash in 11.2%, half-life affected by dose
Topiramate	100–400	2	Many interfere with OCs
Tigabine	8–56	2–4	Does not interfere with OCs

(OCs: oral contraceptives)

■ The fetal anomaly scan at 18–20 weeks of gestation can identify major cardiac defects in addition to neural tube defects.

■ No studies have assessed the role of routine fetal echocardiography in detecting congenital heart disease in babies of WWE taking AEDs compared with the 20-week detailed scan that is currently offered.

■ Based on the current evidence, routine monitoring of serum AED levels in pregnancy is not recommended although individual circumstances may be taken into account.

■ At subsequent visits after the booking appointment, the following need to be evaluated: the mother's well-being, including the ability to cope, memory, concentration and sleep; symptoms such as tiredness and dizziness; the AEDs being taken, including dose and dosing schedule; and seizure frequency and type, including auras.

- Serial growth scans are required for detection of small-for-gestational-age babies and to plan further management in WWE exposed to AEDs.
- There is no role for routine antepartum fetal surveillance with cardiotocography in WWE taking AEDs.

Vitamin K supplementation: Most of the AEDs can inhibit vitamin K transport across the placenta. Enzyme-inducing anticonvulsants can cause hemorrhagic problems in neonates due to deficiency of vitamin K-dependent clotting factors: II, VII, IX, X. This results in decrease in vitamin K-dependent clotting and increases risk of fetal hemorrhage in the first 24 hours after birth.

All babies born to WWE taking enzyme-inducing AEDs should be offered 1 mg of intramuscular vitamin K to prevent hemorrhagic disease of the newborn. There is insufficient evidence to recommend routine maternal use of oral vitamin K to prevent hemorrhagic disease of the newborn in WWE taking enzyme-inducing AEDs.

■ MANAGEMENT OF LABOR

Women with epilepsy should be reassured that most will have an uncomplicated labor and delivery. Tonic-clonic seizures occur in about 1–2% of WWE in labor and within 24 hours of delivery in a further 1–2%.[22]

- The diagnosis of epilepsy per se is not an indication for planned cesarean section or induction of labor.
- In WWE with no underlying obstetric risk factors whose seizures are well-controlled seizures, there is no indication for early delivery. In a small proportion of women with significant deterioration of seizures, which are recurrent and prolonged, and who are at a high risk of status epilepticus, elective cesarean section may be considered. There is no evidence on the optimal timing and mode of delivery in WWE.
- Tertiary care center is an ideal place for delivery, with the team of an obstetrician, anesthesiologist and a neonatologist. The physician/neurophysician should be in consultation for any emergency situation. If delivery is not possible at a higher center, at least prompt transport facility should be available.

Stages of Labor

First Stage of Labor

- Psychological support by hospital staff and family members is extremely beneficial during labor.
- Management of anticonvulsant medication during labor presents a challenge. AED intake should be continued during labor.
- Sleep deprivation and nonintake of AEDs are risk factors for seizures in labor, and it is thought that pain, tiredness, stress, and dehydration may be factors as

well.[23] Adequate hydration and pain relief with an epidural will minimize the risks of seizures in labor and provide maximum safety in the event of a seizure. Healthcare professionals will need to ensure that doses of AEDs are not missed during labor and delivery and should consider parenteral alternatives in cases of excess vomiting. AEDs may be given parenterally (this includes phenytoin, phenobarbital, sodium valproate, and levetiracetam). If the patient has seizures or a preseizure aura, the usual loading dose of phenytoin, 10–15 mg/kg, should be given intravenously at a rate not faster than 50 mg/min.

- Continuous fetal monitoring is recommended in women who are at high risk of a seizure in labor and following an intrapartum seizure.

Second Stage of Labor

Safe vaginal delivery is the aim, and all measures of labor are the same as for a normal woman. The mode of delivery and assisted delivery such as forceps, ventouse, and cesarean section are indicated as for any other labor.

Third Stage of Labor

Manage as in other delivery cases. Watch for postpartum hemorrhage and seizures.

■ GENERALIZED TONIC-CLONIC SEIZURE DURING LABOR

In pregnant women presenting with seizures in the second half of pregnancy which cannot be clearly attributed to epilepsy, immediate treatment should follow the existing protocols for eclampsia management until a definitive diagnosis is made by a full neurological assessment. Other cardiac, metabolic, and intracranial conditions should be considered in the differential diagnosis. Neuropsychiatric conditions including a nonepileptic attack disorder should also be considered.

Immediate treatment should be as follows:

- Oxygen inhalation
- Left lateral position which increases uterine blood flow and decreases the risk for maternal aspiration
- In those with intravenous access, lorazepam given as an intravenous dose of 0.1 mg/kg (usually a 4-mg bolus, with a further dose after 10–20 minutes) is preferred. Diazepam 5–10 mg administered slowly intravenously is an alternative. If there is no intravenous access, diazepam 10–20 mg can be administered rectally and repeated once in every 15 minutes later if there is a continued risk of status epilepticus, or midazolam 10 mg as a buccal preparation are suitable.
- Any seizure lasting more than 5 minutes is unusual and represents a high risk of progressing to convulsive status

epilepticus, a life-threatening medical emergency which affects around 1% of pregnancies in WWE.[24] Treatment should be initiated as soon as reasonably possible before status epilepticus is established.[25,26]

- After the mother is stabilized, continuous electronic fetal monitoring should be commenced. If the fetal heart rate does not begin to recover within 5 minutes or if the seizures are recurrent, expedite delivery. This may require cesarean delivery if vaginal delivery is not imminent.

- The neonatal team should be informed, as there is a risk of neonatal withdrawal syndrome with the maternal use of benzodiazepines and AEDs.[27]

■ BREASTFEEDING AND THE PUERPERIUM

- Breastfeeding is to be generally encouraged.
- WWE should be advised to continue their AEDs in the postnatal period. Nausea and vomiting should be treated and if there is no oral intake, consideration should be given to parenteral administration of AEDs.
- Mothers should be well supported so that trigger of seizure deterioration such as sleep deprivation, stress, and pain are minimized. Sleep deprivation-related seizures could be reduced by arranging help for the mother, especially for night-time feeds. If the mother breastfeeds, storage of breast milk pumped during the day might be beneficial.
- If the AED dose was increased in pregnancy, it should be reviewed within 10 days of delivery to avoid postpartum toxicity.
- Babies born to mothers taking AEDs may have adverse effects such as lethargy, difficulty in feeding, excessive sedation, and withdrawal symptoms with inconsolable crying. Individualized assessment should be made for the level of postdelivery monitoring required for withdrawal symptoms and for any signs of toxicity. This is especially important in premature babies, and serum levels of AEDs in the baby should be checked where appropriate.[28]
- WWE should be screened for depressive disorder in the puerperium.

■ CONTRACEPTION FOR WOMEN TAKING ANTIEPILEPTIC DRUGS

- WWE should be offered effective contraception to avoid unplanned pregnancies.
- Copper intrauterine devices (IUDs), levonorgestrel-releasing intrauterine system (LNG-IUCD), and medroxyprogesterone acetate injections should be promoted as reliable methods of contraception that are not affected by enzyme-inducing AEDs.

- Women taking enzyme-inducing AEDs (carbamazepine, phenytoin, phenobarbital, primidone, oxcarbazepine, topiramate, and eslicarbazepine) should be counseled about the risk of failure with some hormonal contraceptives.
- All methods of contraception may be offered to women taking nonenzyme-inducing AEDs (e.g., sodium valproate, levetiracetam, gabapentin, vigabatrin, tiagabine, and pregabalin).
- In women who are taking enzyme inducers and choose to use oral contraception, the contraceptive efficacy may be improved by increasing the estrogen component to 50 μg (maximum 70 μg), reducing the pill-free interval from 7 to 4 days and tricycling (taking 3 packs back to back).[29]
- Barrier contraception should be additionally used if WWE taking enzyme-inducing AEDs use oral contraceptives (combined hormonal contraception or progestogen-only pills), transdermal patches, vaginal rings, or progestogen-only implants.[30]
- Women taking lamotrigine monotherapy and estrogen-containing contraceptives should be informed of the potential increase in seizures due to a fall in the levels of lamotrigine.
- For emergency contraception for WWE taking enzyme-inducing AEDs, only the copper IUD is recommended. It is unclear whether a higher dose of levonorgestrel or ulipristal acetate is a sufficiently effective strategy. A double dose of levonorgestrel (3 mg as a single dose within 120 hours of unprotected sexual intercourse) may be used pragmatically.

KEY POINTS

- Epilepsy is not a curse but a treatable disease.
- A patient of epilepsy also has a right to marry.
- Pregnancy is not contraindicated in case of epileptic women.
- Preconception counseling of patient about the risks of teratogenesis and possible adverse effects of uncontrolled seizures to maternal health and pregnancy is recommended.
- Preconception review of AEDs aims for minimal effective monotherapy of active epilepsy; consider drug withdrawal if seizure-free.
- AEDs control epilepsy effectively during pregnancy; carbamazepine is the drug of choice and monotherapy is the best.
- Continuous research has been producing safer and better drugs to control epilepsy without adversely affecting fetal development.
- Folic acid supplementation is beneficial for the pregnant woman and the fetus; it should be started preconceptionally.

- Counseling during various stages from preconception to pregnancy and puerperium is mandatory.
- Screen malformation.
- Maternal and fetal monitoring and AED concentrations through pregnancy.
- Risk for fetal and maternal complications can be reduced considerably with effective preconceptional planning and careful management during pregnancy and postpartum period.
- Vitamin K administration in the newborn is recommended.
- Reassure the patient and the family that >90% pregnancies proceed with no problem in WWE.

REFERENCES

1. Helbig KL, Bernhardt BA, Conway LJ, Valverde KD, Helbig I, Sperling MR. Genetic risk perception and reproductive decision making among people with epilepsy. Epilepsia. 2010;51:1874-7.
2. Shostak S, Ottman R. Ethical, legal, and social dimensions of epilepsy genetics. Epilepsia. 2006;47:1595-602.
3. Battino D, Tomson T, Bonizzoni E, Craig J, Lindhout D, Sabers A, et al. Seizure control and treatment changes in pregnancy: observations from the EURAP epilepsy pregnancy registry. Epilepsia. 2013;54:1621-7.
4. Vajda FJ, Hitchcock A, Graham J, O'Brien T, Lander C, Eadie M. Seizure control in antiepileptic drug-treated pregnancy. Epilepsia. 2008;49:172-6.
5. Gjerde IO, Strandjord RE, Ulstein M. The course of epilepsy during pregnancy: a study of 78 cases. Acta Neurol Scand. 1988;78:198-205.
6. Tomson T, Lindbom U, Ekqvist B, Sundqvist A. Epilepsy and pregnancy: a prospective study of seizure control in relation to free and total plasma concentrations of carbamazepine and phenytoin. Epilepsia. 1994;35:122-30.
7. Tomson T, Palm R, Källén K, Ben-Menachem E, Söderfeldt B, Danielsson B, et al. Pharmacokinetics of levetiracetam during pregnancy, delivery, in the neonatal period, and lactation. Epilepsia. 2007;48(6):1111-6.
8. Kaplan PW, Norwitz ER, Ben-Menachem E, Pennell PB, Druzin M, Robinson JN, et al. Obstetrics risk for women with epilepsy during pregnancy. Epilepsy Behav. 2007;11:283-91.
9. Swartjes JM, Van Gejin HP. Pregnancy and epilepsy. Eur J Obstet Gynecol Reprod Biol. 1998;79:3-11.
10. Yerby MS, Kaplan P, Tran T. Risk and management of pregnancy in women with epilepsy. Cleve Clin J Med. 2004;71(2):S25-37.
11. Fairgrieve SD, Jackson M, Jonas P, Walshaw D, White K, Montgomery TL, et al. Population based, prospective study of the care of women with epilepsy in pregnancy. BMJ. 2000;321:674-5.
12. Tomson T, Battino D, Bonizzoni E, Craig J, Lindhout D, Sabers A, et al. Dose-dependent risk of malformations with antiepileptic drugs: an analysis of data from the EURAP epilepsy and pregnancy registry. Lancet Neurol. 2011;10:609-17.
13. Mawhinney E, Craig J, Morrow J, Russell A, Smithson WH, Parsons L, et al. Levetiracetam in pregnancy: results from the UK and Ireland epilepsy and pregnancy registers. Neurology. 2013;80:400-5.
14. Hernández-Díaz S, Werler MM, Walker AM, Mitchell AA. Folic acid antagonists during pregnancy and the risk of birth defects. N Engl J Med. 2000;343:1608-14.
15. Meador K, Reynolds MW, Crean S, Fahrbach K, Probst C. Pregnancy outcomes in women with epilepsy: a systematic review and meta-analysis of published pregnancy registries and cohorts. Epilepsy Res. 2008;81:1-13.
16. Campbell E, Kennedy F, Russell A, Smithson WH, Parsons L, Morrison PJ, et al. Malformation risks of antiepileptic drug monotherapies in pregnancy: updated results from the UK and Ireland Epilepsy and Pregnancy Registers. J Neurol Neurosurg Psychiatry. 2014;85:1029-34.
17. Bromley R, Weston J, Adab N, Greenhalgh J, Sanniti A, McKay AJ, et al. Treatment for epilepsy in pregnancy: neurodevelopmental outcomes in the child. Cochrane Database Syst Rev. 2014;10: CD010236.
18. Meador KJ, Baker GA, Browning N, Cohen MJ, Bromley RL, Clayton-Smith J, et al. Fetal antiepileptic drug exposure and cognitive outcomes at age 6 years (NEAD study): a prospective observational study. Lancet Neurol. 2013;12:244-52.
19. Bromley RL, Mawer GE, Briggs M, Cheyne C, Clayton-Smith J, García-Fiñana M, et al. The prevalence of neuro-developmental disorders in children prenatally exposed to antiepileptic drugs. J Neurol Neurosurg Psychiatry. 2013;84:637-43.
20. Christensen J, Grønborg TK, Sørensen MJ, Schendel D, Parner ET, Pedersen LH, et al. Prenatal valproate exposure and risk of autism spectrum disorders and childhood autism. JAMA. 2013;309:1696-703.
21. Nadel AS, Green JK, Holmes LB, Frigoletto FD Jr, Benacerraf BR. Absence of need for amniocentesis in patients with elevated levels of maternal serum alpha-fetoprotein and normal ultrasonographic examinations. N Engl J Med. 1990;323:557-61.
22. Bardy A. Epilepsy and pregnancy: a prospective study of 154 pregnancies in epileptic women [thesis]. Helsinki, Finland, University of Helsinki; 1982.
23. Schmidt D, Canger R, Avanzini G, Battino D, Cusi C, Beck-Mannagetta G, et al. Change of seizure frequency in pregnant epileptic women. J Neurol Neurosurg Psychiatry. 1983;46:751-5.
24. EURAP Study Group. Seizure control and treatment in pregnancy: observations from the EURAP epilepsy pregnancy registry. Neurology. 2006;66:354-60.
25. DeLorenzo RJ, Garnett LK, Towne AR, Waterhouse EJ, Boggs JG, Morton L, et al. Comparison of status epilepticus with prolonged seizure episodes lasting from 10 to 29 minutes. Epilepsia. 1999;40:164-9.
26. Alldredge BK, Gelb AM, Isaacs SM, Corry MD, Allen F, Ulrich S, et al. A comparison of lorazepam, diazepam, and placebo for the treatment of out-of-hospital status epilepticus. N Engl J Med. 2001;345:631-7.
27. McElhatton PR. The effects of benzodiazepine use during pregnancy and lactation. Reprod Toxicol. 1994;8:461-75.
28. Davanzo R, Dal Bo S, Bua J, Copertino M, Zanelli E, Matarazzo L. Antiepileptic drugs and breastfeeding. Ital J Pediatr. 2013;39:50.
29. Faculty of Sexual and Reproductive Healthcare. Faculty of Sexual & Reproductive Healthcare Clinical Guidance: Combined Hormonal Contraception. London: FSRH; 2011 (updated 2012).
30. Faculty of Sexual and Reproductive Healthcare. Faculty of Sexual & Reproductive Healthcare Clinical Guidance: Drug Interactions with Hormonal Contraception. London: FSRH; 2011 (updated 2012).

CHAPTER 11

Acquired Coagulation Disorders in Pregnancy

Pankaj Desai, N Palaniappan

■ INTRODUCTION

Rudolf Virchow in 1856 postulated the prerequisite triad that invites venous thrombosis as[1]

1. Stasis
2. Local trauma to the vessel wall
3. Hypercoagulability

This triad is shown in **Figure 1**.

Any mild risk factor which triggers one of these three along with pregnancy (which in itself is a risk factor) can lead to venous thrombosis or a coagulation disorder. This chapter, in particular, will deal with only acquired coagulation disorders such as:

- Disseminated intravascular coagulation (DIC)
- Thrombocytopenia
- Inherited coagulopathies
- *Miscellaneous:* Liver disorder, warfarin therapy, acquired hemophilia

■ DISSEMINATED INTRAVASCULAR COAGULATION

Disseminated intravascular coagulation is the rapid activation of intravascular coagulation leading to the deposition of fibrin within the circulatory system. Consumption of coagulation factors would lead to bleeding diathesis, although a minor percentage of individuals may go on to develop widespread thrombosis with peripheral organ ischemia. Usually, the greater risk of coagulopathy comes from the consumption of clotting factors and platelets secondary to massive hemorrhage. DIC may arise from various situations in obstetrics but is usually a secondary phenomenon to a "trigger" of coagulation activity. It would be a prudent move to identify these trigger factors, anticipate DIC, and act wisely in the beginning. A failure to anticipate DIC is cited as a major deficiency in the care of women who die from obstetric hemorrhage.

Trigger Mechanisms

- Vascular endothelial injury
  - Pre-eclampsia
  - Hypovolemic shock
  - Septicemic shock
- Release of thromboplastins
  - Abruptio placenta
  - Amniotic fluid embolism (AFE)
  - Retained dead fetus
  - Hydatidiform mole
  - Chorioamnionitis
  - Placenta accreta
  - Acute fatty liver
  - Hypertonic saline to induce abortion
- Production of procoagulant
  - Fetomaternal hemorrhage
  - Incompatible blood transfusion
  - Phospholipids
  - Intravascular hemolysis
- More than one trigger

Once DIC sets in, there is a potential for a vicious cycle, with further consumption of clotting factors and platelets and bleeding justifying the terminology of "consumption coagulopathy" as shown in **Flowchart 1**.

Risk Factors

Placental Abruption

Placental abruption remains the most common cause of coagulation failure in obstetrics and is related directly to the degree of placental separation and hypovolemic shock. In severe placental abruption with a dead fetus, profound

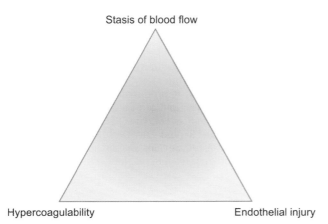

Fig. 1: Virchow's triad

Stasis of blood flow

Hypercoagulability

Endothelial injury

Flowchart 1: Mechanism of consumptive coagulopathy.

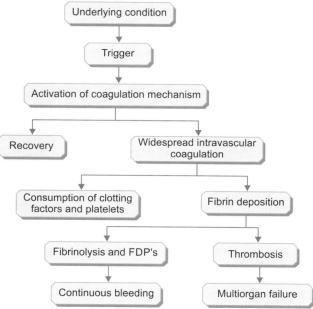

(FDPs: fibrin degradation products)

hypofibrinogenemia has been reported in about one-third of cases but is much less common if the fetus is alive.[2,3] This initial mechanism is due to the release of thromboplastins, but in severe abruption hypovolemic shock, large volume transfusion and high levels of fibrin degradation products (FDPs) that act as anticoagulants themselves will accentuate the situation.

Accidental hemorrhage is now accepted as an obstetric vasculopathy. As a result, the pathophysiology involved in the process of accidental hemorrhage has to be at the fetomaternal interface. The anchoring cytotrophoblasts are responsible to affix the placenta within the uterus. The entire process occurs following implantation at that point in the uterus where the implantation window opens at the time of arrival of the zygote in the uterine cavity. Following a complex process where intricate immunology and apoptosis get involved, the placenta affixes itself and remains so until that time as the delivery of the newborn occurs. Following some strange and hitherto unknown signals, once the baby is born, the placenta senses that its role is over and it readily separates from the uterus and is expelled from the uterine cavity. In accidental hemorrhage, however, this process of separation and expulsion of the placenta occurs much earlier even before the baby is born. Like any premature process in nature, this can lead to devastating complications.[4]

Amniotic Fluid Embolism

Amniotic fluid embolism may lead to maternal death as a result of severe pulmonary hypertension following embolization of the pulmonary vessels by fetal squams. But if the mother survives this acute event, there may be an anaphylactoid reaction to the presence of the fetal tissues in the maternal circulation, pulmonary edema, and the development of an intractable bleeding diathesis due to severe DIC. In most cases, maternal death is unpredictable and unavoidable. The coagulopathy that is part of the AFE syndrome ranges from minor disturbances in laboratory coagulation studies to severe DIC.[5] Any or all of the following hematologic laboratory abnormalities may be present: Elevated fibrin split products of D-dimer products, decreased fibrinogen, thrombocytopenia, and prolonged partial thromboplastin and prothrombin times. The exact incidence of coagulopathy with AFE is unknown, but it is common among those who survive the initial event. On rare occasions, it is the only manifestation present. The incidence of coagulopathy in the analysis of the national registry was 83%.[6]

Retained Dead Fetus

The release of thromboplastic substances from the dead fetus into the maternal circulation is thought to be the trigger for DIC. Approximately 80% of patients with a retained dead fetus will go into spontaneous labor within 3 weeks, but 30% of patients who remain undelivered for more than 4 weeks will develop DIC, usually of a mild degree.[7]

Pre-eclampsia

Pre-eclampsia is associated with endothelial perturbation currently thought to be due to oxidative stress and the release of reactive oxygen species by the ischemic placenta.

Sepsis

Endotoxic shock can be associated with chorioamnionitis, septic abortion, or postpartum sepsis. The bacterial endotoxin produces severe endothelial damage leading to fibrin deposition and DIC.

Management Options

Goals of Management

The aims of the management of DIC are:

- To manage the underlying disorders in order to remove the initiating stimulus
- To maintain the circulating blood volume
- To replace clotting factors and red blood cells

Relevant blood investigations are critical for deciding the management and prognosis of a subject with DIC. These have been given in **Box 1**.

Fluid Replacement in Coagulation Failure

The impending necessity in the initial stages is to maintain circulatory volume and tissue perfusion, and resuscitation

TABLE 1: Blood and components for consumptive coagulopathy.

Fresh whole blood (500 mL)	All components	Difficult to obtain
Packed erythrocytes (250 mL)	Red cells	Increase hematocrit by 3–5% per unit
Fresh frozen plasma (200–250 mL)	All clotting factors	Increase fibrinogen by 100 mg/dL per unit
Platelets (50 mL)	Platelets	Increase platelets 7,500/mm³
Cryoprecipitate (24–40 mL)	I, V, VIII, XIII	Increase fibrinogen 10 mg/dL per unit

with a crystalloid and a colloid solution should be undertaken as early as possible. Dextran solutions should not be used because they interfere with platelet function and can aggravate bleeding and DIC as well as invalidate the laboratory investigations.[8,9]

Replacement of Blood Products

Fresh frozen plasma (FFP) and stored red blood cells provide all the needed components. The use of fresh whole blood should not be encouraged, as it cannot be screened for possible infections. It is occasionally necessary to give extra fibrinogen in the form of cryoprecipitate, although sufficient amounts are usually there in FFP, which also contains factors V, VIII, and antithrombin III. Platelets are not found in FFP, and their functional activity rapidly deteriorates in stored blood. The platelet count reflects both the degree of DIC and the response to transfused blood. If there is persistent bleeding and the platelet count is <50,000/mm³, then the patient may be given concentrated platelets, but these are not usually necessary to gain hemostasis. This is given in **Table 1**.

Other Treatment Options

Heparin

Heparin therapy has been used often, but there is no evidence to suggest that its use confers any benefits over supportive therapy. Heparin is contraindicated if there is hypovolemia and obviously this would include that secondary to abruptio placenta.[10] Also, in a comprehensive review paper, treatment with heparin is recommended in those with the nonsymptomatic type of DIC.[11]

Activated Protein C

In the case of sepsis, recombinant protein C confers advantages in terms of prevailing fibrin deposition and stimulating the immune responses.[10] It has to be started within 24 hours of the onset of first organ dysfunction and is not routinely indicated in DIC in the absence of sepsis. Its use has been restricted due to its exorbitant cost. Activated protein C inhibits the generation of thrombin by inactivating factors Va and VIII.[12,13] Treatment with this agent decreased inflammation, as indicated by a decrease in interleukin-6 levels, a finding consistent with the known anti-inflammatory activity of activated protein C. Furthermore, this agent has direct anti-inflammatory properties, including the inhibition of neutrophil activation, production of cytokines by lipopolysaccharide-challenged monocytes, and E selectin-mediated adhesion of cells to vascular endothelium. Activated protein C is given as an intravenous infusion at a dose of 24 µg per kg body weight per hour for 96 hours.

Recombinant Factor VIIa

Recombinant activated factor VII (rFVIIa) is a recombinant form of the naturally occurring protease. Since 1998, rFVIIa has been approved and used extensively for the control of bleeding or surgical prophylaxis in patients with hemophilia who have inhibitors to coagulation factors.[14] rFVIIa has been approved for use only in Glanzmann thrombasthenia and factor VII deficiency. Other than in these indications, any other use is considered as "off-label" use. Owing to the cost of this novel drug, its use needs to be well justified before prescription. The existing literature does not support its routine use. It is to be given to patients with postpartum hemorrhage only as a last resort after routine medical and surgical therapies have been done just before a hysterectomy. It is given as 90 µg/kg as a single bolus over 3–5 minutes. Check after 20 minutes for temperature, acidaemia, serum calcium, platelet, and fibrinogen. If there is no improvement, administer a second dose of 90 µg/kg.[15]

■ THROMBOCYTOPENIA

Thrombocytopenia complicates up to 10% of all pregnancies and may result from a number of causes **(Table 2)**. Some of these are unique to pregnancy, while others may occur with increased frequency during gestation and still others bear no relationship to pregnancy per se. While some thrombocytopenic disorders are not associated with adverse pregnancy outcomes, others are associated with significant maternal and/or neonatal morbidity and mortality.[16]

Antiphospholipid Antibody Syndrome

S Habeebullah

INTRODUCTION

The antiphospholipid antibody syndrome (APLAS), also known as antiphospholipid syndrome (APS), "sticky blood" or Hughes syndrome, first described in the 1980s, is a complex autoimmune disorder in which autoantibodies are produced against phospholipids and phospholipid-binding proteins.

Normally, the immune system helps in attacking antigens such as viruses and bacteria by producing antibodies. But in some, the immune system wrongly produces antibodies against its own substances called autoantigens. In APS, the body produces antiphospholipid antibodies (aPLs) which may affect some parts of normal cells. More than 20 aPLs have been identified. Some of them may be involved in the pathogenesis of the disease. But the three major aPLs that are of significance during pregnancy are lupus anticoagulant (LA), anticardiolipin antibodies (aCLsz), and antibodies to β2-glycoprotein-I (β2-GP-I). LA is a misnomer. In vitro these antibodies prolong the coagulation tests such as activated partial thromboplastin time (aPTT), but in vivo they are actually prothrombotic by interacting with platelet membrane phospholipids, increasing adhesion and aggregation of platelets. They also may not be associated with systemic lupus erythematosus (SLE). β2-GP-I, which is involved in the coagulation pathway, seems to be the target for most aPLs.

In the presence of persistent aPLs, it manifests as recurrent arterial or venous thrombosis involving multiple organs and recurrent pregnancy loss. The association of aPLs with hypercoagulation was recognized more than half a century ago, but its association with the adverse pregnancy outcome is a relatively recent one.

PREVALENCE

The true prevalence of aPLs positivity is unknown as there are no population-based studies. aPLs are seen in 3–6% of healthy nonpregnant women and in 2% of obstetric population in general but 15% in women with recurrent miscarriage. In women with "early onset" preeclampsia and in SLE persistent antibodies may be found in 30%. It may be noted that a positive test for aPLs may not be clinically significant as transient positivity is known to occur in infections and due to problems with sample collection and processing.

CLASSIFICATION OF ANTIPHOSPHOLIPID SYNDROME

- *Primary APS:* It occurs in the absence of other related disorders. It rarely progresses to SLE.
- *Secondary APS:* It is secondary to other immune derangements such as SLE, infections, malignancies, and drugs. The clinical presentation is similar to that of primary, but the risk of thrombosis in SLE is much higher.
- *Familial APS:* The exact mode of inheritance is not well understood.
- *Catastrophic APS (CAPS):* It is a rare condition characterized by vascular thrombosis at multiple small vascular beds in the body. It can occur in persons with primary or secondary APS.

Diagnosis is suspected when three organ systems are affected in less than a week. Kidney, lung, liver, gastrointestinal (GI), and other organ involvement is seen resulting in multiorgan failure and high mortality. Histologically, evidence of thrombosis without inflammation of the vessel wall will be present. Infection, trauma, and surgery may trigger this condition. It is a medical emergency, and half of the patients do not survive the first episode.

PATHOGENESIS

The exact pathogenesis is not known. Genetic factors such as mutations of coagulation factors have been implicated. The aPLs are prothrombotic. Activation of complements, platelets, and endothelial cells by the anticardiolipin-β2GP-1 complex seems to play a major role in pathogenesis. A number of mechanisms are proposed which include:

- Endothelial cell and monocyte activation
- Inhibition of endothelial prostacyclin production
- Procoagulant effect on platelets (platelet aggregation)
- Inhibition of fibrinolysis
- Interference with activity of protein S

- Activation of complement pathways and inflammatory response
- Direct effect on placental trophoblast affecting invasion of trophoblast
- Thrombosis in utero-placental vessels.

On long-term follow-up, some cases of primary APS may progress to SLE.

PREGNANCY LOSS

Antiphospholipid syndrome is associated in the first trimester with pre-embryonic and embryonic loss, and in the second and third trimesters with preeclampsia, fetal growth restriction (IUGR), and intrauterine fetal death.

Complement activation seems to be required for pregnancy failure as evidenced by increased complement deposition in placentas in women with aPLs. Fetal loss may be due to narrowing of spiral arterioles, intimal thickening, thrombosis of placental bed, infarction, and necrosis:

- aPLs can directly damage the trophoblast leading to defective trophoblastic invasion resulting in early abortion independent of the thrombotic process.
- aPLs may damage the trophoblast resulting in reduced placental hormone production.
- Inflammation also seems to play a role as per the recent data.

CLINICAL MANIFESTATIONS

Depending on the presentation, APS patients can be:
- Carriers (asymptomatic)
- Classical APS (with arterial or venous thromboses)
- Those with recurrent pregnancy loss (otherwise healthy)
- APS with nonthrombotic effects (mild-to-moderate thrombocytopenia, hemolytic anemia, livedo reticularis)
- Catastrophic APS (<1% of all APS).

The manifestations include peripheral thrombosis, neurological, pulmonary, cardiac, GI, and cutaneous manifestations. A 5-year follow-up of 1,000 APS patients (Euro-Phospholipid project) showed thrombocytopenia (3.7%), livedo reticularis (2.6%), stroke (2.4%), transient ischemic attacks (2.3%), deep vein thrombosis (DVT; 2.1%), pulmonary embolism (2.1%), epilepsy (1.7%), cardiac valve vegetations (1.4%), and myocardial infarction (1%). Other reported conditions are valvular heart disease, hemolytic anemia, nephropathy, and cognitive dysfunction.

DIAGNOSIS

International consensus criteria adopted in 2006 are shown below. At least one of the two clinical criteria (vascular thrombosis or pregnancy morbidity) and at least one laboratory criterion [positive LA or medium-to-high titer of β2-GP-I-dependent immunoglobulin G (IgG) or IgM or aCLs] should be present on two occasions >12 weeks apart. This is because transient positive results for aPLs may be seen in various viral infections, etc.

A revised classification of the criteria for APS (revised Sapporo criteria, also called the Sydney criteria)[1] is given in the following text.

Clinical Criteria

- *Vascular thrombosis:* One or more episodes of an arterial, venous, or small vessel thrombosis confirmed by imaging or Doppler studies or histopathology, without significant vasculitis.
- *Obstetric morbidity:* (1) One or more unexplained deaths of a morphologically normal fetus at or beyond 10 weeks of gestation, or (2) one or more premature births of a morphologically normal neonate at or before 34 weeks of gestation, caused by severe preeclampsia/eclampsia or severe placental insufficiency, or (3) three or more unexplained, consecutive miscarriages of <10 weeks of gestation. Other known factors associated with recurrent miscarriage (chromosomal, anatomic, and hormonal) should be excluded.

Laboratory Criteria

- aCL IgG and/or IgM in blood, measured by a standardized ELISA (enzyme-linked immunosorbent assay) in medium or high titers (>40 GPL or MPL or> 99th percentile) on two or more occasions at least 12 weeks apart.
- Anti-β2-GP-I antibody of IgG and/or IgM isotype in blood (>99th percentile) measured by a standardized ELISA on two or more occasions at least 12 weeks apart.
- LA present in plasma, on two or more occasions at least 12 weeks apart, detected according to the guidelines of the International Society on Thrombosis and Hemostasis.

The usual test for syphilis, Venereal Disease Research Laboratory (VDRL), may give false-positive result in the presence of aPLs.

POOR PROGNOSTIC FACTORS

The prognosis of a pregnancy outcome depends on the presence of LA and other aPLs. In one retrospective multicentric study of primary APS treated with low-dose aspirin and low-molecular-weight heparin (LMWH) starting from the first trimester, it was seen that when only LA was positive the live birth rate was 80%. With aCL positivity it was 56% and with anti-β2-GP-I it was 48% and was associated with all pregnancy complications. When aCL and anti-β2-GP-I were positive but LA was negative, the live birth rate was 43%. When all the three aPLs were positive, it was 30% and was associated with placental insufficiency.[2]

Neonatal Antiphospholipid Syndrome

Antiphospholipid antibodies from the mother may reach the fetus through the placenta and may remain in the infant till the age of 6–12 months. Neonatal APS in babies born to APS mothers is extremely rare and is diagnosed by the presence of one clinical feature (venous or arterial thrombosis or thrombocytopenia) along with the presence of at least one aPL.

Antiphospholipid Syndrome and Fertility

There are conflicting reports regarding the role of aPLs in IVF (in vitro fertilization) failure; some studies[3,4] reported "no effect on IVF success" whereas others considered it as a factor associated with IVF failure.[5]

Prevention of Thrombosis

In nonpregnant women with aPL, low-dose aspirin for primary prevention of thrombosis is controversial as there is no evidence for that. For patients of APS with venous thrombosis, heparin (LMW or unfractionated) is started initially followed by warfarin on a long-term basis. For arterial thrombosis prevention, warfarin is usually advocated keeping international normalized ratio (INR) 2 or 3. If warfarin fails, low-dose aspirin can be added.

Obstetric Antiphospholipid Syndrome

For the prevention of pregnancy complications in APS, low-dose aspirin and a prophylactic dose of unfractionated or LMWH is given. The combination has been found to reduce the miscarriage rate by 54% compared to aspirin alone. Similarly, in the absence of APS this combination will not be effective in recurrent miscarriage. Prophylactic low-dose heparin is continued till 6 weeks' postpartum. In thrombotic APS in pregnancy, along with low-dose aspirin, a therapeutic dose of heparin should be given. In the absence of other risk factors for thrombosis, antithrombotic therapy is not continued in patients of obstetric APS.

Treatment[6,7]

- *Only lab criteria, no clinical criteria, no pregnancy morbidity, no thrombosis:* Low-dose aspirin or anticoagulants not recommended unless they are at an increased risk of thrombosis.
- *History of (H/O) thrombosis, ± pregnancy morbidity:* Low-dose aspirin + LMWH followed by lifelong warfarin.
- *Lab criteria, early pregnancy losses but no thrombosis:* Low-dose aspirin + Prophylactic LMWH—both continued for 6 weeks after delivery.
- *Lab criteria, preterm delivery/preeclampsia/placental insufficiency but no thrombosis:* Low-dose aspirin (if it fails LMWH). Following vaginal delivery, aspirin alone/ after cesarean section, add LMWH for 6 weeks.
- *Pregnancy, aPL +ve, with H/O thrombosis:* Therapeutic LMWH + aspirin. Post delivery, warfarin continued for indefinite period.

Low-dose aspirin: Thromboxane is known to cause platelet aggregation and vasoconstriction. Aspirin blocks the conversion of arachidonic acid to thromboxane A2 without affecting the prostacyclin production from endothelial cells. This has been advocated as soon as the pregnancy is confirmed in doses of 60–80 mg daily orally. However, there are reports of a dosage of 100–150 mg daily which is likely more effective.[8] The side effects of aspirin are minimal in the form of small vessel bleeding at the time of surgery. Aspirin is not effective when aPLs are positive without the complete syndrome.

Heparin: The rationale for prophylactic heparin therapy is to prevent arterial and venous thrombosis and thrombosis in microcirculation and at the decidual–trophoblastic interface. It also prevents cellular damage by preventing the binding of aCL and anti-β2-GP-I antibodies to their surfaces. Heparin is started in the first trimester as soon as the pregnancy is confirmed by USG. Since heparin does not cross the placenta, there is no risk of fetal anomalies or fetal hemorrhage. Heparin can cause complications such as maternal hemorrhage, hypersensitivity reaction, and rarely heparin-induced thrombocytopenia, osteopenia and vertebral fractures. There is no difference in the safety and efficacy of unfractionated heparin and LMWH. LMWH is less likely to cause thrombocytopenia and osteoporosis. Besides, it can be administered once daily.

Prophylactic heparin: The LMWH enoxaparin 40 mg (SC) OD or dalteparin 5,000 U (SC) OD is used. Alternatively, unfractionated heparin 5,000–7,500 U twice daily (SC) in the first trimester; 7,500–10,000 U twice daily (SC) in the second trimester; and 10,000 U twice daily (SC) in the third trimester can be given.

Therapeutic dose of heparin: LMWH, enoxaparin 1 mg/kg 12 hourly SC or dalteparin 200 U/kg (SC) OD, is administered. Alternatively, unfractionated heparin 10,000 U 12 hourly SC is given to maintain aPTT about twice the normal range at 6 hours after injection.

Glucocorticoids are not useful in primary APS and may add to the complications but in APS secondary to lupus they are indicated. However, the dosage should be at the lowest effective level to prevent flares.

Immunoglobulin therapy is controversial and reserved for those who fail to respond to first-line therapies and in those who develop heparin-induced thrombocytopenia. Intravenous immunoglobulin (IVIG) is administered at a dose of 0.4 g/kg daily for 5 days. This is repeated monthly. It is expensive and of unproven value.

Other therapies which have the potential in refractory obstetric APS are hydroxychloroquine, statins, biological therapies [anti-tumor necrosis factor α (TNFα) agents], and plasma exchange.

■ PREGNANCY AND LABOR MANAGEMENT OF ANTIPHOSPHOLIPID SYNDROME

A combination of low-dose aspirin and heparin significantly improves the live birth rate, but these pregnancies are at a high risk for early pregnancy failure, early onset preeclampsia, placental insufficiency, and preterm birth. Accordingly, antenatal care should be carefully planned. Besides early pregnancy dating and anomaly scans, growth scans in the late second and third trimesters every 4 weeks, detection of early preeclampsia, and tests for fetal well-being [nonstress test (NST), fetal biophysical profile] weekly or twice weekly, especially in the presence of fetal growth restriction, are carried out. Doppler studies are carried out as indicated in IUGR.

Delivery should be carefully planned at 38–39 weeks depending on the clinical situation. Those receiving LMWH should be changed over to unfractionated heparin to reduce the risk of bleeding during delivery and to facilitate administration of epidural anesthesia. Heparin is stopped 24 hours before induction of labor. If there is no history of thrombosis, aspirin can be stopped by 36 weeks. Even if aspirin is continued, the risk of bleeding is very small.

During the postpartum period in those with a past history of thrombosis, heparin or warfarin can be continued as they are not contraindicated in breast-feeding women. Contraception has to be carefully chosen as estrogen-containing pills add to the risk of thrombosis.

Catastrophic Antiphospholipid Syndrome

This life-threatening emergency condition needs aggressive supportive therapy in the form of anticoagulant therapy (heparin), antihypertensives, corticosteroids, IVIG, and plasmapheresis with or without rituximab though there is no good-quality evidence for their use.[9]

KEY POINTS

- Antiphospholipid syndrome is an autoimmune thrombophilic condition that is marked by the presence in blood of antibodies that recognize and attack phospholipid-binding proteins, rather than phospholipid itself.
- The clinical manifestations of APS include vascular thrombosis and pregnancy complications, especially recurrent spontaneous miscarriages and, less frequently, maternal thrombosis.
- Presence of antiphospholipid antibody (aPL) alone, in the absence of typical clinical complications, does not indicate a diagnosis of APS; long-term asymptomatic

aPL-positive patients exist. When diagnosed in patients with underlying autoimmune disease (usually systemic lupus erythematosus, or SLE), APS is termed secondary APS; in otherwise healthy persons it is termed primary APS.

- The three known APLA are:
  1. Anticardiolipin antibodies IgG or IgM (ELISA)
  2. Anti-beta-2-glycoprotein-I antibodies IgG or IgM (ELISA)
  3. Lupus anticoagulants (Functional assays)
- Laboratory criteria for diagnosis include :
  - aCL IgG and/or IgM in blood, measured by a standardized ELISA in medium or high titers (>40 GPL or MPL or> 99th percentile) on two or more occasions at least 12 weeks apart.
  - Anti-β2-GP-I antibody of IgG and/or IgM isotype in blood (>99th percentile) measured by a standardized ELISA on two or more occasions at least 12 weeks apart.
  - LA present in plasma, on two or more occasions at least 12 weeks apart.
- VDRL may give false-positive result in the presence of aPLs.
- Treatment options include low dose heparin or aspirin

■ REFERENCES

1. Miyakis S, Lockshin MD, Atsumi T, Branch DW, Brey RL, Cervera R, et al. International consensus statement on an update of the classification criteria for definite antiphospholipid syndrome (APS). J Thromb Haemost. 2006;4:295-306.
2. Saccone G, Berghella V, Maruotti GM, Ghi T, Rizzo G, Simonazzi G, et al. Antiphospholipid antibody profile based obstetric outcomes of primary antiphospholipid syndrome: the PREGNANTS study. Am J Obstet Gynecol. 2017;216:5:525-e1-525.e12.
3. Hornstein MD, Davis OK, Massey JB, Paulson RJ, Collins JA. Antiphospholipid antibodies and in vitro fertilization success: a meta analysis. Fertil Steril. 2000;73:330-3.
4. Lacroix O, despierres L, Courbiere B, Barden N. Antiphospholipid antibodies in women undergoing in vitro fertilization treatment: clinical value of IgA anti-β2glycoprotein I antibodies determination. J Biomed Biotechnol. 2014:314704.
5. Kaider B, Price DE, Roussev R, Coulam CB. Antiphospholipid antibody prevalence in patients with IVF failure. Am J Reprod Immunol. 1996;35(4):388-93.
6. American College of Obstetricians and Gynecologists' Committee on Practice Bulletins–Obstetrics. ACOG Practice Bulletin No. 197: Inherited thrombophilias in pregnancy. Obstet Gynecol. 2018;132(1):e18-e34.
7. Danowskia A, Regob J, Kakehasic AM, Funke A, de Carvalho JF, Lima IVS, et al. Guidelines for the treatment of antiphospholipid syndrome. Rev Bras Reumatol. 2013;53(2):184-92.
8. Roberge S, Nicolaides K, Demers S, Hyett J, Chaillet N, Bujold E. The role of aspirin dose on the prevention of preeclampsia and fetal growth restriction: systematic review and meta-analysis. Am J Obstet Gynecol. 2017;216:110.
9. Asherson RA, Cervera R, de Groot PG, Erkan D, Boffa MC, Piette JC, et al. Catastrophic antiphospholipid syndrome: international consensus statement on classification criteria and treatment guidelines. Lupus. 2003;12(7):530-4.

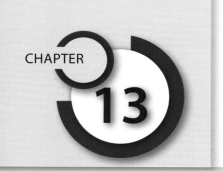

CHAPTER 13

Human Immunodeficiency Virus in Pregnancy

Ambarisha Bhandiwad, Achanta Vivekanand

■ INTRODUCTION

A large number of people have been affected globally with the acquired immunodeficiency syndrome (AIDS) epidemic, since its identification in the early 1980s. As per the statistics published by the Joint United Nations Programme on HIV/AIDS (UNAIDS), World Health Organization (WHO), and United Nations Children's Fund (UNICEF) in December 2012, 34 million people were living with human immunodeficiency virus (HIV)/AIDS in 2011. 50% of adults living with HIV/AIDS were women, and 3.3 million children were living with HIV/AIDS in 2011. The growing epidemic has come to a halt in recent years as the annual number of new HIV cases has steadily declined owing to a large number of cases receiving antiretroviral therapy (ART). Even the mortality related to AIDS has reduced.

South and South-east Asia had 4 million adults and children living with HIV/AIDS by the end of 2011, accounting to a prevalence of 0.3%. Sub-Saharan Africa had a prevalence of 4.9%.

The prevalence of HIV is 0.27% in adults (2011), and around 2.1 million (2011) people are living with HIV (PLHIV) in our own country. Of these PLHIV nationwide, women constitute 39% cases while children < 15 years of age constitute 7%.

■ ETIOLOGY AND PATHOGENESIS

HIV is a retrovirus whose structure is shown in **Figure 1**. It has a core and an envelope. The bullet-shaped capsid is made from protein 24 and contains the enzymes required for HIV replication—reverse transcriptase, integrase, and protease. The genetic material consists of two strands of ribonucleic acid (RNA) and is also contained in the capsid.

HIV can be transmitted by various routes—sexual intercourse, blood/blood-contaminated products, and mother-to-child transmission (MTCT).

On entering the body, HIV attaches to the CD4 cells of the body's immune system and releases its contents into the cell. This leads to the weakening of the person's immune system resulting in AIDS.

The incubation period varies from days to weeks depending upon the exposure to clinical presentation. The acute phase of illness is short and similar to any viral syndrome. Patients often present with fever and night sweats, fatigue, rash, headache, lymphadenopathy, pharyngitis, arthralgias, myalgias, nausea, vomiting, and diarrhea. After subsidence of symptoms, the phase of chronic viremia is set in. The median time for progression from asymptomatic viremia to AIDS is about 10 years. However, the stimuli that cause further progression to AIDS are presently unclear.

Generalized lymphadenopathy, oral hairy leukoplakia, aphthous ulcers, and thrombocytopenia are common clinical findings of an advanced disease. A number of co-existing opportunistic infections (OIs) include esophageal or pulmonary candidiasis, persistent herpes simplex or zoster lesions, condyloma accuminata, tuberculosis (TB), cytomegaloviral pneumonia, retinitis or gastrointestinal disease, molluscum contagiosum, pneumocystis pneumonia, toxoplasmosis, and others. Neurological features are commonly seen in about half of patients. A CD4 count of <200/mm^3 is also considered definitive for the diagnosis of AIDS.

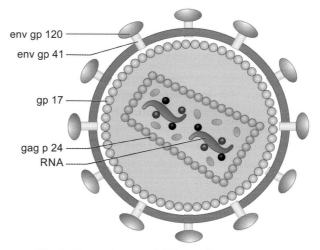

Fig. 1: Human immunodeficiency virus—structure.

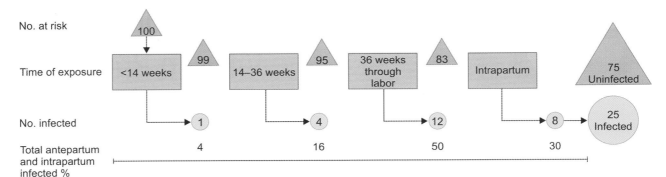

Fig. 2: Mother-to-child transmission of HIV.

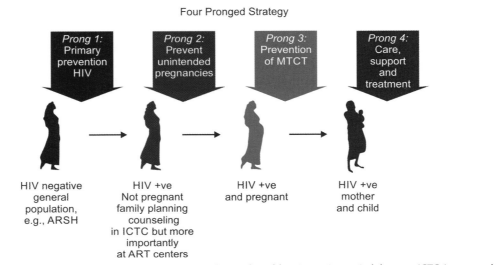

Fig. 3: Four-pronged strategy. (ARSH: Adolescent Reproductive and Sexual Health; ART: antiretroviral therapy; ICTC: Integrated Counselling and Testing Centers; MTCH: mother-to-child transmission)

■ HIV AND PREGNANCY

Pregnancy does not have significant effect on the clinical or immunological course of viral infection.

Mother-to-child transmission of HIV is the primary route of transmission for HIV among children. This transmission is known to occur during pregnancy, delivery, and breastfeeding period **(Fig. 2)**.

It is estimated that the risk of MTCT of HIV is significantly reduced with effective use of antiretroviral (ARV) drugs; however, the risk is 20–45% without drugs. Clinically advanced HIV disease in the mother, high plasma viral load, maternal injectable drug use during pregnancy, preterm delivery, failure to receive ART, and breastfeeding increase the likelihood of transmission during pregnancy.

Prevention of Mother-to-child Transmission

To address the burden of HIV among children, the Prevention of Parent to Child Transmission (PPTCT) of HIV services was launched in 2002 by the National AIDS Control Programme (NACP). As a result, HIV testing services are available to all pregnant women in an antenatal clinic (ANC). It also made accessible the ARV prophylaxis with a single dose of Nevirapine (SD-NVP) at the time of delivery to mother and baby. The ARV prophylaxis using SD-NVP is highly effective in reducing the risk of MTCT from about 45 to <10%. The pediatric HIV can be effectively reduced and eliminated if the currently available drugs are used effectively. The WHO has been recommending the use of multiple drugs for more efficacious ARV regimens, for reducing the transmission to <5% in PPTCT. For more effect, the ARV should be started early in pregnancy and continued throughout the period of delivery and breastfeeding.

According to the new WHO guidelines (June 2013), the Department of AIDS Control has been providing lifelong ART (triple-drug regimen) to all pregnant and breastfeeding women living with HIV, regardless of the CD4 count or the WHO clinical stage across the country from January 1, 2014. This provides early protection against MTCT for future pregnancies and avoids drug resistance.

The overall goals of the PPTCT program are represented by four prongs shown in **Figure 3**.

The vital package of PPTCT services includes the following:

- All pregnant women attending antenatal care are routinely offered HIV counseling and testing with "opt out" option.
- Adopting a family-centric approach involving the spouse and other family members
- Counseling on choices of continuation of pregnancy or Medical Termination of Pregnancy (MTP)—to undertake within the first 3 months of pregnancy only
- Do CD4 testing and WHO staging.
- Linkage to ART services and provide ART regardless of the clinical stage and CD4 count
- Provision of institutional deliveries for all HIV-infected pregnant women.
- Provision of care for OIs and other associated conditions [sexually transmitted infection (STI)/reproductive tract infection (RTI), TB]
- Provision of nutritional counseling and psychosocial support
- Provide counseling and support for breastfeeding
- Provision of ARV prophylaxis for newborn up to a minimum period of 6 weeks
- Integrated follow-up of HIV-exposed infants into routine healthcare visits with immunization
- Ensure initiation of cotrimoxazole prophylactic treatment and early infant diagnosis (EID) using HIV DNA polymerase chain reaction (PCR) at 6 weeks of age; repeat testing at 6 months, 12 months, and 6 weeks after cessation of breastfeeding.
- Safe sex counseling and HIV testing of spouse and other living children
- Confirmation of HIV status of all babies at 18 months using rapid antibody tests
- Strengthen the outreach through auxiliary nurse midwives (ANMs), accredited social health activists (ASHAs), and district-level workers to support and follow up the HIV-infected pregnant women and their families.

Diagnosis During Pregnancy

Universal counseling and voluntary testing for HIV infection are recommended for all pregnant women at the booking visit. Retesting in the third trimester is recommended for women known to be at high risk of acquiring HIV, e.g., those who have a history of sexually transmitted diseases, multiple sex partners during pregnancy, use of illicit drugs.

Three rapid antibody tests are done for confirmation of HIV along with pre-test and post-test counseling. The negative predictive value of a single rapid test is high and hence does not require further testing. However, the positive predictive value is low and hence a reactive rapid test must be confirmed by a supplemental test such as western blot or immunofluorescence assay (IFA). Confirmation of HIV is linked with rapid plasma reagin (RPR) test, done for confirmation of syphilis and screening for TB. Recently, it has been reported that maternal TB increases the risk of HIV transmission from mother to child by 2.5 times.

Management During Pregnancy

Management during pregnancy actively involves the clinical and paramedical team at the health facility constituted by the obstetricians, pediatricians, physicians, medical officers, nurses, ANMs, ASHAs, lab technicians, counselors, and outreach workers. District-level networks, self-help groups (SHGs), and community-based organizations should help support the HIV-infected mother and her family.

On detection of HIV during the antenatal visit, the pregnant woman is initiated on ART [Tenofovir (TDF) + Lamivudine (3TC) + Efavirenz (EFV)] regardless of the clinical stage or CD4 count, although it is important to know the CD4 counts and values of other baseline tests before starting ART. However, one must not delay starting the ART for want of CD4 count results.

If a woman is screen positive (by one test kit) during active labor, she should be initiated on ART but confirmation of the HIV status should be done at the earliest. She must be linked to the ART center, if confirmed positive.

HIV-infected pregnant women require all components of good antenatal care, which include iron–folate supplementation, anemia management, baseline CD4 count, screening of TB, prevention and management of OIs, STI treatment, counseling on nutrition, rest, warning signs, ART linkages-CD4 testing if HIV positive, and starting on ART. It also includes institutional delivery, exclusive breastfeeding within an hour of delivery, postpartum counseling regarding safe sex, HIV-specific advice, and contraception.

Clinical signs of underlying OIs including weight loss during pregnancy require detailed assessment, and the patient may be started with co-trimoxazole prophylactic therapy (CPT) if CD4 $\leq$ 250 cells/mm^3 and continued through delivery and breastfeeding. (Dose: Double-strength tablet—once daily.)

If there is no prior exposure to non-nucleoside reverse transcriptase inhibitors (NNRTIs) (NVP/EFV) at any gestational age, then a combination of TDF (300 mg) + 3TC (300 mg) + EFV (600 mg) is the first-line regimen of choice for HIV-infected pregnant women. In those with previous exposure to SD-NVP (or EFV) for PPTCT prophylaxis in prior pregnancies, an NNRTI-based ART regimen such as TDF + 3TC + EFV may not be fully effective due to persistence of

TABLE 1: Recommendations for HIV-exposed infants.

Infant's birth weight	NVP daily dose (in mg)	NVP daily dose (in mL) (10 mg Nevirapine in 1 mL suspension)	Duration
Birth weight < 2,000 g	2 mg/kg once daily. In consultation with a pediatrician trained in HIV care	0.2 mL/kg once daily	Up to 6 weeks irrespective of whether exclusively breastfed or exclusive replacement fed
Birth weight 2,000–2,500 g	10 mg once daily	1 mL once a day	
Birth weight > 2,500 g	15 mg once daily	1.5 mL once a day	

(NVP: nevirapine)

archived mutation to NNRTIs. Hence, a protease-inhibitor-based ART regimen, namely TDF + 3TC + LPV/r (Lopinavir/Ritonavir), is required in such women.

Routine assessments of hemoglobin or liver function tests (LFTs) and renal function tests (RFT) are performed as and when warranted by clinical signs and symptoms.

Management During Labor

Delivery should be by the vaginal route and cesarean section should be preferred for obstetric indications only.

In some countries such as the UK, cesarean section is recommended before the woman goes into labor if the woman is not taking combination therapy or if the virus can be detected in the blood (a detectable viral load).

The MTCT risk is increased by premature rupture of membranes (PROM), repeated per vaginal examinations, instrumental delivery (forceps/ventouse), invasive fetal monitoring procedures (scalp/fetal blood monitoring), episiotomy, and prematurity. Hence, it is prudent to avoid all these risk factors. Artificial rupture of membranes is avoided and done only in cases with fetal distress or delay in progress of labor. Suctioning of newborn with a nasogastric tube should be avoided unless there is meconium staining of liquor.

While doing cesarean section, early cord clamping is done and membranes should be left intact until the head is delivered through the surgical incision.

Strict universal precautions to prevent any skin and mucous-membrane contact with blood and other body fluids during vaginal delivery or cesarean section should be practiced. One must wear double gloves, surgical masks, protective eyewear or face shields, shoe covers, and plastic aprons (or gowns made of materials that provide an effective barrier). One must also ensure that all the health-care workers who assist in vaginal or cesarean deliveries wear proper gloves and gowns when handling the placenta or the newborn until blood and amniotic fluid have been removed from the newborn's skin. The universal precautions should also be followed during postdelivery care of the umbilical cord.

Postpartum Follow-up and Care

Assessment of maternal healing after delivery and counseling on effective postpartum contraceptive methods form a part of postpartum care. Condom should be consistently used by all HIV-infected males despite following any other family planning method.

Exclusive replacement feeding may be considered in situations where breastfeeding cannot be done (such as maternal death and severe maternal illness). It should be done only when the AFASS (Affordable, Feasible, Acceptable, Sustainable, Safe) criteria are fulfilled. Mixed feeding (both breastfeeding and replacement feeding) should not be done at any cost within the first 6 months.

Infant Care

Recommendations for HIV-Exposed Infants

These recommendations are given in **Table 1**.

Irrespective of whether the infant is on replacement feeding or breastfeeding, all the HIV-exposed infants must receive a minimum of 6 weeks of daily NVP. As per the national recommendations, DNA PCR (dried blood spot) is collected for EID, at 6 weeks (during the first immunization visit at ICTC).

Cotrimoxazole is provided for all HIV-exposed infants after 6 weeks. If in EID, the infant is HIV positive, it is referred to the ART center for whole blood testing and further management. ARV is started as per the national guidelines. Infants may be breastfed up to an year, but exclusive breastfeeding is to be done till 6 months. If the EID results are negative, parents/caregivers are advised that continued monitoring and follow-up of the infant are necessary. If the infant becomes sick, medical attention is to be sought immediately. Confirmation of HIV status is only at 18 months of age.

> (**KEY POINTS**)
> - Women will commence ART treatment as soon as possible after diagnosis, in the second trimester, or earlier if the viral load is >174,000 IU/mL (>100,000 HIV RNA copies /mL).

- Women may have stopped treatment following delivery previously whereas, they will now be advised to remain on HAART for life.
- Although breastfeeding is still not recommended there is advice included on how to support a low risk mother whose viral load is well controlled and who chooses to breastfeed against advice.
- The following women remain a higher risk group and should still be transferred to the regional unit for ongoing care (a) Co-infection with hepatitis B or C. (b) 12 weeks on HAART with no significant reduction in viral load. (c) Non-compliance with medication. (d) Late booking (>30 weeks) with very high viral load. (e) Other maternal/fetal indications that would warrant delivery in the regional unit, e.g., fetal anomaly. (f) Patient request for the purpose of confidentiality.
- Previous recommendations were that all babies would have been treated with postexposure prophylaxis (PEP) for 4 weeks postnatally whereas new advice is that babies born to very low risk mothers may stop PEP after 2 weeks. This will be dependent on the initial HIV PCR result being negative.
- Factors that increase the risk of HIV transmission via breast milk include:
  - Detectable HIV viral load:
  - Advanced maternal HIV disease
  - Longer duration of breastfeeding
  - Breast and nipple infection/inflammation or cracked nipples
  - Infant mouth or gut infection/inflammation
  - Mixed feeding, in particular solid food given to infants less than 2 months of age. HIV positive women should be advised against breastfeeding. However the woman's wishes should be respected and advice and support should be offered should she decide against recommendations to breastfeed.
- Women on HAART (<80IU/mL;<50HIV RNA copies) with no identified obstetric high risk factors should be allowed vaginal delivery like noninfected women. If PROM occurs in them, IOL/augmentation should be done.
- If the woman's viral load is ≥80 IU/mL (≥50 RNA copies) or unknown:
  - Viral load 80–690 IU/ml—consider planned CS at 38–39 weeks
  - Viral load >690 IU/mL or unknown VL or women on Zidovudine monotherapy—elective CS at 38–39 weeks is recommended or emergency CS if admitted in labour. IV Zidovudine should be continued until cord clamped.
  - In preterm labor/PPROM (with viral load >690IU/ml or unknown VL or women on Zidovudine monotherapy) prescribe and start the following ASAP: Nevirapine 200mg stat, Tenofovir 490mg stat, Raltegravir 400 mg BD (if not already started). IV Zidovudine throughout labor and delivery until cord clamped

■ SUGGESTED READING

1. American College of Obstetrics and Gynecologists. Reducing HIV/AIDS Infection in babies and improving the health of pregnant women with HIV/AIDS.
2. Cunningham FG, Leveno KJ, Bloom SL, Hauth JC, Gilstrap LC, Wenstrom KD. Williams Obstetrics, 22nd edition. New York: McGraw Hill; 2005.
3. Misra R (Ed). Ian Donald's Practical Obstetric Problems, 6th edition. New Delhi: BI Publications; 2007.
4. NACO Guidelines 24th December 2012.
5. National AIDS Control Organisation. (2012). NACO Operational Guidelines for ART Services. [online] Available from http://naco.gov.in/sites/default/files/Operational%20guidelines%20for%20ART%20services.pdf [Last accessed September, 2020].
6. National AIDS Control Organisation. (2013). Operational Guidelines for Lifelong ART for all Pregnant Women Living with HIV for Prevention of Parent-to-Child Transmission (PPTCT) of HIV in India. [online] Available from http://naco.gov.in/sites/default/files/National_Guidelines_for_PPTCT.pdf [Last accessed September, 2020]
7. Revised January 2014 PPTCT Regimen.

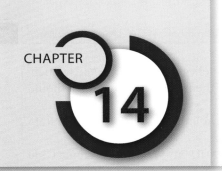

Liver Diseases in Pregnancy

Shikha Seth, Ritu Sharma

◼ INTRODUCTION

Liver is the next most important vital organ after heart, brain, and kidney as it receives 25–35% of cardiac output outside pregnancy. Liver does not increase in size during pregnancy but the workload in the form of metabolic, excretory, and synthetic functions definitely increases under the effect of pregnancy hormones estrogen and progesterone. Some of the fetal products reach maternal circulation through the transplacental route and are excreted through the maternal hepatic system. So, prior to understanding the liver diseases, it is really important to know the significant changes in liver function that occur during pregnancy.

◼ LIVER IN PREGNANCY

During pregnancy, no major changes occur in liver physiology. Classical signs of liver disease such as spider angioma and palmer erythema are often being noted during pregnancy. Anatomically, liver is pushed up by enlarging gravid uterus and becomes less appreciable at term on clinical examination. The biliary system has cholestatic as well as lithogenic tendency during pregnancy under the effect of steroid hormones.[1] Among the liver function tests (LFTs), two levels remarkably change; the first is the alkaline phosphatase (AP) which particularly gets raised in the second half (rises 3–4-fold) as it is released from the placenta and the second is serum albumin which gets lowered due to hemodilution while rest all show only mild deviations.[2]

Clotting factors, specially I, II, V, VII, VIII, X, and XII, increase along with ceruloplasmin and transferrin levels during pregnancy, while the albumin, total proteins, antithrombin III and protein S levels decrease, an adaptation to control the bleeding during delivery. In this chapter, we will be discussing the major liver disorders which are commonly encountered by obstetricians.

◼ VIRAL HEPATITIS

Viral hepatitis is the most common cause of jaundice in pregnancy. It affects not only the mother but also the fetus. The pathogens responsible for viral hepatitis are Hepatitis A, B, C, E viruses, Epstein–Barr virus (EBV), Herpes simplex virus (HSV), and human immunodeficiency virus (HIV). The highest maternal mortality is associated with Hepatitis E virus (HEV) while Hepatitis B virus (HBV) is associated with the maximum risk of vertical transmission and subsequently persistence as chronic infection. A woman presents with general vague symptoms, and diagnosis of hepatitis is made by derangements in LFTs such as bilirubin, liver enzymes, serum proteins, and coagulation profile, the most important being elevated alanine aminotransferase (ALT). Definitive diagnosis is made by serological testing.

Hepatitis A Virus

Hepatitis A virus (HAV), a single-stranded ribonucleic acid (RNA) virus, is transmitted via the feco-oral route and has an incidence of 1:1000 in pregnancy. T-cell-mediated immune response is responsible for the underlying pathogenesis, and thus this infection provides lifelong immunity.[3] Common complications include preterm labor (PTL), premature rupture of membranes (PROM), and abruption.[4,5] There are no fetal effects. *Universal screening for HAV is not recommended during pregnancy. Diagnosis is made by detecting serum anti-HAV immunoglobulin M (IgM) antibodies.* HAV infection can be prevented by improving the sanitary conditions and vaccinating the high-risk pregnant women.[5-7] Treatment is supportive, i.e. maintaining adequate nutrition and avoiding alcohol and hepatotoxic drugs. Breastfeeding is not contraindicated.

Hepatitis B Virus

Hepatitis B virus is a double-stranded DNA virus acquired by vertical transmission as well as horizontal transmission through sexual contact, intravenous drug usage, and blood transfusion. The patient may be asymptomatic or presents with general symptoms such as abdominal pain, nausea, vomiting, loss of appetite, tiredness, pain in muscles and joints, and jaundice. Chronic persistent infection mostly affects young children and can progress to cirrhosis, hepatocellular carcinoma, and early death in 25% of cases. Severe HBV liver disease can lead to intrauterine demise (IUD), stillbirth, diabetes, gestational hypertension, and abruption. Regular monitoring of liver function is required to detect maternal decompensation at the earliest.

TABLE 1: Interpretation of serology in HBV infection.[8]

Status	HBsAg	Anti-HBs (HBsAb)	Anti-HBc (HBcAb)	IgM anti-HBc
Nonimmunized Never infected, risk case *(must be vaccinated)*	–	–	–	–
Immune (acquired by vaccination)	–	+	–	–
Immune (acquired by natural infection) *Recovered case/Vaccination not required*	–	+	+	–
Acute infection	+	–	+	+
Chronic infection	+	–	+	–
Status unclear (resolving/ resolved/false +)	–	–	+	–

(HBsAg: surface antigen; anti-HBs: antibody against HBV surface antigen: anti-HBc = antibody against HBV core antigen: IgM anti-HBc: acute antibody M type against core antigen)
Note: HBeAg if positive is suggestive of a high infectivity stage.

Universal screening with "HBsAg" is recommended at the first antenatal visit regardless of previous vaccination (grade 1A).[5,8] Diagnosis is made by LFTs and serological tests measuring various antigens and antibodies **(Table 1)**. The average incubation period is 90 days but varies from 6 weeks to 6 months.

Alanine aminotransferase and HBV DNA levels are done initially and then at 28 weeks to assess for the need of antiviral therapy (grade 2B).[8] Once a pregnant woman is tested HBV positive, the World Health Organization (WHO) recommends testing for hepatitis D virus (HDV) as coinfection can result in increased mortality. Counseling and screening of close contacts are also recommended.[6]

Universal vaccination of all infants has played an important role in decreasing the global burden.[5] Maternal-to-child transmission (MTCT) rates have been drastically reduced to around 10% because of both active and passive immune-prophylaxis given to newborn within 12–24 hours of birth (grade 1A).[8] High viral load (HBV DNA > 10⁶ copies/mL or > 200,000 IU/mL) and high infectivity proven by envelop antigen (HBeAg) are responsible for this 10% ineffective immunoprophylaxis,[7] and therefore these two tests should be done in the third trimester of all HBsAg-positive cases. The antiviral therapy is recommended in these cases by the American Association for the Study of Liver Diseases. *Tenofovir (300 mg/d) is the first-line drug,* while Telbivudine (600 mg/d, moderate resistance) and Lamivudine (100 mg/d, high resistance) can be used by starting at 28–30 weeks till 3 months' postpartum (grade 2B).[8] To reduce MTCT, one should avoid invasive procedures such as amniocentesis and internal electronic

fetal monitoring during labor[3] **(Flowcharts 1A and B)**. Maternal Fetal Medicine and WHO state that the mode of delivery and breastfeeding do not affect the perinatal transmission.

Hepatitis B immune globulin (HBIG) is given 0.5 mL (0.06 mL/kg, IM) along with the first dose of 0.5-mL vaccine (10 µg) IM in the anterolateral aspect of the thigh ideally within 12 hours of birth at separate sites. The second and third doses of vaccine are given at 1 and 6 months of age, respectively. Serological testing of the baby is done between 9 and 12 months of age by HBsAg and anti-HBs titers to confirm the baby's status as per **Table 1**. The value of anti-HBs (HBsAb) > 10 mIU/mL is considered to be a protective level; booster doses of vaccine should be provided if the value is low.

Hepatitis C Virus

Hepatitis C virus (HCV) is a double-stranded RNA virus which undergoes continuous mutations, as a result of which humoral immunity is ineffective; however, cellular immunity plays a vital role in the pathogenesis. The route of infection is the same as that of HBV with a 60% chance of persisting to chronic hepatitis, and out of them 20% have a probability of developing cirrhosis and hepatocellular carcinoma. The risk of vertical transmission is 3–5%.[5] The Centers for Disease Control and Prevention (*CDC*) *recommends anti-HCV testing for pregnant females with a high risk for infection.*[8-11] Similar to HBV, invasive procedures such as amniocentesis and internal electronic fetal monitoring should be avoided to reduce MTCT.[3] The modes of delivery and breastfeeding do not affect the perinatal transmission in HCV; however, elective cesarean is recommended in cases having coexisting HIV infection.[12] Pegylated interferon (PEG-IFN) and Ribavirin are effective but contraindicated in pregnancy because of adverse fetal effects. Serological testing of the baby is done on two occasions—between 2 and 6 months and 18 months, respectively.

Hepatitis E Virus[13]

Hepatitis E virus (HEV) is a single-stranded RNA virus transmitted via the feco-oral route and *is associated with severe fulminant hepatitis and high maternal mortality up to 20%* due to its effect on the kidneys and suppressed cellular immunity as well as high fetal mortality. Infection is diagnosed by detecting IgM antibodies and HEV RNA. Improving sanitation and avoiding travel to endemic areas can prevent this infection. PEG-IFN and Ribavirin are effective but contraindicated in pregnancy.

Autoimmune Hepatitis

Autoimmune hepatitis (AH) is noninfective but a progressive liver disease that can manifest anytime during gestation

Flowcharts 1A and B: Management plan for HBV in pregnancy.

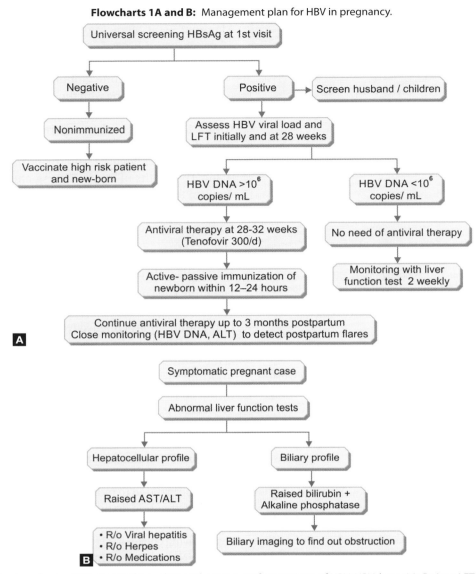

(ALT: alanine aminotransferase; DNA: Deoxyribonucleic acid; HBsAg: surface antigen of HBV; HBV: hepatitis B virus; LFT: liver function test; AST: aspartate aminotransferase; R/o: rule out)

and postpartum. Being autoimmune, the disease activity is subdued during pregnancy under the effect of increased steroid hormones, and therefore dosages of medication can be reduced because of increased immune-tolerance induced in pregnancy. Flares are often seen in the postpartum period in approximately 25% of cases. AH is associated with prematurity, low birth weight, and fetal loss. Immunosuppressive drugs such as Prednisolone and Azathioprine, although a Food and Drug Administration (FDA) category D drug, at low dosage are considered safe and can be continued in pregnancy as well as lactation.

Cholestasis of Pregnancy

Cholestasis, as the name suggests, means stasis (decrease in flow) of bile. It can be "intrahepatic" involving bile ducts, ductules, and canaliculi and "extrahepatic" affecting bile channels outside liver. Extrahepatic cholestasis is mainly due to obstruction of the bile duct tree by stones. *Obstetric cholestasis is the term generally used for intrahepatic cholestasis of pregnancy (IHCP).* The prevalence is 1.2–1.5% and more common in Asian population. It is a multifactorial condition which resolves spontaneously after delivery but clinically important because it can have serious fetal risks such as preterm birth and intrauterine fetal demise.

Presentation

Jaundice and generalized pruritis in absence of rash are the most common presenting symptoms. Association of the right upper quadrant pain is more suggestive of an extrahepatic obstructive lesion. One can easily find scratch marks, especially on limbs and abdomen secondary to pruritis. One must enquire about any development of rashes to differentiate from viral conditions causing marks and itching. Differential diagnosis (D/D) includes pruritis and raised LFT conditions. Any pruritic conditions such as allergy/atopy and skin diseases such as eczema, fungal infections, scratch mark injuries, or folliculitis secondary to pruritis should be examined clearly. Preeclampsia and acute fatty liver of pregnancy (AFLP) are two pregnancy-specific conditions associated with abnormal LFT; they are also the part of D/D which can be differentiated with BP measurements and other biochemical parameters along with liver sonography. *Obstetric cholestasis typically affects palms and soles and worsens at night.*[14] It is more common in multiple pregnancy, recurs in future pregnancies, and has familial tendency also. One can ask for pale stool and dark-colored urine and look for jaundice in few cases. Women with gallstones and carriers of hepatitis C are especially vulnerable to cholestasis.

Diagnostic Investigations

Raised liver enzymes are the characteristic feature of cholestasis such as AP, 5' nucleotidase or gamma glutaryl transferase (GGT), and transaminases [serum glutamic oxaloacetic transaminase (SGOT) and serum glutamic pyruvic transaminase (SGPT)]. Rise in bilirubin is minimal and depends on the extent to stasis. AP in pregnancy is usually of placental origin and therefore must not be singly relied for cholestasis. LFT is the first test to be ordered to diagnose the condition if the above-mentioned symptoms are there. While interpreting the enzyme values, one must remember that for transaminases and GGT, the upper limit of normal throughout pregnancy is approximately 20% less compared to nonpregnant values.[15] Second, the ultrasonography (USG) must be done to evaluate the cause of cholestasis, specially obstructive one where the stone can be easily identified along with dilatation of the ductal system, and also to rule out other hepatic diseases.

Some women may have unexplained persistent pruritis without any biochemical change in LFT; in such cases, the LFT should be repeated after 2 weeks. Viral screen should be done to detect hepatitis B and C and if possible Herpes, EBV, and cytomegalovirus (CMV). Preeclampsia and acute fatty liver are pregnancy-specific conditions responsible for cholestasis.

Pathophysiology

As the pregnancy advances, specially in the second half (i.e., after 20 weeks), cholesterol secretion increases relative to bile acids which makes the bile supersaturated and thick. It will not be wrong to say that pregnancy makes the bile lithogenic, and therefore cholestasis is the disease of the second half of the pregnancy. In the third trimester, pregnancy hormones peak; progesterone especially adds to the stasis part in smaller ducts and is responsible for worsening or unmasking the intrahepatic cholestasis. Severe cholestasis is defined when bile acids are > 40 μmol/L and mild when they are <20 μmol/L. It has also been reported that chances of passage of meconium linearly increase with total bile acid concentration.[16,17]

Follow-up

Once diagnosed, the LFT should be measured weekly until delivery. If the LFT escalates rapidly, other diagnoses should be considered though it is rare with obstetric cholestasis; a coagulation screen should also be performed.

Symptoms and biochemical parameters resolute after delivery, which secures the diagnosis of obstetric cholestasis. Here, it is important to remember that LFT measurement must be deferred in the first 10 days after delivery as it is commonly found to be raised.

Medical Management

Ursodeoxycholic acid (UDCA) is the drug of choice for cholestasis in the second half of pregnancy prescribed at the dose of 150–300 mg daily PO.

Surgical management of secondary cholecystitis, secondary to cholelithiasis in pregnancy confirmed on sonography, should be reserved only for those who are nonresponsive to general and medical management or complicated ones. Literature suggests that 73–90% of acute cholecystitis responds to medical management in pregnancy.[18,19] If required, laparoscopic cholecystectomy can be safely done in the second trimester. In the first trimester, it should be avoided to reduce the risk to the developing fetus and must be delayed till the second trimester while in the third trimester surgery becomes technically challenging.[20-23]

Fetal Risks

Stillbirth/fetal death is the major concern involved with obstetric cholestasis. It is usually sudden without any evidence of placental vascular insufficiency, growth restriction, or oligohydramnios; therefore, Doppler, cardiotocography/nonstress test, biophysical profile, fetal movement count, etc., measures are not useful in predicting fetal death. There is increased likelihood of meconium passage, preterm delivery, fetal distress, more cesarean incidences, and postpartum hemorrhage (PPH).[24-27] Prematurity is mainly iatrogenic resulting from an early decision to deliver in view of suspected complications or mother's anxiety for pruritis and sleepless nights.

Recommendations

- Induction of labor should not be done prior to 37 completed weeks, as early intervention is associated with higher perinatal morbidity.
- To have a better outcome, continuous fetal monitoring in labor should be offered.
- There is no evidence of specific management but the following is advised. Topical emollients, calamine lotion, or aqueous cream provide temporary relief of pruritis and are safe in pregnancy.
- UDCA is the drug of choice for cholestasis in pregnancy. It displaces endogenous bile salts and enhances bile acid clearance across the placenta. Bile-chelating agents such as cholestyramine and in severe cases chlorphenamine that provides sedation at night can be added. Use of dexamethasone at a dose of 10 mg PO for 7 days can be tried if all other measures fail.
- Vitamin K: It can be given as 5–10 mg daily in cases when prothrombin time (PT) is prolonged and prophylactically to cholestasis with normal PT as there may be reduced absorption of this fat-soluble vitamin. Water-soluble preparation (menadiol sodium phosphate) is preferred 10 mg daily which improves both maternal and fetal levels and thus reduces the chances of PPH and neonatal bleeding. Postnatal vitamin K is to be given to babies in the usual manner.
- It has a high recurrence rate (45–90%) with family preponderance also.

CIRRHOSIS AND PORTAL HYPERTENSION

Pregnancy is difficult in cirrhosis, but it is not a contraindication to pregnancy. Cirrhotic women are mostly anovulatory, but with proper treatment they may have regular cycles as well as conception. Maternal mortality, chances of preterm delivery, spontaneous abortion, stillbirth, and perinatal mortality are said to be increased with liver disorders.[28] Cirrhosis is an irreversible disease where the liver develops fibrosis, loses its capacity to metabolize toxins, and blood is shunted away from the liver leading to high pressure in the portal system. The common causative factors associated with cirrhosis are excessive alcohol use (65%), hepatitis B and C infections (10–15%), hepatotoxic medications, etc. Complications of cirrhosis in pregnancy are the same as those in nonpregnancy cases, such as encephalopathy, liver failure, variceal bleeding, and malnutrition. Because of low prevalence of cirrhosis in women of reproductive age and associated reduced fertility, not much data is available.

SYMPTOMS

Early cases with mild portal hypertension (PHT) are asymptomatic, but severe cases may present with hemoptysis due to esophageal variceal bleeding toward the end of the second or third trimester due to increased pressure on inferior vena cava. Acute bleeding not recognized timely may lead to mortality. With advancement of disease, women may present with hypoglycemia, confusion, mental disorientation, encephalopathy, coma, coagulopathy, etc.

Diagnosis

Diagnosis is reached based on the history of risk factors and common findings of liver disease such as spider angiomas, ascites, palmer erythema, and splenomegaly.

Investigations

Liver function test will be deranged along with hypoalbuminemia, raised PT, and thrombocytopenia. Sonography is helpful in diagnosing and biopsy is not usually done, specially during pregnancy. Portosytemic collateral on Doppler along with splenomegaly helps in diagnosing the advanced stage of the disease. Cases with liver stiffness and low platelet count (<1,00,000) should undergo endoscopy to rule out gastroesophageal varices, a feature of the advanced disease. Hepatic pressure gradient measurement is the gold standard method for assessing PHT with pressure > 10 mm Hg. The American Association of Study of Liver Disease (AASLD) recommends that one should avoid the main etiological agent (alcohol) as mainstay of therapy.

Nonselective beta-blockers (propranolol, carvedilol) are recommended for women with a high risk of esophageal varices, i.e., clinically advanced disease, as primary prevention. Variceal ligation is recommended if hemorrhage is reported or medium-to-large varices are found on endoscopy.

Monitoring

Antenatal women can be monitored with LFTs, albumin, and PT every 2–4 weeks based on severity. Cardiotocography should be started at 32 weeks. Those with recurrent hematemesis or on immune-suppressants should have frequent fetal growth assessment.[29] Coagulation, platelet, or hematocrit abnormalities should be managed in the usual way and treated with blood products if required. If there is no evidence of maternal deterioration, growth restriction or fetal distress, then labor can be conducted normally.

In known esophageal varices cases, a Sengstaken–Blakemore tube can be placed in consultation with the gastroenterologist. Early epidural analgesia is helpful, and the second stage must be curtailed with application of forceps or vacuum. In cases with acute variceal bleeding, packed cell transfusion is required and hemoglobin is maintained between 7 and 9g%. Antibiotic prophylaxis is given, i.e., IV ceftriaxone 1 g for 7 days along with vasoactive drugs (somatostatin, octreotide, vasopressin, or its analog). Endoscopy must be performed when the patient is hemodynamically stable, and endoscopic variceal ligation (EVL) can be done if the source is identifiable. A combination of nonselective beta-blockers and EVL is first-line therapy to prevent bleeding.[30] Patients who had a successful transjugular intrahepatic portosystemic shunt (TIPS) during an acute episode do not require beta-blockers. Ideally known varices should be ligated or sclerosed endoscopically prior to pregnancy to prevent hemorrhage in pregnancy. As such, treatment of bleeding varices in pregnancy is the same as in nonpregnant women which includes basic care, monitoring, transfusion, balloon tamponade, endoscopy, and drugs.

GALL STONES/CHOLELITHIASIS AND PREGNANCY

The most common surgical problem associated with pregnancy is gall stones and sometimes this is diagnosed for the first time along with antenatal sonography, the incidence being 10% out of which only 0.2% are symptomatic. Rarely the stone obstructs the bile duct and acute symptomatic cholecystitis develops. The main risk group for cholelithiasis is obesity.

Pathophysiology

Cholesterol secretion increases during pregnancy leading to supersaturated bile; furthermore, the clearance is reduced/slowed under the effect of pregnancy hormone progesterone which leads to sludge or stone formation.

Symptoms

Right upper quadrant pain, nausea, vomiting, indigestion, etc., are the common complaints of cholelithiasis while fever and leukocytosis are the manifestations of acute cholecystitis.

Diagnosis

Ultrasound is the primary modality for diagnosis, which should be done on an empty stomach when the gall bladder is full. Biliary sludge is also called microlithiasis which is also confirmed by seeing low-level echoes that shift with change in position. Gall stone is diagnosed as high-level echoes with postacoustic shadowing. Choledocolithiasis is diagnosed with evidence of gall stones in common bile duct (CBD) on sonography or on endoscopic retrograde cholangiopancreatography (ERCP).

Management

Both medical and surgical options are there. Asymptomatic cholelithiasis is managed by lifestyle changes and dietary modifications, but colic or acute cholecystitis is treated conservatively with IV fluids, antibiotics, antispasmodics, and bowel rest. This treatment is successful in 80% cases during pregnancy. But the recurrence rate is quite high and for such cases second trimester is the best time to go for cholecystectomy (surgical management). While doing laparoscopy in pregnancy one must do open cannulation by the Hasson technique for the umbilical port, keeping intra in peritoneal pressure of 10–12 mm Hg, placing the patient in left lateral position.

LIVER TRANSPLANT

It is rare to have a disease which needs liver transplantation in the reproductive age, but literature mentions successful pregnancy after the liver transplantation and also successful transplant during pregnancy. Ideally in such situations conception should be planned after 2 years because a lot of immune-suppressants are prescribed during this time to prevent the graft rejection.

Regular normal cycles are resumed in 6–8 months.[31]

Effect of Transplant on Pregnancy and Vice Versa

Transplant increases the risk of opportunistic infections which not only complicate maternal prognosis but also can be deadly and morbid for the developing fetus. Apart from the risk of infection following immune-suppression, pregnancy after a transplant has a higher risk of chronic hypertension, preeclampsia, preterm delivery, preterm PROM (PPROM), and anemia.[32] As such, pregnancy in itself does not increase the risk of allograft rejection after transplant.

Managing Pregnancy after Transplant

Apart from routine antenatal care (ANC) investigations, complete blood count, electrolyte, CMV titers, and renal or LFTs should be done. The immuno-suppressive medication is usually continued during pregnancy with some dose adjustments.[8] Corticosteroids are safe in pregnancy but can lead to fetal adrenal axis suppression, fetal growth restriction, and PROM.[33] Azathioprine, the common drug, can be continued as it is not found to be associated with teratogenicity but as it crosses the placenta it is associated with growth restriction, fetal immune-suppression, and bone marrow toxicity. Another commonly prescribed drug is cyclosporine which inhibits T-cell clonal expansion.

Consultation with a maternal-fetal medicine specialist must be taken. Such cases must receive stress dose corticosteroid during labor and delivery. An elevated transaminase level may be found in such cases secondary to drug effects as cyclosporine. Growth scans be done every 4–6 weekly after 24 weeks. Nonstress test and biophysical profile can be started from 28 weeks.[34] The mode of delivery should be planned based on the obstetric condition. Congenital CMV infection can lead to neonatal death.

■ ACUTE FATTY LIVER OF PREGNANCY

It is the condition where fatty infiltration of liver occurs which can even lead to liver failure.[8] The prevalence is 1/15,000 pregnancies. It is a chronic disease and usually complicates the second trimester or third trimester of pregnancy. D/D: Fulminant viral hepatitis, HEV, drug-based hepatoxicity, HELLP (hemolysis, elevated liver enzymes, low platelet count) syndrome, Reye syndrome, and cholestasis of pregnancy.

Pathophysiology

High-risk groups are old primigravidas, multiple gestation, preeclamptics, and history of AFLP. It has genetic preponderance which affects the maternal mitochondrial fatty acid oxidation pathway or an in utero fetus with LCHAD (long-chain 3 hydroxyacyl-coenzyme A dehydrogenase) deficiency. Here, the liver is unable to oxidize the long-chain fatty acids from the fetus, which accumulate and impair the liver functions.[35] Common symptoms are nausea, vomiting, anorexia, pain in abdomen, ascites, and jaundice. Disease if not diagnosed in time secondarily gets complicated with acute renal failure, hepatic encephalopathy, and ultimately mortality.

Diagnosis

Markedly raised aminotransferase levels in the range of 300–500 U/L, bilirubin up to 5 mg/dL or more, leukocytosis (neutrophilia), thrombocytopenia, hypoglycemia, coagulopathy, and later renal dysfunction in combination help in diagnosis.[36,37] On contrast tomography (CT), demonstration of diffuse low density signals and ascites is a good diagnostic finding. Sonography is not much diagnostic as fatty infiltration in AFLP is mainly microvesicular. Definitive diagnosis needs liver biopsy but is not advocated in pregnancy. Biopsy demonstrates microvesicular steatosis and fat droplets around the nucleus.

"Swansea criteria" are a combination of clinical and laboratory values for diagnosis of AFLP.[38]

Six or more criteria are required to be positive to diagnose AFLP among the following:

Vomiting, abdominal pain, polydipsia/polyuria, encephalopathy, elevated bilirubin (>14 μmol/L), hypoglycemia (<4 mmol/L), elevated urea (>340 μmol/L), leukocytosis (>11 × 10[6] cells/L), ascites on sonography, and elevated transaminases (>42 IU/L). It is basically designed to obviate the need of liver biopsy in clinical management.[38]

Management

An AFLP case needs hospitalization as it is a progressive disease. It needs complete assessment of condition and supportive measures such as glucose infusion, blood products transfusion, and others, as required. *The case should be delivered promptly to stop the fatty acid overload on liver*, and the woman and neonate should be tested for LCHAD molecular testing. In confirmed cases, pregnancy should be terminated at completion of 34 weeks. Induction of labor can be done if smooth vaginal delivery is expected, as cesarean section increases the maternal morbidity. General anesthesia must be preferred if coagulopathy is suspected to avoid hematoma with regional blocks if cesarean section is required. The condition improves within 48–72 hours of delivery with normalization of enzyme levels over 2 weeks' time, so supportive treatment should be continued.[36] Major causes of mortality are PPH, renal failure, hypoglycemia, disseminated intravascular coagulation, pulmonary edema, hepatic encephalopathy, etc.[39,40]

■ HEPATIC ADENOMA AND HEMANGIOMA

Adenomas develop in women on long-term use of oral contraceptive pills. Such benign tumors remain undiagnosed but during pregnancy they start growing and have chances of rupture if present near surface. *Ideally, large hepatic adenomas (>5 cm) must be resected if identified before pregnancy if they are large and present near surface.* Hepatic adenoma first diagnosed during pregnancy should be monitored with sonography for growth.

■ ALCOHOL AND PREGNANCY

With the change in the lifestyle, now more and more women of childbearing age are using alcohol. Alcohol use has been found to be associated with menstrual disturbance, infertility, abortions, and miscarriage. Ideally, abstinence from alcohol should be maintained by women planning pregnancy at conception and the whole gestational period as no safe levels have been defined yet. Alcoholism in pregnancy is commonly associated with prematurity, stillbirth, neonatal alcohol withdrawal, and fetal alcohol syndrome. Fetal alcohol syndrome is diagnosed by dysmorphic facial features, growth deficit, and central nervous system (CNS) abnormalities and seen in 10–50% offsprings of moderate-to-heavy drinker women (1–2 oz/day of absolute alcohol) and chronic alcoholics.

■ HYPEREMESIS GRAVIDARUM

Hyperemesis gravidarum is a condition where an uncontrollable vomiting during early months of pregnancy results in dehydration, ketosis, weight loss (>5% of prepregnancy weight), and secondary complications.

The incidence is 0.3–2% of all pregnancies.[41] Nausea and vomiting is common in the first trimester and has been labeled as one of the diagnostic symptoms of pregnancy due to rapid rise of beta subunit of human chorionic gonadotropin (βHCG). Vomiting corresponds with the HCG levels and commonly starts at the 5th week, peaks at 9/10th week (when HCG levels are maximum), and usually disappears at around 16–18 weeks.[42] Vomiting is more in morning; therefore, it is also called morning sickness. Two to three episodes of vomiting and nauseating feeling daily are not worrisome as women continue to gain weight, and there is no effect on fetal growth. As the name suggests, hyperemesis is an extreme form of vomiting where the woman is not able to eat or digest even liquids and lands up into dehydration, weight loss, ketosis, and electrolyte disbalance. If not treated in time or if it persists beyond 16–18 weeks, it causes fatty degeneration and necrosis of liver, esophageal perforation, Wernicke's encephalopathy, coma, seizures, and acute kidney injury. Risk groups are obese, twin pregnancy, trophoblastic disease, nulliparity, and history in previous pregnancy.

Diagnosis is completely clinical and includes vomiting along with dysgeusia, anxiety, sleep disturbance, depression, and need of admission to the hospital, where vitals, weight, LFT, kidney function test (KFT), and electrolytes are regularly checked and treatment is provided accordingly. Ultrasound should be done to rule out a hydatidiform mole or multiple gestation as in these two situations βHCG levels are high and also to screen pancreas and biliary tree. It should be differentiated from acute gastroenteritis, hepatitis, appendicitis, cholecystitis, peptic ulcer, bowel obstruction, diabetic ketoacidosis, benign intracranial hypertension, and migraine. Thyroid, abdominal, and neurological evaluation is must.[43]

Management

The woman is kept nil orally for some time with fluids and electrolytes in the form of intravenous fluids beginning with 1 L/h or to maintain a urine output of >100 mL/h. Ringer's solution is best in the sense that it contains potassium, magnesium phosphorus, etc. Thiamine and multivitamin injection can be added as supplements to avoid deficiency and prevent Wernicke's encephalopathy. The FDA-approved drug for pregnancy is a combination of Pyridoxine and Doxylamine. Antiemetics, if required, can be added in the form of Ondansetron (8 mg IM 12 hourly), Metoclopramide (5–10 mg IV 8 hourly), or Promethazine. Electrolyte deficiency, identified on investigations, should be corrected soon. Once the acute vomiting stops, oral intake in the form of fluids is gradually started and accordingly IV fluids are tapered. Diet is slowly expanded as tolerated, preferably semisolid bland meals. In cases of intractable vomiting, steroids can also be added as methylprednisolone 16 mg 8 hourly for 3 days and tapered over 15 days. In rare, extreme nonrespondent cases parenteral nutrition (TPN) is required. Termination of pregnancy is rarely considered in refractory cases if maternal survival is threatened.[44]

■ HELLP SYNDROME

HELLP syndrome is the complicated form of liver abnormality seen in approximately 20% cases of severe preeclampsia or eclampsia.[45] It is more commonly seen in multiparous, older age gravidas in the third trimester of pregnancy. It must be differentiated from hemolytic uremic syndrome (HUS), thrombotic thrombocytopenic purpura (TTP), and AFLP. It commonly presents with nausea, vomiting, headache, epigastric pain, raised liver enzymes, and mild jaundice along with raised BP. There are two systems which classify HELLP syndrome—"Tennessee" and "Mississippi" based on enzymes and platelet values, respectively. It is a systemic vascular disease characterized by microangiopathic hemolysis and endothelial injury which secondarily can get complicated in the form of subcapsular hematoma, rupture, DIC, pulmonary edema, retinal detachment, placental abruption, acute liver, and renal failure responsible for maternal mortality and intrauterine or peripartum fetal death. Pregnancy should be terminated after completion of 34 weeks if reports remain abnormal.

CONCLUSION

The signs and symptoms of liver diseases are very vague, but specific disorders have both maternal and fetal effects; therefore, a pregnant case must be kept on regular monitoring. A coordinated team approach is often required that involves primary care physician, obstetrician, hepatologist, and surgeon to provide best maternal and fetal outcomes.

■ COMMON LIVER DISEASE PRESENTATIONS

For easy identifications, common liver disease presentations during pregnancy are described:

Right Upper Quadrant Pain in Abdomen

It has a good number of D/D.

Acute colic pain (intermittent) at the site of liver can be because of cholelithiasis which is not uncommon in pregnancy and can result in cholecystitis, choledocholithiasis, or pancreatitis. *Severe unremitting liver site pain* has the possibility of capsular rupture or subcapsular hematoma secondary to preeclampsia or liver adenoma. *Dull ache* is a sign of liver enlargement leading to stretching of capsule. Tenderness is present on liver

TABLE 2: Differentiating features of systemic syndromes.

Reports	HELLP	AFLP	TTP	PE	HUS
Jaundice (%)	5–10%	40–90%	Rare	Mild	Rare
Urine	Proteinuria	Proteinuria	Proteinuria	Proteinuria	Proteinuria
Thrombocytopenia	+	+	+	+	+
Hemolysis (%) LDH	50–100% raised	15–20% normal	100% raised	30% mild	100% raised
Anemia	Mild	No	Yes	Hemoconcentration	Yes
DIC (%)	<20%	50–100%	Uncommon	Uncommon	Uncommon
Hypoglycemia	No	Common	No	No	No
Transaminase	High	High	Mild	High	Mild
Elevated bilirubin	Sometimes	Always	Always	Mild	Always
Impaired renal function (%)	50% mild/moderate	90–100% moderate	30% mild	30% mild	100% severe
Management	Delivery and recovery	Delivery and recovery	Plasma infusion/ exchange	Delivery and recovery	Plasma infusion/ exchange

(AFLP: acute fatty liver of pregnancy; DIC: disseminated intravascular coagulation; HELLP: hemolysis, elevated liver enzymes, low platelet count; HUS: hemolytic–uremic syndrome; LDH: lactate dehydrogenase; PE: preeclampsia; TTP: thrombotic thrombocytopenic purpura)

palpation and seen in cases of viral hepatitis, AFLP, and Budd-Chiari syndrome.

Jaundice During Pregnancy

Icterus can be identified on sclera of eye when the bilirubin reaches 2 mg%. *Direct hyperbilirubinemia:* Conjugated bilirubin is raised in liver damage and biliary obstruction cases. Viral hepatitis is the most common D/D, followed by IHCP. Other causes can be choledocholithiasis, pancreatitis, AFLP, and preeclampsia, all of which present with pain at the epigastrium or liver site as mentioned above **(Table 2)**. *Indirect hyperbilirubinemia* (unconjugated bilirubin) is seen in hemolytic anemia, injuries, genetic Gilbert's syndrome, and newborn, and the bilirubin level rarely crosses 5 mg/dL unless associated with renal insufficiency.

KEY POINTS/SUMMARY[8]

A pregnant case presenting with abnormal liver function is a risk patient and should undergo standard workup. The incidence of abnormal liver tests in pregnancy is around 3–5%. As such there is no gross change in liver test reports during pregnancy except those produced by placenta as AP or as a result of hemodilution as albumin. Sonography is the safe first-line noninvasive diagnostic modality in assessment of abnormal liver functions suggesting biliary disease. MRI may be used without gadolinium in the second and third trimesters if required.

In cases of a symptomatic biliary disease such as pancreatitis, choledocholithiasis and cholangitis, ERCP can be performed. Symptomatic cholecystitis can be managed with laparoscopic cholecystectomy.

Women with chronic hepatitis B infection with high viral load of 10^6 log copies/mL (2,00,000 IU/mL) should be offered antiviral medication Tenofovir or Telbivudine in the third trimester to reduce perinatal transmission. In chronic HBV cases, elective caesarean section is not recommended for preventing MTCT and such females can breastfeed their babies normally

All pregnant high-risk women should be screened with anti-HCV antibody. Invasive procedures such as fetal scalp sampling and amniocentesis should be avoided. Similar to HBV, elective cesarean is not performed just to prevent fetal infection and the women are allowed to breastfeed. Antiviral therapy for HCV is ideally not prescribed in pregnancy.

Autoimmune hepatitis cases should continue their steroid treatment with immune-suppressive drugs such as Azathioprine. Endoscopy can be simply done in the second trimester safely if required.

In cases of IHCP, early delivery at 37 completed weeks is recommended and UDCA should be given at 10–15 mg/kg for symptomatic improvement.

AFLP and HELLP syndromes are two progressive diseases which can be managed promptly by delivering the cases at 34 weeks' completion. If cesarean is planned, then platelets should be transfused to attain the value of 40,000–50,000 cells/μL.

■ REFERENCES

1. Braverman DZ, Johnnson MC, Kern F Jr. Effects of pregnancy and contraceptive steroids on gall bladder function. N Engl J Med. 1980:302;362.
2. Bacq Y, Zarca O, Weill J, Brechot JF, Mariotte N, Vol S, et al. Liver function tests in normal pregnancy: A prospective study of 102 pregnant women and 103 matched controls. Hepatology .1996;23:1020.
3. Shao Z, al Tibi M, Wakim-Fleming J. Update on viral hepatitis in pregnancy. Clevel Clin J Med. 2017;84(3):202-6.

4. Elinav E, Ben-Dov IZ, Shapira Y, Daudi N, Adler R, Shouval D, et al. Acute hepatitis A infection in pregnancy is associated with high rates of gestational complications and preterm labor. Gastroenterology. 2006;130:1129-34.

5. American College of Obstetricians and Gynecologists. ACOG Practice Bulletin No. 86: Viral hepatitis in pregnancy. Obstet Gynecol. 2007;110:941-56.

6. World Health Organization (WHO). Hepatitis A fact sheet. [online] Available from www.who.int/mediacentre/factsheets/fs328/en/ [Last accessed September, 2020].

7. US Centers for Disease Control and Prevention (CDC). (2013). Viral hepatitis—statistics & surveillance. [online] Available from www.cdc.gov/hepatitis/statistics/2013surveillance/commentary.htm#hepatits A [Last accessed September, 2020].

8. Society for Maternal-Fetal Medicine (SMFM), Dionne-Odom J, Tita ATN, Silverman NS. #38: Hepatitis B in pregnancy screening, treatment and prevention of vertical transmission. Am J Obstet Gynecol. 2016;214:6-14.

9. Zou H, Chen Y, Duan Z, Zhang H, Pan C. Virologic factors associated with failure to passive-active immune-prophylaxis in infants born to HBsAg positive mothers. J Viral Hepat. 2012;19:e18-e25.

10. Tran TT, Ahn J, Reau N. ACG clinical guideline: liver disease and pregnancy. Am J Gastroenterol. 2016;111:176-94.

11. Schillie S, Wester C, Osborne M, Wesolowski L, Ryerson AB. CDC Recommendations for Hepatitis C Screening Among Adults — United States, 2020. MMWR Recomm Rep. 2020;69(No. RR-2):1-17.

12. Moyer VA; US Preventive Services Task Force. Screening for hepatitis C virus infection in adults: US Preventive Services Task Force Recommendation Statement. Ann Intern Med. 2013;159:349-57.

13. US Centers for Disease Control and Prevention (CDC). Viral hepatitis— hepatitis E information. Hepatitis E FAQs for health professionals. [online] Available from www.cdc.gov/hepatitis/hev/hevfaq.htm. [Last accessed September, 2020].

14. Kenyon AP, Tribe RM, Nelson-Piercy C, Girling JC, Williamson C, Seed PT, et al. Pruritus in pregnancy: a study of anatomical distribution and prevalence in relation to the development of obstetric cholestasis. Obstet Med. 2010;3:25-9.

15. Girling JC, Dow E, Smith JH. Liver function tests in preeclampsia: importance of comparison with a reference range derived for normal pregnancy. Br J Obstet Gynaecol. 1997;104:246-50.

16. Glantz A, Marschall HU, Mattsson LA. Intrahepatic cholestasis of pregnancy: relationships between bile acid levels and fetal complication rates. Hepatology 2004;40:467-74.

17. Lee RH, Kwok KM, Ingles S, Wilson ML, Mullin P, Incerpi M, et al. Pregnancy outcomes during an era of aggressive management for intrahepatic cholestasis of pregnancy. Am J Perinatol. 2008;25:341-5.

18. Date RS, Kausahal M, Ramesh A. A review of management of gall stone disease and its complications in pregnancy. Am J Surg. 2008;196(4):599-608.

19. Ghumman E, Barry M, Grace PA. Management of gall stone in pregnancy. Br J Surg. 1997;84:1646.

20. Dhupar R, Samaldone GM, Hamad GG. Is there a benefit to delaying cholecystectomy for symptomatic gall bladder disease during pregnancy? Surg Endosc. 2010;24(1):108-12.

21. Lee S, Bradley JP, Ludmir J, Mele MM, Sehdev HM. Cholelithiasis in pregnancy: Surgical versus medical management. Obstet Gynecol. 2000;95:70.

22. Barone JE, Bears S, Chen S, Tsai J, Russel JC. Outcome study of cholecystectomy during pregnancy. Am J Gynaecol. 1999;177:232.

23. Chong VH, Jalihal A. Endoscopic management of biliary disorders during pregnancy. Hepatobiliary Pancreat Dis Int. 2010;9(2):180-5.

24. Kenyon AP, Piercy CN, Girling J, Williamson C, Tribe RM, Shennan AH. Obstetric cholestasis, outcome with active management: a series of 70 cases. BJOG. 2002;109:282-8.

25. Bacq Y, Sapey T, Bréchot MC, Pierre F, Fignon A, Dubois F. Intrahepatic cholestasis of pregnancy: a French prospective study. Hepatology. 1997;26:358-64.

26. Reid R, Ivey KJ, Rencoret RH, Storey B. Fetal complications of obstetric cholestasis. Br Med J. 1976;1:870-2.

27. Fisk NM, Storey GN. Fetal outcome in obstetric cholestasis. Br J Obstet Gynaecol. 1988;95:1137-43.

28. Borhanmanesh F, Haghighi P. Pregnancy in patients with cirrhosis of the liver. Obstet Gynecol. 1970;36(2):315-24.

29. Russell MA, Craigo SD. Cirrhosis and portal hypertension in pregnancy. Semin Perinatol. 1998;22(2):156-65.

30. Garcia-Tsao G, Abraldes JG, Berzigotti A, Bosch J. Portal hypertensive bleeding in cirrhosis: Risk stratification, diagnosis, and management: 2016 practice guidance by the American Association for the study of liver diseases. Hepatology. 2017;65(1):310-35.

31. Laifer SA, Abu-Elmagd K, Fung JJ. Hepatic transplantation during pregnancy and the puerperium. J Matern Fetal Med. 1997;6(1):40-4.

32. Deshpande NA, James NT, Kucirka LM, Boyarsky BJ, Garonzik-Wang JM, Cameron AM, et al. Pregnancy outcomes of liver transplant recipients: a systematic review and meta-analysis. Liver Transpl. 2012;18(6):621-9.

33. Scantlebury V, Gordon R, Tzakis A, Koneru B, Bowman J, Mazzaferro V, et al. Childbearing after liver transplantation. Transplantation. 1990;49(2):317-21.

34. Casele HL, Laifer SA. Pregnancy after liver transplantation. Semin Perinatol. 1998;22(2):149-55.

35. Benjaminov FS, Heathcote J. Liver disease in pregnancy. Am J Gastroenterol. 2004;99(12):2479-88.

36. Nelson DB, Yost NP, Cunningham FG. Acute fatty liver of pregnancy: clinical outcomes and expected duration of recovery. Am J Obstet Gynecol. 2013;209(5):456.e1-7.

37. Browning MF, Levy HL, Wilkins-Haug LE, Larson C, Shih VE. Fetal fatty acid oxidation defects and maternal liver disease in pregnancy. Obstet Gynecol. 2006; 107(1):115-20.

38. Geol A, Ramakrishna B, Zachariah U, Ramachandran J, Eapen CJ, Kurian G, et al. How accurate are the Swansea criteria to diagnose acute fatty liver of pregnancy in predicting hepatic microvesicular steatosis? Gut. 2011;60:138-9.

39. Knight M, Nelson-Piercy C, Kurinczuk JJ, Spark P, Brocklehurst P, for the UK Obstetric Surveillance System. A prospective national study of acute fatty liver of pregnancy in the UK. Gut. 2008;57(7):951-6.

40. Sibai BM. Imitators of severe preeclampsia. Obstet Gynecol. 2007;109(4):956-66.

41. Goodwin TM. Hyperemesis gravidarum. Obstet Gynecol Clin North Am. 2008;35(3):401-17.

42. Bailit JL. Hyperemesis gravidarum: Epidemiologic findings from a large cohort. Am J Obset Gynecol. 2005;193(3):811-4.

43. Tan JY, Loh KC, Yeo GS, Chee YC. Transient hyperthyroidism of hyperemesis gravidarum. BJOG. 2002;109(6):683-8.

44. Poursharif B, Korst LM, Macgibbon KW, Fejzo MS, Romero R, Goodwin TM. Elective pregnancy termination in a large cohort of women with hyperemesis gravidarum. Contraception. 2007;76(6):451-5.

45. Saphier CJ, Repke JT. Hemolysis, elevated liver enzymes, and low platelets syndrome: a review of diagnosis and management. Semin Perinatol. 1998:169;1000.

CHAPTER 15

Febrile Illness in Pregnancy

Deepa Lokwani Masand

■ INTRODUCTION

Maternal death and poor birth outcomes are the major public health issues across the world. Febrile illness in pregnancy is often linked to the undesirable pregnancy and fetal outcomes. The World Health Organization (WHO) has also considered pregnant women to be "priority risk group" as the chances of mortality and morbidity amplify in association with infectious diseases due to various physiological changes of pregnancy. Globally, febrile illness during pregnancy (FIDP) is a recognized clinical problem with a significantly elevated fetomaternal risk.

India is a developing nation with endemicity to various infectious agents. A wide range of fetomaternal medical complications follow pyrexia in pregnancy due to various *preventable* etiologies such as malaria and dengue with <1% mortality and <3% hospitalization rate if all basic treatment protocols are followed. However, H1N1 leads to higher mortality up to 20% if treatment is not started within the first 5 days. Though varicella and enteric are less common, they lead to serious fetal abnormalities.

■ MALARIA

Malaria during pregnancy is a major public health concern and an important contributor to maternal and infant morbidity and mortality in endemic countries. Data from 2016 shows ongoing malaria transmission in 91 countries and territories **(Fig. 1)**. Malarial infection continues to be a major public health problem in India, particularly because of *Plasmodium falciparum* which is prone to complications. Globally, *P. vivax* causes 4% of estimated cases which increase to 41% outside the African continent and mainly four countries (Ethiopia, India, Indonesia, and Pakistan) account for 78% of *P. vivax* cases. In India, about 21.98% population live in high-transmission (>1 case/1,000 population) areas and about 67% in low-transmission (0–1 case/1,000 population) areas for malaria.

Pregnant women are three times more likely to suffer from severe disease as a result of malarial infection compared with their nonpregnant counterparts. They are also at a higher risk for severe anemia, maternal death, and adverse obstetric outcomes such as abortion, premature labor, intrauterine death, low-birth-weight neonates, and neonatal death.

Etiopathogenesis (Fig. 2)

Malaria is a parasitic infection caused by the protozoans *P. falciparum, P. vivax, P. malariae,* and *P. ovale* (extremely rarely *P. knowlesi*). The transmission is by the bite of a

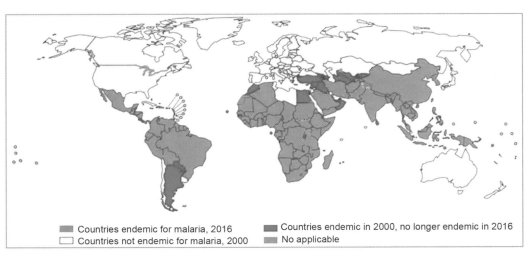

Fig. 1: Countries endemic for malaria in 2000 and 2016. Countries with 3 consecutive years of zero indigenous cases are considered to have eliminated malaria. No country in the WHO European region reported indigenous cases in 2015 but Tajikistan has not yet hod 3 consecutive years of zero indigenous cases, its last case being reported in July 2014.
Source: WHO database

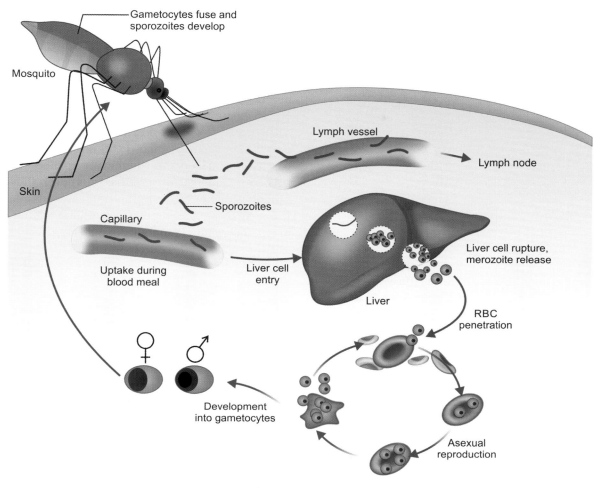

Fig. 2: Life cycle of malaria infection.
Source: Rev Obstet Gynecol. Summer. 2009;2(3):186-92.

sporozoite-bearing female anopheles mosquito; therefore, factors influencing mosquito breeding such as temperature, humidity, and rainfall affect malaria incidence. After a period of pre-erythrocytic development in the liver, parasitic invasion of the erythrocyte occurs that consumes hemoglobin and alters red cell membrane, thus facilitating *P. falciparum*-infected erythrocytes to cytoadhere (or stick) into small blood vessels of brain, kidney, and other organs which interfere with microcirculatory flow and metabolism in vital organs. The hallmarks of the falciparum malaria parasite in pregnancy are sequestration into placenta and evading host defense mechanisms such as splenic processing and filtration. Sequestration does not occur in benign malarias due to *P. vivax*, *P. ovale*, and *P. malariae*. Clinically, malaria is categorized into two types:

1. *Uncomplicated malaria:* It is characterized by two stages:
   a. Cold stage with cold sensation and shivering
   b. Hot stage with fever, headache, sweating, and occasionally seizures

BOX 1: Manifestation of severe malaria.

- Impaired consciousness/coma
- Repeated generalized convulsions
- Renal failure
- Pulmonary edema
- Acute respiratory distress syndrome
- Circulatory shock
- Disseminated intravascular coagulation
- Spontaneous bleeding
- Acidosis
- Hemoglobinuria
- Jaundice

Symptoms occur every 2–3 days and last for 6–10 hours depending upon the infecting species.

2. *Severe malaria:* It is a medical emergency due to severe *P. falciparum* infection characterized by a parasitemia level of >5% and clinical features of organ damage/serological findings **(Box 1)**.

Pregnant females in areas of low transmission are nonimmune and may be symptomatic at very low parasite

TABLE 1: Comparison of occurrence of complications in areas of high and low transmission.

Complication	High transmission	Low transmission
Hypoglycemia	–	++
Severe anemia	+++	+++
Pulmonary edema	–	++
ARF	–	++
Hyperpyrexia	+	+++
Placental malaria	+++	+++
LBW babies	+++	+++
Abortions	–	+++
Congenital malaria	–	+++

(ARF: acute renal failure; LBW: low birth weight)
Courtesy: Kakkilaya BS. Malaria and pregnancy. 2018.

levels and carry high risk for severe malaria which can result in spontaneous abortion and maternal death in up to 60% of cases whereas in high endemic areas pregnant females may have asymptomatic malarial infection with incidental placental parasitemia due to high acquired immunity **(Table 1)**. Placental sequestration of malaria leads to increased prevalence of severe maternal anemia and low-birth-weight babies that contribute to infant mortality. Such problems are more common during the first and second pregnancies as the parasitemia level decreases with an increasing number of pregnancies.

Management

The WHO recommends confirmation of every suspected malaria case by microscopy or rapid diagnostic test (RDT) before initiating treatment. Accurate diagnosis improves the management of febrile illnesses and ensures that antimalarial medicines are given when necessary. Only those areas where diagnostic testing for the parasite is not possible, the treatment for malaria should be initiated solely on clinical suspicion.

Microscopic examination of Giemsa-stained peripheral thick blood smears is more sensitive in detecting malarial parasite as a greater volume of concentrated blood is examined. The WHO considers it as the standard method for detection. Thin smear aids in parasite species' identification and quantification. Diagnosis of malaria is unlikely if three consecutive blood smears taken 12–24 hours apart are negative.

Diagnosing placental malaria in women during pregnancy remains a major challenge.

Rapid diagnostic test detects circulating parasite antigens with a simple dipstick format. Several RDT types are available; some detect only *P. falciparum* while others can detect other parasites also. Erythrocytes infected with *P. falciparum* release Plasmodium lactate dehydrogenase

(pLDH) and histidine-rich protein-II (HRP-II) that can be detected in peripheral blood using monoclonal antibody-based RDTs. RDTs based on one-step malaria HRP-II may be an important tool to detect placental *P. falciparum* infection during pregnancy, and pLDH-based RDT can be used to monitor effective antimalarial therapy which is the product of viable parasites.

Molecular techniques are highly sensitive with polymerase chain reaction (PCR) detecting as low as 1–5 parasites/μL of blood. Techniques are expensive and highly trained technicians are needed; moreover, they are not advantageous in high malaria transmission areas where submicroscopic parasitemia is prevalent among humans to maintain natural immunity to malaria parasites.

Treatment

Treatment of malaria in pregnancy needs to be energetic, anticipatory, and careful.

Admission is advised for all pregnant women with uncomplicated malaria to hospital and with severe malaria to an intensive care unit.

It involves the following aspects and needs equal importance:
- Treatment of malaria and complications
- Management of labor

Treatment of Uncomplicated Malaria

Efficacious and prompt treatment of malaria in a woman reduces the systemic effects of parasitemia and the adverse effects on the fetus.

The aim is to treat the illness along with prevention of complications which are as follows:
- Assess severity—general condition, BP, temperature, pallor, jaundice
- Blood sugar every 4–6 hourly as hypoglycemia can be profound and persistent and may be exacerbated by quinine
- Hemoglobin and parasite count 12 hourly
- Serum creatinine; serum bilirubin
- Intake/output chart daily

Antimalarial treatment is given after accurate diagnosis according to **Tables 2 to 4**.

Uncomplicated malaria during pregnancy is not an indication for induction of labor.

Up till delivery, screening of blood film is done weekly for early positive detection.

Regular antenatal care for maternal health and fetal growth assessment is advised that include periodic blood counts, blood sugar, and fetal growth scans.

The patient should be counseled about the risk of relapse and symptoms of recurrence.

TABLE 2: Management in uncomplicated malaria.

Uncomplicated malaria/ P. falciparum or species not identified (P. vivax, P. ovale, P. malariae, or P. knowlesi malaria)	Chloroquine-resistant or unknown resistance	*First trimester of pregnancy* 7 days of quinine + clindamycin Quinine sulfate: 542 mg base (= 650 mg salt) po tid Clindamycin: 20 mg base/kg/day po divided tid × 7 days OR quinine monotherapy if clindamycin is not available <div align=center>OR</div> An ACT or oral artesunate + clindamycin is an alternative if quinine + clindamycin is not available or fails The antimalarial medicines considered safe in the first trimester of pregnancy are quinine, chloroquine, clindamycin, and proguanil *Second and third trimesters of pregnancy* Standard six-dose artemether + lumefantrine regimen 1 tablet = 20 mg artemether/120 mg lumefantrine A 3-day treatment schedule with a total of six oral doses is recommended. Dihydroartemisinin–piperaquine had the best efficacy and an acceptable safety profile, with an additional benefit of a longer post-treatment prophylactic effect, which supports its suitability as a chemoprophylaxis or chemoprevention agent. (England Journal of Medicine)
Uncomplicated malaria/ P. falciparum or species not identified (P. vivax, P. ovale, P. malariae, or P. knowlesi malaria)	Chloroquine-sensitive	*All trimesters* Chloroquine phosphate 600 mg base (= 1,000 mg salt) po immediately, followed by 300 mg base (= 500 mg salt) po at 6, 24, and 48 hours <div align=center>OR</div> Hydroxychloroquine 620 mg base (= 800 mg salt) po immediately, followed by 310 mg base (= 400 mg salt) po at 6, 24, and 48 hours <div align=center>OR</div> Standard ACT regimen

(ACT: artemisinin-based combination therapy)
Courtesy: WHO, CDC.

TABLE 3: Management of malaria in cases of relapse.

Preventing relapse in P. vivax or P. ovale malaria, pregnant, and breastfeeding women	Only P. vivax and P. ovale form hypnozoites, which are dormant parasite stages in the liver that cause relapses of infection weeks to years after the primary infection	Weekly chemoprophylaxis with chloroquine until delivery and breastfeeding are completed, chloroquine phosphate is 300 mg base (= 500 mg salt) orally <div align=center>OR</div> Primaquine postnatally after checking G6PD status of the infant

(G6PD: glucose-6-phosphate dehydrogenase)
Courtesy: WHO, CDC.

TABLE 4: Management of severe malaria.

Severe malaria	Intravenous (IV) artesunate available under investigational new drug (IND) protocol: Give 2.4 mg/kg per dose. Administer one dose at 0, 12, 24, and 48 hours for a total of four doses. <div align=center>AND</div> Follow artesunate by one of the following: Artemether lumefantrine regimen as above <div align=center>OR</div> Clindamycin Slow infusion of 10 mg base/kg IV loading dose followed by 5 mg base/kg IV every 8 hours for 7 days <div align=center>OR</div> Switch to oral clindamycin (oral dose as above) as soon as the patient can take oral medication (administration via the nasogastric tube or after an antiemetic)

Courtesy: WHO, CDC.

Peripartum malaria is an indication for placental histology and blood films from placenta and cord to detect congenital malaria at an early stage, and neonates should be screened weekly till 28 days.

Management of Severe Malaria

Severe malaria is characterized by *P. falciparum* asexual parasitemia and complications due to organ dysfunction and fetal compromise.

The WHO recommends parenteral antimalarial medicines in pregnancy with severe malaria. Treatment must be prompt and immediate in full doses. Parenteral artesunate is the treatment of choice in all trimesters; intramuscular artemether is the alternative.

Management of Complications

Optimal management can be planned with a multidisciplinary team of intensive care specialist, infectious disease specialist, obstetrician, and neonatologist.

Cerebral malaria is assessed using Glasgow Coma Score. The main aim is to maintain airway and to prevent convulsions. Treatable causes of coma such as hypoglycemia, bacterial meningitis, and hyperpyrexia should be managed promptly.

Septicemic shock (algid malaria) due to secondary bacterial infections such as urinary tract infection and pneumonia may present with hypotension initially. Corrective measures under full monitoring of vital parameters and intake and output include fluid replacement for hemodynamic stability and administration of parenteral broad-spectrum antimicrobials after sending blood culture.

Severely anemic women (hemoglobin < 8 g/100 mL or packed cell volume < 24%) should be transfused slowly, preferably with packed cells and intravenous frusemide 20 mg.

Acute malaria results into *thrombocytopenia* which usually recovers within 1–2 weeks of antimalarial treatment.

Disseminated intravascular coagulation is a known complication of severe malaria but pharmacological thromboprophylaxis should be withheld till the platelet count is low, for risk of hemorrhage.

Careful fluid balance and observation of jugular venous pressure (JVP)/central venous pressure (CVP) by central venous access help optimize fluid balance and avoid complications such as acute pulmonary edema and renal failure.

In severe malaria, cardiotocograph monitoring may reveal fetal tachycardia, bradycardia, or late decelerations in relation to fever; signs of fetal distress diminish as the maternal temperature falls.

Stillbirth and premature delivery in malaria in pregnancy are best preventable with prompt and effective antimalarial treatment.

Prevention

According to the WHO latest estimates, many countries with ongoing malaria transmission significantly reduced their disease burden. On a global scale, the rate of new malaria cases declined by 21% between 2010 and 2015 and malaria death rates declined by 29% in the same 5-year period.

In India, the incidence and deaths due to malaria have reduced significantly in recent years. During the period of 2000–2017, cases declined by 58.63% from 2.03 to 0.84 million and deaths declined by 88.85% from 932 to 104 million annually. The *P. falciparum* percentage remained around 50% from 2000 to 2013 but rose to 65.6% in 2016 due to increased *P. falciparum* detection through widespread use of RDTs by trained accredited social health activists (ASHAs).

Closing gaps in access to proven malaria control tools is top priority for the WHO Global Malaria Program. It is divided into two parts:
1. Core vector-control measures
2. Preventive treatment strategies for the most vulnerable groups

In areas with high malaria transmission, young children and pregnant women are particularly vulnerable to malaria infection and death. Apart from high-transmission areas, wherein populations do not acquire significant immunity to malaria, risk is present for all age groups.

Vector-control Measures

- Insecticides-treated nets (ITNs) are the mainstay of malaria-prevention efforts, particularly in sub-Saharan Africa. Long-lasting insecticidal nets (LLINs) have been recommended by the WHO for high-risk population featured to kill mosquitoes for 3 years and then replaced.
- Indoor residual spraying (IRS) is another powerful way to rapidly reduce malaria transmission. It involves spraying of insecticides over indoor walls and ceilings where malaria-carrying mosquitoes are likely to rest after biting household occupants. IRS is effective for 3–6 months and depends upon the insecticide formulation used and type of surface sprayed.

These two core vector-control interventions—use of ITNs and IRS—are considered to have made a major contribution in reduction of malaria burden since 2000.

In specific settings and circumstances, core vector-control tools can be supplemented with other methods:
- Larval source management
- Personal protection measures

Larviciding is recommendable only in areas with few fixed habitats such as in urban and periurban areas of sub-Saharan Africa or rural areas of Asia and the America. At present, 14 formulations are recommended by the WHO Pesticide Evaluation Scheme (WHOPES) for larval control.

Personal protection measures are required to reduce contact between mosquitoes and humans. Supplementary measures may include window screens, insecticide-treated blankets, hammocks, window curtains, repellents, and protective clothing (yet to be formally recommended by WHO).

Intermittent Preventive Treatment of Malaria in Pregnancy

In malaria-endemic areas of Africa, intermittent preventive treatment for all pregnant women with sulfadoxine-pyrimethamine (IPTp-SP) is recommended. The dose is given during the second trimester at a minimum of 1-month interval, with the administration of at least three doses. IPTp reduces maternal and infant mortality, anemia, and other adverse effects of malaria during pregnancy.

Malaria Vaccine

A number of malaria vaccine research projects are underway, but the only vaccine to have completed phase 3 testing is RTS-S/AS01, which reduced clinical incidence by 39% and severe malaria by 31.5% among children aged 5–17 months who completed four doses.

In November 2016, the WHO announced that the RTS-S vaccine would be piloted to three countries in sub-Saharan Africa **(Fig. 3)**.

In India, the Malaria Group at International Centre for Genetic Engineering and Biotechnology (ICGEB), New Delhi, has undertaken efforts to develop vaccines for both *P. vivax* and *P. falciparum* malaria. An ideal malaria vaccine, besides being stable, easily administrable, inexpensive to manufacture, and affordable in poor malaria-endemic countries, should also be safe, highly effective, and provide long-term immunity.

■ DENGUE

Dengue is an emerging vector-borne disease caused by single-stranded ribonucleic acid (RNA) flavivirus. There are four serotypes of dengue virus—DEN1, DEN2, DEN3, and DEN4 transmitted to human by mosquito *Aedes aegypti*. All the four serotypes have been isolated in India, but at present DENV1 and DENV2 serotypes are widespread.

The WHO has estimated that 2.5 billion people live in countries with a high risk for dengue fever, 50 million people are infected annually, and 22,000 deaths result from dengue fever.

In India, the risk of dengue has shown an increase due to rapid urbanization, lifestyle changes, and improper water storage practices in urban, periurban, and rural areas resulting into proliferation of mosquito-breeding areas. During 2017, about 157,996 cases were reported with 253 deaths.

Pregnant women are vulnerable to this disease, which is associated with maternal and neonatal morbidity and mortality. As most of the states in India are dengue endemic, dengue fever should be the differential diagnosis in any FIDP.

Early detection and access to proper medical care reduce fatality from 20 to <1%. Dengue fever is a notifiable disease; every dengue patient should be notified to the Medical Officer of Health (MOH) of that region.

Clinical Course

After the incubation period, the illness begins abruptly and, in patients with moderate-to-severe disease, is followed by three phases clinically: febrile, critical, and recovery. Lack of early recognition and progression leads to complications such as dengue hemorrhagic fever (DHF) and dengue shock syndrome (DSS) **(Fig. 4 and Table 5)**.

Tourniquet test: Positive [inflate BP cuff to midpoint between systolic BP (SBP) and diastolic BP (DBP) for 5 minutes. The test is positive when >10 petechial spots appear/1 sq inch area.]

The Centers for Disease Control and Prevention (CDC) and WHO classification according to severity:

- *Dengue fever (without warning signs):* Fever with two other symptoms such as nausea, vomiting, rashes, myalgia, leukopenia, and positive Tourniquet test
- *Dengue with warning signs:* Abdominal pain, persistent vomiting, ascites, pleural effusion, mucosal bleeding, hepatosplenomegaly, decrease in platelet count, and increased hematocrit (HCT)
- *Severe dengue fever:* Includes DHF and DSS.
  Criteria for severe dengue:
  - Severe plasma leakage leading to shock (DSS), fluid accumulation with respiratory distress
  - Severe bleeding
  - Severe organ involvement
    - *Liver:* Aspartate aminotransferase or alanine aminotransferase > 1,000 IU/L
    - *Central nervous system:* Impaired consciousness
    - Heart and other organs

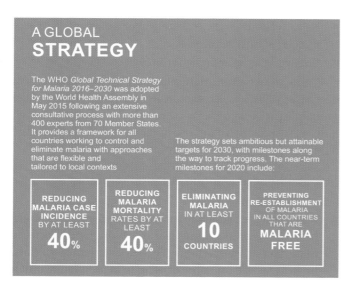

Fig. 3: WHO global strategy to control malaria.
Source: WHO

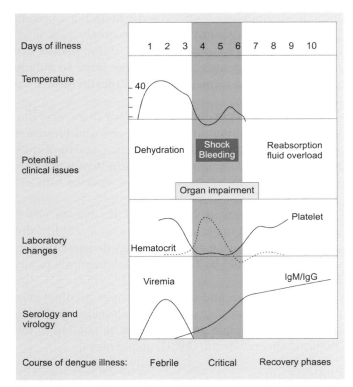

Fig. 4: Course of dengue illness. (IgM = immunoglobulin M; IgG = immunoglobulin G. Temperature is given in degrees Celsius [°C]) Adapted from Yip WCL. Dengue Haemorrhagic Fever: Current Approaches to Management. Medical Progress October 1980. *Courtesy:* WHO, 2009.

TABLE 5:	Symptoms and complications of all three phases of dengue.		
	Febrile phase	*Critical phase*	*Recovery phase*
Symptoms	Fever with headache/ arthralgia/myalgia Tourniquet test +	Fever starts subsiding Warning signs appear	Afebrile
Potential complication	Dehydration	Shock Bleeding Multiorgan involvement	Volume overload
Lab change	WBC low	Platelet low HCT rise	HCT: Stable/ normal WBC increase Platelet increase
	1–4 days	3rd to 6th day	7th to 10th day

(HCT: hematocrit; WBC: white blood cells)

The *new revised classification* given by the Indian Medical Association in December 2015 aims to distinguish confidently between mild, moderate, and severe dengue infection for better use in clinical practice and management **(Flowchart 1)**.

Dengue fever may be due to primary or secondary infection. In primary infection, there is a slow and low titer

of immunoglobulin M (IgM) antibody response. During secondary infection, antibody titers rise dramatically even in acute phase and over the preceding 2 weeks.

Laboratory Diagnosis

A diagnosis of dengue infection is confirmed by the detection of the viral NS1 antigen or seroconversion of IgM or IgG-specific antibody titer.

Rapid NS1 antigen: The government of India recommends use of ELISA (enzyme-linked immunosorbent assay)-based antigen detection test (NS1) 1st day onward.

Dengue IgM: Detected after day 5 of fever by IgM antibody capture ELISA (MAC-ELISA).

Full blood count/complete blood count (FBC/CBC): HCT as a baseline as well as to monitor progress of disease is the most important tool.

Misdiagnosis or delayed diagnosis is very common in pregnancy due to some of the overlapping clinical and/ or laboratory features with better recognized conditions mimicking dengue disease and plasma leakage **(Table 6)**.

- Hyperemesis gravidarum during the first trimester of pregnancy resembles the warning signs of severe dengue, and this may delay the recognition of severe dengue.
- Lower baseline HCT after the second trimester (establishing the baseline HCT during the first 2–3 days of fever is essential for early recognition of plasma leakage)
- Plasma leakage signs such as pleural effusion and ascites could be difficult to elicit in the presence of a gravid uterus.
- Eclampsia or pre-eclampsia
- HELLP (hemolysis, elevated liver enzymes, and low platelet count) syndrome
- Pneumonia, pulmonary embolism

The earliest abnormality in the FBC is a progressive decrease in WBC, which should alert the physician to a high probability of dengue. Clinicians need to maintain a high index of suspicion to diagnose pregnant women with febrile illness living in dengue-endemic areas.

Management of Dengue During Pregnancy (Flowchart 2)

- Management of dengue infection in pregnancy should be taken seriously to reduce morbidity and mortality in mother as well as fetus. The clinical manifestations, treatment, and outcome of dengue in pregnant women are similar to those in nonpregnant women.

Flowchart 1: Revised classification for mild, moderate, and severe dengue (by Indian Medical Association).

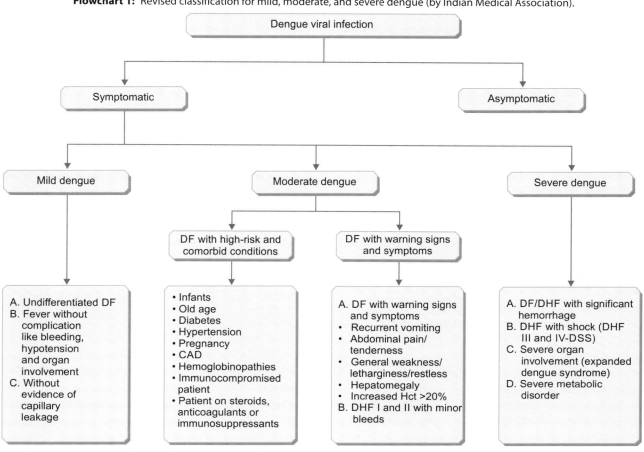

(CAD: coronary artery disease; DF: dengue fever; DHF: dengue hemorrhagic fever; DSS: dengue shock syndrome; Hct: hematocrit)

TABLE 6: Similarities and differences between dengue, pregnancy, and HELLP syndrome.

	Normal pregnancy	*Dengue*	*Hellp*
Fever	Blunted febrile response	+	–
Bleeding	Bleeding can be due to obstetrical cause	+ (mild to severe)	– (DIVC in severe disease)
Abdominal pain	+/–	+/–	+/–
Ascites, pleural effusion	–	+ in plasma leakage	–
WBC	Elevated	Leukopenia	No specific changes
Thrombocytopenia	+	+ unique FBC changes	+
Hematocrit	↓ (hemodilution after the second trimester)	↑ in plasma leakage	Maybe normal/↓
Hemolysis	–	–	+
Liver enzymes	Mild ↑	Mild to severe ↑	Mild to moderate ↑

DIVC = disseminated intravascular coagulopathy, FBC = full blood count HELLP = hemolysis, elevated liver enzymes and low platelet count; WBC = white blood cell

- Conservative medical and obstetrical management is the treatment of choice.
- Early admission and close follow-up with FBC daily is very important.

- The gestation and the phase of dengue are important factors in determining the management. A discussion with the team of obstetrician, physician, and pediatrician about the management is mandatory.

Flowchart 2: Dengue case management.

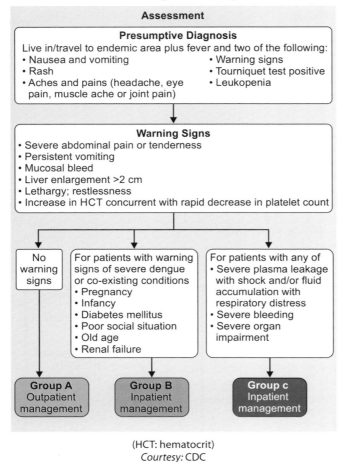

(HCT: hematocrit)
Courtesy: CDC

- Consultation with and explanation to the family members about the course of DHF and its management are also important for decision-making.

Dengue Fever without Warning Signs (Group A)

- Monitor vital parameters and intake–output charting 4 hourly.
    - *Labs:* Daily CBC, other investigations if necessary
- *Treatment:*
    - Paracetamol and tepid sponging for fever
    - Plenty of fluids and routine food advised (2.5 L of liquids) in case of nausea/vomiting of pregnancy; IV fluid [normal saline (NS)] 100 cc/h is given.
    - Watchful vigilance for warning sign, especially when fever starts subsiding
    - Rise in HCT (20% of baseline) (if baseline is not known, consider 36 as baseline)

Dengue Fever with Warning Signs (Group B)

- Monitor vitals (BP/P/pulse pressure, capillary refill) hourly.

- Catheterize to know precise urine output hourly (aim 0.5 mL/kg/h).
- Intense fluid resuscitation (NS). Bolus of 5–10 mL/kg/h × 2 hours given followed by 3–5 mL/kg/h as maintenance. This is monitored by urine output and pulse pressure.
- The fluid volume for the critical period (M + 5%) for a pregnant mother should be calculated based on the weight prior to pregnancy.

Pearls for Obstetric Management

The risk of bleeding is at its highest during the period of plasma leakage (critical phase). Therefore,

- Tocolytic agents and measures to postpone labor to a suitable time may be considered.
- Avoid induction of labor/planned surgery in this phase.
- If delivery is inevitable, it should take place in a hospital where blood/blood components and a team of skilled obstetricians and a neonatologist are available.
- Operative delivery for obstetric indications only
- Blood and blood products should be cross-matched and saved in preparation for delivery.
- Prophylactic platelet transfusion is not recommended unless obstetrically indicated.
- There is NO role of steroid/IVIG/prophylactic antibiotics.
- Trauma or injury should be kept to the minimum if possible.
- Ergotamine and/or oxytocin infusion as per the standard obstetrical practice should be commenced to contract the uterus after delivery to prevent postpartum hemorrhage.
- It is essential to check for complete removal of the placenta after delivery.
- If severe hemorrhage occurs, replacement with transfusion of fresh whole blood/fresh packed red cells should be promptly instituted.

Risk of Vertical Transmission

The risk of vertical transmission is well established among women with dengue during the perinatal period. After delivery, the newborn may go into shock and severe fetal or neonatal dengue illness, and death may occur when there is insufficient time for the production of protective maternal antibodies which may be confused with septic shock or birth trauma. History of FIDP is important, which may help to diagnose DSS among neonates and infants. Close observation and symptomatic and supportive treatment are the mainstay of management. Congenital infection could eventually be suspected on clinical grounds and then confirmed in the laboratory.

Adverse Pregnancy Outcome

It is still uncertain whether dengue is a significant factor for adverse pregnancy outcomes such as preterm birth, low birth weight, and cesarean deliveries.

Convalescent Phase

- Rise of WBC count followed by rise of platelet count and stabilization of HCT are features of the convalescent phase.
- Signs of fluid overload—cough, wheeze, and tachypnea should be monitored.
- Rise of both SBP and DBP is observed.

Discharge from Hospital

- When the patient becomes afebrile for 24 hours without antipyretics with improved appetite
- Rising trends of WBC and platelets seen along with normal HCT at baseline value

Dengue Fever with Shock on Admission (Group C)

A patient's transfer to a critical care unit with a multidisciplinary approach is advised for further management. While transferring this patient, recent CBC, HCT, electrolytes, and other investigations along with fluid bolus before and during transfer should be done with all reports. Further management in a critical care unit is done according to standard protocols given by CDC and WHO with the help of algorithms **(Flowcharts 3 to 6)** as per the condition of the patient.

■ H1N1 (SWINE FLU)

H1N1 is an emerging global concern and needs a close vigilance as over the period, potential worldwide epidemics and pandemic outbreaks have been witnessed.

Epidemiology

According to WHO, H1N1 caused pandemic in 2009 which got over in August 2010. It had origination from Mexico on March 18, 2009, spreading across all origin. The first case reported in India was on May 13, 2009, and postpandemic affected individuals from all age groups in 2017–2018.

India reported 937 cases of H1N1 and 218 deaths with a case fatality rate of 23.2% in the year 2014. According to the latest report by the Ministry of Health and Family Welfare, H1N1 affected 8,543 people between 2010 and October 2017 and a 20-fold rise in the number of cases was seen in the year 2017. The states worst affected were Gujarat and Rajasthan followed by Delhi and Tamil Nadu with lesser death toll in the latter due to awareness and a developed healthcare sector **(Fig. 5)**.

H1N1 During Pregnancy

Among the general population, pregnant women are four to five times more likely to develop influenza-associated complications, increased severity of disease, and death, especially if they have comorbidities.

The complications are increased due to alterations in the heart rate, lung function and immunological function, preterm labor pain, and severe pneumonia.

If the woman develops hyperthermia during the early pregnancy, then found to be associated with congenital anomalies such as neural tube defects. If fever develops during labor, then the infant may get predisposed to neonatal seizures, cerebral palsy, newborn encephalopathy, and death.

Complications during the pregnancy are spontaneous fetal loss, nonreassuring fetal heart rate (commonly fetal tachycardia), febrile morbidity, and preterm delivery. In infants, the complications are prolonged vomiting, diarrhea, or inability to feed leading to poor nutritional status.

Pathogenesis

H1N1 is a subtype of influenza A, an orthomyxoviridae RNA virus classified on the basis of surface proteins Hemagglutinin (H) and Neuraminidase (N). H1N1 is also referred to as "swine flu" which is a misnomer. At times, it is denoted as Influenza A(H1N1)pdm09 as this pandemic was caused in the year 2009. The time-to-time epidemic or pandemic outbreaks occur due to antigenic drift and shift of the virus.

- Transmission—airborne from human to human via:
  - Large droplets (expulsion while speaking, sneezing, or coughing)
  - Direct or indirect contact by contaminated hands and surfaces
- Incubation period—ranges from 1 to 4 days
- Period of communicability—1 day before to 7 days after the onset of symptoms

Clinical Presentation

- Mild symptoms—fever, rhinitis, sore throat, cough, tachypnea, headache, fatigueness, diarrhea, and vomiting
- Severe/danger symptoms—shortness of breath, breathlessness, chest pain, altered mental state, and hypotension
- Common causes of death—respiratory failure and refractory shock (secondary to severe pneumonia with multiorgan failure)

Flowchart 3: Group B—inpatient management for dengue patients with warning signs.

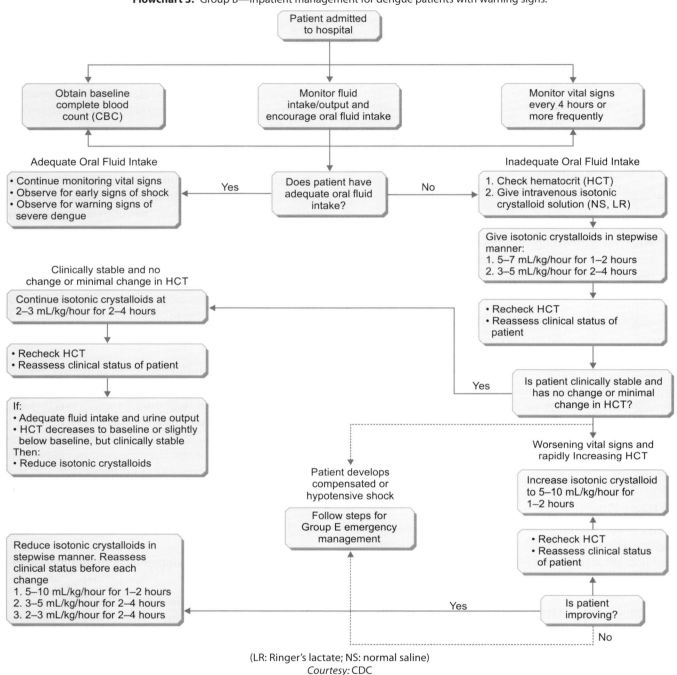

(LR: Ringer's lactate; NS: normal saline)
Courtesy: CDC

Diagnosis

- *Definition by CDC*
  - *Confirmed case:* Individuals with influenzae-like illness and laboratory-confirmed H1N1 subtype of influenza A either by real-time (RT) –PCR or by culture
  - *Probable case:* Individuals with influenza-like illness and test positive for influenza A by RT-PCR

or in whom the strain of infection has not been determined
- *Routine investigations:* CBC, liver function test, renal function test, chest X-ray, and coagulation profile
- *Specific investigations:*
  - Rapid influenza diagnostic tests (RIDTs) which detect viral antigen-stimulating immune response and provide results within 10–15 minutes

Flowchart 4: Management of hemorrhagic tendencies.

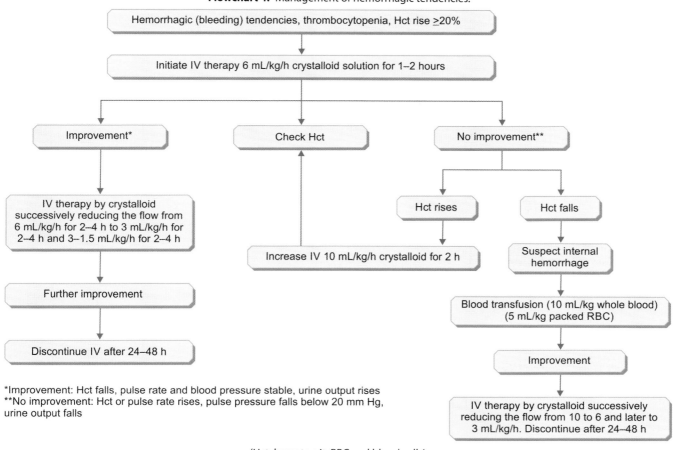

(Hct: hematocrit; RBC: red blood cells)
Courtesy: CDC

– *Other flu tests:* Rapid molecular assay which detects genetic material of virus produces results in 15–20 minutes and is more accurate than RIDTs

■ *Investigations for confirmation of diagnosis:* Samples obtained before antiviral therapy, i.e., swabs from nasopharyngeal or throat or nasal, tracheal aspirate from intubated patients

– RT-PCR

– Cultures

– Specific antibody titer—about 4-fold rise

Management

Antepartum

■ Implementation of infection control measures such as isolation of infected case, well-ventilated wards with beds at 1 m apart, restricted entries of people inside ward, dispose waste as biohazardous

■ Wear masks, gowns, gloves, caps, and shoe-covers before entering the ward.

Supportive Therapy (Table 7 and Flowchart 7)

■ Intravenous fluids, parenteral nutrition, oxygen therapy, ventilator support, paracetamol, treating coinfection, and corticosteroids in preterm cases. Aspirin is contraindicated as it causes Reye's syndrome.

■ *Specific:* Oseltamivir at a dose of 75 mg twice daily for 5 days is recommended as a safe drug for prophylaxis and treatment.

■ Oseltamivir (oral drug) and zanamivir (inhaled as dry powder) are neuraminidase inhibitors.

– *Mechanism of action:* Viral surface glycoprotein (hemagglutin) binds to sialic acid residues over respiratory epithelial surface glycoproteins, necessary for the initiation of infection. As the virus replicates, it attaches to the host cell in the same way until neuraminidase cleaves the link and free the new virions.

– *Side effects:* Nausea and vomiting but respiratory distress is the matter of concern.

Flowchart 5: Management of compensated shock.

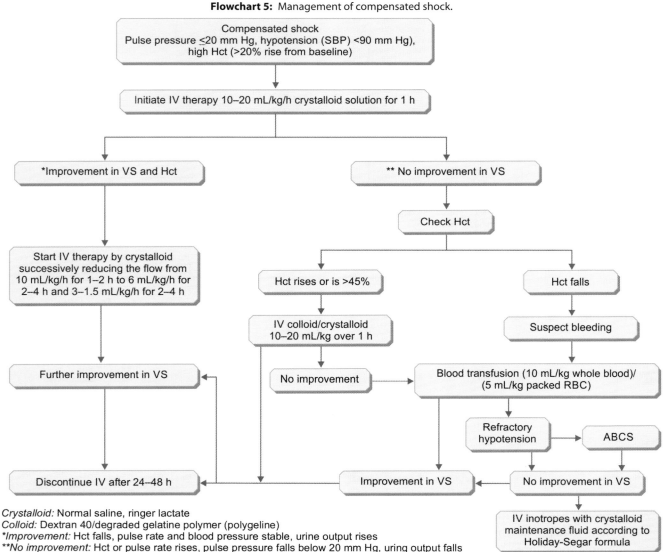

Crystalloid: Normal saline, ringer lactate
Colloid: Dextran 40/degraded gelatine polymer (polygeline)
*Improvement: Hct falls, pulse rate and blood pressure stable, urine output rises
**No improvement: Hct or pulse rate rises, pulse pressure falls below 20 mm Hg, uring output falls
• *Unstable vital signs:* Urine output falls, signs of shock
• In cases of acidosis, hyperosmolar or Ringer's lactate solution should not be used
• *Serial platelet and Hct determinations:* Drop in platelets and rise in Hct are essential for early diagnosis of DHF
• Cases of DHF should be observed every hour for vital signs and urine output

(DBP: diastolic blood pressure; DHF: dengue hemorrhagic fever; Hct: hematocrit; RBC: red blood cells; SBP: systolic blood pressure; ABCS: acidosis, bleeding, calcium (Na^{++} and K$^+$), sugar; VS: volemic status)
Courtesy: CDC
Source: Journal of the Indian Medical Association. 2015;113:12.

Vaccine

- The WHO and Indian Council of Medical Research (ICMR) recommend vaccination yearly.
- Vaccine is given to healthcare workers in hospitals and institutions, team in contact with infected cases, pregnant women (irrespective of gestation), persons with immunodeficiency or immunocompromised status, and persons with systemic diseases such as chronic obstructive pulmonary disease, bronchial asthma, diabetes, and heart disease.

- H1N1 monovalent vaccine (FDA approved) can be given as intramuscular (inactivated) to individuals > 6 months old and pregnant women and also as intranasal spray (live).
- Live intranasal vaccine is contraindicated in pregnant women, individuals < 2 years old and > 50 years old, and in presence of systemic disease while inactivated vaccine is contraindicated in cases of anaphylaxis.
- Pregnant women (of any trimester) and breastfeeding mothers should receive recommended, age-appropriate, licensed, inactivated influenza vaccine.

Flowchart 6: Management of profound shock.

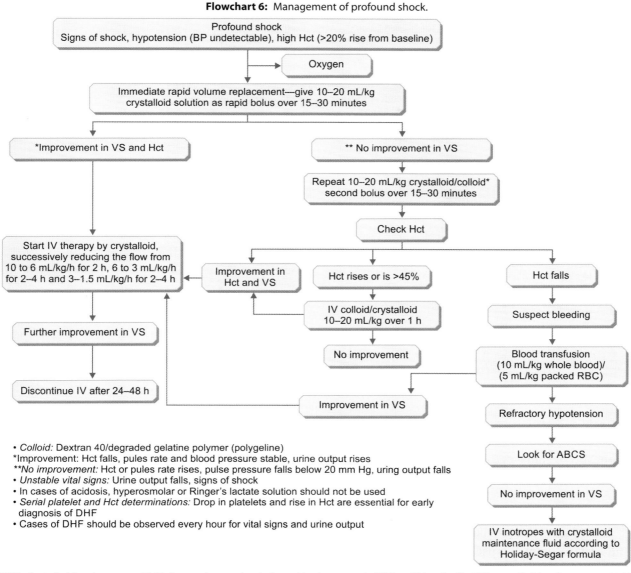

- *Colloid:* Dextran 40/degraded gelatine polymer (polygeline)
- *Improvement: Hct falls, pules rate and blood pressure stable, urine output rises
- **No improvement:* Hct or pules rate rises, pulse pressure falls below 20 mm Hg, uring output falls
- *Unstable vital signs:* Urine output falls, signs of shock
- In cases of acidosis, hyperosmolar or Ringer's lactate solution should not be used
- *Serial platelet and Hct determinations:* Drop in platelets and rise in Hct are essential for early diagnosis of DHF
- Cases of DHF should be observed every hour for vital signs and urine output

(DBP: diastolic blood pressure; DHF: dengue hemorrhagic fever; Hct: hematocrit; RBC: red blood cells; SBP: systolic blood pressure; ABCS: acidosis, bleeding, calcium (Na^{++} and K$^+$), sugar; VS: volemic status)
Courtesy: CDC
Souce: Journal of the Indian Medical Association. 2015;113:12.

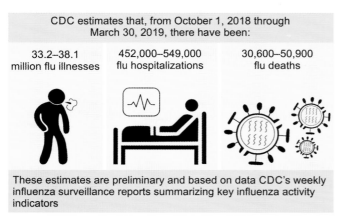

CDC estimates that, from October 1, 2018 through March 30, 2019, there have been:

33.2–38.1 million flu illnesses

452,000–549,000 flu hospitalizations

30,600–50,900 flu deaths

These estimates are preliminary and based on data CDC's weekly influenza surveillance reports summarizing key influenza activity indicators

Fig. 5: CDC data of flu illnesses from October 1, 2018, to March 30, 2019.

TABLE 7: Antiviral medication dosing recommendations for treatment or chemoprophylaxis of novel influenza A (H1N1) infection.		
Agent, group	*Treatment*	*Chemoprophylaxis*
Oseltamivir		
Adults	75 mg capsule twice per day for 5 days	75 mg capsule once per day for 10 days
Zanamivir		
Adults	Two 5 mg inhalations (10 mg total) twice per day for 5 days	Two 5 mg inhalations (10 mg total) once per day for 10 days

Courtesy: CDC

Flowchart 7: Suspected influenza A infection.

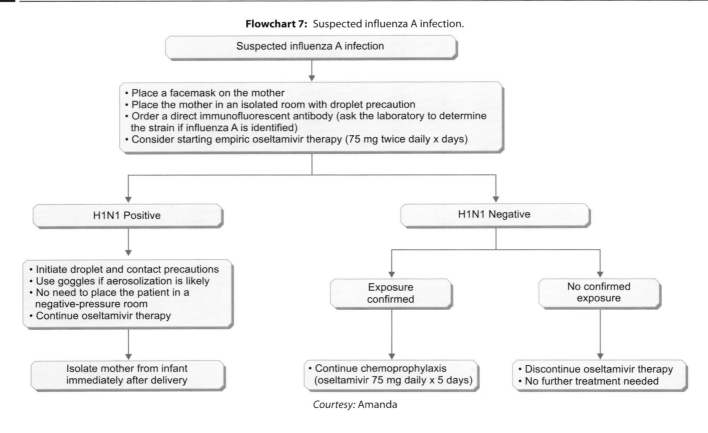

Courtesy: Amanda

- It is safe and effective for administration with (Tdap) vaccine during the same antenatal visit.
- The ICMR recommended trivalent vaccine for 2017–2018 constituting of the following strains:
  - A/Michigan/45/2015 (H1N1)pdm09-like virus
  - A/Hong Kong/4801/2014 (H3N2)-like virus
  - B/Brisbane/60/2008-like virus
- The WHO recommends use of quadrivalent vaccines in 2018–2019 in the northern hemisphere constituting of the following strains:
  - A/Michigan/45/2015 (H1N1)pdm09-like virus
  - A/Singapore/INFIMH-16-0019/2016 (H3N2)-like virus
  - B/Phuket/3073/2013-like virus (B/Yamagata/16/88 lineage)
  - B/Colorado/06/2017-like virus (B/Victoria/2/87 lineage)
- The efficacy of the vaccine is about 70–80% and helps in prevention of severe complications of influenza.
- It takes about 2–3 weeks for development of immunity by the use of vaccine.
- Influenza immunization prevents one to two hospitalizations per 1,000 pregnant women and reduces stillbirth by 50%.

Chemoprophylaxis

- Recommended for contact with cases, pregnant women, within 2 weeks postpartum, family members, workplace or school mates, co-travelers, and health care personnel
- *Drug of choice:* Oseltamivir 75 mg once a day for 10 days and is effective till 10 days after the last exposure

Intrapartum

- Protection of infant against infected secretions by usage of face mask by the mother, using the respirator within 6 feet of the infectious patient, and universal precautions at the time of delivery
- Upon delivery, the newborn is immediately separated from the mother and kept in a warmer at a distance of >6 feet.
- Infected women are prone to higher risk of fetal distress and operative delivery.
- Antivirals for 15 days are recommended for all pregnant women and within 2 weeks postpartum.
- Bathe the newborn once the temperature stabilizes.

Postpartum

- Temporary separation of newborn is considered.
- *Contact criteria (between mother and baby):* If the mother received antiviral medication for minimum

48 hours, has no temperature spikes for 24 hours without antipyretics, and has control over cough with respiratory secretions

Newborn

- A newborn during delivery may be exposed to infected respiratory secretions and also lacks immunologic competence which gradually develops over the first few months.
- Prevention against exposure to virus from the infected persons at home.
- Antiviral chemoprophylaxis is not indicated up till 3 months of infancy, but antivirals may be required in cases of severe or deteriorating illness.
- Human milk is considered noninfectious unlike other body secretions; hence, breastfeeding is not contraindicated once the criteria for the close contact are met.
- *To infants < 14 days old:* Oseltamivir 3 mg/kg/dose once daily for 5 days
- *To older infants:* Oseltamivir 3 mg/kg/dose twice daily for 5 days

■ VARICELLA/CHICKENPOX

Varicella or chickenpox is an acute infection caused by varicella zoster virus (VZV), a DNA virus of the herpes family which is highly contagious. It is a self-limiting primary infection seen mainly during childhood. Herpes zoster is the reactivation of VZV that occurs in immunosuppression, old age, or hormonal changes.

Epidemiology

Varicella has worldwide distribution. In temperate countries, most of the cases can be seen during winter and spring with higher prevalence among children leading to immunity in about 90% pregnant women excluding the migrants from tropic countries. In the tropic countries, the older age group is vulnerable to infection leading to adverse outcomes **(Fig. 7)**.

During the year 2013 in India, about 28,090 chickenpox cases with 61 deaths were reported with a case fatality rate of 0.21%. Kerala was reported with the highest chickenpox cases (12,168) while West Bengal had the maximum number of deaths (68) from chickenpox.

The incidence of varicella in pregnancy is 1–7 cases per 10,000 pregnancies while herpes zoster is less common, 0.5 per 10,000 pregnancies.

Pathogenesis

- Exposure to antigen produces host immunoglobulins (IgG, IgM, and IgA). IgG leads to cell-mediated immune response limiting the duration of primary infection.
- VZV remains latent in dorsal sensory nerve ganglion cells by immune response but upon reactivation it causes herpes zoster.
- The average incubation period of varicella is 14–16 days.
- Human is the only source.
- Entry of virus is via conjunctiva and mucous membranes of the nasopharynx. Transmission occurs through droplet nuclei, direct contact, and transplacental to fetus.
- One attack of varicella results in permanent immunity with 95% predictive value.

Clinical Presentation (Fig. 8)

- Short prodromal period of 1–2 days characterized by fever and malaise
- Disease is infectious— 48 hours of rash appearance until vesicles crust over within 5 days
- Pruritic rashes develop into maculopapules which turn into vesicular and crust upon healing.
- The rash appears first on head progressing to trunk and extremities with the highest concentration over the trunk.

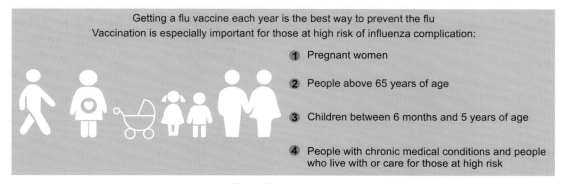

Getting a flu vaccine each year is the best way to prevent the flu
Vaccination is especially important for those at high risk of influenza complication:

1. Pregnant women
2. People above 65 years of age
3. Children between 6 months and 5 years of age
4. People with chronic medical conditions and people who live with or care for those at high risk

Fig. 6 Flu vaccination.
Source: WHO 2019.

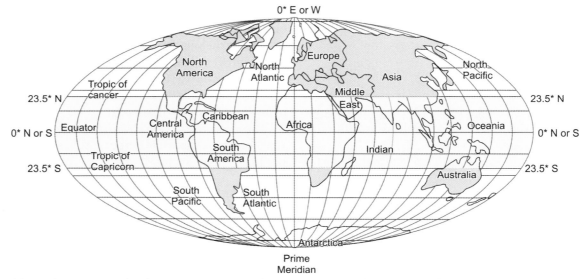

Fig. 7: World map showing tropical and temperate zone. Topical zones are shown within the Tropic of Cancer and Tropic of Capricorn. Tropical climates have high temperatures throughout the year. Subtropical climates are found adjacent to the tropics. Temperate climates have mild to warm summers and cool winters (most European countries). Some countries have a mixture of climates. Map reproduced with kind permission of: www.worldatlas.com
Courtesy: NHS guidelines.

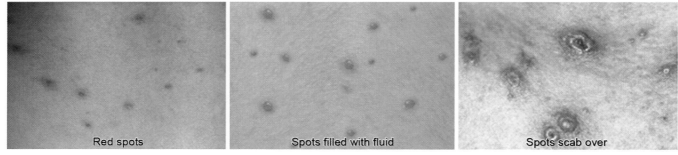

Fig. 8: Clinical presentation of varicella zoster virus.

- New lesions are seen throughout the course of infection with variable clinical presentations present at the same time, i.e., pleomorphism.

Maternal and Fetal Outcomes

- Pregnant women have higher systemic complications such as hepatitis, pneumonia, encephalitis, cerebellar ataxia, and sepsis
- Maternal pneumonia complicates 10–20% of cases in pregnancy which increase with increasing gestational age and also result in higher mortality.
- The vertical transmission rate during the first and second trimesters is about 8–9%.
- If maternal infection occurs before 20 weeks of gestation, then the congenital varicella in fetus accounts to nearly 10% cases.
- Congenital varicella/fetal varicella syndrome features are skin lesions (70%), limb hypoplasia (46–72%), muscle hypoplasia, neurological-like microcephaly, cortical atrophy, hydrocephaly and ventriculomegaly, mental retardation (48–62%), ocular defects such as microphthalmia, chorioretinitis and cataract (44–52%), developmental delay, intrauterine growth restriction (IUGR), placental anomalies, and hydrops fetalis
- If a woman delivers 5 days before or 2 days after the onset of rash, the newborn is at risk for neonatal varicella with mortality about 30% which has reduced to about 7% due to use of VZV immunoglobulin (VZV Ig).

Differential Diagnosis (for Varicella Infection)

Insect bites, impetigo, dermatitis herpetiformis, smallpox, drug eruptions

Diagnosis

- Primary diagnosis is based upon clinical presentation.
- The diagnosis is confirmed by detection of IgM or isolation of VZV by PCR. PCR is the most sensitive test

and samples obtained are vesicle fluid, cerebrospinal fluid, serum, tissues, and amniotic fluid.

- Direct fluorescent assay (DFA) is another rapid test that replaced Tzanck test and is performed on scrapings from base of skin lesion.
- Serological tests are not used to diagnose acute infection as they provide false-negative results among immune-compromised patients and early infections while false positives following blood transfusion.

- Antenatally, fetal varicella can be diagnosed using ultrasound after 5 weeks following the maternal primary infection.

Management (Flowchart 8)

Antenatal

- Symptomatic treatment, hygiene, counseling about risks and consequences, routine antenatal care, and fetal monitoring

Flowchart 8: Algorithm for the management of varicella-zoster contact in pregnancy.

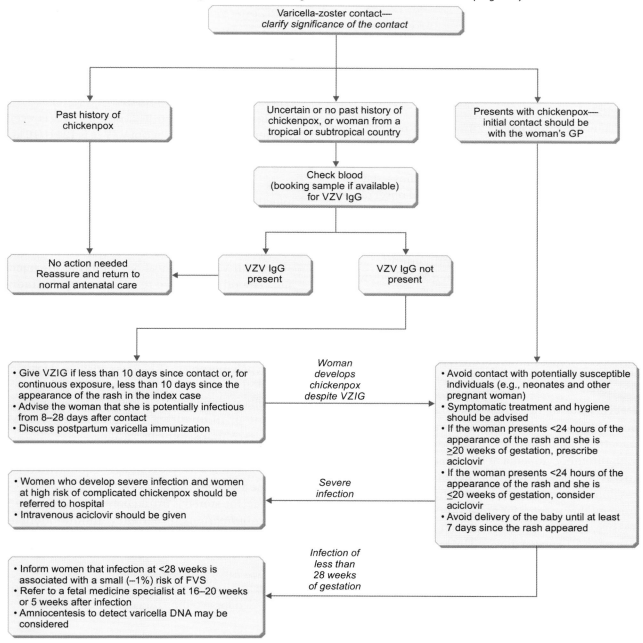

(FVS: fetal varicella syndrome; GP: general practitioner; IgG: immunoglobulin G; VZIG: varicella-zoster immunoglobulin; VZV: varicella-zoster virus)

Courtesy: RCOG Green Top Guideline No. 13 & NHS- Varicella Zoster Virus (VZV) (Chickenpox) and Shingles in Maternity / 08072/ 5.0

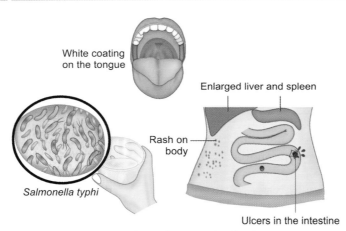

White coating
on the tongue

Enlarged liver and spleen

Rash on
body

Salmonella typhi

Ulcers in the intestine

Fig. 9: Clinical features of typhoid.

- Pregnant women having respiratory discomfort or immune-compromised are referred to a tertiary care hospital.
- Varicella infection before 28 weeks of pregnancy to be referred to a fetal medicine specialist 5 weeks after infection or at 16–20 weeks for detailed ultrasonography.
- Oral Acyclovir of dosage 800 mg five times a day for 7 days is recommended within 24 hours of onset of rash, if the gestation period is ≥20 weeks.
- If <20 weeks of gestation, use of acyclovir is to be considered.
- Intravenous Acyclovir is recommended in severe chickenpox cases—dosage 10–15 mg/kg of body weight intravenously every 8 hours for 5–10 days, started within 24–72 hours of developing rash.
- Acyclovir is a synthetic nucleoside analog of guanine highly specific to VSV-infected cells and inhibits viral DNA polymerase hindering the replication of virus.

Intrapartum
- Delivery during the viremia or when the vesicles are active can be extremely hazardous and can precipitate maternal hemorrhage or coagulopathy in association with thrombocytopenia or hepatitis.
- Intravenous acyclovir is recommended for rash resolution, immune recovery, and transfer of antibodies from mother to fetus for protection.
- Passive transfer of immunoglobulins to baby occurs 7 day relapse between the onset of rash and delivery.
- The needle placement site for epidural or spinal anesthesia is to be devoid of cutaneous lesions.
- Keep the neonatologist prior informed about maternal infection.

Postpartum
- Mothers having chickenpox within 7 days before or after delivery have to be administered VZV Ig ± Acyclovir.

- Breastfeeding is not contraindicated.
- Infant requires monitoring of 14–16 days for signs of infection and is treated with acyclovir if infected.

Prevention
Control

The measures taken are notifying the disease, case isolation, and disinfection of articles soiled with nasal and throat discharges. Contact with the infected cases has to be avoided.

Varicella Zoster Virus Immunoglobulin
- VZV Ig is effective if received within 72–96 hours of exposure to VZV but can be administered within 10 days of contact.
- Nonimmune pregnant females are considered potentially infectious from 8 to 21 days after exposure if VZV Ig is not received and 8–28 days if VZV Ig is received.
- The recommended dosage of VZV Ig is 125 U/10 kg to a maximum of 625 U or alternatively 1 mg/kg body weight.
- The second dose is administered in cases of lapse of 3 weeks from the last dose continuing to be exposed to infection.
- The intravenous route of administration demonstrated to have rapid attaining of optimal serum levels over the intramuscular route. The most common adverse effect with VZV Ig is local discomfort at the injection site. The other adverse reactions are pain, redness, gastrointestinal symptoms, headache, rash, etc.

Vaccine
- VZV DNA classification based upon restriction fragment length polymorphism (RFLP) is considered for vaccine selection.
- Varicella vaccine can be administered as monovalent vaccine or in quadrivalent form along with MMR (Measles, Mumps, Rubella) vaccine.
- The children of age group 1–12 years require one dose while children > 12 years of age require two doses of vaccine 4–6 weeks apart.
- This vaccine stored is frozen between –58°F and +5°F.
- *Contraindications:* Pregnancy, immunodeficiency state, high steroid therapy, allergy to neomycin, active tuberculosis, severe systemic disease, aspirin intake, recent blood transfusion
- All the nonimmune women should be vaccinated and counseled for avoiding pregnancy for 1 month.

■ TYPHOID

Typhoid fever, also known as enteric fever, is a systemic infection caused by gram-negative bacterium *Salmonella enterica* serotype Typhi (typhoid fever) or *S. enterica* serotype paratyphi A, B, or C (paratyphoid fever) and is a major public-health problem in developing countries.

According to WHO data sheet 2018, the estimated global typhoid disease burden is 11–20 million cases with 128,000–161,000 deaths annually, the maximum number of cases being from Asia. The disease is now uncommon in the developed countries where majority of the disease burden is acquired through travelers to and from endemic areas.

Typhoid fever is endemic in India. Reported data for the year 2017 shows 2.22 million cases and 493 deaths. The incidence of infection with *Salmonella* in pregnant patients is similar to the general population (0.2%).

Etiopathogenesis

Human carriers are the only known reservoir of the disease.

The common mode of transmission is by ingestion of an infecting dose of the organism via the fecal-oral route or urine-oral routes. This may take place directly through soiled hands contaminated with feces or urine of cases or carriers or indirectly by the ingestion of contaminated water and food/milk or through flies.

The incubation period usually lasts for 10–14 days. But it may be as short as 3 days or as long as 3 weeks depending upon the dose of the bacilli ingested.

Salmonellae are gram-negative, nonsporulating, flagellate, facultative intracellular, anaerobic bacilli. *S. enterica* typhi is the most common etiological agent and *S. enterica* paratyphi A, B, or C accounts for a very much lower number of cases (around 3–17%) of enteric fever. *S. typhi* has three main antigens: 0, H, and Vi. *S. typhi* is an intracellular bacterium that resides within the modified phagosomes of antigen-presenting cells (APCs) in the tissues of various organs. A recurrent febrile response is usually seen after the bacteria invade the mucosa of the small intestine which, in turn, causes a transient bacteremia. This is followed by continued multiplication of organisms within phagocytic cells and sustained episodes of secondary bacteremia. These microbes disseminate via the hematogenous route and have at least partially intracellular life cycles.

The clinical presentation of human salmonellosis usually ranges from an asymptomatic, chronic carrier state to acute gastroenteritis, septicemia, or even death in untreated cases.

The onset of bacteremia is accompanied by malaise, vague abdominal discomfort, cough, myalgia, and fever usually without rigors, a syndrome easily mistaken for a viral illness at its onset, or cholecystitis. The characteristic feature is high temperature (39–40°C) persistent uptill the second week. The erythematous "rose spot" rash is present in 5–30% cases.

Cell-mediated (innate) immunity is important in curtailing infection during the first week of infection when CD4 T-cells response is detectable. CD8 T-cells response is delayed until the second week postinfection.

Serious complications are reported in 10–15% of patients who have been ill for more than 2 weeks due to delayed diagnosis and treatment in underprivileged regions with gastrointestinal bleeding and hepatic dysfunction. Perforation of necrotic Peyer's patches occurs in 1–3% of hospital inpatients. Confusion and obtundation may obscure intestinal perforation and are often accompanied by septic shock.

Pregnant females are at a higher risk of severe infection due to:
- Modulation of cell-mediated immunity (type 1) with a shift to humoral immunity (type 2) that is even more pronounced at the fetomaternal interface.
- Nausea and vomiting of pregnancy and decreased gastrointestinal motility result into delayed diagnosis and reduced response through antibiotic treatment.

Enteric fever during pregnancy can result in miscarriage (65–80%), stillbirth, preterm labor, and neonatal sepsis. The incidence of fetal loss in untreated typhoid can be as high as 80%.

Vertical transmission in enteric fever occurs through:
- Fetomaternal interface (transplacental)
- Ongoing bacteremia during labor
- Fecal contamination of birth canal

Management

It is of paramount importance that the diagnosis of enteric fever should be considered in FIDP with prompt institution of antibiotic therapy which is necessary for improved maternal and fetal prognosis.

Laboratory Diagnosis of Typhoid

Microbiological Procedures

The definitive diagnosis of typhoid fever depends on the isolation of *S. typhi* from blood, bone marrow, and stools prior to antibiotic treatment. Blood cultures are positive early in the course of infection, while stool cultures are positive later in the course of the infection. Cultures of multiple sites (urine, amniotic fluid, skin scrapings, bone marrow) improve the yield of a positive culture in a pregnant female.

Serological Procedure

The Felix-Widal test measures agglutinating antibody levels against O and H antigens. Usually, O antibodies appear on days 6–8 and H antibodies on days 10–12 after the onset of disease. Though having moderate sensitivity and specificity, the Widal test provides a fast and affordable option for testing typhoid fever in endemic areas with limited resources.

New Diagnostic Tests

The recent advances for quick and reliable diagnostic tests for typhoid fever as an alternative to the Widal test include the following:

IDL Tubex® test detects IgM09 antibodies within a few minutes

Typhidot® detects specific IgM and IgG antibodies against a 50-kD antigen and takes 3 hours; a newer version of Typhidot-M® detects specific IgM antibodies only.

The *dipstick test* is based on the binding of *S. typhi*-specific IgM antibodies in samples to *S. typhi* lipopolysaccharide (LPS) antigen and the staining of bound antibodies by an antihuman IgM antibody conjugated to colloidal dye particles.

General Principles for the Management of Typhoid

There should be rapid diagnosis and institution of appropriate antibiotic treatment.

Adequate rest, hydration, and correction of fluid-electrolyte imbalance are recommended.

Antipyretic therapy is given as required (such as paracetamol 120–750 mg taken orally every 4–6 hours)

Adequate nutrition: A soft, easily digestible diet should be continued unless the patient has abdominal distension or ileus.

Close attention should be paid to hand washing and limitation of close contact with susceptible individuals during the acute phase of infection

Ampicillin or amoxicillin is considered the first-line drug during pregnancy. Ceftriaxone is the preferred drug in pregnancy followed by oral cephalosporins. The treatment should continue for 7–14 days' duration.

Surgery may be required in the case of internal bleeding or splits in sections of the digestive system; however, these complications are rare after appropriate treatment with antibiotics.

Successful antibiotic treatment should be followed by stool cultures in pregnant patients to monitor persistent shedding of the bacteria as they are at an increased risk of relapse due to altered biliary motility and bone marrow activity, especially in inadequately treated patients.

Prevention

Protection and purification of drinking water supplies, improvement of basic sanitation, and promotion of food hygiene are essential measures to interrupt transmission of typhoid fever. Salmonellosis, in spite of being a dreadful illness in pregnancy, can easily be prevented by simple measures, such as hand hygiene, and avoidance of eating contaminated food, water, and animal products as the causative organism can be killed by drying, pasteurization, and common disinfectants.

While ultimately, control of typhoid fever must take the form of improved sanitation and domestic and personal hygiene, these are long-term objectives in many developing countries. A complementary approach to prevention is immunization, which is the only specific preventive measure, likely to yield the highest benefit for the money spent.

Immunization against typhoid does not give 100% protection, but it definitely lowers both the incidence and the seriousness of the infection. It is recommended to (1) those living in endemic areas, (2) household contacts, (3) groups at risk of infection such as school children and hospital staff, (4) travelers proceeding to endemic areas, and (5) those attending melas and yatras.

Two safe and effective vaccines are now licensed and available. Typhoid vaccines (both polysaccharide and live vaccine) are category C drugs during pregnancy.

Vi Polysaccharide Vaccine

The Vi capsular polysaccharide vaccine provides effective immunity for 2 years with a single dose administered subcutaneously or intramuscularly. It is safe to use during pregnancy since it is a purified Vi capsular polysaccharide bacterial component from the Ty2 *S. typhi* strain and not a live vaccine. Frequent travelers or long-term residents in high-risk areas need boosters every third year.

Ty2 la Vaccine

The oral live attenuated bacterial vaccine (Ty21a) strain of *S. typhi* is available as enteric-coated capsules. A three-dose regimen is recommended every alternate day, 1st, 3rd, and 5th day, without simultaneous consumption of antibiotic or antimicrobial medication. The oral Ty21a vaccine is not recommended for pregnant patients because of their diminished gastrointestinal motility and frequent nausea and vomiting. The recommendation is to repeat every 3 years for people living in endemic areas and every year for individuals travelling from nonendemic to endemic countries.

Salmonellosis in the mother should be considered as a differential diagnosis in febrile FIDP, to prevent fetal and maternal morbidity. Only a high index of suspicion depending on the clinical presentation, along with proper laboratory diagnostics, can help in initiation of appropriate therapy in pregnancy to save the lives of these fetuses.

■ SUGGESTED READING

Malaria

1. AIIMS. National Anti-Malaria Programme. [online] Available from http://www.rfhha.org/images/pdf/national_health/NATIONAL_ANTI_MALARIA_CONTROL_PROG.pdf. [Last accessed September, 2020]

2. Center for Disease Control and Prevention. (2019). CDC Treatment Guidelines. [online] Available from https://www.cdc.gov/malaria/resources/pdf/clinicalguidance.pdf [Last accessed September, 2020]

3. Centers for Diseases Control and Prevention. (2019). CDC guidelines for treatment of malaria in the United States. [online] Available from https://www.cdc.gov/malaria/resources/pdf/treatmenttable.pdf [Last accessed September, 2020]

4. Dunn JS, Nour NM. Malaria and pregnancy: A global health perspective. Rev Obstet Gynecol. 2009;2(3):186-92.

5. Gaillard T, Boxberger M, Madamet M, Pradines B. Has doxycycline, in combination with anti-malarial drugs, a role to play in intermittent preventive treatment of Plasmodium falciparum malaria infection in pregnant women in Africa. Malaria J. 2018;17:469.

6. Jagannathan P. How does malaria in pregnancy impact malaria risk in infants. BMC Med. 2018;6:212.

7. Megnekou R, Djontu JC, Nana BC, Bigoga J. Accuracy of one step malaria rapid diagnostic test (RDT) in detecting Plasmodium falciparum placental malaria infection in women living in Yaoundé, Cameroon. Malaria J. 2018;17:450.

8. National Health Mission. (2019). National vector borne disease control programme (India). [online] Available from https://nvbdcp.gov.in/index1.php?lang=1&level=1&sublinkid=5784&lid=3689 [Last accessed September, 2020]

9. Park K. Park's Textbook of Preventive and Social Medicine, 25th edition. Jabalpur: Banarsidas Bhanot; 2019.

10. Rao VB, Jensen TO, Jimenez BC, Robays J, Lasry E, Sterk E, et al. Malaria in pregnancy: a call for a safe, efficient, and patient-centred approach to first-trimester treatment. Lancet. 2018. [online] Available from https://www.thelancet.com/journals/langlo/article/PIIS2214-109X(18)30228-6/fulltext [Last accessed September, 2020]

11. Royal College of Obstetricians Gynaecologists. (2018). Malaria in Pregnancy, Diagnosis and Treatment (Green-top Guideline No. 54B). [online] Available from https://www.rcog.org.uk/en/guidelines-research-services/guidelines/gtg54b [Last accessed September, 2020]

12. Tarning J. Treatment of malaria in pregnancy. N Engl J Med. 2016;374(10):981-2.

13. van Loon, Gai PP, Hamann L, Addo GB, Mockenhaupt FP. MiRNA-146a polymorphism increases the odds of malaria in pregnancy. Malaria J. 2019;18:7.

14. WHO Reproductive Health Library. (2016). WHO recommendation on intermittent preventive treatment of malaria in pregnancy. [online] Available from https://extranet.who.int/rhl/topics/preconception-pregnancy-childbirth-and-postpartum-care/antenatal-care/who-recommendation-intermittent-preventive-treatment-malaria-pregnancy [Last accessed September, 2020].

15 World Health Organization. (2017). World Malaria Report. Malaria Prevention Works. Geneva: World Health Organization; 2017. [online] Available from https://apps.who.int/iris/bitstream/handle/10665/254991/WHO-HTM-GMP-2017.6-eng.pdf [Last accessed September, 2020]

16. World Health Organization. Guidelines for the Treatment of Malaria, 3rd edition. Geneva: World Health Organization; 2015. [online] Available from http://apps.who.int/iris/bitstream/10665/162441/1/9789241549127_ eng.pdf [Last accessed September, 2020].

Dengue

1. Biswas A, Pangtey GS, Devgan V, Singla P, Murthy P, Dhariwal AC, et al. Indian national guidelines for clinical management of dengue fever. J Ind Med Assoc. 2015;113:196-206.

2. FOGSI. (2015). Dengue in pregnancy: management protocols. [online] Available from https://www.fogsi.org/wp-content/uploads/2015/11/dpmp.pdf [Last accessed September, 2020]

3. Friedman EE, Dallah F, Harville EW, Myers L, Buekens P, Breart G, et al. Symptomatic dengue infection during pregnancy and infant outcomes: A retrospective cohort study. PLoS Negl Trop Dis. 2014;8(10):e3226.

4. JIMA. 2015;113(12) [online] Available from http://module.ima-india.org/ima/JIMA/2015/dec/index.html [Last accessed September, 2020]

5. National Health Mission. (2019) National Vector Borne Disease Control Programme (NVBDCP): Dengue. [online] Available from https://nvbdcp.gov.in/index1.php?lang=1&level=1&sublinkid=5776&lid=3690 [Last accessed September, 2020]

6. Paixão ES, Teixeira MG, Costa MDCN, Rodrigues LC. Dengue during pregnancy and adverse fetal outcomes: a systematic review and meta-analysis. Lancet Infect Dis. 2016;16(7):857-65.

7. Park K. Park's Textbook of Preventive and Social Medicine, 25th edition. Jabalpur: Banarsidas Bhanot; 2019.

8. Pavanaganga A, Sailakshmi MPA, Rekha BR. 2017. Dengue fever during pregnancy: Maternal and fetal complications. SAFOG. 2017;9(2):88-91.

9. Schilling S, Ludolfs D, Van An L, Schmitz H. Laboratory diagnosis of primary and secondary dengue infection. J Clin Virol. 2004;31(3):179-84.

10. World Health Organization. (2012). WHO Handbook for Clinical Management of Dengue [online] Available from http://www.wpro.who.int/mvp/documents/handbook_for_clinical_management_of_dengue.pdf [Last accessed September, 2020]

11. Xiong YQ, Mo Y, Shi TL, Zhu L, Chen Q. Dengue virus infection during pregnancy increased the risk of adverse fetal outcomes? An updated meta-analysis. J Clin Virol. 2017;94:42-9.

H1N1 (Swine FLU)

1. AAFP Foundation. (2019). 2018-2019 Influenza Vaccine Is Effective, Says CDC. [online] Available from https://www.aafp.org/news/health-of-the-public/20190220fluvaccine.html [Last accessed September, 2020]

2. Al-Husban N, Obeidat N, Al-Kuran O, Al Oweidat K, Bakri F. H1N1 infection in pregnancy; A retrospective study of fetomaternal outcome and impact of the timing of antiviral therapy. Mediterranean J Hematol Infect Dis. 2019;11(1):e2019020.

3. Carlson A, Thung SF, Norwitz ER. H1N1 influenza in pregnancy: What all obstetric care providers ought to know. Rev Obstet Gynecol. 2009;2(3):139-45.

4. Centers for Disease Control and Prevention. (2010). CDC 2018-2019 U.S. Flu Season: Preliminary burden estimates. [online] Available from https://www.cdc.gov/flu/about/burden/preliminary-in-season-estimates.htm [Last accessed September, 2020]

5. Centers for Disease Control and Prevention. (2010). H1N1 flu. [online] Available from https://www.cdc.gov/h1n1flu/guidance/obstetric.htm [Last accessed September, 2020]

6. Centers for Disease Control and Prevention. (2018). Diagnosing flu. [online] Available from https://www.cdc.gov/flu/symptoms/testing.htm [Last accessed September, 2020]

7. Centers for Disease Control and Prevention. (2019). Flu & pregnant women. [online] Available from https://www.cdc.gov/flu/protect/vaccine/pregnant.htm [Last accessed September, 2020]

8. Centers for Disease Control and Prevention. (2019). Influenza (flu). [online] Available from https://www.cdc.gov/flu/season/flu-season-2018-2019.htm [Last accessed September, 2020]

9. Centers for Disease Control and Prevention. (2019). Recommendations for obstetric health care providers related to use of antiviral medications in the treatment and prevention of influenza. [online] Available from https://www.cdc.gov/flu/professionals/antivirals/avrec_ob.htm [Last accessed September, 2020]

10. Centers for Disease Control and Prevention. (2020). Influenza antiviral medications: Summary for clinicians. [online] Available from https://www.cdc.gov/flu/professionals/antivirals/summary-clinicians.htm [Last accessed September, 2020]

11. FOGSI. (2014). H1N1 in pregnancy. [online] Available from http://www.fogsi.org/wp-content/uploads/2015/11/h1n1_in_pregnancy.pdf [Last accessed September, 2020]

12. Health Protection Surveillance Centre. (2018). Guidelines on the management of pregnant women with suspected influenza. [online] Available from http://www.hpsc.ie/a-z/respiratory/influenza/seasonalinfluenza/guidance/pregnancyguidance) [Last accessed September, 2020]

13. Indian College of Obstetricians & Gynaecologists (ICOG). (2018). Maternal infection exposure to expression. [online] Available from www.icogonline.org (Issue no. 3) [Last accessed September, 2020]

14. Influenza vaccination during pregnancy. ACOG Committee Opinion No. 732. American College of Obstetricians and Gynecologists. Obstet Gynecol. 2018;131:e109-14.

15. Jain A, Sharma R, Nagar MK, Kaushik PB. A death audit of H1N1 influenza cases in a tertiary care hospital in Southern Rajasthan. Current outbreak—2017. Natl J Community Med. 2018;9(5):380-4.

16. Management Guideline for pregnant women and neonates born to women with suspected or confirmed pandemic H1N1 influenza (swine flu A/H1N1 influenza). (2011). [online] Available from http://www.perinatalservicesbc.ca/Documents/Guidelines-Standards/HealthPromotion/H1N1ManagementGuideline.pdf [Last accessed September, 2020]

17. Ministry of Health and Family Welfare Directorate General of Health Services. (2017). Seasonal influenza: Guidelines for vaccination with influenza vaccine. [online] (2019) Available from (https://mohfw.gov.in/sites/default/files/Seasonal%20Influenza%20-%20Guidelines%20for%20vaccination%20with%20Influenza%20Vaccine%20%28updated%29.pdf [Last accessed September, 2020]

18. Park K. Park's Textbook of Preventive and Social Medicine, 25th edition. Jabalpur: Banarsidas Bhanot; 2019.

19. Ravindran M, Gowtham S, Mehta P, Narayanan P. Retrospective analysis of maternal and foetal outcome of H1N1 influenza amongst antenatal mothers at a tertiary care hospital. J Patient Saf Infect Control. 2017;5:69-72.

20. Silasi M, Cardenas I, Racicot K, Kwon JY, Aldo P, Mor G. Viral infections during pregnancy. Am J Reprod Immunol. 2015;73(3):199-213.

21. World Health Organization (South-East Asia). (2019). Flu facts. [online] Available from http://www.searo.who.int/india/topics/influenza/flu-fact-sheet-2019.pdf [Last accessed September, 2020]

22. World Health Organization. (2010). Pregnancy and pandemic influenza A (H1N1) 2009: Information for programme managers and clinicians. [online] Available from https://www.who.int/csr/resources/publications/swineflu/h1n1_guidance_pregnancy/en/ [Last accessed September, 2020]

23. World Health Organization. (2018). Recommended composition of influenza virus vaccines for use in the 2018-2019 northern hemisphere influenza season. [online] Available from https://www.who.int/influenza/vaccines/virus/recommendations/2018_19_north/en/ [Last accessed September, 2020]

Varicella/Chickenpox

1. Ayoade F, Kumar S. Varicella Zoster (Chickenpox). Treasure Island (FL): StatPearls Publishing; 2020. [online] Available from https://www.ncbi.nlm.nih.gov/books/NBK448191/ [Last accessed September, 2020]

2. Centers for Disease Control and Prevention. (2018). CDC Vaccine Information Statements (VISs): Chickenpox VIS. [online] Available from www.cdc.gov/vaccines/hcp/vis/vis-statements/varicella.html [Last accessed September, 2020]

3. Centers for Disease Control and Prevention. Chickenpox (Varicella). [online] Available from www.cdc.gov/chickenpox/hcp/index.html [Last accessed September, 2020]

4. Centers for Disease Control and Prevention. Varicella. In: CDC Epidemiology and Prevention of Vaccine Preventable Disease. 2018. [online] Available from https://www.cdc.gov/vaccines/pubs/pinkbook/varicella.html[Last accessed September, 2020]

5. Duff P. Diagnosis and management of varicella infection in pregnancy. Perinatology. 2010;1:6-12.

6. FOGSI. (2016). Good clinical practice recommendations on preconception care-India. [online] Available from https://www.fogsi.org/gcpr-preconception-care/ [Last accessed September, 2020]

7. Indian College of Obstetricians & Gynaecologists (ICOG). (2018). Maternal infection exposure to expression. [online] Available from www.icogonline.org (Issue no. 3) [Last accessed September, 2020].

8. Institute of Obstetricians and Gynaecologist, Royal College of Physicians of Ireland. (2018). Clinical practice guideline no. 19; chickenpox in pregnancy [online] Available from https://rcpi-live-cdn.s3.amazonaws.com/wp-content/uploads/2016/05/35.-Chicken-Pox-in-Pregnancy.pdf [Last accessed September, 2020]

9. Lamont R F, Sobel JD, Carringtton D, Tovi SM, Kusanovic JP, Vaisbuch E, et al. Varicella zoster virus (chickenpox) infection in pregnancy. BJOG. 2011;118(10):1155-62.

10. NHS. (2017). Chickenpox guideline (GL805). [online] Available from https://www.nhs.uk/conditions/chickenpox [Last accessed September, 2020]

11. Park K. Park's Textbook of Preventive and Social Medicine, 25th edition. Jabalpur: Banarsidas Bhanot; 2019.

12. Pergam SA, Limave AP and the AST Infectious Diseases Community of Practice. Varicella zoster virus (VZV). Am J Transplant. 2009;9(Suppl 4):S108-15.

13. Royal College of Obstetricians and Gynaecologists. (2015). Chickenpox in Pregnancy (Green-top Guideline No. 13). [online] Available from https://www.rcog.org.uk/en/guidelines-research-services/guidelines/gtg13/ [Last accessed September, 2020]

14. Sahay R, Yadav PD, Majumdar T, Patil S, Sarkale P, Shete AM, et al. Clinico-epidemiological investigation on Varicella Zoster Virus indicates multiple clade circulation in Maharashtra state, India. Heliyon. 2018;4(8):e00757.

15. Silasi M, Cardenas I, Racicot K, Kwon JY, Aldo P, Mor G. Viral infections during pregnancy. Am J Reprod Immunol. 2015;73(3):199-213.

Typhoid

1. Banerjee T, Shukla BN, Filgona J, Anupurba S, Sen MR. Trends of typhoid fever seropositivity over ten years in north India. Indian J Med Res. 2014;140:310-3.

2. Bhutta ZA. Current concepts in the diagnosis and treatment of typhoid fever. BMJ. 2006;333:78-82.

3. Centers for Disease Control and Prevention. (2017). Typhoid fever and paratyphoid fever. [online] Available from https://www.cdc.gov/typhoid-fever/index.html [Last accessed September, 2020]

4. Centers for Disease Control and Prevention. CDC Health Information for International Travel: 2008. Atlanta: US Department of Health and Human Services; 2008:345-9.

5. Centers for Disease Control and Prevention. Updated recommendations for the use of typhoid vaccine advisory committee on immunisation practices, United States, 2015. Weekly. 2015;64(11):305-8.

6. Chandel DS, Chaudhry R, Dhawan B, Pandey A, Dey AB. Drug-resistant Salmonella enterica serotype paratyphi A in India. Emerg Infect Dis. 2000;6:420-1.

7. Gluck B, Ramin KD, Ramin SM. Salmonella typhi and pregnancy: A case report. Infect Dis Obstet Gynecol. 1994;2:186-9.

8. Hasbun J, Osorio R, Hasbun A. Hepatic dysfunction in typhoid fever during pregnancy. Infect Dis Obstet Gynecol. 2006; 64828:1-2.

9. Kanungo S, Dutta S, Sur D. Epidemiology of typhoid and paratyphoid fever in India. J Infect Developing Countries. 2008;2(6):454-60.

10. Ministry of Health Fiji Islands. (2010). Guidelines for the diagnosis, management, and prevention of typhoid fever. [online] Available from https://www.health.gov.fj/wp-content/ uploads/2014/05/Typhoid-Guideline_-Long-Version_-2010.pdf [Last accessed September, 2020]

11. National Institute for Communicable Diseases. (2016). Typhoid: NICD recommendations for diagnosis, management and public health response. [online] Available from http://www.kznhealth.gov.za/family/Typhoid_Guidlines.pdf [Last accessed September, 2020]

12. NHS. (2018). Typhoid fever. [online] Available from https://www.nhs.uk/conditions/typhoid-fever/. [Last accessed September, 2020]

13. Park K. Park's Textbook of Preventive and Social Medicine, 25th edition. Jabalpur: Banarsidas Bhanot; 2019.

14. Poonia S, Satia MN, Torame VP, Natraj G. Vertical transmission of Salmonella typhi. J Postgrad Gynecol Obstet. 2015;2. [online] Available from www.jpgo.org/2015/01/vertical-transmission-of-salmonella.html [Last accessed September, 2020]

15. Sethi S, Gautam V, Gupta K, Suri V, Angrup A. Vertical transmission of Salmonella enterica serotype Paratyphi A leading to abortion. JMM Case Reports. 2017;4.

16. The Philippine Clinical Practice Guidelines on the Diagnosis, Treatment and Prevention of Typhoid Fever in Adults. (2017). [online] Available from https://psmid.org.ph/index.php/public-resources/117-diagnosis-treatment-and-prevention-of-typhoid-fever-in-adults-2017 [Last accessed September, 2020]

17. Touchan F, Hall JD, Lee RV. Typhoid fever during pregnancy. Obstet Med. 2009;2:161-3.

18. Vigliani MB, Bakardikev AI. First Trimester Typhoid Fever with Vertical Transmission of Salmonella Typhi, an Intracellular Organism. Case Rep Med. 2013; 2013: 973297.

19. World Health Organization. (2018). Typhoid fever (Salmonella typhi) Investigation Guideline. [online] Available from https://www.who.int/immunization/monitoring_surveillance/burden/vpd/WHO_SurveillanceVaccinePreventable_21_Typhoid_R1.pdf?ua=1 [Last accessed September, 2020]

20. Zaki SA, Karande S. Multidrug-resistant typhoid fever: a review. J Infect Dev Ctries. 2011;5(5):324-37.

21. Zoppi L. (2018). Typhoid treatment. [online] Available from https://www.news-medical.net/health/Typhoid-Treatment.aspx [Last accessed September, 2020]

Skin Diseases in Pregnancy

Hemant Talnikar, Hemant Deshpande

■ INTRODUCTION

Many skin changes occur during pregnancy. These changes may be a cause of worry for a pregnant woman.

The cutaneous changes during pregnancy can be divided broadly into three major categories:

1. *Physiological changes:* Changes that occur normally with almost all pregnancies
2. *Common skin diseases:* Skin conditions or diseases that are not at all related to gestation and may improve or worsen during pregnancy
3. *Pregnancy-associated dermatoses:* These are specific for the gestational state.

Prospective mothers are worried about their skin changes during the gestational period—usually about cosmetic appearance or doubt about the chances of recurrence of the same problem during the next pregnancy or about any adverse effect on the fetus regarding morbidity or mortality.

Due to marked changes in estrogen and progesterone levels during the gestational period, profound skin changes occur. Knowledge of changes in skin is very important. Recognition of physiological changes from that of true skin diseases separates the conditions that need immediate and prompt treatment to reduce morbidity and mortality.

In the pathogenesis of pregnancy-specific dermatoses, interaction of hormonal factors with the immune system plays a very important role in hormonal changes during pregnancy-specific cutaneous diseases. Significant and complex physiological skin changes occur during the period of pregnancy.

During pregnancy, a fetoplacental unit produces a variety of protein hormones—such as human chorionic gonadotropin (HCG), human placental lactogen (HPL), human somatomammotropin (HSM), human chorionic thyrotropin (HCT), and human chorionic corticotropin (HCC).

During the gestational period, the activities of maternal pituitary, thyroid, and adrenal glands also increase.

Along with protein hormones, steroid hormones such as estrogen and progesterone play a very important role in cutaneous changes.

The production and serum levels of these hormones are dynamic. The HCG level remains elevated throughout pregnancy, but peak is achieved during 10–12th week of gestation. The levels of estrogen and progesterone rise during the first and second trimesters but attain plateau during the third trimester of pregnancy.

Classification of Pregnancy-associated Specific Dermatoses

The most recent classification defined by Ambros Rudolph et al. (2006) is given in the following text.

This classification involved four main categories: pemphigoid gestationis (PG), pruritic folliculitis of pregnancy (PFP), intrahepatic cholestasis of pregnancy (ICP), and atopic eruption of pregnancy (AEP). Atopic eruption of pregnancy is the new umbrella term to encompass eczema in pregnancy, PP, and PFP **(Table 1)**.

■ PHYSIOLOGICAL SKIN CHANGES DURING PREGNANCY

Due to hormonal, metabolic, and immunologic factors, physiological changes in pigmentation, vascularity, nevi, connective tissues, glands, hair, nails, and mucous membranes occur.

TABLE 1: Classification of pregnancy-associated specific dermatoses.

Class	Synonyms
Pemphigoid gestationis (PG)	Herpes gestationis (HG)
Polymorphic eruption of pregnancy (PEP)	• Pruritic urticarial papules and plaques of pregnancy (PUPPP) • Toxic erythema of pregnancy • Toxemic rash of pregnancy • Late-onset prurigo of pregnancy
Intrahepatic cholestasis of pregnancy (ICP)	• Cholestasis of pregnancy • Obstetric cholestasis • Jaundice of pregnancy • Pruritus/prurigo gravidarum
Atopic eruption of pregnancy (AEP)	• Prurigo of pregnancy • Prurigo gestationis • Early onset prurigo of pregnancy • Pruritic folliculitis of pregnancy • Eczema in pregnancy

Pigmentation

Pigmentary changes are the most common in gravid females. A generalized increase in skin pigmentation (hyperpigmentation) is very commonly seen in them. Pigmentation is prominently seen in darker skin types. Hyperpigmentation often fades after delivery but may not resolve completely. Estrogen, progesterone and melanocyte-stimulating hormones derived from Proopio melanocortin stimulates melanocytes. But the exact mechanism of hyperpigmentation and pathogenesis of its distribution are not known completely. The density of melanocytes in epidermis increases and there is upregulation of tyrosinase. Human placental lipids also contribute in the process of hyperpigmentation.

Areas that are already pigmented become darker, e.g., nipples, around areola (also called secondary areola), genital area, perineum, axillae, inner thighs, neck, newly formed scars, freckles, and lentigines. Linea alba in the midline of the abdominal wall becomes darker and is called linea nigra (vertical band of pigmentation that extends from the xiphoid process to pubic symphysis).

During the second half of pregnancy, >70% of pregnant women and especially dark-skinned pregnant women develop melasma (chloasma or mask of pregnancy).

Macular, irregularly shaped, sharply marginated, symmetrically patterned pigmentation appears over forehead, temples, cheeks, upper lip, and sometimes over chin.

The epidermal type of melasma is found in approximately 70% of cases, mixed type in about 24% of cases, and dermal type in only 6% of cases.

During pregnancy, only broad-spectrum sunscreen is prescribed along with avoidance of sunlight. This will help to prevent additional darkening. Melasma may fade after delivery, but many women need treatment. Actual treatment is recommended after delivery to avoid potential fatal risk.

Melanocytic nevi may increase in number and by size during pregnancy.

Transition lines between tip and lighter pigmented areas are called pigmentary demarcation lines. Such types of lines on the posteromedial portion of lower extremities are called type B pigmentary demarcation lines and are commonly associated with pregnancy.

Pruritus

Itching in pregnancy is called pruritus gravidarum. It occurs in almost 20% of all pregnancies. It may be due to underlying skin diseases such as eczema and urticaria or may be due to hepatic, renal, or thyroid systemic diseases.

But intense pruritus without any primary cutaneous sign is called pruritus gravidarum.

Pruritus is a mild variant of IHC and perceived over abdomen during the third trimester of pregnancy when the skin is stretched maximally. Along with abdomen, itching also occurs over scalp, perianal, and perivulval regions.

Striae Distensae

Striae distensae are also called striae gravidarum or stretch marks and commonly seen in the second and third trimesters of pregnancy. Approximately 90% pregnant women develop striae over abdomen, breast, thighs, and buttocks. Striae develop at right angles to the skin tension lines. Physical factors and hormones (relaxin, estrogen, and corticosteroids) cause thinning of elastin fibers and fibrillin microfibrils in dermis, causing linear pink or erythematous, purple or violaceous atrophic bands or streaks and later on develop into linear depressions with hypopigmentation having fine wrinkles over it.

Striae gravidarum are similar to striae seen in Cushing syndrome, corticosteroid therapy, and rapid changes in body weight.

Familial predisposition, history of striae, excess weight gain, and younger age are risk factors for the development of striae gravidarum.

Various creams, moisturizers, emollients, and oils are used to prevent occurrence of striae during pregnancy, but no treatment is effective in preventing them. In the postpartum period, striae may shrink and may fade to flesh-colored lines but never disappear completely. In this period, topical tretinoin and pulsed dye laser (585 nm) are prescribed.

Vascular Changes

Vascular changes are due to sustained high levels of circulating estrogen. These changes are similar to vascular changes seen in hyperthyroidism and cirrhosis.

"Spider nevi" or "spider angiomas" occur secondary to dilatation and proliferation of blood vessels. They appear as red lesions with branches extending outward from central puneta. These lesions usually appear during the second trimester, and all lesions regress within 3 months of delivery.

Spider angiomas usually develop around eyes, neck, face, upper chest, arms, or hands.

Palmar erythema is commonly seen in skin types I and II. It is seen in approximately 70% of pregnant women and in darker skin types it is seen in 30% of pregnant women. It is seen in the first trimester of pregnancy and usually resolves in the postpartum period. It may involve the whole palm with pink mottling or involve only thenar and hypothenar eminences. Fingers are usually spared.

In the third trimester, edema and hyperemia of gingiva are seen. It may lead to gingivitis and bleeding gums if oral hygiene is poor.

In the first or second trimester, due to proliferation of vessels within hypertrophied gums, granuloma gravidarum (pyogenic granuloma, pregnancy tumors, pregnancy epulis) may develop. These lesions are smooth, soft, red or purple, friable, either sessile or pedunculated nodules. Granulomas usually regress during the postpartum period. If bleeding occurs, excision is required.

Small hemangiomas occur in about 5% of pregnant women. Hemangiomas are usually seen over head, neck, and digits.

Hemangioendotheliomas and glomangiomas (glomus tumor) are also seen as vascular changes during pregnancy.

In about 40% of pregnant women, varicosities of saphenous, vulvar, and hemorrhoidal veins may appear due to increased venous pressure on veins by the gravid uterus. Varicosities are seen during the late first trimester and resolve in the postpartum period. Rarely deep vein thrombosis may occur. It is a serious condition leading to permanent damage to leg veins. Occasionally, death due to pulmonary embolism may occur.

In nearly half of the pregnant women, nonpitting edema of the face, eyelids, feet, and hands may appear. Edema is most obvious in early morning and disappear at the end of the day. No treatment is available for this condition, but it is important to recognize and differentiate this edema from the edema seen in cardiac, renal, and preeclamptic states.

Pain, numbness, and swelling of the hand, sparing the little and ring fingers, are seen in carpal tunnel syndrome. Carpal tunnel syndrome is due to compression neuropathy of the median nerve as it passes beneath the flexor retinaculum. Increased soft-tissue mass caused by a hormonally mediated edema condition resolves in the postpartum period.

After delivery scalp hair enter the telogen (resting) phase of the hair growth cycle, causing more shedding (telogen effluvium) of scalp hair. This stage lasts for a few months to at least 1 year; spontaneous recovery within 12 months is usual.

In later stages of pregnancy, mild frontoparietal recession (androgenetic alopecia) may occur.

Hirsutism, acne, and other evidence of virilization occur rarely during the third trimester of pregnancy. Virilization results from androgen-secreting tumor, luteoma, lutein cyst or polycystic ovarian disease (PCOD). A female fetus may get masculinized.

Nails

Nail growth is more during pregnancy but nails become brittle, soft, and dystrophic with transverse grooves (Beau's lines). Distal onycholysis, subungual hyperkeratosis, and longitudinal melanonychia may be seen in pregnant women.

Sore Nipples

Many women develop fissuring and irritation of nipples with discomfort in breast feeding, in the early puerperium period. Mastitis and deep abscesses may develop due to secondary bacterial infections of the cracked nipples.

Eccrine, Apocrine, and Sebaceous Gland Activity

Eccrine glands activity is increased during pregnancy. This along with increased thyroid activity causes hyperhidrosis and increased frequency of miliaria. But in some women, palmar sweating may be decreased during pregnancy.

Apocrine glands activity is reduced leading to improvement in Fox–Fordyce disease and hidradenitis suppurativa.

Sebaceous glands become hyperactive and hypertrophied. But their effect on acne is unpredictable. Formation of Montgomery tubercles is increased. Sebum excretion increases during pregnancy and comes to a normal level after delivery. This is due to the result of rising maternal progesterone and androgen levels along with sebotrophic stimulus from the maternal pituitary sebum level that remains raised during lactation.

Hair

Due to hormonal changes during pregnancy, progression of hair from the anagen phase to the telogen phase is slowed down. More and more hairs are retained in the anagen phase. So, hair growth on the scalp is more pronounced during pregnancy. Scalp hair becomes thick or dense. Hypertrichosis (hirsutism) may be seen on face, arms, legs, back, and suprapubic area. This is due to increased levels of androgens from ovarian and placental origin, acting on pilosebaceous units.

■ PEMPHIGOID GESTATIONIS (HERPES GESTATIONIS/GESTATIONAL PEMPHIGOID DERMATITIS MULTIFORMIS GESTATIONIS)

Pemphigoid gestationis is a rare, extremely pruritic, recurrent, autoimmune subepidermal bullous dermatosis occurring usually in the second trimester or late pregnancy and immediate postpartum period.

Pemphigoid gestationis can occur in association with trophoblastic tumors, e.g., choriocarcinoma and hydatidiform mole.

The incidence of PG varies from 1:2000 to 1:60,000 pregnancies, depending on the prevalence of human leukocyte antigen (HLA) haplotypes DR3 and DR4. Nearly half of the cases develop during the first pregnancy.

Etiopathogenesis

The pathogenesis of PG is not known completely. It is an autoimmune disease. PG may be associated with other autoimmune diseases such as vitiligo, Graves' diseases, alopecia areata, hypothyroidism, and autoimmune thrombocytopenia. PG most probably results from breakdown of the protective immunity of the fetoplacental unit from maternal allogenic recognition. Autoantibodies against two hemidesmosomal proteins are developed, e.g., BP180 and less commonly BP230. Out of these two proteins, BP180 is the major target antigen. It is found in the basement membrane of skin and amniotic epithelium of placenta.

"Silencing" or nonexposure of major histocompatibility complex (MHC) class II antigen on trophoblast protects the fetus from recognition by the immune system of the mother, in normal pregnancy. When MHC class II antigens are aberrantly expressed in trophoblast and amniochorionic stromal cells, as in PG, they lead to exposure of BP180 (collagen XVII) to the immune system of the mother. Presentation of aberrant self-antigen leads to antibody production. Cross-reaction of these antibodies with collagen XVII forms immune complexes and activates complement. Complement promotes infiltration of inflammatory cells. These inflammatory cells release mediators of inflammation. These mediators course tissue damage and formation of blisters.

In the last few weeks of pregnancy, the level of progesterone is increased. Progesterone decreases antibody formation and estrogen increases it. So improvement of PG, just before delivery, and again flare-up in the postpartum period are seen. Recurrence of PG in the premenstrual period is seen due to a decreased level of progesterone in the premenstrual phase. The oral contraceptive pill contains estrogen. So, use of contraception induces recurrence of PG.

Clinical Features

Itching (pruritus) is intense and may precede skin lesions. Initially, skin lesions are erythematous, pruritic urticarial papules and plaques. Later on, vesicles are formed around the umbilicus over the abdomen. Then lesions spread to cover the entire skin surface except the face and mucous membrane. In the early prebullous stage, it is very difficult to differentiate between PG and PEP, clinically and histopathologically. Diagnosis of PG becomes clear when tense blisters, just like those seen in bullous pemphigoid, appear.

Etiology

The natural course of PG is characterized by exacerbation and remissions. Improvement in late pregnancy and flare-up at the time of delivery are seen. Lesions resolve after delivery within weeks or months and again exacerbate at the time of menstruation and the use of hormonal contraception. Rarely PG can recur with persistence of lesions over several years.

Fetal prognosis is generally good, but chances of prematurity and small-for-date babies are more. This risk correlates with disease severity. Antibodies may get transferred passively from mother to fetus. About 10% of newborns may develop mild skin lesions (neonatal PG). As maternal antibodies are cleared from a neonate's circulation within days to weeks, lesions over neonatal skin get resolved spontaneously.

No active treatment but just conservative line of treatment is required in neonates.

Pemphigoid gestationis can recur in subsequent pregnancies and with the use of oral contraceptives. In successive recurrences, lesions may appear at an earlier period of gestation and with more severity. Counseling of women, when planning the next pregnancy, should be done.

Investigations

Findings of histopathology depend on the stage of the disease and its severity. In the prebullous stage, the edema of the upper and mid-dermis with perivascular inflammatory infiltrate of lymphocytes, histiocytes, and a variable number of eosinophils is seen.

In the bullous stage, subepidermal blisters at the level of lamina lucida at the dermoepidermal junction are seen.

Direct immunofluorescence (DIF) of perilesional skin is the gold standard in the diagnosis of PG. It shows linear deposition of C3 along the dermoepidermal junction in all cases. Along with C3, additional deposition of immunoglobulin G (IgG) is seen in 30% cases. In 30–100% cases, circulating IgG antibodies may be detected by indirect immunofluorescence, binding to roof of salt-split skin. For monitoring disease activity, the level of antibody may be measured using ELISA (enzyme-linked immunosorbent assay) and immunoblot techniques.

Treatment

Treatment depends on the stay and severity of the disease. It aims to control pruritus and prevent blister formation.

In the prebullous stage, topical corticosteroids and oral antihistamines are sufficient.

In the bullous stage, oral corticosteroids (prednisolone: 0.5–1 mg/kg/day) along with topical corticosteroids and oral antihistamines are prescribed.

Cases not responding to systemic corticosteroids may get benefit from azathioprine, IV immunoglobulins, and plasma exchange therapy.

■ INTRAHEPATIC CHOLESTASIS OF PREGNANCY

Generalized pruritus, with or without jaundice and without hepatitis or hepatotoxic medicines and having no primary skin lesions but biochemical abnormalities, is present in ICP. Symptoms disappear spontaneously after delivery, but the condition recurs in subsequent pregnancies.

Etiology and Pathogenesis

The etiology of ICP is multifactorial involving genetics, hormones, diet, and underlying hepatic, biliary, or pancreatic conditions. It is a reversible form of hormonally triggered cholestasis that develops in genetically predisposed pregnant women in late pregnancy.

Origin of intrahepatic cholestasis of pregnancy is familial. Maternal prognosis is good. Pruritus disappears spontaneously within days to week after delivery to recur in subsequent pregnancy or with the use of oral contraceptives.

Increased risk of intra- and postpartum hemorrhage is seen in both the mother and the child when the woman is having jaundice and vitamin K deficiency. Fetal prognosis can be impaired with increased risk of prematurity, fetal distress, and stillbirth. As toxic bile acids pass into fetal circulation, they may cause acute placental anoxia and cardiac depression.

Intrahepatic cholestasis of pregnancy is more commonly seen in women over 35 years of age, having twin pregnancy, having a female fetus, and who conceived via in vitro fertilization.

Clinical Features

Itching begins in the second and third trimesters. Initially, it is localized to abdomen, palms, and soles. In some cases, itching is widespread. Jaundice is present in about 10% cases. Primary cutaneous lesions are not seen. Secondary skin lesions in the form of excoriations, erosions, scabbing, and severe prurigen nodules due to scratching are present.

Intense pruritus during the third trimester without jaundice is pruritus gravidarum and intense pruritus with jaundice is intrahepatic jaundice of pregnancy. Pruritus worsens with advancing gestation, but jaundice does not increase. Pruritus may worsen at night.

Intrahepatic cholestasis of pregnancy is the second most common cause of gestational jaundice after viral hepatitis. The risk of ICP increases in hepatitis C seropositive patients. It is associated with early onset of ICP.

Differential Diagnosis

Viral hepatitis, other pruritic dermatoses of pregnancy, and other courses of generalized pruritus should be considered while diagnosing ICP.

Diagnosis

Liver function tests are normal. Alkaline phosphatase may be raised (due to placental production of alkaline phosphatase, elevated levels are considered to be normal during pregnancy). Levels of serum total bile acids are elevated. Conjugated fraction of bile acid is most sensitive and suitable for ICP monitoring.

Treatment

Ursodeoxycholic acid (UCDA) (15 mg/kg/day; 450–1200 mg/day) is the drug of choice. It reduces itch and serum bile acid levels. It decreases biliary secretion of endogenous and toxic levels of bile acid. It protects cholangiocytes from apoptosis caused by bile acids.

When compared with cholestyramine, UDCA is safe and works faster. UDCA has a sustained effect on pruritus and improves liver function abnormalities of ICP. Other drugs are antihistamines (loratadine and cetirizine), S-adenosyl-L-methionine, dexamethasone (for fetal lung maturity), and cholestyramine. But it has not shown to improve fetal prognosis and may contribute to malabsorption of vitamin K leading to bleeding complications. So, cholestyramine should be avoided.

Along with UDCA treatment, close obstetric check-up is needed with weekly fetal cardiotocographic monitoring from 34 weeks' gestation onward to detect early signs of fetal distress.

Vitamin K is given to mother if jaundice is present.

Topical emollients, aqueous cream with 1–2% menthol, are given.

Early induction of labor may be considered at 36 weeks of gestation in severe cases and 38 weeks of gestation in mild cases. Rest and low-fat diet are recommended.

Prognosis

Maternal pruritus resolves rapidly after delivery. But ICP is related to increased risk of meconium staining and premature labor (fetal distress). Toxic bile acids affect fetal cardiomyocytes causing sudden fetal death.

■ POLYMORPHOUS ERUPTION OF PREGNANCY

Polymorphous eruption of pregnancy is the term proposed by Holmes. This term is favored in the UK. In other parts of the world, the lengthy terms proposed by Lawly in 1979, "pruritic urticarial papules" and "plaques of pregnancy", are favored.

Polymorphous eruption of pregnancy is a common, benign, intensely pruritic self-limiting inflammatory disorder that usually occurs in the third trimester of pregnancy in primigravidas. The incidence of PEP is 1:160

TABLE 6: Ultrasound features of TORCH infection.

Infecting agent	CNS anomalies	Craniofacial anomalies	CVS anomalies	GIT anomalies	Musculoskeletal anomalies	Growth anomalies	Misc.
CMV	Ventriculomegaly, microcephaly, intracranial calcification	Cataract, microophthalmia	Cardiomegaly, pericardial effusion, SVT	Echogenic bowel, ascites	–	IUGR	Hydrops
Rubella	Microcephaly	Cataract, microophthalmia	ASD/VSD, pulmonary stenosis	Hepatosplenomegaly	–	IUGR	–
HSV	Ventriculomegaly	–	Myocardial calcification	Hepatic calcification	Persistent leg flexion	IUGR	–
Toxoplasma	Hydrocephalus, microcephaly, intracranial calcification	Cataract, microophthalmia	–	Hepatosplenomegaly, abdominal calcification	–	–	Hydrops, placentomegaly .

(ASD: atrial septal defect; CMV: cytomegalovirus; CNS: central nervous system; CVS: cardiovascular system; GIT: gastrointestinal tract; HSV: herpes simplex virus; IUGR: intrauterine growth restriction; SVT: supraventricular tachycardia; VSD: ventricular septal defect)

in amniotic fluid. A PCR quantifies parasite load; hence, it helps in both diagnosis and prognosis of infection. A positive PCR with structural abnormalities in scan is associated with poor outcome and without abnormalities requires long follow-up postnatally. A negative PCR rules out infection.[10] Invasive procedure should be carried out 6 weeks after maternal infections or to wait till 20 weeks of gestation because viral shedding by fetal kidneys is reduced in the first 20 weeks of pregnancy due to reduced fetal diuresis.[11,12]

Role of Ultrasound

Ultrasound plays an important role in the diagnosis of infection and management strategy, because it has prognostic value also. There are disease-specific anomalies which are detected in ultrasound in early pregnancy **(Table 6)**.

■ MANAGEMENT PROTOCOLS OF TORCH

Management protocols of TORCH are given in **Table 7**.

■ TOXOPLASMA INFECTION IN PREGNANCY

Toxoplasmosis is a zoonotic disease caused by an obligate intracellular protozoan *Toxoplasma gondii*. Its life cycle comprises sexual phase and asexual phase. Sexual phase occurs only in cats while asexual phase takes place in warm-blooded animals including humans.

Epidemiology

Mother acquires infection by consumption of undercooked or raw meat which contains toxoplasma cyst. Water or food contaminated by oocysts which are excreted in the feces of infected cats are another source of infection.[13,14] Maternal

infections are mostly asymptomatic. It is a self-limiting disease.

Primary infection in immunocompromised females confers immunity; however, secondary infection due to reactivation may be severe leading to encephalitis.

Fetal Effects

Maternal infection is transmitted to the fetus only in cases of primary infection (except in immunocompromised patients). The rate of vertical transmission increases with gestational age, but the affection rate decreases. Majority of infected fetuses are asymptomatic. Few may exhibit neurological symptoms and may present with the classical triad (congenital toxoplasmosis) which comprises chorioretinitis, intracranial calcifications, and hydrocephalus.

Diagnosis

Serological conversion in serology testing is a gold standard test but is not possible in a single serum sample. The presence of specific antitoxoplasma IgG and IgM in maternal serum is most commonly used for detection of maternal infection. Positive IgG with negative IgM suggests infection before pregnancy but in the third trimester, interpretation is difficult as the infection might be present in the prepregnancy period or the mother might have encountered active asymptomatic infection in the first and second trimesters. Amniocentesis, cordocentesis, and PCR assay are used for diagnosis of fetal infection. A high PCR quantitative parasite load before 20 weeks has the greatest risk for a poor fetal outcome.[15] The outcome is worse in the fetus in whom structural abnormalities are detected in scan. Berrebi reported that the outcome of fetuses at 2 years of age whose mothers acquired the infection during

TABLE 7: Management of TORCH.

Infection	Prepregnancy	Pregnancy	Labor	Postpartum
Toxoplasma	–	Maternal infection screened by serology followed by amniotic PCR for fetal infection. If +ve, then spiramycin orally till delivery is done	–	–
Rubella	Routine screening recommended. Vaccination for nonimmune women. Immune women require no action. Women having acute infection should avoid pregnancy for 3 months	Seroconversion in the first trimester—MTP advised. Fetal infection: (1) in first trimester—termination, (2) in second trimester—decision according to the timing of infection, (3) in the third trimester only—counseling	–	Nonimmune women are given vaccination
CMV	–	Fetal infection positive—consider MTP when appropriate	Routine care	Neonatal evaluation and follow-up
Herpes	Avoid pregnancy in active lesions	Acyclovir 200 mg 5 times a day for 10 days or until clinical resolution	Active genital lesion—cesarean indicated. Vaginal delivery when no active lesions. In PPROM individualize patient management	Evaluation of newborn and neonatal prophylaxis. Acyclovir when active maternal lesions seen.

(CMV: cytomegalovirus; MTP: Medical Termination of Pregnancy; PPROM: preterm premature rupture of the membranes)

the first trimester of pregnancy with no detectable structural abnormalities in scan was not significantly different from that of fetuses whose mothers were infected in late pregnancy.[16]

Ultrasound Findings in Congenital Toxoplasmosis (Figs. 1 to 5)

Ventriculomegaly, microcephaly, intracerebral calcification scattered in the whole brain, cataract, hepatomegaly, splenomegaly, ascites, and placental thickening.

Management

Prevention

At present, no vaccine is available for toxoplasmosis. Prevention is possible by avoiding contact of pregnant females with cats and not touching feces of cats with bare hands.

Treatment

The drug of choice is spiramycin 1g (3 million IU) two to three times daily orally for 3 weeks followed by 2 weeks of drug-free interval until delivery, in case of infection before 18 weeks of gestation.[8] Mothers acquiring infection in late pregnancy without fetal infection are treated using pyrimethamine and sulfonamide.[17] These drugs are not prescribed until 18 weeks of gestation because they cause fetal bone marrow suppression. If fetal infection is diagnosed, then pyrimethamine 25 mg orally daily with oral sulfadiazine 1 g four times a day for 3 weeks is given alternately with 3 weeks of spiramycin till delivery.

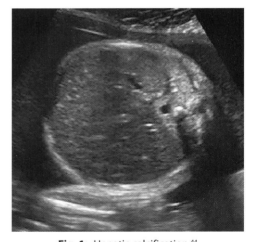

Fig. 1: Hepatic calcification.[44]

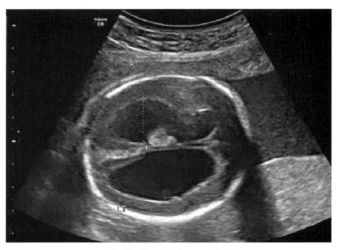

Fig. 2: Ventriculomegaly.[45]

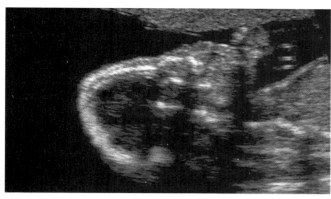

Fig. 3: Microcephaly.[46]

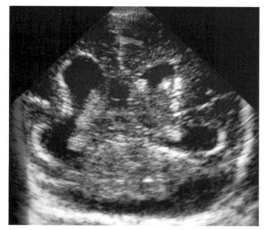

Fig. 4: Intracranial calcification.[47]

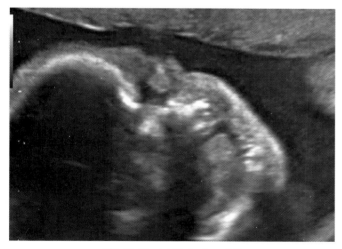

Fig. 5: Congenital cataract.[45]

■ RUBELLA (GERMAN MEASLES) IN PREGNANCY

Rubella is a viral disease caused by ribonucleic acid (RNA) toga virus. It infects only human beings.

Epidemiology

Rubella was an endemic infection before the introduction of the vaccination program. In countries where rubella immunization is routinely offered, the occurrence of congenital rubella syndrome is rare.[18,19] The incubation period is of 12–24 days.

Infection occurs via respiratory droplets with the infection period ranging from 7 days before to 5–7 days after the onset of rash.

Maternal Effects

Rubella infection has a characteristic maculopapular rash which begins on face and spreads to trunk and extremities. It usually resolves within 3 days in the same order in which it appeared (first face and then body).[20]

Fetal Effects

Rubella is one of the most teratogenic agents. The risk of malformation after 16 weeks is almost negligible. Beyond 20 weeks, it usually causes fetal growth restrictions.[21] The risk of transmission of infection to fetus is 80% in the first trimester which decreases to 25% in the second trimester and increases in the third trimester from 35% at 27–30 weeks to 100% beyond 36 weeks' gestation.[20]

Rubella causes multiple organ disease in a fetus which is known as congenital rubella syndrome (CRS). It includes one or more of the following:

- *Heart:* Patent ductus arteriosus, pulmonary artery stenosis
- *Central nervous system (CNS):* Microcephaly, mental retardation, developmental delay
- *Eye:* Cataract, glaucoma
- *Sensorineural deafness:* It is the most common single defect.
- Purpura
- *Gastrointestinal tract (GIT):* Hepatosplenomegaly, jaundice
- Radiolucent bone disease

Extended rubella syndrome occurs in the second and third decades of life. It also occurs in newborns who were asymptomatic at birth. It is characterized by progressive panencephalitis and diabetes.

Diagnosis

Clinical diagnosis of rubella is not reliable. Hence, every nonimmune woman, woman who presents with rubella-like symptoms, or a woman who was exposed to an infected individual during pregnancy should undergo serological testing. In case of seronegative result, the mother should be tested weekly for up to 4 weeks from the date of contact. In such cases, the rubella avidity test is useful.[22]

Ultrasound Findings

Early gestational age at fetal infection has a higher risk of congenital malformation in the fetus.[23,24] Hence, ultrasound examination is must in women who had been diagnosed rubella infection in the first trimester of pregnancy. Various ultrasound findings in CRS are as follows:

- *CNS:* Microcephaly, intracranial calcification
- *CVS:* Atrial septal defect/ventricular septal defect (ASD/VSD), pulmonary artery stenosis
- Hepatosplenomegaly
- *Craniofacial:* Cataract, micro-ophthalmia
- Intrauterine growth restriction (IUGR) Hydrops, polyhydramnios, ascites, etc.

APCR is a technique of choice for fetal infection. Positive PCR with structural abnormalities in scan are associated with poor outcome and without abnormalities requires long follow-up postnatally. Negative PCR rules out infection.[10]

Management

Prevention

Every woman of child-bearing age who is nonimmune to rubella should be given MMR (measles, mumps, rubella) vaccine 0.5 mL. Rubella vaccine is a live attenuated vaccine; hence, pregnancy must be avoided for 1 month after vaccination. In case vaccine is given inadvertently to a pregnant female, then termination is not advised as the risk of malformation in the fetus is only theoretical and not evidence based. If a pregnant woman is found nonimmune to rubella, then the MMR vaccine should be given after delivery.[25] Breastfeeding is not contraindicated in vaccination.

Treatment

No treatment is available in present for maternal and fetal rubella infection. Termination of pregnancy is advisable in case of maternal infection in early pregnancy.

■ CYTOMEGALOVIRUS IN PREGNANCY

Cytomegalovirus is a deoxyribonucleic acid (DNA) virus of herpes family which affects only humans. It is found in body secretions. The main feature of the virus is its capacity to establish a permanent state of latent infection after primary infection in host throughout life which may occasionally get reactivated by environmental stimuli and lead to reinfection.[26] Primary infection does not confer immunity for reinfection; however, the chances of vertical transmission are negligible.

Epidemiology

Cytomegalovirus is the most common cause of intrauterine infection in developed countries (about 0.5–2% of live birth) and a common cause of sensorineural hearing loss and mental retardation.[27] CMV is transmitted by coming in contact of saliva, semen, cervical secretions, or nasopharyngeal secretion of the infected persons.

The mother usually acquires infection from children. The fetus may be affected intrauterine, intrapartum, and postpartum by breastfeeding. The risk of fetal infection is 30–40% in case of primary infection and <1% in cases of reactivation of infection from the latent phase.

Fetal Effects

The risk of transmission of primary CMV infection in a fetus is 30–40% and is a cause of severe morbidity in the fetus.[28] The risk of transmission following primary infection increases progressively from the periconceptional period (3 months before conception) to term. In case of secondary infection, the risk of transmission is 1% but once infected the course of fetal infection is similar and severe abnormalities have been reported.[29] CMV has a particular tropism for neuronal cells of the periventricular zone of brain. During early pregnancy, the damage of neurons of the peri ventricular zone results in extensive damage of brain. In late pregnancy, white matter abnormalities are more common.[30]

10% of infected neonates have symptoms at birth. 20–30% of them will die. Rest are asymptomatic at birth out of which 5–15% of them will develop sequelae such as sensorineural hearing loss, delay of psychomotor development, and visual impairment.[31] Congenital fetal CMV infection presents as acute infection involving multiple organ systems with 30% mortality rate. Cytomegalovirus causes:

- Petechiae, purpura (79%)
- Hepatosplenomegaly (74%)
- Jaundice (63%)
- Blueberry muffin spots reflecting extramedullary hematopoiesis
- IUGR

Diagnosis

Maternal infection is diagnosed by documenting CMV-specific IgM antibodies or seroconversion to critical titer of IgG. Avidity test is used to distinguish the type of infection. Amniocentesis and PCR are used to detect viral DNA in amniotic fluid and fetal blood.

Ultrasound Findings

Cytomegalovirus affinity toward neuronal cells causes various congenital brain abnormalities.[32-36] Ventriculomegaly is a common finding. However, the rate of CMV infection with isolated ventriculomegaly is 6% so serological testing is advised in such cases. Intracranial calcification around the periventricular zone is also common. In toxoplasma, it is scattered throughout the brain. Other signs include intraventricular hemorrhage, intraventricular adhesions, subependymal cysts, periventricular leukomalacia, microcephaly, lissencephaly, porencephaly, cerebellar agenesis, hypogenesis, and hypoplasia.

Extracerebral abnormalities include echogenic bowel, bowel dilatation, hepatosplenomegaly, multiple liver calcification, cardiomegaly, pericardial effusion, and nonimmune hydrops.

Management

Prevention

At present, no CMV vaccine is available. The Centre for Disease Control recommends regular hand washing practices with soap and water after contact with diapers and oral secretions and not sharing food, utensils, and toothbrushes. The presence of CMV from cervix or urine near term does not warrant cesarean section.

Treatment

No definitive intrauterine therapy is available which is 100% effective. Hence, termination of pregnancy is offered. CMV hyperimmune globulin has been found to be safe and effective in treatment and prevention of congenital CMV infection.

■ GENITAL HERPES IN PREGNANCY

Genital herpes is caused by herpes simplex virus (HSV) which is a DNA virus of Herpesviridae family.

Epidemiology

Out of the two types of HSV, HSV-2 causes genital herpes and is transmitted through the sexual route while HSV-1 causes oral virus and is transmitted by the nonsexual route. They infect the mucosal epithelial cells, nerves and persist in the latent phase and causes recurrent infection.[37]

However, the epidemiology of HSV is changing with increasing genital infections with HSV-1 virus. Approximately 70% of neonatal HSV cases are due to HSV-2 and 30% are due to HSV-1.[38]

Maternal Effects

About 70% of new HSV infections in pregnant women are asymptomatic; however, the severity is more. Symptomatic women may present with fever, headache, ulcers at genitalia, cervix, vaginal discharge, and inguinal lymphadenopathy. Severe complications include meningitis, encephalitis, disseminated skin lesions, and hepatitis. Asymptomatic patients are infectious between 1 week and 3 months after infection.

Fetal Effects

Neonatal infection is acquired in three ways: (1) intrauterine (5%), peripartum (85%), and postnatal (10%).[39] Infection acquired before 20 weeks of gestation causes miscarriage, still birth and congenital malformation involving CNS, skin, and eye.[40]

After 20 weeks, it is associated with an increased risk of preterm labor.

Newborn infection may manifest as:

- Local infection involving eye, mouth, and skin lesion
- CNS disease manifesting as lethargy, poor feeding, and seizures. It has the worst prognosis.
- Disseminated disease involving multiple major organs (25%)

Diagnosis

Serology is important for assessment of pregnant women with genital infection. It differentiates between HSV-1 and HSV-2 antibodies. Viral culture, PCR, and cytology are definitive tests for diagnosing HSV infection but do not differentiate between primary and recurrent infection. They have low sensitivity as viral shedding is intermittent and the sample may be taken when the virus is not shed.

Ultrasound Signs

The most common ultrasound features are as follows:

- *CNS:* Severe ventriculomegaly, hydranencephaly, microcephaly, enlarged cisterna magna
- Nonimmune hydrops
- Abdominal calcification, especially within the liver
- Skin scarring

Management

Disseminated HSV infection is treated by intravenous acyclovir 5–10mg/kg every 8 hours for 2–7 days followed by oral acyclovir therapy for 10 days.[41]

Vertical transmission should be prevented in women at risk by means of viral suppressive therapy after 36 weeks of gestation. The American College of Obstetricians and Gynecologists (ACOG) recommends acyclovir 400 mg orally thrice daily or valaciclovir 500mg orally twice daily as suppressive therapy after 36 weeks.

Mode of Delivery

If primary genital infection is acquired during the third trimester within the last 4–6 weeks of delivery, elective cesarean section is recommended. In case of recurrent HSV infection, cesarean section is performed only if there are clinical symptoms or viral cultures are positive. There is no absolute duration of membrane rupture beyond which the fetus would not benefit from cesarean delivery. Such a mother should wash her hands thoroughly and avoid contact between lesions, hands, and infant. Breastfeeding is not contraindicated.

■ RECENT ADVANCES IN TORCH MANAGEMENT

- The ACOG (2017) does not recommend prenatal screening for toxoplasmosis in areas of low prevalence.
- Prenatal treatment of toxoplasma is based on two regimens—spiramycin alone or a pyrimethamine-sulfonamide combination given with folinic acid (ACOG 2017).
- Transmission rates of primary infection of CMV:
  - *30–36%:* First trimester
  - *34–40%:* Second trimester
  - *40–72%:* Third trimester
- Paired serological tests are most useful only when the first sample has been drawn during clinical illness. The second sample is drawn 4 weeks later, and rise in titer or otherwise is used to interpret the test results and diagnose infection.[42]
- Cesarean section should be recommended to all women presenting with a primary episode of genital herpes lesion at the time of delivery or within 6 weeks of the expected date of delivery.[43]

KEY POINTS

- TORCH is a group of infections caused by bacteria, viruses, and protozoans in the mother and the fetus.
- TORCH agents causes miscarriage, congenital malformations, preterm labor.
- TORCH has been excluded from the causes of recurrent pregnancy loss.
- Routine screening is not recommended in India
- The serologic test is a fundamental test for diagnosing acute infection in pregnant females. Serological conversion in serology testing is a gold standard test but is not possible in a single serum sample.
- Fetal Infection is diagnosed by invasive procedures including PCR which quantifies parasite load.
- Ultrasound plays an important role in the diagnosis and management of TORCH infection.
- Rubella causes multiple organ disease in a fetus which is known as congenital rubella syndrome (CRS).
- Cytomegalovirus affinity toward neuronal cells causes various congenital brain abnormalities.
- 70% of neonatal HSV cases are due to HSV-2 and 30% are due to HSV-1.
- If primary genital infection is acquired during the third trimester within the last 4–6 weeks of delivery, elective cesarean section is recommended. In case of recurrent HSV infection, cesarean section is performed only if there are clinical symptoms or viral cultures are positive.

■ REFERENCES

1. Thellin O, Henin E. Pregnancy and the immune system: Between tolerance and rejection. Toxicology. 2003;185:179.
2. Ledger WJ. Perinatal infection and fetal/neonatal brain injury. Curr Opin Obstet Gynecol. 2008;20(2):120-4.
3. World Health Organization. Hepatitis B. Emergencies preparedness, response. [online] Available from https://www.who.int/csr/don/archive/disease/hepatitis/en/ [Last accessed September, 2020].
4. Radhakrishnan G, Srivastava H. Maternal infection. Practical Obstetric Problems. 2015;269-5.
5. Abdel- Fattah SA, Bhat A, Illanes S, Bartha JL, Carrington D. TORCH test for fetal medicine indications: only CMV is necessary in the United Kingdom. Prenat Diagn. 2005;25(11):1028-31.
6. Capuzzo E, Spinillo A. Genital infections as a cause of abortion in the first trimester of pregnancy. Review of the literature. Minerva Ginecol. 1995;47:557-60.
7. American College of Obstetricians and Gynecologists. Perinatal viral and parasitic infections. Number 20, September 2000. Int J Gynaecol Obstet. 2002;76(1):95-107.
8. Montoya JG, Remington JS. Management of Toxoplasma gondii infection during pregnancy. Clin Infect Dis. 2008;47:554566.
9. Many A, Koren G. Toxoplasmosis during pregnancy. Can Fam Physician. 2006;52:29-32.
10. Mace M, Cointe D, Six C, Levy-Bruhl D, du Châtelet IP, Ingrand D, et al. Diagnostic value of reverse transcriptase- PCR of amniotic fluid for prenatal diagnosis of congenital rubella infection in pregnant woman with confirmed primary rubella infection. J Clin Microbiol. 2004;42:4818-20.
11. Guerra B, Lazzarotto T, Quarta S, Lanari M, Bovicelli L, Nicolosi A, et al. Prenatal diagnosis of symptomatic congenital cytomegalovirus infection. Am J Obstet Gynecol. 2000;183:476-82.
12. Donner C, Liesnard C, Brancart F, Rodesch F. Accuracy of amniotic fluid testing before 21 weeks gestation in prenatal diagnosis of congenital cytomegalovirus infection. Prenat Diagn.1994;14:1055-9.
13. Tondury G, Smith DW. Fetal rubella pathology. J Pediatr.1966;68(6):867-79.
14. Banatvala JE, Brown DW. Rubella. Lancet. 2004;363:1127-37.
15. Thalib L, Gras L, Roman S, Prusa A, Bessieres M-H, Petersen E, et al. Prediction of congenital toxoplasmosis by polymerase chain reaction analysis of amniotic fluid. BJOG. 2005;11:567.
16. Berrebi A, Bardou M, Bessieres MH, Nowakowska D, Castagno R, Rolland M, et al. Outcome for children infected with congenital toxoplasmosis in the first trimester and with normal ultrasound findings: a study of 36 cases. Eur J Obstet Gynecol Reprod Biol. 2007;135:53-7.
17. Romand S, Wallon M, Frank J, Thulliez P, Peyron F, Dumon H. Prenatal diagnosis using polymerase chain reaction on amniotic fluid for congenital toxoplasmosis. Obstet Gynecol. 2001; 97: 296-300.
18. Miller E, Cradock-Watson JE, Pollock TM. Consequences of confirmed maternal rubella at successive stages of pregnancy. Lancet. 1982;2:781-4.
19. Rosa C. Rubella and rubeola. Semin Perinatal. 1998;22:318-22.
20. Gappe SG, Niebyl JR, Simpson JL (Eds). Obstetrics: Normal and Problem Pregnancies, 4th edition. New York : Churchill Livingstone; 2002. pp. 1328-30.
21. Dontigny L, Arsenault MY, Martel MJ, Clinical Practice Obstetrics Committee. Rubella in pregnancy. J Obstet Gynaecol Can. 2008;30(2):152-8.
22. Rousseau S, Hedman K. Rubella infection and reinfection distinguished by avidity of IgG. Lancet. 1988;1:1108-9.
23. Migliucci A, Di Fraja D, Sarnol, Acampora E, Mazzarelli LL, Quaglia F, et al. Prenatal diagnosis of congenital rubella infection and ultrasonography: a preliminary study. Minerva Ginecol. 2011; 63(6):485-9.

24. Tang JW, Aarons E, Hesketh LM, Strobel S, Schalasta G, Jauniaux E, et al. Prenatal diagnosis of congenital rubella infection in second trimester of pregnancy. Prenat Diagn. 2003;23:509-12.

25. Centres for Disease Control and Prevention (CDC). Rubella. In: Epidemiology and Prevention of Vaccine-Preventable Diseases. he Pink Book: Course Textbook - 12th Edition.; Georgia: CDC; 2012.

26. Mocarski ES, Sherk T, Pass RF. Cytomegaloviruses. In: Knipe DM, Howley PM (Eds). Fields Virology, 5th edition. Philadelphia, PA: Lippincott Williams and Wilkins;2007. pp. 2701-72.

27. Kenneson A, Cannon MJ. Review and meta- analysis of the epidemiology of congenital cytomegalovirus (CMV) infection. Rev Med Virol. 2007;17:253-76.

28. Yinon Y, Farine D, Yudin MH. Screening, diagnosis, and management of cytomegalovirus infection in pregnancy. Obstet Gynecol Surv. 2010;65(11):736-43.

29. Zalel Y, Gilboa Y, Berkenshtat M, Yoeli R, Auslander R, Achiron R, et al. Secondary cytomegalovirus infection can cause severe fetal sequelae despite maternal preconceptional immunity. Ultrasound Obstet Gynecol. 2008;31:417-20.

30. Gressens P. Pathogenesis of migration disorders. Curr Opin Neurol. 2006;19:135-40.

31. SOGC Clinical Practice Guideline. Cytomegalovirus infection in pregnancy. No 240, April 2010.

32. Guerra B, Simonazzi G, Puccetti C, Lanari M, Farina A, Lazzarotto T, et al. Ultrasound prediction of symptomatic congenital cytomegalovirus infection. An J Obstet Gynecol. 2008;198: 380 .e1-7.

33. Benoist G, Salmon LJ, Jacquemard F, Daffos F, Ville Y. The prognostic value of ultrasound abnormalities and biological parameters in blood of foetuses infected with cytomegalovirus. BJOG. 2008;115:823-39.

34. Malinger G, Lev D, Zahalka N, Ben Aroia Z, Watemberg N, Kidron D, et al. Fetal cytomegalovirus infection of the brain: the spectrum of sonographic findings AJNR Am J Neuroradiol. 2003;24:28-32.

35. Bailao LA, Osborne NG, Rizzi MC, Bonilla-Musoles F, Duarte G, Bailão TCRS. Ultrasound markers of fetal infection part 1: viral infections. Ultrasound Q. 2005;21:295-308.

36. Crino JP. Ultrasound and fetal diagnosis of perinatal infection. Clin Obstet Gynecol. 1999;42:71-80.

37. Nyholm JL, Schleiss MR. Prevention of maternal cytomegalovirus infection: current status and future prospects. Int J Womens Health. 2010;2:23-35.

38. Gupta R, Warren T, Wald A. Genital herpes. Lancet. 2007; 370(9605):2127-37.

39. Whitley R, Davis EA, Suppapaya N. Incidence of neonatal herpes simplex virus infections in a managed-care population. Sex Transm Dis. 2007;34:704-8.

40. Kimberlin DW. Neonatal herpes simplex infection. Clin Microbiol Rev. 2004;17:1-13.

41. Sauerbrei A, Wutzler P. Herpes simplex and varicella-zoster virus infections during pregnancy: current concepts of prevention, diagnosis and therapy. Part1: herpes simplex virus infection. Med Microbial Immunol. 2007;196(2):89-94.

42. http://www.fogsi.org/smtp.

43. http://www.rcog.org.uk/gtg30.

44. http://radiopaedia.org/articles/fetal-intrahepatic calcification

45. http://obgyn.onlinelibrary.wiley.com

46. http://www.thelancet.com

47. http://onlinelibrary.wiley.com/pdf/dmcn

Preterm Labor

Vidya Gaikwad, Hemant Deshpande

■ INTRODUCTION

In the era of modern obstetrics, where there has been a rapid advancement in all specialties, preterm labor still remains an enigma for the obstetricians today and is the leading cause of neonatal mortality and morbidity. Perinatal mortality among preterm Indian babies has been reported to be two to seven times higher than in term babies.

■ DEFINITION

Preterm labor is defined as the onset of labor with regular, painful, frequent uterine contractions causing progressive effacement and dilation of the cervix occurring before 37 completed weeks with intact membranes.

According to the World Health Organization, *preterm delivery* is defined as delivery before 37 weeks' gestation or 259 days.

Threatened preterm is defined as the onset of labor in patients with intact membranes before 37 weeks of gestation without any change in cervical effacement and dilatation.

These criteria for the diagnosis of preterm labor, defined by the onset of increasingly frequent and painful uterine contractions with progressive effacement and dilatation of the cervix, can be assessed most accurately once contractions occur at least once every 10 minutes. There is 80% cervical effacement and the cervix is at least 3 cm dilated.

■ INCIDENCE

The incidence of preterm birth ranges from 5 to 18% the world over and 13 to 15% in India.

■ CAUSES OF PRETERM LABOR

Socioeconomic Causes

There is a relationship between factors such as low socioeconomic class, limited antenatal care, inadequate nutrition, early marriage and teenage pregnancy, unmarried, low maternal weight, and preterm labor.

Maternal smoking and alcohol intake: Women smoking 6–10 cigarettes daily had three times high risk of preterm birth as compared to nonsmokers. Fetal alcohol syndrome related to material intake does include preterm birth.

Occupational factors such as prolonged walking or standing, strenuous working conditions, and long weekly working hours have been implicated in preterm birth.

Psychological stress and higher levels of maternal cortisol have been associated with spontaneous preterm birth.

Previous preterm birth and abortions: History of previous preterm birth is the most important predictor of the likelihood of preterm delivery in the multiparous women. The risk can be up to 70%, if there have been two or more previous spontaneous preterm births. Spontaneous second-trimester abortion is also a significant risk factor. The higher the gestation-induced abortions, the higher the risk of preterm labor. First-trimester abortion is not a significant factor.

Specific Causes of Preterm Labor

Lower Genital Tract Infections

Microbial colonization of the fetal membranes or the amniotic fluid, or alterations in the vaginal flora such as those seen in patients with bacterial vaginosis, has been associated with spontaneous labor and preterm delivery.

Chorioamnionitis

Clinical and epidemiologic evidence implicates systemic and intrauterine infection in the etiology of premature labor and delivery; maternal chorioamnionitis occurs when several protective mechanisms of the urogenital tract and uterus fail during pregnancy or when increased numbers of microbial floral or highly pathogenic flora are introduced into the genital environmental.

Infections

Periodontitis, urinary tract infection (UTI), and pyelonephritis are responsible for causing preterm labor.

Maternal Medical Disorders

Anemia during pregnancy was found to be the most common association in preterm labor.

with this drug has made other β-agonists a more popular choice for treatment for preterm labor.

Dose: Injection isoxsuprine HCl 40 mg as infusion in 5% dextrose (concentration of 0.08 mg/mL) and started at 0.08 mg/min in a patient diagnosed with preterm labor. The dose is increased every 10 minutes while monitoring uterine contractions to a maximum dose up to 0.24 mg/min until contractions decrease or occurrence of side effects and maintained for a period of 12 hours. The patient is then given injection isoxsuprine HCl 10 mg IM 8 hourly for 24 hours and then switched on to oral therapy of tablet isoxsuprine HCl 10 mg 8 hourly till necessary.

Mechanism of action: Isoxsuprine interacts with β2-receptors on the myometrial cell membrane to release adenyl cyclase within the cell. It catalyzes the intracellular formation of cyclic adenosine monophosphate (cAMP), which subsequently leads to relaxation of the uterine musculature due to changes in calcium availability.

Pharmacology: The onset of action is about 1 hour (oral) and 10 minutes (IV). It belongs to pregnancy category C. β-agonists should be used to delay delivery for 24–48 hours in order to administer corticosteroids to promote fetal lung maturity.

Ritodrine

Ritodrine is the first United States Food and Drug Administration (US FDA) approved tocolytic agent for preterm labor. Ritodrine decreases the intensity and frequency of uterine contractions in women with preterm labor. It appears to be equally efficacious to other tocolytics. The incidence of cardiovascular side effects with ritodrine is reported to be lower than with less-selective β2-agonosits such as isoxsuprine.

Dose: Intravenous infusion of injection ritodrine is started with 50–150 mg in crystalloid at a rate of 0.1 mg/min and increased every 15 minutes by 0.05 mg/min until contractions cease or up to a maximum rate of 0.35 mg/min provided side effects do not occur. Once an adequate dose is reached, it should be maintained for 12 hours after contractions stop. Fluid balance is maintained. Intravenous infusion is not tapered or stopped until oral treatment is started. Tablet ritodrine 10 mg is given 30 minutes before discontinuing the infusion, and one tablet (10 mg) every 2 hourly for the first 24 hours as long as the pulse rate dose not exceed 120 bpm is given. The dose is then adjusted to 10–20 mg every 4–6 hours as necessary.

Mechanism of action: Ritodrine is a sympathomimetic agent with predominantly β2 activity. It increases the concentration of cAMP which causes relaxation of the uterine musculature.

Pharmacology: Orally administered ritodrine is rapidly absorbed in the gastrointestinal tract. Ritodrine belongs to pregnancy category B.

Monitoring of the Patient on Intravenous β-Sympathomimetics

- Monitor maternal pulse; if >120 bpm, stop the drip immediately.
- Monitor blood pressure; if systolic BP < 90 mm Hg, discontinue the drip.
- Auscultation of lung fields is done every 20–30 minutes.
- Monitoring of uterine contractions is done every half hourly.
- Fluid balance should be watched closely.

Adverse Effects of Intravenous β-Sympathomimetics

- *Cardiac symptoms:* Palpitation, tremors, chest pain, tightness, tachycardia, tachypnea, arrhythmias, ischemia
- Hypotension
- *Pulmonary edema:* Twin pregnancies with a higher maternal blood volume maybe at increased risk. The exact cause of pulmonary edema is not known. The administration of corticosteroids, with their mineralocorticoid activity causing salt and fluid retention, may add to the effect of β-sympathomimetic drugs.
- Hyperglycemia is caused due to glycogenolysis with the possibility for neonatal hypoglycemia.
- Hypokalemia due to shift of circulating potassium into cells
- Lipolysis leading to increased serum lactate
- Fetal cardiac effects can occur with long-term exposure and may include hypertrophy of the intraventricular septum and myocardial cell necrosis.
- Anaphylactic shock
- Erythema and rash

Prostaglandin Synthetase Inhibitors

Indomethacin

Mechanism of action: Indomethacin involves primarily inhibition of prostaglandin (PG) synthesis. These arachidonic acid derivatives are important mediators in the cascade leading to preterm labor. Although the exact sites of synthesis and action of these compounds have not yet been elucidated, recent reports indicate that the uterus and cervix are probably the major target organs for PG synthetase inhibition.

Dosage: 100–200 mg is given as rectal suppositories or 50–100 mg orally and repeated after 1 hour if necessary.

A maintenance dose of 25–50 mg 4–6 hourly is given for 2–3 days.

Pharmacology: Indomethacin is rapidly absorbed after oral administration with peak plasma concentration seen in 1–2 hours.

Adverse effects: Maternal indomethacin treatment is known to reduce the amount of amniotic fluid. Fetal ductal constriction is the side effect associated with maternal indomethacin treatment. This effect is more common after 32 weeks of gestation; indomethacin therapy is not usually recommended after 32 weeks. Recent reports also have suggested increased risks of neonatal intraventricular hemorrhage and necrotizing enterocolitis with indomethacin exposure.

Role of Progesterone Preterm Labor

Progesterone is the most potent anti-PG agent. It is a vital hormone for maintaining pregnancy till term. Micronization of progesterone increases the bioavailability by reducing the particle size and increasing the surface area. The role of progesterone is in prevention of preterm labor than treating it and its key action appears to be in the cervix.

Progesterone can be given as a weekly intramuscular administration of 17α hydroxyprogesterone caproate or a 250-mg daily vaginal micronized progesterone (200–400mg) from 24 to 34 weeks in patients at risk of preterm birth or with short cervix. The peak blood concentration is better achieved with the intramuscular route. However, the vaginal route bypasses the first-pass hepatic metabolism and results in sustained plasma levels with high bioavailability. The systemic side effects seen with the parental route are alteration in lipid profile, glucose metabolism, sedation, dizziness, nausea, and constipation. These are not seen with the vaginal micronized form. The side effects of the vaginal route are nausea, drowsiness, pruritus, and discharge. Progesterone vaginal gel 8%—dose 90 mg every night—is better accepted than suppository and has minor side effects such as discharge and vaginal irritation in few patients.

The ACOG guidelines (2012) state that women with history of prior preterm birth or cervical length < 20 mm before 24 weeks can be treated with vaginal or intramuscular progesterone from 16 to 34 weeks. Thus, progesterone is cheap, easily available, safer for both mother and fetus, and therefore can be continued to maintain quiescence in patients of preterm birth who had successful acute tocolysis.

Antenatal Corticosteroids

Antenatal glucocorticoid therapy can prevent several life-threatening complications of preterm delivery such as the respiratory distress syndrome and intraventricular hemorrhage and necrotizing enterocolitis. Women with expected labor in the next 7 days should receive a single course of antenatal steroids. Steroid efficacy is at its maximum when delivery occurs 24 hours after the last dose and with 7 days. Both betamethasone and dexamethasone are equally effective in promoting the acceleration of lung maturation.

Mechanism of Action

Corticosteroids circulating in the free form in maternal circulation cross the placenta and stimulate the differentiation of pulmonary epithelial cells into type II pneumocytes to synthesize and release surfactant into alveolar spaces and acceleration of structural development.

Dosage

The recommended glucocorticoid regimens consist of the administration of the mother of either two 12-mg doses of betamethasone given intramuscularly 24 hours apart or four 6-mg doses of dexamethasone given intramuscularly 12 hours apart. At this dose, it occupies steroid receptors at the maximum level. Beyond this dose, there is a possibility of adverse effects (neurotoxicity, demyelination of neurons, etc.). It reaches fetal plasma 1–2 hours after administration; half-life is 12 hours. The RCOG guideline on antenatal corticosteroids has concluded that there is no evidence to recommend multiple courses of antenatal corticosteroids.

Steroid administration may raise the WBC count by 30% which will return to baseline by 3 days. Hyperglycemia can occur as early as 3–8 hours which will return to normal within 24 hours in nondiabetic patients but may be raised for up to 5 days in diabetic patients. Hence, close blood sugar monitoring is advised and may require adjustment of insulin dosage. Mothers with PROM and PPROM without overt chorioamnionitis do not exhibit increased chances of sepsis after a single course of steroids.

Corticosteroids are effective only when given by the parental route. Oral administration is not recommended. Recent studies have found that early onset neonatal sepsis, chorioamnionitis, and neonatal death are associated with multiple courses of betamethasone therapy.

■ INTRAPARTUM MONITORING

First Stage

The patient is confined to bed to prevent early rupture of membranes. Epidural anesthesia can be given, which by relaxation of pelvic floor offers less soft-tissue impact on the presenting part and hence less trauma. Labor should be watched by intensive clinical monitoring or continuous electronic monitoring. Variable decelerations are frequently (55–75%) associated in continuous electronic monitoring of a preterm fetus, but there is a poor correlation with pH. The avoidance of hypoxia and hypothermia after delivery is extremely important in reducing morbidity and mortality. Asphyxia and prematurity are not a good combination.

Second Stage of Labor

Birth should be gentle and slow to avoid rapid compression and decompression of head. A carefully controlled spontaneous delivery of head with an appropriate episiotomy to release soft-tissue resistance should be done. The tendency to delay is curtailed by low forceps, but routine use of forceps is not indicated. The cord should be clamped immediately after birth to prevent hypervolemia and hyperbilirubinemia. A skilled neonatal resuscitation team should be ready.

Cesarean Section

In cases of preterm infants weighing 900–1,500 g, cesarean section should be performed before the active phase of labor. Also, cesarean section should be considered if the fetus is a breech presentation and <34 weeks' gestation.

KEY POINTS

- Preterm birth is not only the leading cause of neonatal mortality and morbidity but has long term consequences for the health of the child.
- It is a huge financial and emotional burden for the society.
- Preterm labor is defined as onset of labor with regular painful, frequent uterine contractions causing progressive effacement and dilatation of the cervix occurring before 37 completed weeks with intact membranes.
- Previous preterm birth is the most important predictor of preterm delivery.
- Lower genital tract infections like bacterial vaginosis has been associated with preterm labor and delivery.
- Many studies have shown an increased risk of preterm birth if fetal fibronectin is positive after 24 weeks of gestation and decreased risk if this protein is negative in cervical secretions.
- Preventive strategies for preterm labor include – early identification of risk factors, correction of anemia, treatment of asymptomatic bacteriuria, urinary tract infections, maternal periodontal disease, progesterone therapy and management of cervical incompetence.
- Management of preterm labor includes administration of corticosteroids, tocolysis, magnesium sulfate for fetal neuroprotection and progesterone therapy.

- Progesterone therapy can be both preventive as well as for maintenance of uterine quiescence following successful acute tocolysis.
- Atosiban, an oxytocin receptor antagonist is recommended as a first line agent by RCOG. Compared to other tocolytics, it has a more favorable safety profile.
- Despite all efforts if preterm labor progresses, the delivery should be carried out with all safety precautions.
- Preterm labor should be preferably monitored by continuous electronic fetal monitoring.
- Avoidance of hypoxia and hypothermia after delivery is extremely important in reducing morbidity and mortality.
- Preterm birth is associated with both short-term and long-term complications in the child.

SUGGESTED READING

1. Berghella V, Saccone G. Fetal fibronectin testing for prevention of preterm birth in singleton pregnancies with threatened preterm labor: a systematic review and metaanalysis of randomized controlled trials. Am J Obstet Gynecol. 2016;215(4):431-8.
2. Eduardo B da Fonseca, Roberto E Bittar, et al. Prophylactic administration of progesterone by vaginal suppository to reduce the incidence of spontaneous preterm birth in women at increased risk: a randomized placebo-controlled double-blind study. Am J Obstet Gynecol. 2003;188(2):419-42.
3. Jobe AH, Goldenberg RL. Antenatal corticosteroids: an assessment of anticipated benefits and potential risks. Am J Obstet Gynecol. 2018;219(1): P62-74.
4. Klein LL, Gibbs RS. Use of microbial cultures and antibiotics in the prevention of infection-associated preterm birth. Am J Obstet Gynecol. 2004;190(6):1493-1502.
5. Leitich H, Bodner-Adler B. Bacterial vaginosis as a risk factor for preterm delivery: A meta-analysis. Am J Obstet Gynecol. 2003;189(1):139-47.
6. Leitich H, Kaider A. Fetal fibronectin—how useful is it in the prediction of preterm birth? BJOG. 2003;110 (Suppl. 20):66-70.
7. Romero R, Sibai BM, Sanchez-Ramos L, Valenzuela GJ, Veille JC, Tabor B, et al. An oxytocin receptor antagonist (atosiban) in the treatment of preterm labor: randomized, double-blind, placebo-controlled trial with tocolytic rescue. Am J Obstet Gynecol. 2000;182(5):1173-83.
8. Sanchez-Ramos L, Roeckner J. 79: Vaginal progesterone: agent of choice for preterm delivery prevention in singleton pregnancies with short cervix. Am J Obstet Gynecol. 2019;220(1):S62-S63.
9. Valenzuela GL, Sanchez-Ramos L, et al. Maintenance treatment of preterm labor with the oxytocin antagonist atosiban. Am J Obstet Gynecol. 2000;182(5):1184-90.
10. Zephyrin LC, Hong KN, et al. Gestational age–specific risks vs benefits of multicourse antenatal corticosteroids for preterm labor. Am J Obstet Gynecol. 2013;209(4): 330.e1-330.e7.

Prelabor Rupture of the Membranes

RP Rawat

INTRODUCTION

The term "prelabor rupture of membrane" (PROM) is used when the amniotic membranes rupture before the onset of labor.[1] The incidence is 8–10% in term pregnancies and 5–10% of all pregnancies besides a strong association with high maternal and perinatal morbidity and mortality.[2] Chorioamnionitis is bound to occur in long-standing cases of PROM. The incidence of chorioamnionitis varies from 6 to 10% and occurs in 40% of prolonged PROM (persisting > 24 hours).[3] It occurs in 2.0-3.5% of preterm pregnancies and the most common cause of preterm birth[4] along with fatal consequences on maternal health and high rates of neonatal sepsis and mortality in <5 years' age group.[5]

PATHOPHYSIOLOGY OF FETAL MEMBRANES

Amnion, which is the inner layer, is further composed of five layers. These layers include (1) inner amniotic epithelial layer, (2) basement membrane, (3) compact layer, (4) fibroblast layer, and (5) intermediate layer, coming from the innerside closest to the fetus to the outer side adjacent to the maternal uterine cavity. The amnion is totally avascular in humans and has no nerves. The innermost amniotic epithelial cells secrete collagen types III and IV as well as the glycoproteins laminin and fibronectin which form the attachment to the next amniotic layer—the basement membrane. The compact layer is formed by types I and III collagen secreted by the adjacent fibroblast layer. The fourth layer (fibroblast layer) is the thickest and toughest of all and comprises mesenchymal cells and macrophages. The intermediate layer (all known as spongy layer or *zona spongiosa*), composed of type III collagen, proteoglycans and glycoproteins, is in contact with chorion and forms a junction between it and the amnion. These junctions are very fine and not clearly established **(Fig. 1)**. The chorion comprises a reticular layer with collagen types I, III, IV, V, and VI; basement membrane (collagen type IV, fibronectin, and laminin); and trophoblast cells with polarity directed toward the maternal decidua.[6-8] Although chorion is thicker than amnion, its tensile strength is less.

Marked swelling and disruption of the collagen network within the compact, fibroblast, and spongy layers result in PROM. By measuring the concentration of enzymes in the amniotic fluid with immunoassays and enzymatic methods, many studies have implicated matrix metalloproteinase-1 (MMP-1), MMP-8, and MMP-9 in the mechanisms of membrane rupture. MMPs, by acting preferentially on collagen type I, degrade the interstitial collagens.

In cases of preterm PROM (PPROM), Maymon et al. described increase in concentrations of MMP-1 in the amniotic fluid. Elevated amniotic fluid concentrations of MMP-8 have been demonstrated in cases of PPROM. Athayde et al. found that patients with PPROM had higher MMP-9 concentrations compared with preterm labor and intact membranes, who were delivered at term.[9-12] Vadillo-Ortega et al. suggested activation of MMP-9, a 92-kDa type IV collagenase in these cases.

ETIOLOGY

Urogenital infection and microbial colonization lead to preterm labor by causing an increase in local cytokines

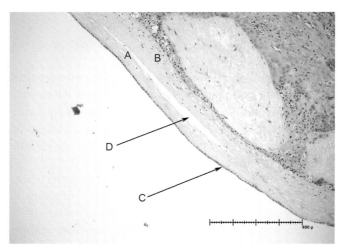

Fig. 1: Chorioamniotic membranes. (A) Amniotic membrane; (B) chorionic membrane; (C) amnion epithelium; (D) very fine fibrous network developing after overlapping of the membranes during the 12–15th weeks' gestation.
Source: Tchirikov M, Schlabritz-Loutsevitch N, Maher J, Buchmann J, Naberezhnev Y, Winarno AS, et al. Mid-trimester preterm premature rupture of membranes (PPROM): etiology, diagnosis, classification, international recommendations of treatment options and outcome. J Perinatal Med. 2017;46(5). [online] Available from: https://doi.org/10.1515/jpm-2017-0027 [Last accessed September, 2020]

BOX 1: Risk factors of PROM.

- *Systemic and environmental:*
  - Cigarette smoking
  - Drug abuse
  - Anemia
  - Low socioeconomic status
  - Unmarried status
  - History of PROM/ preterm birth (PTB) in previous pregnancy
- *Genetical:*
  - Collagen vascular disorders (Ehler-Danlos syndrome, SLE)
  - Hyaluronic acid disorder involving fibrillin I gene (Marfan syndrome)
  - Chronic corticosteroid therapy
- *Nutritional:*
  - Low body mass index
  - Malnutrition
- *Uterine:*
  - Ascending bacterial infection
  - Antepartum hemorrhage
  - Abdominal trauma
  - Uterine anomalies
  - Cervical insufficiency
  - Previous cervical dilatation
- *Fetal and uteroplacental:*
  - Polyhydramnios
  - Multiple pregnancy
  - Decidual hemorrhage, placental abruption
  - Chorioamnionitis
- *Invasive diagnostic:*
  - Amniocentesis
  - Chorionic villous sampling
  - Cardiocentesis
- *Infection:*
  - Sore throat, caries, sinusitis, UTI
  - Group B streptococcus
  - Inflammation

(PROM: prelabor rupture of membranes; SLE: systemic lupus erythematosus; UTI: urinary tract infection)

or an imbalance between MMPs and tissue inhibitors of metalloproteinases (TIMPs). The organisms implicated are *Chlamydia trachomatis*, *Trichomonas vaginalis*, group B beta-hemolytic streptococci (GBS), and *Neisseria gonorrhoeae*. Bacterial vaginosis also predisposes to PROM and preterm labor. Amniotic fluid cultures are positive in 25–35% of women with PROM. Several risk factors have been known to be associated with PROM, which may be either present prior to pregnancy or identified during pregnancy. Previous preterm birth with or without PROM is an important risk factor. Cervical cerclage, amniocentesis, cordocentesis, and fetoscopy are well-recognized risk factors for mid-trimester PROM. In most cases of PROM, no etiological factor is identified. The risk factors for PROM are given in **Box 1**.[13-20]

DIAGNOSIS OF PROM

The diagnosis of PROM can be made from the clinical history and physical examination mainly, requiring laboratory examination in some cases:

- Visualization of amniotic fluid lying in vaginal pool or leaking from cervical canal.
- Nitrazine test—performed from posterior fornix, with pH > 6-6.5.
  False-positive result may be seen with blood and semen contamination, alkaline aseptic, and bacterial vaginosis. False-negative result may be due to prolonged leaking with minimal residual fluid on inspection and fern testing.
- Fern test—fluid obtained from posterior fornix with a sterile swab shows microscopic-arborized crystal on smear, due to interaction of amniotic fluid protein and salt with dried vaginal secretions.
- Test detecting amniotic fluid proteins:
  - *Immunoassay of placental alpha macroglobulin 1 (Amnisure):* The US Food and Drug Administration (FDA) has recently approved the use of placental alpha macroglobulin 1 (PAMG-1), for the diagnosis of PPROM. It is a 34-kDa placental glycoprotein synthesized by the deciduas and is found in abundance in amniotic fluid (2000–25,000 ng/mL), but its concentration is very low in maternal blood (5–25 ng/mL) and in cervix (0.005–0.2 ng/mL). This test is already in clinical use in some hospitals although its prospective usefulness as an adjunct test for PPROM still remains to be validated in clinical trials. The PAMG-1 immunoassay in vaginal fluid yields results that are comparable to those of the instillation of indigo carmine into the amniotic cavity. Sosa et al. described that the PAMG-1 test in patients with PROM and positive amnio-dye test after 12 hours from intra-amniotic transabdominal dye injection had a sensitivity of 100.0%, specificity of 99.1, positive predictive value of 96.3%, negative predictive value of 100.0%, and ± likelihood ratios of 74.6. The predictive values of diagnostic tests are summarized in **Table 1**.[21-26]
  - Fetal fibronectin test
  - β-human chorionic gonadotropin (b-hCG)
  - Prolactin
  - Lactate (Amnolect)
  - Insulin-like growth factor binding protein 1 (IGFBP1)
  - IGFBP1/alpha-fetoprotein (Amnioquick Duo+).
- Amino infusion with indigo carmine dye (1 mL dye + 9 mL sterile saline): Passage of indigo carmine on to the perineal pad within 30 minutes of administration is suggestive of PROM. The test has good sensitivity but usually not needed. The urine is also colored due to dye.
- Ultrasound—oligohydramnios in absence of any fetal urinary tract malformation or fetal growth retardation may be suggestive of PROM.

TABLE 1: Predictive value of the diagnostic test based on the detection of amniotic fluid protein in PROM.

Test/references	Name of test	Cutoff	Sensitivity (%)	Specificity (%)	PPV	NPV
Nitrazine (pH)		Positive/negative	90–97	16–70	63–75	80–93
Ferning and/or pooling		Positive/negative	51–98	70–88	84–93	87–97
AFP	ROM check	>30 µg/L	90–94	95–100	95–100	91–94
Fetal fibronectin		>50 ng/mL	97–98	70–97	74–90	98–100
IGFBP-1	PROM test	>3 µg/L	74–97	74–97	72–92	56–87
Prolactin		>30–50 µIU/mL	70–95	76–78	72–94	75–93
b-hCG		>40–65 µIU/mL	68–95	70–95	73–91	78–97
Urea and creatinine		>0.12–0.6 mg/dL	90–100	87–100	94–100	91–100
Lactate	Lac test	≥4.5 mmol/L	79–86	88–92	88–92	78–87
PAMG-1	Amnisure	>5.0 ng/mL	98–99	88–100	98–100	91–99
IGFBP-1/alpha fetoprotein	Amnioquick duo+		97–6%	97–9%	74–93	97.9%

(AFP: alpha fetoprotein; β-hCG: beta-subunit of human chorionic gonadotropin; IGFBP-1: insulin-like growth factor binding protein 1; NPV: negative predictive value; PAMG-1: placental alpha-microglobulin 1; PPV: positive predictive value.

Source: Tchirikov M, Schlabritz-Loutsevitch N, Maher J, Buchmann J, Naberezhnev Y, Winarno AS, et al. Mid-trimester preterm premature rupture of membranes (PPROM): etiology, diagnosis, classification, international recommendations of treatment options and outcome. J Perinatal Med. 2017;46(5). [online] Available from: https://doi.org/10.1515/jpm-2017-0027 [Last accessed September, 2020]

■ MANAGEMENT OF PROM

According to the Royal College of Obstetricians and Gynaecologists (RCOG) and Royal Australian and New Zealand College of Ophthalmologist (RANZCOJ), the American College of Obstetricians and Gynecologists (ACOG) guidance update 2017 PROM should be managed as follows.

Initial Assessment

- Confirmation of PROM diagnosis and gestational age.
- Fetal presentation and assessment of maternal and fetal well-being.
- In situation of diagnostic uncertainty, a nitrazine test (pH based) and a sterile speculum examination should be performed. Digital examination has been shown to increase the rate of neonatal infection and should be avoided unless immediate induction is planned.

Term and Late Preterm PROM (>37 Weeks and >34–37 Weeks)

- A single course of betamethasone may be considered between 34 and 36 weeks.
- Acute and severe neonatal complications are uncommon after 34 weeks' gestation.
- Risk of chorioamnionitis increases by waiting.
- Expectant management prolongs pregnancy by only a few days.
- If delivery is recommended, induction by oxytocin drip.
- Induction with prostaglandins is equally effective as oxytocin but may have a higher rate of chorioamnionitis.

It should be considered in cases with poor Bishop's score.

Currently, the data is insufficient to recommend for or against cervical ripening with mechanical methods such as Foley's balloon.

Further the data is also insufficient for recommendation of antibiotic prophylaxis beyond group B streptococcus (GBS) indication. A recent meta-analysis revealed that in cases those who received antibiotic with latency >12 hours had a lower rate of chorioamnionitis (2.9 vs. 6.1) and endometritis (0% vs. 2.2%) compared with control group. In these cases, administration of prophylactic antibiotics is associated with a significantly lower rate of chorioamnionitis by 51% and endometritis by 88%.

Active management with induction of labor in term PROM is associated with lower maternal infective morbidity and increased maternal satisfaction without any rise in operative deliveries. The incidence of neonatal intensive care unit (NICU) admissions and requirement of postnatal antibiotic is also reduced. However, some clinicians may opt for a short trial of expectant management (e.g., up to 24 hours) in highly selected and well-supervised cases after initial assessment.[27-29]

Use of tocolysis: Therapeutic tocolysis is not recommended.

Expected Management

The following situations may be considered for expectant management:

- Cephalic presentation with fixed head in a case with term PROM.

- Cases with high vaginal swab negative for GBS.
- No clinical signs of infection to the mother—tachycardia, fever, uterine tenderness.
- Normal cardiotocography (CTG) tracing.
- No history of repeated digital examination or cervical cerclage.
- Regular maternal assessment of temperature, evaluation of vaginal loss, and assessment of fetal well-being.
- Adequate resources/staff support in inpatient department (IPD).

PPROM between 28 Weeks and 33[+6] Weeks

- Expectant management in a hospital setting is recommended, provided there is no maternal/or fetal indication for early termination.
- Proceed to delivery at 34 weeks.
- Single course of corticosteroids is recommended.
- Latency antibiotics are recommended—NICHD-MFMU (*Eunice Kennedy Shriver* National Institute of Child Health and Human and Maternal-Fetal Medicine Units Development) recommendation:
  - Ampicillin 2 g IV 6 hourly + erythromycin 250 mg 6 hourly for 48 hours followed by oral amoxycillin 250 mg 8 hourly + erythromycin 333 mg 8 hourly for 5 days.
  - If allergic to β-lactam antibiotic, erythromycin only may be used as an alternative.
  - Amoxicillin–clavulanic acid is not recommended due to an increased risk of necrotizing enterocolitis in newborn.
- There is no clinical evidence to support the use of serial WBC counts or other infectious markers.
- Sometimes, the membranes may reseal spontaneously leading to good outcomes.
- If PROM occurs before 32 weeks and imminent delivery is expected, fetal neuroprotective treatment with magnesium sulfate is recommended.

The Oxford Patient Safety Collaboratives (PSC)/ Academic Health Science Network (AHSN) maternity network recommends magnesium sulfate for neuro-protection before preterm birth[29,30] (**Flowchart 1**): 22 + 6 weeks, <32 weeks.[1,2]

▇ FETAL COMPLICATIONS OF PROM

- Prematurity
- Respiratory distress syndrome
- Necrotizing enterocolitis
- Intraventricular hemorrhage
- Pulmonary hypoplasia
- Limb deformities
- Fetal infection:
  - Septicemia

Flowchart 1: Management of PPROM.

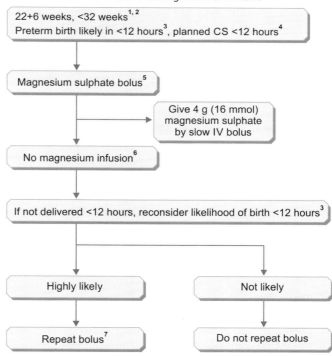

*There is clinical benefit <32 weeks.
*If <26 + 6 (singleton) or <27 + 6 (multiple) or estimated fetal weight (EFW) < 800 g, transfer to level 3 neonatal unit (NNU).

  - Pneumonia
  - Perinatal death
- Cord prolapse and cord compression
- Long-term sequelae:
  - Periventricular leukomalacia
  - Cerebral palsy
  - Hearing and visual defects
  - Mental retardation
  - Chronic lung diseases.

PPROM at <28 Weeks/Mid-trimester Leaking

- Latency 40–50% will deliver within 1 week and 70–80% will deliver within 2–5 weeks.
- Survival with PPROM > 22 weeks is significantly higher (57.7%) than <22 weeks (14.4%).
- Maternal complications—abruption, infection, endometritis, retained placenta, puerperal sepsis.
- Fetal complications—pulmonary hyperplasia, Potter's deformity (presenting with low-set ears, recessed chin, prominent bilateral epicanthal fold, limb contracture, and skeletal malformation).

Management

- Counseling of the patient and family regarding the risk and benefit of expectant versus immediate delivery should be done.

- The option of immediate delivery should be offered.
- Corticosteroid data are limited but they should be recommended once the age of viability is reached or pregnancy > 26 weeks and if the couple opt for expectant management. Management will be on the same line as in 28–32 weeks of gestation. This includes following hospitalization and bed rest, initial assessment of fetal status and uterine contraction, and subsequent monitoring of mother and fetus.
- Latency antibiotic should be given as per NICHD-MFMU similar to PPROM at 34–36 weeks.[27-29]

PROM FOLLOWING AMNIOCENTESIS

- Following amniocentesis, the risk of PROM is only 1%.
- Expectant management can be done in outpatient department with close follow-up.
- Regular monitoring of the patient with ultrasound and careful watch for signs of infection, bleeding, and/or miscarriage.
- Good prognosis with a perinatal survival rate of 91% has been reported in these cases in contrast to spontaneous PROM. The amniotic fluid reaccumulation occurred within 1 month in 72% cases.
- *Other treatment options:* Amino infusion. Tissue sealants are considered experimental at present.

PRETERM PROM AND FUTURE PREGNANCIES

A cohort study done by Aris et al. concluded that a history of PPROM in the first singleton pregnancy was associated with its equal likelihood in the second pregnancy but with an increased incidence of adverse maternal and neonatal outcomes than in the first pregnancy. Complications include a higher incidence of recurrent PPROM, instrumental and cesarean deliveries, preeclampsia (PE) and antepartum hemorrhage (APH) in the mother, and neonatal infection, death, admission to the neonatal unit, preterm delivery and low birth weight (LBW) in the baby. In women in whom there was no recurrence of PPROM, there was still a significant increase in risk of PE, instrumental and cesarean delivery, and neonatal unit admission:[30]

- Progesterone supplementation may be started at 16–24 weeks.[31]
- Cervical length screening should be considered.
- Cerclage may be considered in women with:
  - Current singleton pregnancy
  - Prior spontaneous preterm birth < 34 weeks
  - Cervical length < 25 mm before 24 weeks.

KEY POINTS

- Term PROM is used when the amniotic membranes rupture before the onset of labor.
- The diagnosis of PROM can be made from the clinical history and physical examination.
- Antibiotic prophylaxis reduces the risk of chorio-amnionitis and endometritis.
- Fetal neuroprotective treatment with magnesium sulfateisre commended in PPROM is recommended.

REFERENCES

1. Hnat MD, Mercer BM, Thurnauet G, Iams JD, Peter Van Dorsten J. Perinatal outcomes in women with preterm rupture of membranes between 24 and 32 weeks of gestation and a history of vaginal bleeding. Am J Obstet Gynecol. 2005;193(1):164-8.
2. Surayapalem S, Cooly V, Salicheemala B. A study on maternal and perinatal outcome in premature rupture of membranes at term. IJRCOG. 2017;6(12): 5368.
3. Seaward PG, Hannah ME, Myhr TL, Farine D, Ohlsson A, Wang EE, et al. International Multicentre Term Prelabor Rupture of Membranes Study: evaluation of predictors of clinical chorioamnionitis and postpartum fever in patients with prelabor rupture of membranes at term. Am J Obstet Gynecol. 1997;177(5):1024-9.
4. Yudin MH, van Schalkwyk J, Van Eyk N. No. 233-Antibiotic therapy in preterm premature rupture of the membranes. J Obstet Gynaecol Can. 2017;39(9):e207-12.
5. Bryce J, Boschi-Pinto C, Shibuya K, Black RE. WHO estimates of the causes of death in children. Lancet. 2005;365(9465):1147-52.
6. Maymon E, Romero R, Pacora P, Gervasi MT, Bianco K, Ghezzi F, et al. Evidence for the participation of interstitial collagenase (matrix metalloproteinase1) in preterm premature rupture of membranes. Am J Obstet Gynecol. 2000;183:914-20.
7. Maymon E, Romero R, Pacora P, Gervasi MT, Gomez R, Edwin SS, et al. Evidence of in vivo differential bioavailability of the active forms of matrix metalloproteinases 9 and 2 in parturition, spontaneous rupture of membranes, and intra amniotic infection. Am J Obstet Gynecol. 2000;183:887-97.
8. Malak TM, Ockleford CD, Bell SC, Dalgleish R, Bright N, Macvicar J. Confocal immunofluorescence localization of collagen types I, III, IV, V and VI and their ultrastructural organization in term human fetal membranes. Placenta. 1993;14: 385-406.
9. Goldenberg RL, Culhane JF, Iams JD, Romero R. Epidemiology and causes of preterm birth. Lancet. 2008;371:75-84.
10. Mymon E, Romero R, Pacora P, Gomez R, Athayde N, Edwin S, et al. Human neutrophil collagenase (matrix metalloproteinase 8) in parturition premature rupture of the membranes and intrauterine infection. Am J Obstet Gynecol. 2000;183:94-9.
11. Athayde N, Edwin SS, Romero R, Gomez R, Maymon E, Pacora P, et al. A role for matrix metalloproteinase-9 in spontaneous rupture of the fetal membranes. Am J Obstet Gynecol. 1998;179: 1248-53.
12. Kumar D, Schatz F, Moore RM, et al. The effects of thrombin and cytokines upon the biomechanics and remodeling of isolated amnion membrane, in vitro. Placenta. 2011;32:206.
13. McLaren J, Taylor DJ, Bell SC. Increased concentration of pro-matrix metalloproteinase 9 in term fetal membranes overlying the cervix before labor: implications for membrane remodeling and rupture. Am J Obstet Gynecol. 2000;182:409.
14. Ferguson SESG, Salenieks ME, Windrim R, Walker MC. Preterm premature rupture of membranes: nutritional and socioeconomic factors. Obstet Gynecol. 2002;100(6):1250-6.
15. Williams MAMR, Stubblefield PG, Lieberman E, Schoenbaum SC, Monson RR. Cigarettes, coffee, and preterm premature

rupture of the membranes. Am J Epidemiol. 1992;135(8): 895-903.

16. Workineh Y, Birhanu S, Kerie S, Ayalew E, Yihune M. Determinants of premature rupture of membrane in Southern Ethiopia, 2017: case control study design. BMC Res Notes. 2018;11:927.

17. Aaron B, Caughey Julian N, Robinson ERN. Contemporary diagnosis and management of preterm premature rupture of membranes. Rev Obstet Gynecol. 2008;1(1):11-22.

18. Chandiramani M, Bennett PR, Brown R, Lee Y, MacIntyre DA. Vaginal microbiome-pregnant host interactions determine a significant proportion of preterm labour. Fetal Matern Med Rev. 2014;25(1):73-8.

19. Kanayama N, Terao T, Horiuchi K. The role of human neutrophil elastase in the premature rupture of membranes. Asia Oceania J Obstet Gynaecol. 1988;14(3):389-97.

20. Fortunato SJ, Menon R, Lombardi SJ. Role of tumor necrosis factor-α in the premature rupture of membranes and preterm labor pathways. Am J Obstet Gynecol. 2002;187(5):1159-62.

21. Brown RG, Marchesi JR, Lee YS, Smith A, Lehne B, Kindinger LM, et al. Vaginal dysbiosis increases risk of preterm fetal membrane rupture, neonatal sepsis and is exacerbated by erythromycin. BMC Med. 2018;16:9.

22. Mercer BM. Preterm premature rupture of the membranes. Obstet Gynecol. 2003;101:178-93.

23. Sosa CG, Herrera E, Restrepo JC, Strauss A, Alonso J. Comparison of placental alpha microglobulin-1 invaginal fluid with intra-amniotic injection of indigo carmine for the diagnosis of rupture of membranes. J Perinat Med. 2014;42:611-6.

24. Dorfeuille N, Morin V, Tetu A, Demers S, Laforest G, Gouin K, et al. Vaginal fluid inflammatory biomarkers and the risk of adverse neonatal outcomes in women with PPROM. Am J Perinatol. 2016;33:1003-7.

25. Eleje GU, Ezugwu EC, Eke AC, lkechebelu J, Obiora CC, Ojiegbe N, et al. Comparison of the duo of insulin like growth factor binding protein1/alpha fetoprotein (Amnioquick duo+®) and traditional clinical assessment of diagnosing premature rupture of the fetal membranes. Rev Obstet Gynecol. 2008;1: 11-22.

26. The Royal Australian and New Zealand College of Obstetricians and Gynaecologists (RANZCOG) (2017). Term prelabour rupture of membranes (term PROM). [online] Available from: https:// ranzcog.edu.au/RANZCOG_SITE/media/RANZCOG-MEDIA/ Women%27s%20Health/Statement%20and%20guidelines/ Clinical-Obstetrics/Term-Prelabour-Rupture-of-Membranes-(Term-Prom)-(C-Obs-36)-review-2017.pdf?ext=.pdf [Last accessed September, 2020]

27. Royal College of Obstetricians and Gynaecologists (2017). Preterm prelabour rupture of membranes. (Green-Top Guideline No. 44). [online] Available from: https://www.rcog.org.uk/en/ guidelines-research-services/guidelines/gtg44/ [Last accessed September, 2020].

28. ObG Project (2017). ACOG Guidance Update: Diagnosis and Management of PROM (Prelabor Rupture of Membranes). [online] Available from: https://www.obgproject.com/2017/12/29/ acog-guidance-update-diagnosis-management-prom-prelabor-rupture-membranes/ [Last accessed September, 2020]

29. Royal Berkshire, NHS Foundation Trust (2020). Magnesium sulphate for neonatal neuro-protection (GL868). [online] Available from: https://www.royalberkshire.nhs.uk/Downloads/ GPs/GP%20protocols%20and%20guidelines/Maternity%20 Guidelines%20and%20Policies/Ultrasound%20and%20 Fetal%20Medicine/Magnesium%20sulphate%20for%20NN%20 neuroprotection_V3.0_GL868_APR20.pdf [Last accessed September, 2020]

30. Aris IM, Logan S, Lim C, Choolani M, Biswas A, Bhattacharya S. Preterm prelabour rupture of membranes: a retrospective cohort study of association with adverse outcome in subsequent pregnancy. BJOG. [online] Available from: https://doi. org/10.1111/1471-0528.14462. [Last accessed September, 2020]

31. Combs CA, Garite TJ, Maurel K, Abril D, Das A, Clewell W, et al. 17 hydroxyprogesterone caproate for preterm rupture of the membranes: a multicenter, randomized, double-blind, placebo controlled trial. Am J Obstet Gynecol. 2015;213:364.e1-12.

Cervical Insufficiency

Hemant Deshpande, Manjula S Patil

INTRODUCTION

Early pregnancy loss is an emotionally frustrating event for couples and is a challenge for obstetricians. Cervical insufficiency (CI) is classically defined as "the inability of the uterine cervix to support pregnancy because of a functional or structural defect" and is the most common cause of mid-trimester pregnancy loss.

This syndrome of painless progressive dilatation and effacement of cervix occurs between 16th and 24th weeks of gestation. The basic defect is the weakness of the sphincter mechanism of the internal os. When the content of the gravid uterus attains a critical weight, which exceeds the power of resistance of the internal os, it causes dilatation of the cervical canal, uterine contractions, and delivery of a live fetus. The onset of CI is caused by biochemical and biophysical changes which take place at term but appear earlier in the pregnancy of women with CI.

Cervical insufficiency as a cause of habitual abortion was noticed as early as in 1658 by Cole and Culpepper who described it as "The fault in woman which hindered conception is when the seed is not retained or the orifice of the womb being so slack that it cannot rightly contract itself to keep the seed".

Gream and Lancet were the first to use the term "cervical incompetence" in 1865; Douay from France performed the first operation for incompetent os in 1938 followed by Shirodkar[1] and McDonald[2] in the 1950s. Though there are many changes that are noted in indications for surgery for cervical incompetence, the choice of surgery still remains the same.

INCIDENCE

Golan A Barman (1989) studied the incidence and found that incompetence is seen in:

- 0.5–1% of all pregnancies
- 0.2% of all abortions
- 16–20% of mid-trimester abortions
- 12% of all habitual abortions

DEFINITION

Larry Cousins has defined cervical incompetence as the inability of the uterine cervix to retain an intrauterine pregnancy until term.

In 1960, Wayne has described cervical incompetence as any condition of the uterine cervix that permits sufficient "painless' dilatation to allow spontaneous rupture of membranes and subsequent onset of labor prior to the end of the 36th week of gestation.

David Charles defined an incompetent internal cervical os as one which is incapable of maintaining a normal pregnancy to that time when a viable fetus can be delivered.

Campioni (1998) defined cervical incompetence as an abnormal dilatation of the cervical canal at the body-neck junction with no pain or blood loss and in the absence of uterine contractile activity.

According to the American College of Obstetrician and Gynecologists (ACOG),[3] the term cervical insufficiency is used to describe the inability of the uterine cervix to retain a pregnancy in the absence of the signs and symptoms of clinical contraction or labor or both in the second trimester.

Roman et al.[4] in 2016 have defined CI as "transvaginal ultrasound-cervical length (TVU-CL) < 25 mm before 24 weeks in women with prior pregnancy losses or preterm births at 14–36 weeks or by cervical changes detected on physical examination before 24 weeks of gestation".

Incompetence causes repetitive, painless spontaneous passive dilatation and leaking followed by expulsion of an immature live fetus in the second trimester.

ETIOPATHOGENESIS

The uterine cervix is an essential component in conception, which maintains pregnancy till term and delivery of the baby. Uterine contractions and cervical dilatation and effacement are the unique events responsible for successful expulsion of the fetus, and the exact mechanisms behind these are not completely understood till date. Earlier, uterine contractions are thought to be the primary factor responsible for successful delivery but variable dilatation of cervix noticed in majority of women in the last few weeks before the onset of labor, cervical incompetence, and failure of the cervix to dilate even in the presence of good uterine contractions as in failed induction of labor clearly indicate the role of cervix as an equally important factor.

The length and strength of the cervix in normal circumstances prevent CI and ascent of microorganisms and thus prevent preterm birth. The competence of the cervix is determined by the amount and distribution of the collagen and elastin and smooth muscle in the cervical stroma. Changes in the amount, composition, and orientation of these components lead to cervical ripening prior to labor onset. The cervix is lined by a single layer of tall columnar epithelium which is thrown into folds to form the crypts. Subepithelial stroma is composed mainly of collagen (80%) and matrix and smooth muscle (15–20%) and very minimal elastin. The collagen fibers are densely packed in a nonpregnant cervix giving it firmness and are scattered in full dilatation of the cervix. It is thought that the directionality of the collagen fibers may determine their ability to withstand forces encountered in pregnancy: circumferentially around the cervical canal to prevent dilatation of the cervix and longitudinally to resist those associated with cervical effacement.[5] Elastin plays an important role in cervical remodeling during delivery and postpartum. The components of the matrix are dermatan sulfate, glycosaminoglycans, and hyaluronic acid. At the time of parturition, there is a relative elevation of hyaluronic acid levels in the cervix with a simultaneous drop in dermatan sulfate.

Structural changes in the cervix have also been attributed to the hormones estrogen, progesterone, and relaxin from corpus luteum.

A cervical biopsy specimen in experimental studies in women with an incompetent cervix when compared with a normal cervix has shown to be associated with reduced or absence of elastic fibers, unusually low collagen:muscular ratio, and increased collagen turnover with higher proportion of newly synthesized collagen with lower mechanical strength suggested by increased collagen extractability and collagenolytic activity. The initial case reports of Shirodkar's[1] have confirmed the role of a defect in the cervical internal os (proven by repeated digital examination) as the cause of cervical incompetence at least in cases with risk factors, and cervical stitch strengthens this defect. Since the incompetence begins from the internal os and progresses downward, it may be necessary to reconsider altered anatomy of the internal os as a cause of CI and to possibly consider it as a separate pathology.

Researches using a 3D reconstructive technique[6] may give a promising result in future. In this 3D reconstruction and examination of tissue at microscopic resolution are done. It has significant potential to enhance the study of both normal and disease processes, particularly those involving structural changes or those in which the spatial relationship of disease features is important as in cervix.

Various mechanisms exist for the effacement and dilatation of the uterine cervix:

- Influence of the uterine contractions (intrapartum mechanism)
- Influence of the weight of the contents of the gravid uterus (passive mechanism characteristic of cervical incompetence)
- Influence of the biochemical process on the depolymerization of the collagen

It appears that the onset of cervical incompetence is caused by the biochemical and biophysical changes which are typical of changes taking place at term but appear earlier in the pregnancy of women with cervical incompetence.

Historically, a case series of 70 cases by McDonald[2] and 30 cases by Shirodkar[1] in 1950s had cervical injury as an important predisposing factor caused by either dilatation and curettage (D&C) or by cervical amputation or by birth trauma in almost all the cases of cervical incompetence, but the prevalence of the antecedent obstetric risk factors leading to CI is decreasing in the contemporary practice.[7,] This may be attributable to improved surgical techniques; judicious usage of effective cervical ripening agents prior to procedures such as D&C, mid-trimester abortions and hysteroscopy and reduced incidence of cervical amputation and the fact that all diethylstilbestrol (DES)-exposed women have crossed reproductive age.

The pathophysiology of CI is still poorly understood, and majority of CI occurs in the absence of obvious risk factors. The risk factors include:

- *Acquired causes:* Cervical trauma due to:
  - D&C/dilatation and evacuation
  - Cervical amputation
  - Cervical conization
  - Cervical lacerations and tears in precipitate labor, breech extraction, forceps delivery, delivery of a large baby, Duhrssen's incision
- *Congenital causes*
  - With associated uterine anomalies: Bicornuate uterus, subseptate uterus, septate uterus, hypoplastic uterus
  - Without associated uterine anomalies, it is seen where the connective tissue and fibrous tissue content of the cervix are sparse.
- Relative or functional incompetence seen in twins (it is no more being considered as CI).
- *Dysfunctional incompetence:* Hunter (1961) described dysfunctional incompetence where there is a typical history of incompetence, but the cervix shows no abnormality till miscarriage is inevitable. It is believed

that the majority of failures of encirclage come from this group.

Grades of Incompetence

Baden and Baden graded the incompetence in four grades, depending upon the time of termination. Grading of CI is of only theoretical importance.

- *Grade 1:* Mildest from those occurring from 30th to 36th week
- *Grade 2:* From 24th to 30th week
- *Grade 3:* From 18th to 24th week
- *Grade 4:* All those earlier than 18th week

◼ DIAGNOSIS

The diagnosis of CI depends on the past obstetric performance.

Clinical Presentation

In majority of the cases, CI is diagnosed following ≥1 pregnancy loss and a detailed history regarding the events leading to such loss plays a major role in diagnosing CI and to rule out all other causes of preterm labor (PTL). Women remain asymptomatic till advanced cervical dilatation and then notice pain for short duration followed by rupture of membranes and expulsion of a live previable fetus. The treating physician in the index pregnancy should inform the patient regarding the need for early intervention in successive pregnancy to prevent recurrence.

In a woman without a history of pregnancy loss, diagnosis of CI depends on clinical presentation, physical examination, and ultrasound findings. Mostly women remain asymptomatic and rarely present with symptoms such as pelvic pressure, premenstrual-like cramping or backache, and increased vaginal discharge for days or weeks. Speculum examination may show variable cervical dilatation with or without a bulging bag of membranes at or beyond the external os.

Ultrasound done in these women shows varying degrees of internal os dilatation (ranging from Y, V, U) with shortening of the cervical length (CL) and ballooning of the membranes.[8]

Diagnostic Tests

Preconceptional Diagnosis

Most of these tests assess the functional anatomy of the internal os and are of historical importance. None of these tests has been validated in the rigorous scientific studies and should not be used to diagnose CI[3] or to place history-indicated cerclage.[9]

- *Hegar test:* Passage of number 8 Hegar dilator through the cervical canal without resistance is diagnostic of incompetence (Graig and Jenings).

- Dr VN Shirodkar suggested that if there is absence of closing snap when dilatators are being withdrawn, it is diagnostic of incompetence.
- *Bergman's balloon test:* If Foley's catheter containing 1 mL of water can be pulled through the internal os of the nonpregnant patient using <600 g of pull, then diagnosis of incompetence is probable.
- *Compliance test:* Neuman and Merkataz studied cervical resistance by filling a Foley's catheter balloon with water within the cervical canal. With normal competence, the resistance was 131 mm Hg as opposed to 21.4 mm Hg in women with incompetence.
- *Hysterosalpingography (HSG):* HSG in the postmenstrual phase shows that funneling of cervix, disappearance of the uterocervical angle, and canal width of >8 mm at the level of internal os are diagnostic of incompetence.

Screening for Cervical Insufficiency During Pregnancy

Ultrasound is the most important and noninvasive tool to screen women for CI and prediction of preterm birth. In 1979, Sarti described use of ultrasound to visualize the lower uterine segment and cervical canal and dilatation at the level of internal os, and the diagnosis of an incompetent cervix based on ultrasound findings was reported in 1983. The first report on the use of TVU to measure the length of cervix was made in 1986, the publication which gave the Y-V-U phenomenon.[8]

Measurement of CL plays a key role in the diagnosis of CI. A short cervix is one of the strongest risk factors for PTL.[4,8,10] CL screening should be done in all women using TVU at 19–23 weeks of pregnancy.[9] TVU-CL is the "gold standard" for measurement of CL as recommended by the ACOG,[10] Society of Maternal and Fetal Medicine (SMFM) and Society of Obstetricians and Gynaecologists of Canada (SOGC); other approaches may be considered where it is not available or feasible.

All high-risk women (singleton pregnancy with a previous history of PTL) should undergo CL screening every fortnight from 16 to 23/6 weeks of pregnancy and low-risk women during a routine anomaly scan between 18 and 24 weeks of pregnancy.[4,9,10] CL measurement strategies and the management based on CL are shown in **Flowchart 1**.

Technique

Cervical length measurement with ultrasound can be done by:

- Transabdominal ultrasound (TAU)
- Transvaginal ultrasound (TVU)
- Transperineal ultrasound (TPU)

A proper technique is essential for accurate and reproducible measurement of CL and is precisely given by

Flowchart 1: Cerclage algorithm.[4]

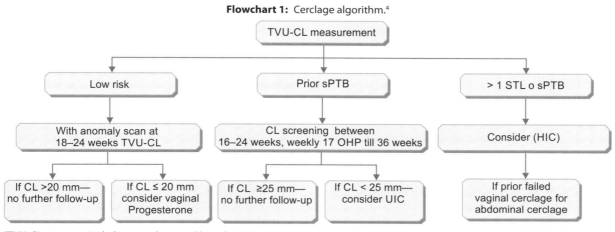

(TVU-CL: transvaginal ultrasound cervical length; sPTB: spontaneous preterm birth; STL: second trimester loss; 17 OHP: 17 hydroxy progesterone; HIC: history indicated cerclage; UIC: ultrasound indicated cerclage)

CLEaR (Cervical Length Education and Review)[11] program and Fetal Medicine Foundation (FMF) task force criteria of CL measurement, which include the following:

- Empty maternal bladder and place woman in dorsal lithotomy position.
- Transvaginal sonography with a high-frequency probe of 5–7 MHz
- Ultrasound probe introduced in the vagina and directed to the anterior fornix with no undue force (this may increase the CL)
- Sagittal view of the cervix obtained. Optimal field (cervix should occupy two-third of the screen)
- Anterior width = posterior width
- Cervical internal os seen (endocervical mucosa is used as a guide).
- Cervical external os seen
- Cervix canal visible throughout
- Correct placement of caliper (linear distance between triangular echodensity at the external os and V-shaped notch at the internal os)
- Each examination should be performed over 2–3 minutes and at least three measurements should be obtained; at least one of these measurements should be obtained while applying either suprapubic or uterine fundal pressure to detect asymptomatic cervical incompetence (Guzman cervical stress test). The shortest best measurement should then be used.

Since the cervix is a dynamic organ, a single snapshot of cervix does not give accurate result. The bladder should be emptied just prior to the scan since a full bladder can increase the CL by 5 mm and even the dilated internal os may appear closed.

Findings to be Noted

Length of cervix (Fig. 1): The average CL in pregnancy at 20–24 weeks of gestation is 34 mm while in the nonpregnant

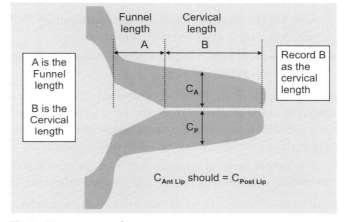

Fig. 1: Measurement of cervix.
Sources: Berghella V, Kuhlman K, Weiner S, Texeira L, Wapner RJ. Cervical funneling: sonographic criteria predictive of preterm delivery. Ultrasound Obstet Gynecol. 1997; 10(3):161-6; Burger M, Weber-Rössler T, Willmann M. Measurement of the pregnant cervix by transvaginal sonography: an interobserver study and new standards to improve the interobserver variability. Ultrasound Obstet Gynecol. 1997;9(3):188-93.

cervix it is 25 mm. The length of a pregnant cervix is rarely >6 cm. CL remains stable between 14 and 28 weeks of pregnancy and is not significantly affected by race/ethnicity, parity, and maternal height. It undergoes gradual shortening thereafter.

A cervical length of 26 mm represents 26th percentile and 35 mm 50th percentile. CL ≤ 25 mm (below 10th percentile) is associated with 75% risk of PTL.[4] Other findings on ultrasound include separation of fetal membranes, debris in the amniotic fluid, rapid rate of decrease of CL over time, and short cervix before 20 weeks which are associated with an increased risk of PTL.

- *Cervical score:* Cervical length—internal OS diameter if less than 0.5 cm risk of preterm birth is more. Average cervical internal OS diameter in normal pregnancy ranges from 1 to 4 mm and a diameter of more than 9 mm is high risk for mid trimester loss and preterm birth.

- *Cervical index:* By GOMEZ

$\dfrac{1 + \text{funnel length}}{\text{cervical length}}$ if more than 0.5 cm, risk of preterm birth is more.

Cervical consistency index (CCI):

- CCI is based on the observation that the cervix undergoes softening, i.e., change in the consistency well before change in the cervical length (CL) and few studies have shown CCI as the better and earlier predictor of CI and PTB in high risk population.
- It is calculated as AP'/ AP x 100 where anteroposterior diameter of the cervix before is AP and at maximal compression is AP' are used.
- Lower the CCI higher the compressibility and softness and higher chances of cervical insufficiency and premature birth even when CL is normal.
- This method still needs to be validated by larger prospective RCTs in future.

Funneling of the cervix: Presence or absence of the funneling should be noted and is designated by T-Y-V-U.[8] These letters are a pictorial representation of the shape of the interface between the internal os and the lower uterine segment.

T—normal cervical appearance, Y—early opening of internal os, V—funneling of cervix, U—ballooning of cervix

Intra-amniotic debris: Hyperechoic particles in the amniotic fluid, which indicate inflammatory material, are associated with an increased risk of PTL.

Digital examination of cervix: Not indicated to diagnose CI.

■ MANAGEMENT

Treatment of the incompetent internal os of the cervix aims to restore the normal caliber of the isthmus by closure of the defect.

Prevention of Incompetence

- Judicious use of cervical-ripening agents before D&C, hysteroscopy, etc.
- The cervical dilatation preceding diagnostic curettage should not exceed No. 9 Hegar dilatator.
- Avoiding traumatic instrumental deliveries
- Timely and meticulous repair of cervical tears

Treatment

Nonsurgical Treatment

Certain nonsurgical measures tried till date include activity restriction, bed rest, and pelvic rest, but none of these has been proven to be effective and are thus not recommended.[3,9,10]

Progestational agents (medical cerclage): Progesterone causes narrowing of the cervical canal in addition to suppression of myometrial contractile activity and can raise the electrical sensitivity threshold of the smooth muscle of the uterus and lower the contractility of the myometrium. It is a patent antiprostaglandin agent. Various indications for progesterones based on the available evidence are as follows:

- Vaginal progesterone (200 mg or 90 mL gel) is offered to women without previous history of preterm birth or mid-trimester loss, and TVU-CL at 16[+0] and 24[+0] weeks of pregnancy is <25 mm.[4,10]
- Previous history of PTL—intramuscular injection of 17-hydroxyprogesterone from 14 to 36 weeks of pregnancy[4,10]
- As an adjunct with cervical cerclage in high-risk women with short CL[10]

Pessary: Cervical Pessary has a promise as an alternative treatment for CI since its it is non-invasive, easy to use, low cost, does not require anesthesia and can be done in outpatient department. Its efficacy as a primary treatment than as an adjunctive needs to be proven by larger randomized studies. It may be beneficial in asymptomatic women with a short cervix with no prior history of spontaneous preterm birth, in pregnant women with twin gestation with CL 25–38 mm, short cervix beyond 24 weeks of gestation or with continued cervical shortening.[10] Pessary is used as an adjuct to progesterone in majority of these indications. Multicenter open-label randomized controlled trial (RCT) conducted in Spain between 2007 and 2010 [PEPCEP (Pesario Cervical Para Evitor Prematurida)][12] enrolling 385 patients found significant reduction in the spontaneous preterm birth rate in the pessary group (6% vs. 27%), but the Cochrane database systematic review in 2013 did not recommend pessary. So, presently data is limited with ongoing trials on the potential benefit of pessary.

Cervical pessary prevents CI by one of the following mechanisms: The bag of water acts as a hydraulic wedge. The cervix with its axis directly and centrally aligned with the relatively nonresistant vagina leads itself of its own dissolution. Pessary accentuates the resistance to this hydrostatic force. The Hodge or Smith pessary works by changing the direction of inclination of the cervical canal and prevents the gravitational dilatation of the cervix. There is distribution of the weight of growing ovum through the lower uterine segment into the cul de sac, the vaginal floor, and the retrosymphyseal osteomuscular structures. Tension exerted on the uterosacral ligaments will have a sling effect on the anterior cervix with their splayed continuity with the cervical fascia and compressing the cervical canal.

Electrocautery: Barnes (1961) used electrocautery in a nonpregnant state. Conization of the cervix is done with cautery. Stenosis of cervix and lacerations are main complications.

Surgical Treatment

The objectives of surgery are to enhance resistance of the cervix to effacement and dilatation by the primary repair of an anatomical defect, reinforcement by a circumferential suture. The procedure which has been attempted to correct the incompetence ranges from the simple cervical cauterization of Barnes to the more complex submucosal placement of the stitch around the circumference of the cervix as advocated by Dr Shirodkar[1] and Dr McDonald[2] in the mid-1950s. The definitive treatment of CI is cerclage.

Cervical Cerclage

Preconceptional Cerclage

A preconceptual procedure is rarely performed. Abdominal cerclage when indicated can be done preconceptionally and may have similar efficacy to postconceptional cerclage.[13]

*Lash and Lash procedure (**Fig. 3**):* Described in 1950 by Lash and Lash, this procedure is done in cases of a defect in the cervix secondary to trauma with extensive cervical lacerations reaching up to the internal os. So, correction should be performed by excising a wedge of the damaged cervix at the cervicoisthmic level in order to preserve the normal width of the endocervical portion and the internal os. This is carried out in the nonpregnant state. Sutures are either of chromic catgut number 2 or polyglactin.

Technique: Reflection of the bladder is accomplished by a semicircular incision through the vaginal wall. The suture is tied anteriorly over number 4 Hegar dilator and the second suture is placed 1–2 cm distal to the first. This operation may be appropriate as an alternative to the postconceptual placement of a transabdominal cervicoisthmic cerclage in

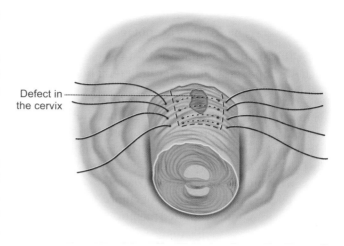

Fig. 3: Lash technique.

a patient with a severely scarred cervix. The success rate is 85%.

External wrapping technique: This technique was described by Page to produce a circular scarring of the cervix. The use of sterile talc wrapped in oxycel gauze produces scarring at the level of internal os.

Cutis graft technique: This technique consists of excision of a wedge of cervical circumference from the external to the internal os. The cervix was then reconstructed and wrapped spirally from the external os to the internal os by a strip of skin which was sutured in place at 1.5–2 cm. This operation does not affect fertility.

Silicone plastic cuff: This was devised in 1971 by Yosowitz. The cuff is a silicone plastic rim with two fluid inflatable balloons attached to the inner and outer surfaces, respectively. The cuff is inserted into the vagina prior to insertion of the speculum and the speculum is then inserted and the cervix is then pulled through with a ring forceps. Inflation of each balloon is done with saline and hoses are then lighted with silk sutures and placed in the vagina. The cuff left is free from complications which the pessary has, such as vaginal necrosis discomfort and adjustment to the variations in cervical size.

Postconceptional Cerclage

History-indicated or prophylactic or elective cerclage:[3,9]
- History of one or more second-trimester pregnancy losses suggestive of CI or
- History of prior physical examination-indicated cerclage
  Conventionally, prophylactic cerclage was liberally used for many indications such as bad obstetric history with second-trimester losses, history of cone biopsy, >2 dilatation and evacuation, Mullerian anomalies, DES exposure, and multiple pregnancies. The beneficial effect

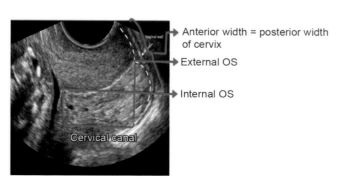

Anterior width = posterior width of cervix
External OS
Internal OS
Cervical canal

Fig. 2

of cerclage for these indications has not been proven in scientific studies; hence, they are not recommended.

Timing: The ACOG recommends 13–14 weeks of gestation though the upper gestational age limit remains obscure.

Physical examination-indicated cerclage:[3,9] Cerclage placement in the setting of cervical dilatation is called "physical examination-indicated cerclage," "rescue cerclage," or "emergency cerclage." This is done regardless of the CL, obstetric history, or risk factors for PTL. Cervical dilatation beyond 4 cm and bulging membrane beyond the external os carry higher chances of failure. Onset of labor, overt chorioamnionitis, ruptured membranes, and bleeding are all absolute contraindications to the procedure.

The risks of emergency cerclage include intraoperative rupture of membranes, infectious morbidity and sepsis, laceration at the surgical site, hemorrhage, and failure, and these have to be thoroughly counseled before decision-making.

A recent systematic review and meta-analysis by Ehsanipoor et al.[14] including 10 studies with 757 women, of which 485 (64%) underwent physical examination-indicated cerclage and 272 (36%) were expectantly managed, have shown that cerclage is associated with a significant increase in neonatal survival (71% compared with 43%) and prolongation of pregnancy of approximately 1 month. In fact, the case series of McDonald's[2] in 1957 including 70 cases of cervical incompetence were all physical examination-indicated cerclage with reasonable success. Thus, emergency cerclage definitely has a role in properly selected patients.

Technique:
- *Position:* Lithotomy with Trendelenburg position will shift the pressure off the bulging membranes before stitch placement.
- *Suture:* Braided sutures are preferred over Mersilene tape and sharp needles are preferred over blunt needles as blunt needles may cause too much distortion of the anatomic relationships while trying to pass the needle.
- *Maneuvers for prolapsed membranes:*
  - Backfilling of bladder with 250–500 mL of saline
  - Displacing the bulging bag of membranes with Foley's catheter with 30 mL of saline or sponge stick or condom catheter on sponge stick
  - Ring forceps on the cervix to gently pull the cervical tissue beyond a prolapsed bag of membranes
  - Placement of stay suture on cervix to hold and pull it down
  - Amnioreduction
- *Amniocentesis:* Amniocentesis prior to cerclage is not routinely indicated but in patients with physical examination-indicated cerclage in the absence of overt chorioamnionitis, it is done to rule out subclinical infection, since many studies have noted worse perinatal outcomes in the presence of subclinical infection. Amniotic fluid markers of inflammation such as positive Gram stain, low glucose concentration (<15 mg/dL), elevated WBC count (>30 cells/mL), increased leukocyte esterase and interleukin-6, and culture and sensitivity are studied and used to guide the treatment.

Ultrasound-indicated cerclage:[3,9] A short cervix is an important risk factor for PTL. Ultrasound-indicated cerclage is placed for a short cervix of <25 mm before 24 weeks of gestation in a singleton pregnancy with prior spontaneous preterm birth between 16 and 34 weeks of gestation. This intervention is shown to reduce the risk recurrence of PTL by 30%.

An ultrasound-indicated cerclage is not recommended for funneling of the cervix (dilatation of the internal os on ultrasound) in the absence of cervical shortening.[9]

No cerclage is indicated "*after the period of viability.*"

Cerclage in Multiple Pregnancies

Prophylactic cerclage was once a very common indication. Current evidence does not support history or ultrasound-indicated cerclage in twins and higher order pregnancies. In fact, cerclage placement may be detrimental and may even increase the risk of PTL.[3,9]

Serial sonographic surveillance with or without ultrasound-indicated cerclage

Women with a history of spontaneous second-trimester loss or preterm delivery who have not undergone a history-indicated cerclage may be offered serial sonographic surveillance for a short cervix and considered for ultrasound-indicated cerclage.[3,9]

Routes of Cerclage Placement

- *Transvaginal route*: It is the preferred route. Shirodkar's cerclage and its modifications, McDonald's cerclage, Wurm's stitch, Hefner stitch
- *Transabdominal route*: Transabdominal cerclage was first introduced 50 years ago as a treatment of choice in those women with failed transvaginal cerclage. Conceptually, it is targeted at closing the upper cervix at or near the internal os to maintain the strength at that level.

Indications

- Failed vaginal cerclage in prior pregnancy
- Cervical attenuation either due to congenital hypoplasia or due to cervical amputation or excisional procedures or extensive cervical tear during delivery
- Radical trachelectomy

Post-Term Pregnancy (Prolonged Pregnancy)

Hemant Deshpande, Sonali Deshpande

INTRODUCTION

Post-term pregnancy is one of the most common, yet challenging, conditions faced by obstetricians in the past as well as today. Post-term gestation still continues to represent a high-risk situation with potentially significant obstetric mortality and morbidity which mandates the obstetrician to accurately diagnose and manage postdatism. The management has to be tailored to suit the facilities available in each center.

In the past, the period from 3 weeks before until 2 weeks after the estimated date of delivery (EDD) was considered "term," with the expectation that neonatal outcomes from deliveries in this interval were uniform and good. Increasingly, however, research has shown that neonatal outcomes, especially respiratory morbidity, vary depending on the timing of delivery within this 5-week gestational age range. To address this lack of uniformity, a work group was convened in late 2012, which recommended that the label "term" be replaced with the designations early term (37 0/7 weeks of gestation through 38 6/7 weeks of gestation), full term (39 0/7 weeks of gestation through 40 6/7 weeks of gestation), late term (41 0/7 weeks of gestation through 41 6/7 weeks of gestation), and post-term (42 0/7 weeks of gestation and beyond) to more accurately describe deliveries occurring at or beyond 37 0/7 weeks of gestation.[1]

The incidence of prolonged pregnancy decreases as the accuracy of the dating criteria employed increases. The incidence of prolonged pregnancy varied from 3 to 10% or more depending on whether it was calculated in a prospective or retrospective manner (in which obviously wrong gestational assessments may have been corrected).[2] It also depends on the history and early clinical examination for confirmation of pregnancy alone or whether early first-trimester ultrasound examination was utilized to calculate the gestation in the first half of pregnancy.

It cannot be relied upon if the woman is not sure of her last menstrual period (LMP) or the period was immediately after discontinuation of hormonal contraceptives or lactation. Also, the length of the menstrual cycle is to be taken into consideration as it will influence the date of ovulation.

The incidence of post-term pregnancy was 7.5% when diagnosis was based on menstrual dating. The incidence was 2.6% when dating was based on early ultrasound examination and 1.1% when the ultrasound and menstrual history coincided. Prolongation of pregnancy beyond 40 weeks occurs more frequently, about 1 in every 10 pregnancies.[3]

ETIOLOGY AND ASSOCIATED RISK FACTORS

The majority of post-term pregnancies have no known etiology. One-third to one-half of the variation in post-term birth in a population can be attributed to maternal or fetal genetic influence on the initiation of parturition.[4] The chance of post-term birth increases with advancing maternal age, higher body mass index, primiparous, or carrying a male fetus. Previous post-term birth and family history increase the risk of post-term pregnancy.

In rare cases, post-term pregnancy has been attributed to defects in fetal production of hormones involved in parturition.[5]

Fetal disorders associated with placental sulfatase deficiency (e.g., X-linked ichthyosis) result in extremely low estriol levels and other hormonal changes compared with normal pregnancies. Anencephaly, which results in absence or hypoplasia of the hypothalamus and pituitary and adrenal hypoplasia, often results in post-term pregnancy when polyhydramnios is absent.[6]

Since pregnancies with anencephaly are now routinely detected antenatally and terminated or induced, post-term duration is no longer observed.

PATHOPHYSIOLOGY

The post-term pregnancy has two basic pictures: One where the fetus grows continuously with more amniotic fluid, more birth weight, big cord, and a large placenta and the other which shows signs of dysmaturity such as less liquor, thin cord, calcified placenta, and baby with a wrinkled face and old man's look. The postdate fetus experiences a range of physiologic changes that predispose it to the development of hypoxia and acidosis.

Amniotic Fluid Volume

The volume of amniotic fluid becomes maximum at or around 24 weeks' gestation and remains constant until approximately 37 weeks' gestation. Then, there begins a slight decline in the amniotic fluid volume (AFV) but during the postdate period, it is estimated that there is a 33% decline in the AFV each week.

The AFV is maximum at 37–38 weeks' gestation, approximately 1,000 mL. It then progressively reduces to 700 mL at 40 weeks, 450 mL at 42 weeks, 250 mL at 43 weeks, and 150 mL at 44 weeks.[7] Also, the vernix content increases markedly. It becomes thick, cloudy, and turbid. The phospholipid content increases so as to change lecithin–sphingomyelin (L/S) ratio to 4:1.

As placental blood flow decreases, the fetus must redistribute a decreased circulating blood volume in an attempt to maintain renal blood flow. Diminished fetal ventricular function may also hamper the fetal efforts to maintain renal perfusion. As renal blood flow decreases, so does fetal urinary output. Eventually, a decrease in amniotic fluid leads to umbilical cord compression. Intermittent cord compression can be diagnosed by identifying the presence of variable deceleration during fetal heart rate (FHR) testing. Cord compression stimulates the passage of meconium by the same vagal reflex that initiates a heart rate deceleration. Meconium passed into a small AFV tends to be thicker, more tenacious, and more difficult to clear after aspiration. A significant amount of compression can lead to hypoxia, acidosis, and fetal distress.

The use of amniotic fluid index is a better predictor of perinatal morbidity and mortality. The decline in AFV has an impact on fetal movement in the potentially compromised fetus.

Decreased fetal movement does represent a sign of potential fetal jeopardy that appears to be related to the presence of oligohydramnios. This finding becomes highly significant in the postdate pregnancy in which amniotic fluid dynamics can occur quickly. Thus, a decline in fetal activity may be the sole manifestation of a decline in AFV and should not be disregarded.

Also, an inverse relationship between the AFV and FHR deceleration is seen.

Placenta

Placental senescence decreases the transfer of oxygen, fuels, and wastes across the placental surface as the number of villous capillaries and intervillous spaces decline.

Grannum and coworkers have advocated using sonography to grade the severity of placental ageing on a scale of 0–3.[8] A grade 3 placenta exhibits sonographic findings of linear echogenic densities, probably representing areas of increased calcium deposition, dividing the placental bed into compartments. Echolucent areas may be seen in the central portion of the compartments. The incidence of grade 3 placentas increased after 40 weeks, but its presence alone cannot be used to predict the occurrence of fetal distress or postmaturity syndrome.

Histopathologically, the placental change shows reduced diameter and length of villi. There are areas of fibrinoid necrosis and atherosis of choriodecidual vessels. It also shows both white and red infarcts. White infarcts are seen in 10–20% of term placenta and increase up to 60% in post-term placenta. The calcium deposits are 2–3 g/100 g placental weight at term and increases to 10 g/100 g in post-term cases.[9]

Umbilical Cord Dimensions

Umbilical cord dimensions, including vessel size, increase with advancing gestation. The size of the umbilical cord and its vessels correlate with the size of the fetus. The larger the fetus, the larger will be the umbilical cord, artery, and vein. These findings suggest that Doppler umbilical flow studies may be unreliable in the postdate pregnancy because of the significantly larger vessels encountered in this population.

■ DIAGNOSIS

The diagnosis of pregnancy ≥ 42 + 0 weeks of gestation is based on the clinician's most accurate estimate of the woman's EDD.

Estimation of Gestational Age

God schedules a birthday, not man! How true and yet nothing in obstetrics creates more anxiety for a pregnant woman and her obstetrician than being "overdue." It has become apparent that clinical methods for estimation of gestational age are inferior to sonographic measurements obtained in early pregnancy.

For most pregnancies, the best estimate of the delivery date is based on sonography. If sonography was performed before 22 + 0 weeks of gestation and this EDD differs from that calculated from menstrual dating by more than expected, the pregnancy is suboptimally dated.

Crown–rump length (CRL) measured in the first trimester, if available, is the most accurate sonographic method of determining the EDD. First-trimester CRL is more accurate than any second-trimester (14 + 0 to 27 + 6 weeks) biometric parameter used for gestational age assessment because there is less biological variation in fetal measurements in the first trimester than later in gestation. It is also more accurate than mean sac diameter.

The EDD derived from the earliest sonographic assessment of gestational age (first-trimester CRL or fetal biometry before 22 weeks) becomes the woman's EDD, and this EDD is not changed by subsequent ultrasound examinations.

■ COMPLICATIONS

Post-term pregnancy is associated with maternal, fetal, and neonatal complications. Many of the complications are sequelae of either excessive fetal growth or placental insufficiency.

Macrosomia

Because of the longer duration of intrauterine growth, post-term fetuses tend to be larger than term fetuses and have a higher incidence of macrosomia ($\geq$4,500 g: 2.5–10% post-term vs. 0.8–1% at term).[10] Macrosomia increases the risks for several adverse sequelae, including abnormal labor progression, cesarean delivery, assisted vaginal delivery, shoulder dystocia, maternal/fetal/newborn birth injury, postpartum hemorrhage, and neonatal metabolic problems.

Dysmaturity

Not all post-term fetuses continue to grow along a normal growth trajectory. Up to 20% of post-term fetuses have "fetal dysmaturity (postmaturity) syndrome," a term used to describe fetuses with characteristics of chronic intrauterine malnutrition.[11] These fetuses are at increased risk of umbilical cord compression due to oligohydramnios, and abnormal antepartum or intrapartum FHR patterns due to placental insufficiency or cord compression. Meconium passage is common and may be related to physiological maturation of the gut, fetal hypoxia, or both. Dysmature neonates have a long thin body, long nails, and are small for gestational age. Their skin is dry (vernix caseosa is decreased or absent), meconium-stained, parchment-like, and peeling; it appears loose, especially over the thighs and buttocks, and has prominent creases; lanugo hair is sparse or absent, while scalp hair is increased. These neonates are at risk for morbidities associated with growth restriction, including hypoglycemia, polycythemia, perinatal asphyxia, meconium aspiration, and persistent pulmonary hypertension. They are also at risk for neurodevelopmental complications (e.g., seizures, cerebral palsy).

Postmaturity Syndrome

Postmaturity syndrome was described in detail by Clifford and advocates. They postulated the use of a staging system to quantify increasingly severe clinical manifestation of placental dysfunction.

- *Stage I:* This stage is typified by a long, lean infant with wrinkled, loss of vernix and subcutaneous fat

- *Stage II:* This stage includes the clinical findings of stage I and adds greenish meconium staining of amniotic fluid, fetal skin, and placental membrane.
- *Stage III:* This stage is characterized by a high incidence of fetal distress and yellow-brown meconium staining, indicative of the presence of meconium for several days.[12]

The incidence of the postmaturity syndrome increases with the length of pregnancy; at 42 weeks, about 20% of fetuses will have stigmata of postmaturity.[13]

Though such a picture is associated with infants born after 42 weeks, they are not the norm or characteristic of prolonged pregnancy. Infants with such features may be born even at 39 and 40 weeks. So, the term "prolonged pregnancy" should be preferred to postmaturity for pregnancies beyond 42 weeks. The term "postdatism" implies pregnancy which exceeds the EDD and is best avoided.

Perinatal Mortality

The perinatal mortality rate at $\geq$42 weeks of gestation is twice the rate at term, increasing fourfold at 43 weeks and five- to sevenfold at 44 weeks.[13]

Neonates born at $\geq$41 weeks of gestation experience a one-third greater risk of neonatal mortality than term neonates born at 38–40 weeks of gestation.[14] Post-term pregnancy is associated with significant risks to the mother. There is an increased risk of (1) labor dystocia (9–12% vs. 2–7% at term); (2) severe perineal lacerations (third- and fourth-degree tears), related to macrosomia (3.3% vs. 2.6% at term); (3) operative vaginal delivery; and (4) doubling in cesarean section (CS) rates (14% vs. 7% at term). Cesarean delivery is associated with a higher incidence of endometritis, hemorrhage, and thromboembolic disease.

Long-term Outcome

Studies that are employed after rigorous pregnancy dating criteria and stratified infants based on their Clifford staging showed that once the infant passed the perinatal period, his/her development was comparable to term-controlled infants.

■ RECURRENCE RISK

After one post-term pregnancy, the risk of a second post-term birth is increased two- to fourfold; the risk of recurrence is even higher after two prior post-term pregnancies.

■ MANAGEMENT

The balance between the likelihood of a successful induction of labor and the risks of expectant management is the major concern while managing prolonged pregnancies.

What is definitely not controversial in the management of prolonged pregnancy is:

- No pregnancy with any high-risk factor such as diabetes mellitus, hypertensive disorders in pregnancy, growth restriction, oligohydramnios, or any other condition known to compromise placental function should be allowed to go beyond 40 weeks. The risk is twice as high in the high-risk women as against the low-risk women.
- If the cervix is favorable with Bishop's score (≥6) and the likelihood of a successful vaginal delivery is sufficiently high, induction of labor should be done as there is no reason to expose the woman to the added risks associated with prolongation of pregnancy.
- It is the otherwise "normal" pregnancy that presents the more difficult decision-making options.
- A logical plan for reducing perinatal mortality and morbidity associated with prolonged pregnancy is to terminate pregnancy before such events occur. There have been doubts about the value of labor inductions mainly because it was feared that this would result in more operative interventions without preventing perinatal deaths. As a result, fetal testing was employed to avoid inductions.
- Numerous randomized-controlled trials have been published on induction of labor versus fetal surveillance in prolonged pregnancy. Contrasting results have been obtained. A 2018 meta-analysis of randomized trials comparing labor induction with expectant management of pregnancies at or beyond term concluded that a policy of labor induction at or beyond term compared with expectant management is associated with fewer perinatal deaths and fewer CSs but more operative vaginal births. Neonatal Intensive Care Unit (NICU) admissions were lower and fewer babies had low Apgar scores with induction. No important differences were seen for most of the other maternal and infant outcomes.[15]

Expectant management is the alternative to induction. Expectantly managed pregnancies typically undergo twice-weekly fetal assessment beginning at 41 + 0 weeks (or shortly thereafter), with intervention if spontaneous labor does not begin by a predefined gestational age or fetal assessment testing is abnormal. Either a nonstress test plus assessment of AFV or the biophysical profile (BPP) can be used for antenatal monitoring; there is no convincing evidence that one method is superior to the other.[16] Routine induction after 41 weeks resulted in reduced perinatal mortality without increased risk of mortality without cesarean or instrumental delivery so that there appears to be good evidence to suggest that no approach is superior and either management scheme is valid. The professional guidelines suggest routine induction between 41 + 0 and 42 + 0 weeks of gestation, with the exact timing during this week determined by the clinician and woman's preferences and local circumstances.[17] The American College of Obstetricians and Gynecologists recommends induction of labor after 42 + 0 weeks and by 42 + 6 weeks but considers induction at 41 + 0 to 42 + 0 weeks reasonable.[18]

Fetal Surveillance

Post-term pregnancy is a universally accepted indication for antenatal fetal monitoring because of the increased risk of antepartum fetal demise with advancing gestational age. Fetal surveillance may be used in an attempt to observe the prolonged pregnancy safely till the onset of labor or spontaneous ripening of cervix, prior to induction (elective). The optimal type and frequency of fetal testing is twice-weekly antepartum fetal surveillance between 41 + 0 and 42 + 0 weeks of gestation. Twice-weekly AFV assessment is important because amniotic fluid can become severely reduced within 24–48 hours.

Various tests that allow surveillance of the fetus in utero are as follows:

- Cardiotocography (CTG) and nonstress tests (NSTs)
- Contraction stress test (CST)
- Ultrasonography (USG)
- Biophysical profile (BPP)
- Fetal kick counts

It is clear that monitoring the post-term fetus with Doppler ultrasonography of the umbilical artery has no proven benefit. Evaluation of pulsatility indices of the uterine arteries, middle cerebral artery, descending aorta, ductus venosus, and inferior vena cava is also not useful.[19]

In clinical practice, optimally lowest perinatal mortality and morbidity is obtained with twice-weekly NST and AFV estimations, though intervention rates are highest with this regime. Of the above, probably the most useful are CTG/NST (with the use of vibroacoustic stimulation to shorten the duration of NST) and USG/BPP (or selectively AFV instead of the entire BPP).

It is important to remember that no perfect strategy for fetal surveillance exists that will completely eliminate the risk of fetal death. Also, false-positive tests may commonly lead to unnecessary interventions which can be potentially hazardous. Since the fetal status at the time the test is performed is known, and since the fetal condition can alter over a short period of time, these tests should be performed at frequent intervals.

The frequency of fetal surveillance must be related to the risk of fetal morbidity and mortality, a risk that rises with gestational age. For that reason, testing should be performed at 40 weeks, 41 weeks, and then twice weekly.

Active Intervention

During the course of fetal surveillance, active intervention is indicated when oligohydramnios or nonreassuring NST is detected.

Oligohydramnios

A definite relationship exists between fetal well-being and AFV. A decrease in fluid causes cord compression which can result in antepartum fetal hypoxia and jeopardy which can cause FHR abnormalities and subsequent intrapartum fetal distress. Amniotic fluid index (AFI) < 5 is critical and indicates the need for pregnancy termination. A decrease in fetal movements could also be the sole manifestation of decreased AFV, so the mother should be asked to keep fetal movement counts. Those post-term pregnancies with normal amniotic fluid are at low risk for fetal compromise.

The cord changes in dysmaturity cases are decreases in Wharton's jelly. The cord becomes thin and vulnerable for compression.

Nonreassuring Nonstress Test

Since the cardinal features of postdate pregnancy are oligohydramnios and cord compression, the commonly seen FHR patterns are as follows:

- Moderate-to-severe variable decelerations with slow recovery
- Episodes of spontaneous fetal bradycardia with loss of beat-to-beat variability
- Baseline *saltatory patterns* with oscillations >20 beats/min are occasionally seen.
- Repetitive late decelerations suggesting placental insufficiency are seen in a minority of patients with small for gestational age babies with dysmaturity.
- Prolonged decelerations may occur prior to or during delivery and precede majority of CSs done for fetal distress. Nonreactivity with decelerations may be the first indication of decreased AFV. Nonreassuring FHR patterns including baseline tachycardia may indicate meconium-stained liquor.

Fetal Biophysical Profile

The BPP is based on the acute and chronic adaptive response of the fetus to hypoxemia. The acute response is measured by assessing the FHR, fetal breathing movements, fetal movements, and fetal tone. It has been found that different CNS centers responsible for various biophysical activities respond in a set pattern to a decreasing level of oxygenation. The CNS center which develops last during fetal life is affected first and the CNS center which develops the earliest during fetal life is affected last. Clinically, acute hypoxemia will be picked up first by the NST and by the time the fetus stops all movements and loses tone, the hypoxemia

TABLE 1: Manning's biophysical profile scoring: Technique and interpretation.[20]

Biophysical variable	Normal score = 2	Abnormal score = 0
Fetal breathing movement	At least 1 episode of FBM of at least 30 seconds duration in 30 minutes observation	Absent or no episode of ≥ 30 seconds in 30 minutes
Gross body movements	At least 3 discrete body/limb movements in 30 minutes	2 or fewer episodes of body/limb movement in 30 minutes
Fetal tone	At least 1 episode of active extension with return to flexion of fetal limbs or trunk. Opening and closing of hand is considered as normal tone.	Either slow extension with return to partial flexion or movements of limb in full extension or absent fetal movements with fetal hand held in complete or partial deflexion
Reactive FHR	At least 2 episodes of FHR acceleration of ≥15 bpm and of 15 seconds' duration associated with fetal movement in 30 minutes	Less than 2 episodes of acceleration of FHR or acceleration of <15 bpm in 30 minutes
Qualitative AFV	At least 1 pocket of AF that measures at least 2 cm in 2 perpendicular planes	Either no AF pockets or a pocket <2 cm in 2 perpendicular planes

(AF: amniotic fluid; AFV: amniotic fluid volume; FHR: fetal heart rate)

TABLE 2: Manning's biophysical profile management protocol.[20]

Score	Interpretation	Recommended management
10	Normal infant, low risk of chronic asphyxia	Repeat testing at weekly intervals, repeat twice weekly in prolonged pregnancy
8	Normal infant, low risk of chronic asphyxia	Repeat testing at weekly intervals, repeat twice weekly in prolonged pregnancy. Deliver if oligohydramnios present
6	Suspected chronic asphyxia	Repeat testing in 4–6 hours. Deliver if oligohydramnios present
4	Suspected chronic asphyxia	If ≥36 weeks and cervix is favorable, then deliver. If <36 weeks and L/S ratio <2, repeat test in 24 hours. If repeat score <4, deliver
0–2	Suspected chronic asphyxia	Extended testing time to 120 minutes, if persistent score is 4 then deliver, provided gestational age is sufficiently advanced to permit possible neonatal survival

(L/S: lecithin–sphingomyelin)

is fairly advanced and perinatal morbidity will be high. In addition, measurement of AFV for assessment of chronic response of the fetus to hypoxemia should also be done.

Manning's biophysical profile scoring and biophysical profile management protocol are given in **Tables 1** and **2**, respectively.

Modified Biophysical Profile

Since the BPP is a time-consuming test, several authors have combined NST with assessment of AFV.[21]

Labor Induction

Induction of labor is recommended for women who are known with certainty to have reached 41 weeks (>40 weeks + 7 days) of gestation. Induction of labor is not recommended for women with an uncomplicated pregnancy at gestational age < 41 weeks. Induction with an unfavorable cervix leads to a two-fold increase in cesarean delivery, a large percentage being for failed induction, relative to those who present in spontaneous labor. Cervical ripening employed prior to induction results in shorter labor, lower CS rates, decreased maternal morbidity, and decreased fetal distress so that ripening of cervix must be employed as part of the induction process. Intracervical prostaglandin E2 (PGE2) gel/intracervical Foley's catheter/membrane sweeping of membranes appears to be the most acceptable method of cervical ripening. With the favorable cervix, amniotomy and oxytocin infusion are the methods of choice. Vaginal Misoprostol is another attractive option in induction of labor. It is more effective than vaginal prostaglandins for cervical ripening and labor induction based on outcomes such as failure rate of delivery within 24 hours.

Intrapartum Monitoring

Cardiotocography must be part of the admission test in every postdated woman admitted in labor. Continuous monitoring is advocated in labor.

An attempt must be made to assess fetal weight due to increased chances of macrosomia. USG estimates of fetal weight have a low predictive value which has a lot of practical implications. Management of suspected fetal macrosomia still remains a subject of debate and includes CS for "established" or prophylactic induction for "impending" macrosomia. Evidence that these interventions are beneficial is lacking. A reasonable policy for management of macrosomia would be to await the onset of spontaneous labor in the absence of other risk factors and careful monitoring of the labor. If vaginal delivery is undertaken, be prepared for complications such as shoulder dystocia, dysfunctional labor, and maternal trauma. Avoid instrumental delivery in the possibly macrosomic fetus with protracted labor.

Use of partograms is advocated for detection of abnormal labor patterns. Anticipate the need for anesthesia/pediatric-neonatology assistance. CS may be the preferred method of termination:

- In the presence of severe maternal or fetal compromise with an unfavorable cervix as ripening will take time

- Woman remote from delivery, especially if cephalopelvic disproportion (CPD) is suspected with hyper- or hypotonic dysfunctional labor
- Nulligravida in early labor with thick meconium. In the above circumstance, the likelihood of a successful vaginal delivery is reduced appreciably.

Reducing Incidence of Post-term Gestation

Sweeping or stripping of membranes is an age-old method still in common use. If done at 38–40 weeks, it has been found to reduce the number of women entering labor beyond 41 or 42 weeks without modifying CS rates or increasing maternal/perinatal infections.

Shoulder Dystocia

Shoulder dystocia is an obstetric emergency. The goal of management is to safely deliver the infant before asphyxia and cortical injury occurring from umbilical cord compression and impeded inspiration, without causing peripheral neurologic injury or other fetal or maternal trauma. Most interventions are intended to disimpact the anterior shoulder from behind the symphysis pubis by rotating the fetal trunk or delivering the posterior arm and shoulder. In general, the operator has up to 5 minutes to deliver a previously well-oxygenated term infant before an increased risk of asphyxial injury occurs. The word DOPE is a reminder for a complication such as macrosomia, D—diabetes, O—obesity, P—post-term, E—excessive weight gain during pregnancy.

Suspected macrosomia is not an indication for termination of pregnancy. Pregnant women with suspected macrosomia should be provided individualized counseling about the risk and benefits of vaginal and cesarean delivery.

Initial Steps

When shoulder dystocia is suspected, the gravida and labor room personnel should be given instructions in a clear and calm manner.

- *Call for help:* Nursing, anesthesia, obstetric, and pediatric staff should be called to the labor room, if not already available, to provide assistance as needed.
- The woman should be positioned with her buttocks flush with the edge of the bed to provide optimal access for executing maneuvers to affect delivery.
- Excessive downward traction, greater than usual head and neck traction, and fundal pressure *should be avoided* because this combination of maneuvers can stretch and injure the brachial plexus. These actions also may further impact the shoulders and cause uterine rupture or other injury.

- A tight nuchal cord, if present, should be released over the fetal head and left intact as umbilical blood flow helps in neonatal resuscitation and transition.
- Performing a mediolateral episiotomy is useful to facilitate delivery of the posterior shoulder and other internal procedures.
- A distended bladder, if present, should be drained, which will facilitate suprapubic pressure and may reduce any space-occupying effects of a full bladder in the vagina.
- Proceed with McRoberts maneuver

McRoberts Maneuver with Suprapubic Pressure

This maneuver requires use of an assistant to apply pressure suprapubically with the palm or fist, directing the pressure on the anterior shoulder both downward (to below the pubic bone) and laterally (toward the baby's face or sternum) in conjunction with the McRoberts maneuver. Suprapubic pressure is supposed to adduct the shoulders or bring them into an oblique plane, since the oblique diameter is the widest diameter of the maternal pelvis. It is most useful in mild cases and those caused by an impacted anterior shoulder. Delivery of the posterior arm almost always relieves impaction of the anterior shoulder and resolves the dystocia. It is an appropriate second maneuver if the less technically demanding and often successful McRoberts maneuver and suprapubic pressure fail. The maneuver, which is best performed under adequate anesthesia, requires introducing a hand into the vagina to locate the posterior shoulder and arm. If the fetal abdomen faces the maternal right, the operator's left hand should be used; if the fetal abdomen faces the maternal left, the right hand is used. The posterior arm should be identified and followed to the elbow. If the elbow is flexed, the operator can grasp the forearm and hand and pull out the arm. If it is extended, pressure is applied in the antecubital fossa. This flexes the elbow across the fetal chest and allows the forearm or hand to be grasped. The arm is then pulled out of the vagina, which also delivers the posterior shoulder and reduces the shoulder diameter by 2–3 cm, as the 13-cm bisacromial diameter becomes a 10–11-cm axilloacromial diameter.[22] If the anterior shoulder cannot be delivered at this point, the fetus can be rotated and the procedure repeated for the anterior (now posterior) arm. A similar procedure is followed if the arm is trapped behind the fetus. In this case, manipulation of the forearm so that it can be swept ventrally and out the vagina may involve deliberate or inadvertent fracture of the humerus.

Secondary maneuvers are as follows:

- *Rubin maneuver:* Under adequate anesthesia, the clinician places one hand in the vagina and on the back surface of the posterior fetal shoulder and then rotates it anteriorly toward the fetal face. If the fetal spine is on the maternal left, the operator's right hand is used; the left hand is used if the fetal spine is on the maternal right.
- *Woods screw maneuver:* Rotate the fetus by exerting pressure on the anterior, clavicular surface of the posterior shoulder to turn the fetus until the anterior shoulder emerges from behind the maternal symphysis
- *Gaskin all-fours maneuver: in this maneuver, introduced by Ina May Gaskin, the mother is placed on her hands and knees.*

The last resort procedures that can be used are Gunn-Zavanelli-O'Leary maneuver (if shoulder dystocia occurs in a labor room and cannot be resolved by the maneuvers, the woman should be moved to an operating room for cesarean delivery after the Gunn-Zavanelli-O'Leary maneuver), abdominal rescue procedure, or symphysiotomy. Clear and complete documentation in the medical record is critically important after deliveries complicated by shoulder dystocia.

Multiple Gestation

There is no defined gestational age cutoff to define a prolonged pregnancy in twins, triplets, or higher order multiples. The average gestation lengths for twin, triplet, and quadruplet pregnancies are 36, 33, and 29 weeks, respectively.

KEY POINTS

A logical and functional protocol for the management of prolonged pregnancy would be as follows:
- Prolonged pregnancy refers to a pregnancy that is ≥42 + 0 weeks of gestation or 294 days from the first day of the LMP.
- The diagnosis of post-term pregnancy is based on the clinician's most accurate estimate of the patient's delivery date, which is based on LMP for some patients and on ultrasound dating for others.
- In pregnancies dated by first-trimester ultrasound examination, the prevalence of post-term pregnancy is less and fewer inductions are performed for post-term pregnancy than in pregnancies dated by LMP.
- Women at the highest risk of post-term pregnancy are those with a previous post-term pregnancy. The risk of a second post-term pregnancy is increased two- to fourfold and is even higher after two prior post-term pregnancies.
- Many of the maternal, fetal, and neonatal complications of post-term pregnancy are sequelae of either excessive fetal growth (macrosomia) or placental insufficiency (fetal/neonatal dysmaturity, growth restriction, oligohydramnios).

- Perinatal mortality increases with increasing gestational age after 40 weeks of gestation.
- For pregnancies that reach 41 + 0 weeks of gestation, induction of labor is suggested rather than expectant management. Induction is associated with lower perinatal mortality than expectant management and does not increase the risk of cesarean delivery. The absolute benefits of routine induction are modest, however, and depending on personal values and preferences, some women may choose to be managed expectantly.
- For women at 41 + 0 weeks who choose expectant management, monitor the fetal well-being by nonstress testing with AFV assessment or by the BPP, twice weekly beginning at 41 + 0 weeks.
- Consider induction of labor at or beyond 41 weeks in patients with a favorable cervix (Bishop's score = 6 or can rupture membranes).
- If any testing is abnormal (API < 5/nonreassuring NST/significant FHR decelerations) and fetal well-being cannot be assured, delivery must be considered the method depending on individual circumstances.
- Consider cervical ripening at 41 weeks.
- Assess fetal weight if macrosomia is suspected.
- Monitor labor very carefully. Anticipate problems so that they can be managed well in time.
- From 42 weeks if they deny induction, meticulous antenatal monitoring is required, i.e., twice-weekly CTG and ultrasound.

■ REFERENCES

1. ACOG Committee Opinion No 579: Definition of term pregnancy. Obstet Gynecol. 2013;122(5):1139-40.
2. Alash AM, Barqawi RA, Bani-Irshid IH. Management of post-date pregnancies with unfavorable cervix in primigravida. JRMS. 2006;13(1):19-22.
3. Boyd ME, Usher PH, McLean FH, Kramer MS. Obstetric consequences of post maturity. Am J Obstet Gynaecol. 1988;158(2):334.
4. Oberg AS, Frisell T, Svensson AC, Iliadou AN. Maternal and fetal genetic contributions to postterm birth: familial clustering in a population-based sample of 475,429 Swedish births. Am J Epidemiol. 2013;177(6):531-7.
5. Liggins GC, Kennedy PC, Holm LW. Maternal and fetal genetic contributions to postterm birth: familial clustering in a population-based sample of 475,429 Swedish births. Am J Obstet Gynecol. 1967;98(8):1080-6.
6. Milic AB, Adamsons K. The relationship between anencephaly and prolonged pregnancy. J Obstet Gynaecol Br Commonw. 1969;76(2):102-11.
7. Trimmer KJ, Leveno KJ, Peters MT, Kelly MA. Observations on the cause of oligohydramnios in prolonged pregnancy. Am J Obstet Gynaecol. 1990;163:1900-3.
8. Grannum PA, Berkowitz RL, Hobbins JC. The ultrasonic changes in the maturing placenta and their relation to fetal pulmonic maturity. Am J Obstet Gynecol. 1979;133:915.
9. Becroft DM, Thompson JM, Mitchell EA. Placental infarcts, intervillous fibrin plaques, and intervillous thrombi: incidences, cooccurrences, and epidemiological associations. Pediatr Dev Pathol. 2004;7(1):26-34.
10. Spellacy WN, Miller S, Winegar A, Peterson PQ. Macrosomia-maternal characteristics and infant complications. Obstet Gynecol. 1985;66(2):158.
11. Vorherr H. Placental insufficiency in relation to postterm pregnancy and fetal postmaturity. Evaluation of fetoplacental function; management of the postterm gravida. Am J Obstet Gynecol. 1975;123(1):67-103.
12. Cliford SH. Postmaturity with placental dysfunction, clinical syndrome & pathological findings. J Pediatr. 1954;44(1):1-13.
13. Feldman GB. Prospective risk of stillbirth. Obstet Gynecol. 1992;79(4):547-53.
14. Bruckner TA, Cheng YW, Caughey AB. Increased neonatal mortality among normal-weight births beyond 41 weeks of gestation in California. Am J Obstet Gynecol. 2008;199(4):421. e1.
15. Middleton P, Shepherd E, Crowther CA. Induction of labour for improving birth outcomes for women at or beyond term. Cochrane Database Syst Rev. 2018;5:CD004945.
16. Alfirevic Z, Walkinshaw SA. A randomised controlled trial of simple compared with complex antenatal fetal monitoring after 42 weeks of gestation. Br J Obstet Gynaecol. 1995;102(8):638-43.
17. Clinical Practice Obstetrics Committee, Maternal Fetal Medicine Committee, Delaney M, Roggensack A. Guidelines for the management of pregnancy at 41+0 to 42+0 weeks. J Obstet Gynaecol Can. 2008;30:800.
18. American College of Obstetricians and Gynecologists. Practice bulletin no. 146: Management of late-term and postterm pregnancies. Obstet Gynecol. 2014;124:390.
19. Kauppinen T, Kantomaa T, Tekay A, Mäkikallio K. Placental and fetal hemodynamics in prolonged pregnancies. Prenat Diagn. 2016;36:622.
20. Manning FA, Platt LD, Sipos L. Antepartum fetal evaluation: development of a fetal biophysical profile. Am J Obstet Gynecol. 1980;136:787.
21. Miller DA, Rabello YA, Paul RH. The modified biophysical profile: antepartum testing in the 1990s. Am J Obstet Gynecol 1996; 174:812.
22. Poggi SH, Spong CY, Allen RH. Prioritizing posterior arm delivery during severe shoulder dystocia. Obstet Gynecol. 2003;101:1068.

- Anterior placenta and placenta previa covering the internal cervical os are independent risk factors [odds ratio (OR) 4.1 and OR 3.5, respectively] for postpartum hemorrhage (PPH) during cesarean section.[25]
- Maternal hemorrhagic morbidity is more common in women with placenta previa (19% vs. 7%, adjusted RR 2.6, 95% CI 1.9–3.5), and main factors accountable for it include predelivery anemia, thrombocytopenia, diabetes, and magnesium use.[26]
- The risk of massive hemorrhage together with the possibility of needing a blood transfusion has been estimated to be approximately 12 times more likely in cesarean section for placenta previa than in cesarean delivery for other indications.[27,28]
- The chances of maternal complications at the cesarean section in such cases increase with an inexperienced surgeon or a trainee.[29]
- The cases are strongly associated with the need for complex intraoperative maneuvers to deliver baby (likely transverse or breech presentation).[30]
- Increased neonatal morbidities including an increased risk of lower 5-minute Apgar scores, neonatal intensive care unit (NICU) admission, anemia, respiratory distress syndrome, mechanical ventilation, and intraventricular hemorrhage.[31]
- High -risk factor of associated placenta accreta[6]

■ PROGNOSIS

Maternal

With good and timely management, it has been shown that maternal mortality can be brought down to zero. This has been achieved because of the availability of blood and blood products in abundance, availability of emergency and timely cesarean section, more expertise of surgeons with new techniques, safe anesthesia, and antibiotics. Good antenatal care with elimination of anemia and routine diagnosis of placenta previa along with/without associated accreta on ultrasound also contributes to lowered mortality.

Fetal

The perinatal mortality still remains high despite the expectant management and available resources.

KEY POINTS

- Painless, sudden, recurrent, causeless bleeding in third trimester is typical of placenta previa.
- Ultrasonography for localization of placenta and color Doppler to rule out placenta accreta syndrome are the mainstay of diagnosis.

- Conservative management improves perinatal morbidity and mortality.
- The patient with anterior placenta previa and previous cesarean delivery are at high risk for morbidly adherent placenta.

■ REFERENCES

1. Reddy UM, Abuhamad AZ, Levine D, Saade GR; Fetal Imaging Workshop Invited Participants. Fetal imaging: Executive summary of a joint Eunice Kennedy Shriver National Institute of Child Health and Human Development, Society for Maternal-Fetal Medicine, American Institute of Ultrasound in Medicine, American College of Obstetricians and Gynecologists, American College of Radiology, Society for Pediatric Radiology, and Society of Radiologists in Ultrasound Fetal Imaging Workshop. J Ultrasound Med. 2014;33:745-57.
2. Silver RM. Abnormal placentation: Placenta previa, vasa previa and placenta accreta. Obstet Gynecol. 2015;126:65468.
3. Vahanian SA, Lavery JA, Ananth CV, Vintzileos A. Placental implantation abnormalities and risk of preterm delivery: a systematic review and metaanalysis. Am J Obstet Gynecol. 2015; 213:S78-90.
4. Cleary-Goldman J, Malone FD, Vidaver J, Ball RH, Nyberg DA, Comstock CH, et al. Impact of maternal age on obstetrics outcome. Obstet Gynecol. 2005;105:983.
5. Babinszki A, Kerenyi T, Torok O, Grazi V, Lapinski RH, Berkowitz RL. Perinatal outcome in grand and great grand multiparity: effects of parity on obstetric risk factors. Am J Obstet Gynecol. 1999;181:669.
6. Silver RM, Landon MB, Rouse DJ, Leveno KJ, Spong CY, Thom EA, et al.; National Institute of Child Health and Human Development Maternal-Fetal Medicine Units Network. Maternal morbidity associated with multiple repeat cesarean deliveries. Obstet Gynecol. 2006;107:1226-32.
7. Grady R, Alavi N, Vale R, Khandwala M, McDonald SD. Elective single embryo transfer and perinatal outcomes: a systematic review and meta-analysis. Fertil Steril. 2012;97:324-31.
8. Korosec S, Ban Frangez H, Verdenik I, Kladnik U, Kotar V, Virant-Klun I, et al. Singleton pregnancy outcomes after in vitro fertilization with fresh or frozen-thawed embryo transfer and incidence of placenta praevia. Biomed Res Int. 2014; 2014:431797.
9. Ananth CV, Demissie K, Smulian JC, Vintzileos AM. Placenta previa in singleton and twin births in the United States, 1989 through 1998: a comparison of risk factor profiles and associated conditions. Am J Obstet Gynecol. 2003;188:275.
10. Hung TH, Shau WY, Hsieh CC, Chiu TH, Hsu JJ, Hsieh TT. Risk factors for placenta accreta. Obstet Gynecol. 1999;93:545.
11. Weis MA, Harper LM, Roehl KA, Odibo AO, Cahill AG. Natural history of placenta previa in twins. Obstet Gynecol. 2012;120: 753-8.
12. Jauniaux ERM, Alfirevic Z, Bhide AG, Belfort MA, Burton GJ, Collins SL, et al. on behalf of the Royal College of Obstetricians and Gynaecologists. (2018). Placenta praevia and placenta accreta: Diagnosis and management (Green-top Guideline No. 27a). [online] https://www.rcog.org.uk/en/guidelines-research-services/guidelines/gtg27a/ [Last accessed October, 2020]
13. Royal College of Obstetricians & Gynaecologists. (2011). Antepartum haemorrhage (Green-top Guideline No. 63) [online] Available from https://www.rcog.org.uk/en/guidelines-research-services/guidelines/gtg63/ [Last accessed October, 2020]

14. Roberts D, Brown J, Medley N, Dalziel SR. Antenatal corticosteroids for accelerating fetal lung maturation for women at risk of preterm birth. Cochrane Database Syst Rev. 2017;3:CD004454.

15. Zlatnik MG, Little SE, Kohli P, Kaimal AJ, Stotland NE, Caughey AB. When should women with placenta previa be delivered? A decision analysis. J Reprod Med. 2010;55:373-81.

16. American College of Obstetricians and Gynaecologists. ACOG committee opinion no. 560: Medically indicated late-preterm and early-term deliveries. Obstet Gynecol. 2013;121:908-10.

17. Spong CY, Mercer BM, D'Alton M, Kilpatrick S, Blackwell S, Saade G. Timing of indicated late-preterm and early-term birth. Obstet Gynecol. 2011;118:323-33.

18. Cho JY, Kim SJ, Cha KY, Kay CW, Kim MI, Cha KS. Interrupted circular suture: bleeding control during cesarean delivery in placenta previa accreta. Obstet Gynecol. 1991;78:876.

19. Diemert A, Ortmeyer G, Hollwitz B, Lotz M, Somville T, Glosemeyer P, et al. The combination of intrauterine balloon tamponade and the B-Lynch procedure for the treatment of severe postpartum hemorrhage. Am J Obstet Gynecol. 2012;206(1):65.e1.

20. Dildy GA, Scott AR, Saffer CS. An effective pressure pack for severe pelvic hemorrhage. Obstet Gynecol. 2006;108(5):1222.

21. Albayrak M, Ozdemir I, Koc O, .Demiraran Y. Post-partum haemorrhage from the lower uterine segment secondary to placenta previa/accreta: successful conservative management with Foley balloon tamponade. Aust N Z J Obstet Gynaecol. 2011;51(4):377.

22. Druzin ML. Packing of lower uterine segment for control of postcesarean bleeding in instances of placenta previa. Surg Gynecol Obstet. 1989;169:543.

23. Zlatnik MG, Cheng YW, Norton ME, Thiet MP, Caughey AB. Placenta previa and the risk of preterm delivery. J Matern Fetal Neonatal Med. 2007;20:719-23.

24. Thomas J, Paranjothy S (Ed). The National Sentinel Caesarean Section Audit Report. London: RCOG Press; 2001.

25. Baba Y, Matsubara S, Ohkuchi A, Usui R, Kuwata T, Suzuki H, et al. Anterior placentation as a risk factor for massive hemorrhage during cesarean section in patients with placenta previa. J Obstet Gynaecol Res. 2014;40:1243-8.

26. Gibbins KJ, Einerson BD, Varner MW, Silver RM. Placenta previa and maternal haemorrhagic morbidity. J Matern Fetal Neonatal Med. 2018;31:494-9.

27. Mavrides E, Allard S, Chandraharan E, Collins P, Green L, Hunt BJ, et al. on behalf of the Royal College of Obstetricians and Gynaecologists. Prevention and management of postpartum haemorrhage. BJOG. 2016;124:e106-49.

28. Royal College of Obstetricians and Gynaecologists. (2015). Blood transfusions in obstetrics (Green-top Guideline No. 47). [online] Available from https://www.rcog.org.uk/en/guidelines-research-services/guidelines/gtg47/ [Last accessed October, 2020].

29. Madsen K, Grønbeck L, Rifbjerg Larsen C, Østergaard J, Bergholt T, Langhoff-Roos J, et al. Educational strategies in performing cesarean section. Acta Obstet Gynecol Scand. 2013;92:256-63.

30. Pelosi MA, Apuzzio J, Fricchione D, Gowda VV. The "intra-abdominal version technique" for delivery of transverse lie by low-segment caesarean section. Am J Obstet Gynecol. 1979;135:1009-11.

31. Lal AK, Hibbard JU. Placenta previa: an outcome-based cohort study in a contemporary obstetric population. Arch Gynecol Obstet. 2015;292:299-305.

Abruptio Placentae

Shilpa Chaudhari

INTRODUCTION

An abruptio placentae is a major cause for antepartum hemorrhage. It contributes almost in 35% of antepartum hemorrhage as an etiological factor. It is associated with high maternal and fetal complications in comparison to placenta previa. Abruptio placentae contribute almost 19% to the maternal mortality caused by hemorrhage.

Edward Rigby in 1776 described abruptio placentae as accidental hemorrhage. In Latin, abruptio placentae means "rending asunder of the placenta" and denotes sudden accident.[1]

DEFINITION

Abruptio placentae is a form of antepartum hemorrhage where bleeding occurs from the uterine wall due to premature separation of a normally implanted placenta, before delivery of the fetus (first stage of labor included).[2]

EPIDEMIOLOGY

Placental abruption complicates around 0.3–1% of births. The incidence varies according to the criteria used for diagnosis. When the placenta is routine examined by a pathologist, a higher incidence of abruption is reported. The incidence is more in black women than white women.

The concealed type of abruptio placentae is seen in 20–30% of all abruptio placenta cases and 65–80% are of revealed type. The incidence of a severe form of abruptio placentae (grades 3 and 4) is 0.2%.

If there is a history of abruption in previous pregnancy, its recurrence rate is 5–16% in the next pregnancy, and if there is a history of abruption in previous two pregnancies the rate of recurrence increases up to 25% in the third pregnancy.

TYPES OF ABRUPTIO PLACENTAE

Types of abruptio placentae are considered according to different factors described below:

- According to the bleeding pattern
  - *Revealed:* Following separation of placenta, blood insinuates downward in between the membrane and the decidua. The blood comes out through the cervical canal, which is visible externally.
  - *Concealed:* Blood gets collected behind separated placenta in between the membrane and the decidua. Collected blood is prevented from coming out of the cervix. At times, blood may percolate into the amniotic sac, causing blood-stained liquor.
  - *Mixed:* Here, a part of abruption is revealed and some amount is concealed.
- *According to the extent of placental separation*
  - *Partial abruptio placentae:* Some part of placenta is separated.
  - *Complete abruptio placentae:* Complete placenta is separated.
- *According to clinical presentation*
  - *Grade 0:* Diagnosed postdelivery on examination of placenta; absence of clinical features of abruptio placentae in antenatal and intranatal periods
  - *Grade 1:* External bleeding is mild; the uterus may be tender; absence of shock; absence of fetal distress
  - *Grade 2:* External bleeding mild to moderate; uterine tenderness is always present; absence of shock; fetal distress or even fetal death may occur.
  - *Grade 3:* Bleeding is moderate to severe; most of the time it is concealed. Uterine tenderness is marked, shock is pronounced, and fetal death is a rule. Coagulation defects are present.

ETIOLOGY

The primary cause of abruption is unknown. The incidence increases with:

- Maternal age
- High parity
- Poor socioeconomical condition
- Race or ethnicity (more in Africans than in Asians and Latin Americans).

COMMONLY ASSOCIATED CONDITIONS WITH PLACENTAL ABRUPTION

Hypertension in Pregnancy

Hypertension is commonly associated with abruption. It includes preeclampsia, gestational hypertension, and chronic hypertension. The association of preeclampsia with placental abruption is 44%. Around 1.5% women with chronic hypertension suffer from placental abruption.[3] There is a threefold increase in abruption with chronic hypertension and a fourfold increase with severe preeclampsia. There is reduction in risk of placental abruption when severe preeclampsia and eclampsia patients are treated with magnesium sulfate.[4]

Premature placental separation in preeclampsia is due to spasm of vessels in utero placental bed (spiral arteries). This leads to anoxic endothelial damage leading to rupture of vessels or extravasation of blood in decidua basalis which is referred to as retroplacental hematoma. In patients with eclampsia, the incidence of abruption is seen around 24%.[5] It has been observed that abnormal uterine artery Doppler velocimetry at 23–24 weeks of gestation may carry an increased risk of abruption later in pregnancy, supporting the concept of a long-standing process in some patients.[6,7]

Women who have preeclampsia, abruption, or intrauterine growth restriction have an increased risk of developing any of these complications in a subsequent pregnancy.[8]

Premature Rupture of Membrane

There is an increased incidence of abruption with premature rupture of membrane (PROM). Karmmer and coworkers found the incidence of abruption to be 3.1% in patients with rupture of membrane for >24 hours.[9] There is a threefold risk of abruption with PROM.

The occurrence of placental abruption in preterm PROM was seen higher than in the term (0 per 1,000 vs. 4.2 per 1,000 live births).[10]

Cigarette Smoking

There is a two-fold increased risk of abruption in smokers.[11] The incidence increases five- to eightfold if there is association of chronic hypertension or preeclampsia in smoker patients.

Smoking increases the incidence by 40% with each additional year of smoking. The risk of abruption is correlated with the number of cigarettes smoked per day and the duration of smoking.[12]

Cocaine Abuse

Cocaine abuse in pregnancy is associated with an increased risk of abruption. It may be due to release of catecholamines and presence of hypertension.

Several studies have documented the association of abruption with cocaine abuse. It is thought that acute vasospasm is the etiology of this placental separation in these cases.[13]

Thrombophilias

Thromboembolic disorders during pregnancy (causing clotting disorders) are associated with placental abruption. Placental abruption occurs in 0.8% of pregnancies in the venous thromboembolism (VTE). Women with VTE are at an increased risk of placenta-mediated complications.[14] There is a significant increase in risk of abruption with factor V Leiden or prothrombin gene mutation.[15]

The American Congress of Obstetricians and Gynecologists guideline recommends that thrombophilias are no longer tested for after placental abruption, as they do not appear to increase the risk of abruption.[16]

Trauma

Major external trauma by road traffic accidents or pelvic fractures increases the incidence of abruption by 1.5–9.4%. Evidence of abruption is also seen with a forceful attempt of external cephalic version and needle puncture injury during amniocentesis. Pregnant women hospitalized with no reported injuries after motor vehicle crashes were at an increased risk of adverse pregnancy outcomes including preterm labor and placental abruption. There is an increased risk for abruption, even in the absence of direct uterine trauma.[17] Shearing forces associated with sudden movement may cause placental separation. This separation may become clinically evident only several hours or days after the trauma. In particular, domestic violence and motor vehicle accidents may be associated with abruption.[18]

Multifetal Pregnancy

One study found the incidence of abruption to be 6.2 per 1,000 singleton births, 12.2 per 1,000 twin births, and 15.6 per 1,000 triplet births.[19]

Sudden Uterine Decompression

Sudden decompression of uterus leads to a diminished surface area of the uterus adjacent to placental attachment resulting in separation of placenta. This usually occurs after delivery of first baby of twins, sudden escape of liquor amnii in polyhydramnios, or PROM.

In the above situations, there is engorgement of uterine and placental vessels resulting in extravasation of blood.

Uterine Leiomyoma

The risk of placental abruption is increased by threefold in women with fibroids. Submucosal fibroids, retroplacental fibroids, and fibroids with volumes > 200 cm are independent risk factors for placental abruption.[20]

One retrospective study reported placental abruption in 57% of women with retroplacental fibroids in contrast with 2.5% of women with fibroids located in alternate sites.[21]

Raised Maternal Serum Alfa Fetoprotein

An increased level of alpha-fetoprotein (AFP), in the absence of congenital anomalies, is associated with placental abruption.[22] Second-trimester maternal serum AFP (MSAFP) levels are higher in women with subsequent placental abruption; however, the clinical usefulness of this test is limited.[23]

- Asymptomatic bacteriuria
- Folic acid deficiency
- Antiphospholipid antibody (APLA) syndrome
- External cephalic version
- Diabetes mellitus

■ PATHOLOGY

There is hemorrhage in decidua basalis, which splits leaving a thin layer adherent to the myometrium. This is called an early stage of decidual hematoma. Decidual hematoma leads to separation, compression, and ultimate destruction of placenta adjacent to it. Up to this stage, the symptoms may not be present. Decidual hematoma is discovered only on examination of freshly delivered placenta. It has circumscribed depression measuring a few centimeters in diameter on the maternal surface and is covered by dark-colored blood. Very recently separated placenta may not appear different from a normal placenta at delivery. The age of retroplacental clots is difficult to determine.

In some cases, a decidual spiral artery ruptures to cause a retroplacental hematoma. When this hematoma expands, it disturbs more vessels to separate more placenta.

As the uterus is still distended by products of conception, it is unable to contract sufficiently to compress the torn vessels. The escaping blood might dissect the membranes from the uterine wall and eventually reveal or may completely retain within the uterus (concealed). Concealed hemorrhage is likely when:

- There is an effusion of blood behind the placenta, but its margins still remain adherent.
- The placenta is completely separated, but the membranes retain their attachment to the uterine wall.
- The blood gets access to amniotic cavity after breaking through the membranes.
- The fetal head (presenting part) is closely applied to the lower uterine segment and blood cannot pass through it.
- Absence of rhythmic uterine contractions plays a significant role for blood to remain concealed.

Bleeding with placental abruption is almost always maternal. In 20% cases, fetal to maternal bleeding is seen. Significant fetal bleeding is seen only in traumatic cases. Fetal bleeding results from placental bleeding than placental separation. On an average, 10–12 mL of fetal to maternal hemorrhage is seen. It can vary from 80 to 100 mL depending on the severity of trauma.

■ CLINICAL FEATURES

Signs and symptoms can vary considerably, as they are dependent on the type of abruption (revealed, concealed, or mixed). Clinical presentation can range from stable to shock with complications (disseminated intravascular coagulation and acute renal failure).

The main symptom is vaginal bleeding with pain in the abdomen as compared to painless bleeding of placenta previa. Presence of uterine tenderness, pallor, hypertension, uterine hypertonicity, fetal distress, and absent fetal heart sound (FHS) are dependent on (**Table 1**):

- Degree of separation of placenta
- Speed with which separation occurs
- Amount of blood concealed inside the uterine cavity.

■ DIAGNOSIS

Abruptio placenta is most of the times diagnosed only on the basis of clinical findings. So, the management should be started on the first clinical suspicion. Diagnosis is confirmed

TABLE 1: Symptoms in revealed and concealed types of abruption.

Symptoms	Revealed	Concealed
Character of bleeding	Acute abdominal pain followed by bleeding. Continuous dark color bleeding	Acute abdominal pain not followed by bleeding. Slight, dark-colored bleeding may be present
General condition	Shock is usually absent; if present, then it is in proportion to visible blood loss	Shock is pronounced, which is out of proportion to visible blood loss
Pallor	Related to visible blood loss	Pallor is severe and out of proportion to visible blood loss
Features of preeclampsia	May be absent	Frequent association is seen
Uterine height	Proportionate to gestational age	May be enlarged compared to period of gestation
Uterine feel	Soft	Tense, tender and rigid
Fetal parts	Can be felt easily	Difficult to feel
Fetal heart sound	FHS usually present	Severe distress, absence of fetal heart (IUD)
Urine output	Adequate	Usually diminished
Coagulation disorder (petechial to bleeding diathesis)	Mostly not associated	Frequency of association is 20%

by ultrasonography only in 25% cases. Sensitivity is low, so the diagnosis remains a clinical diagnosis.

Ultrasonographic findings are inconsistent as both the blood clot and the placenta are hypoechoic and differentiation is difficult.

Findings suggestive of placental abruption are as follows:

- Retroplacental hematoma (hyperechoic, isoechoic, hypoechoic)
- Preplacental hematoma (jiggling appearance with a shimmering effect of the chorionic plate with fetal movement).

Placental Abruption Diagnosis

- Increased placental thickness and echogenicity
- Subchorionic collection
- Marginal collection[18]

So, it is important to note that the negative findings on ultrasonography do not exclude placental abruption.

Detection rates of only 12–25% are generally reported.[24] However, in skilled hands, high rates of diagnosis have been reported.[25] If there is ultrasound evidence of placental abruption, the positive predictive value is high.[24]

■ INVESTIGATIONS

- Hemogram
- Blood group and Rh typing
- Serum HIV antibody test
- Serum HBsAg
- Serum VDRL
- Urine routine and microscopy
- Blood sugar level—random

Specific Investigations

- Renal function test (blood urea, serum creatinine, serum uric acid)
- Liver function test
- Fundoscopy
  - Coagulation profile Bleeding time
  - Clotting time
  - Clot observation test **(Box 1)**
  - Platelet count
  - Prothrombin time (PT) with international normalized ratio (INR)
  - Activated partial thromboplastin time (aPTT)
  - D-dimer

BOX 1: Clot observation test.

- Blood is taken in a test tube. If no clot within 8 min—hypofibrinogenemia
- If no clot forms but retraction of clot in 1 hour—thrombocytopenia
- If clot dissolves in 1 hour –fibrinolysis

- Blood cross matching kept ready
- A Kleihauer–Betke test is often ordered. However, it is rarely positive in cases of abruption and should not be used in trying to diagnose or rule out abruption. Its value mostly is to assess the need for additional Rh immune globulin in Rh-negative women.[26]

■ DIFFERENTIAL DIAGNOSIS

1. Revealed type of abruption can be confused with placenta previa.
2. Concealed type of abruption can be confused with rupture of the uterus, acute appendicitis, intestinal perforation, volvulus, acute hydramnios, and tonic uterine contractions.

■ MANAGEMENT

Treatment of abruptio placenta depends upon the gestational age, status of mother and fetus, and presence or absence of complications (coagulation disorder and acute renal failure).

In preterm pregnancy if the diagnosis is uncertain and the fetus is alive but without evidence of fetal distress, expectant management is done. This needs close observation, and facilities for immediate interventions should be available when needed. The use of tocolysis is controversial. Tower and coworkers did not find any change in perinatal mortality in the patients conservatively managed by tocolysis.[27] However, Stall and Combs found improvement in outcome in highly selected groups of patients.[28,29] The cases with established placental abruption should be considered for termination of pregnancy and are a contraindication to tocolytic therapy, as the disease is associated with a high rate of maternal and perinatal morbidity and mortality.

Definitive Treatment

The course of any type of abruption, especially concealed type, may lead to adverse effect on maternal health, so once the diagnosis of abruptio placenta is confirmed, prompt and fast delivery has to be considered.

General Measures

- Intravenous access with large-bore cannulae in at least two places
- At the same time withdraw the blood for previously mentioned investigations.
- An indwelling urinary catheter
- Central venous line for measurement of central venous pressure in case of shock. Such cases may need intensive care unit management.

- Volume expanders—crystalloids. An infusion of two units of crystalloids, 20% of which retain in circulation. The blood volume change lasts for 30 minutes.
- Continuous monitoring of vitals
- Consultation with an anesthetist and a hematologist (whenever availability of a hematologist is there).

Vaginal Delivery

If the patient is already in labor, then acceleration of labor with amniotomy is done (low rupture of membrane). In extensive placental abruption, the uterus is likely to be hypertonic. The baseline intrauterine pressure may be 50 mm Hg or higher, which rhythmically increases up to 75–100 mm Hg with good contractions. Due to hypertonicity, it is difficult to determine contraction and relaxation on palpation. Rupture of membranes may cause reduction in bleeding from the implantation site and may reduce the entry of thromboplastin in maternal circulation. The intrauterine pressure also gets reduced to some extent and response to oxytocin drip (for augmentation) is also improved upon. The oxytocin drip is given in standard doses (2.5 U in 5% glucose with titration of dose). If there is severe placental separation (grades III and IV) and fetus is dead, vaginal delivery is preferred (unless there is some other obstetrical complication which is contraindicated for vaginal delivery).

Cesarean delivery with an associated coagulation disorder can cause bleeding from abdominal and uterine incisions. In contrast, vaginal delivery causes stimulation of myometrium; uterine contractions also cause constrictions of the vessels, so severe hemorrhage is avoided. The cause of concern is that if the vaginal delivery is going to take >8–10 hours, it can have an adverse effect on the mother.

The maternal outcome depends on the diligence with which adequate fluid and blood replacement therapy is pursued, rather than on the time interval of delivery. Since it is not always possible to have arrangement of blood and blood components urgently, interval of delivery is important to prevent complications.

Cesarean Delivery

A fetus which is alive but in distress always requires cesarean delivery.[30] It is dangerous to perform cesarean delivery in women who are profoundly hypovolemic and have severe consumptive coagulopathy. It is always a dilemma to go for a cesarean delivery in patients who had been previously chosen for vaginal delivery due to delay in progress of labor (exceeding 8–10 hours) or the patient's condition worsens because of complications such as acute renal failure and consumptive coagulopathy. In patients with consumptive coagulopathy stabilizing the patient with fresh frozen plasma, platelet transfusion, cryoprecipitate first and then going forward with cesarean delivery is safer.

After delivery, placental examination should be done to note:
- Completeness of placenta
- Area of abruption
- Presence of clots
- Weight of clot (replace blood loss according to weight of clot ~ 1.5 times more than the weight of clot)
- Send placenta for histopathological examination.

Active Management of Third Stage of Labor (AMTSL)

Antepartum hemorrhage (APH) arising from placental abruption and placenta previa is associated with an increased risk of postpartum hemorrhage (PPH).[31,32] Active versus expectant management of the third stage of labor reduces the risk of PPH (blood loss greater than 1,000 mL) and need for blood transfusion.[33]

A Cochrane review suggests that when combination of ergometrin and oxytocin is used for third stage of labor, then it is associated with small reduction in risk of PPH, as compared with oxytocin used alone for third stage of labor.[34]

◼ COMPLICATIONS OF ABRUPTIO PLACENTAE

Shock

In severe type of abruptio, shock is out of proportion to visible blood loss and is considered true obstetric shock. It is better to start with a fresh whole blood for prompt restoration of circulation. Shock can be pronounced in cases of preeclampsia as there is already hemoconcentration. These patients may have a tendency to go in shock even with a small amount of blood loss. Central venous pressure monitoring is a guideline for fluid infusion. The role of vasoconstriction drug is a debate. The cardinal principle in shock management is to improve tissue perfusion. Shock is always disproportionate to visible loss in mixed and concealed types of abruptio placenta.

Consumptive Coagulopathy

The most common cause of obstetric consumptive coagulopathy is placental abruptio. Its incidence is 20%. The major mechanism is by induction of coagulation intravascularly and to a lesser extent retroplacentally. There is release of thromboplastin in maternal circulation from placenta and decidua tissue. If there is associated preeclampsia, it contributes to the coagulation disorder by exposing the underlying collagen to plasma and coagulation factor by injury to endothelial cells.

The overall effect is hypofibrionogenemia (<150 mg/dL), elevated fibrin degradation product (FDP), variable decrease in D-dimer, and other coagulation factors. These changes are seen in 30% abruption cases and are severe enough to cause fetal demise. Fresh frozen plasma can be given as replacement of clotting factor (15 mg/kg body weight), cryoprecipitate to replace fibrinogen level (4 g of fibrinogen in 1,000 mL of 5% glucose given intravenously). Platelet transfusion is done, if count is <10,000.[35] In case of nonavailability of cryoprecipitate, a large amount of fresh whole blood can be given.

Renal Failure

Renal failure is mostly seen with severe forms of abruption where treatment of hypovolemia is delayed or given incompletely. The incidence of acute renal failure in cases of abruption is 1.2–8.9%. Reversible tubular and cortical necrosis is seen in abruption. Renal ischemia is caused by:

- Hypovolemic shock
- Reflex spasm of vessels due to sudden distention of uterus
- Occlusion of glomerular capillaries by microthrombi in consumptive coagulopathy
- Kidney pathology caused by a hypertensive state of pregnancy.

The early stage of renal ischemia causes renal tubular necrosis which is reversible; later on, irreversible cortical necrosis occurs. Treatment is to wait for 2–3 weeks during which tubular epithelium regenerates. During this period, patients are kept on hemodialysis or peritoneal dialysis. The patient should be prevented from going into irreversible cortical necrosis by correcting hypovolemia in time and maintaining renal perfusion.

Couvelaire Uterus or Uteroplacental Apoplexy

Extravasation of blood often takes place into the uterine musculature, beneath the serosa, and at times into the ovaries, broad ligament, tubes, and even peritoneal cavity. It is seen in severe type of abruption. This was described first time by Couvelaire in 1912 and he named it is as uteroplacental apoplexy. Its incidence cannot be calculated accurately as it is demonstrable only on laparotomy. It should be suspected in severe cases, particularly those associated with renal or coagulation failure. The uterus has bluish purple to coppery discoloration. Typically, ploughing of blood in myometrium and reaching up to the subserosal layer lead to irregular coppery dark brown lining seen mostly at the fundocornual axis, spreading to the anterior or posterior uterine wall.

These myometrial hemorrhages seldom interfere with uterine contractions. It is not sufficient enough to produce postpartum hemorrhage as the uterus retains its contractile power. Presence of Couvelaire uterus is not an indication for hysterectomy.

■ PROGNOSIS

Prognosis depends upon the type and severity of abruption. It also depends upon the time interval between placental separation and delivery of placenta.

Maternal

It is associated with maternal mortality in 19% cases and related to other complications such as:

- Hemorrhage
- Hypovolemic shock
- Consumptive coagulopathy
- Acute renal failure
- Postpartum hemorrhage
- Puerperal sepsis

A severe form of antepartum hemorrhage can lead to necrosis of the anterior pituitary gland causing Sheehan's syndrome.

Fetal

Perinatal consequences include low birth weight, preterm delivery, asphyxia, and still birth. In developed countries, approximately 10% of all preterm birth and 10–20% of all perinatal deaths are caused by placental abruption.[36]

- Intrauterine growth restriction
- *Preterm birth:* Abruption is associated with an increased risk of preterm birth (adjusted relative risk 3.9; 95% CI 3.5–4.4). Thrombin is a powerful uterotonic agent, and intrauterine bleeding may lead to uterine contractions and preterm labor. In addition, bleeding may weaken the chorioamniotic membranes, predisposing to preterm PROM.[37]
- *Neurological impairment in the infant:* It is also associated with an increased risk for periventricular leukomalacia, cerebral palsy, and neurodevelopmental delay.[38]
- *Perinatal death:* Although the incidence is variable, abruption greatly increases the risk of perinatal death, particularly at preterm gestations. Perinatal deaths are seen in 16.5% cases. Placental abruption with disseminated intravascular coagulation (DIC) and blood transfusion had a significant higher incidence of perinatal mortality than other patients.[39]

According to Ananth CV, the perinatal mortality rate is 119 per 1,000 live births (17% compared with 8.2% among all other births); 55% of the excess perinatal deaths with abruption were due to early delivery. Even the babies born at 40 weeks of gestation and with birth weight 3.5–4 kg had a 25-fold higher mortality with abruption.[40]

Subsequent pregnancies should be monitored carefully.[41] It has been suggested that intensive surveillance should be commenced 3 months before the gestational age at which the previous abruption occurred.[42]

■ PREVENTION

- Correcting the folic acid deficiency and anemia during the antenatal period
- Early diagnosis and effective treatment of preeclampsia, asymptomatic bacteriuria, and diabetes mellitus
- Avoidance of trauma
- Avoiding sudden decompression of uterus
- Prompt diagnosis and initiation of treatment of abruptio placenta to minimize the risk of grave complications.

KEY POINTS

- Abruptio placenta is the major cause of still births in an antepartum hemorrhage.
- Diagnosis is mostly clinical; negative USG findings should not rule out abruption.
- Maternal mortality is high.
- Early detection and prevention of complications is the key to reduction of mortality rate.
- Prompt and fast delivery has to be considered once diagnosis is confirmed.
- Hypovolemic shock, acute renal failure, and consumption coagulopathy are major complications.
- In most of the cases of preeclampsia with antepartum hemorrhage, the cause is abruption.
- Couvelaire uterus is not an indication for hysterectomy.
- The risk of recurrence is high with high mortality rates.

■ REFERENCES

1. Rigby E. An Essay on the Uterine Haemorrhage Which Precedes the Delivery of the Full Grown Fetus, 6th edn. London: Burkes and Kinnebrook.
2. Oyelese Y, Ananth CV. Placental abruption. Obstet Gynecol. 2006;108:1005-101.
3. Sibai BM, Lindheimer M, Hauth J, Van Dorsten P, Klebanoff M, MacPherson C, et al. Risk factors for preeclampsia, abruptio placentae, and adverse neonatal outcomes among women with chronic hypertension. N Engl J Med. 1998;339(10):667-71.
4. Magpie Trial Collaborative Group. Do women with pre-eclampsia, and their babies, benefit from magnesium sulphate? The Magpie Trial: a randomised placebo-controlled trial. Lancet. 2002;359(9321):1877-90.
5. Abdell TN, Sibai B, Hays JM, Anderson GD. Relationship of hypertensive disease to abruptio placentae. Obstet Gynecol. 1984;63(3):365-70.
6. Kurdi W, Campbell S, Aquilina J, England P, Harrington K. The role of color Doppler imaging of the uterine arteries at 29 weeks gestation in stratifying antenatal care. Ultasound Obstet Gynecol. 1998;12:339-45.
7. Harrington K, Cooper D, Lees C, Hecher K, Campbell S. Doppler ultrasound of the uterine arteries: the importance of bilateral notching in the prediction of pre-eclampsia, placental abruption or delivery of a small for gestational age baby. Ultrasound Obstet Gynecol.1996;7:182-8.
8. Ananth CV, Peltier MR, Chavez MR, Kirby RB, Getahun D, Vintzielos AM. Recurrence of ischemic placental disease. Obstet Gynecol. 2007;110:128-33.
9. Major CA, de Veciana M, Lewis DF, Morgan MA. Preterm premature rupture of membranes and abruptio placentae: is there an association between these pregnancy complications? Am J Obstet Gynecol. 1995;172:672-6.
10. Markhus VH, Rasmussen S, Lie SA, Irgens LM. Placental abruption and premature rupture of membranes. Acta Obstet Gynecol Scand. 2011;90(9):1024-9.
11. Ananth CV, Smulian JC, Vintzileos AM. Incidence of placental abruption in relation to cigarette smoking and hypertensive disorders during pregnancy: a meta-analysis of observational studies. Obstet Gynecol. 1999;93(4):622-8.
12. Raymond EG, Mills JL. Placental abruption. Maternal risk factors and associated fetal conditions. Acta Obstet Gynecol Scand. 1993;72:633-9.
13. Addis A, Moretti ME, Ahmed Syed F, Einarson TR, Koren G. Fetal effects of cocaine: an updated meta-analysis. Reprod Toxicol. 2001;15:341-69.
14. Hansen AT, Schmidt M, Horvath –Puho E, Pedersen L, Rothman KJ, Hvas AM, et al. Preconception venous thromboembolism and placenta-mediated pregnancy complications. J Thromb Haemost. 2015;13(9):1635-41.
15. Facchinetti F, Marozio L, Grandone E, Pizzi C, Volpe A, Benedetto C. Thrombophilic mutations are main risk factor for placental abruption. Haematologica. 2003;88(7):785-8.
16. American College of Obstetricians and Gynecologists Women's Health Care Physicians. Practice Bulletin No. 138. Inherited Thrombophilias in Pregnancy. Obstet Gynecol. 2013;122:706-17.
17. Schiff MA, Holt VL. Pregnancy outcomes following hospitalization for motor for motor vehicle crashes in Washington state from 1989-2001. Am J Epidemiol. 2005;161:503-10.
18. Yinka O, Vintzileos AM. BMJ Best Practice Topics. [online] Available from Bestpractice.bmj.com.updated [Last accessed October, 2020].
19. Salihu HM, Bekan B, Aliyu MH, Rouse DJ, Kirby RS, Alexander GR et al. Perinatal mortality associated with abruptio placenta in singletons and multiples. Am J Obstet Gynecol. 2005;193:198-03.
20. Exacoustòs C, Rosati P. Ultrasound diagnosis of uterine myomas and complications in pregnancy. Obstet Gynecol. 1993;82:97-101.
21. Burton CA, Grimes DA, March CM. Surgical management of leiomyomata during pregnancy. Obstet Gynecol. 1989;74:707-9.
22. Bartha JL, Comino-Delgado R, Arce F. Maternal serum alpha-fetoprotein in placental abruption associated with preterm labor. Int J Gynaecol Obstet. 1997;56(3):231-6.
23. Tikkanen N, Hamalainen E, Nuutila M, Paavonen J, Vlikorkala O, Hiilesmaa V. Elevated maternal second trimester serum alpha-fetoprotein as a risk factor for placental abruption. Prenat Diagn. 2007;27(3):240-3.
24. Kikutani M, Ishihara K, Araki T. Value of ultrasonography in the diagnosis of placental abruption. J Nippon Med Sch. 2003;70(3):227-33.
25. Yeo L, Ananth C, Vintzileos A. Placental abruption. In: Sciarra J (Ed). Gynecology and Obstetrics. Hagerstown, MD: Lippincott, Williams & Wilkins; 2004.
26. Atkinson A, Santolaya-Forgas J, Matta P, Canterino J, Oyelese Y. The sensitivity of the Kleihauer-Betke test for placental abruption. J Obstet Gynaecol. 2015;35:139-41.
27. Tower CV, Pircon RA, Heppaed N. Is tocolysis safe in the management of third trimester bleeding? Int J Obstet Gynecol. 1999;180:1572-8.
28. Sholl JS. Abruptio placentae clinical management in nonacute cases. Am J Obstet Gynaecol. 1987;156(1):40-51.

29. Combs CA, Nyberg DA, Mack LA, Smith JR, Benedetti TJ. Expectant management after sonographic diagnosis of placental abruption. Am J Perinatol. 1992;9(3):170-4.

30. Kayani SI, Walkinshaw SA, Preston C. Pregnancy outcome in severe placental abruption. BJOG. 2003;110:679-83.

31. Stones RW, Paterson CM, Saunders NJ. Risk factors for major obstetric haemorrhage. Eur J Obstet Gynecol Reprod Biol. 1993;48(1):15-8.

32. Schuurmans N, MacKinnon C, Lane C, Etches D. Prevention and management of postpartum haemorrhage. J Soc Obstet Gynaecol Can. 2000;22:271-81.

33. Begley CM, Gyte GM, Murphy DJ, Devane D, McDonald SJ, McGuire W. Active versus expectant management for women in the third stage of labour. Cochrane Database Syst Rev. 2010;(7):CD007412.

34. McDonald S, Abbott JM, Higgins SP. Prophylactic ergometrine oxytocin versus oxytocin for the third stage of labour. Cochrane Database Syst Rev. 2004;(1):CD000201.

35. World Health Organization, UNICEF, United Nations Population Fund. Managing Complications in Pregnancy and Childbirth. WHO Guidelines, 2nd edition; 2018.

36. Tikkanen M. Placental abruption: epidemiology, risk factors and consequences. Acta Obstet Gynecol Scand. 2011;90(2):140-9.

37. Lockwood CJ, Toti P, Arcuri F, Paidas M, Buchwalder L, Krikun G, et al. Mechanisms of abruption-induced premature rupture of the fetal membranes: thrombin-enhanced interleukin-8 expression in term decidua. Am J Pathol. 2005;167:1443-9.

38. Gibbs JM, Weindling AM. Neonatal intracranial lesions following placental abruption. Eur J Pediatr. 1994;153:195-7.

39. Pitaphrom A, Suckcharoen N. pregnancy outcome in placental abruption. J Med Assoc Thia. 2006;89(10):1572-8.

40. Anant CV, Wilcox AJ. Placental abruption and perinatal mortality in the united states. Am J Epidemiol. 2001;153(4):332-7.

41. Furuhashi M, Kurauchi O, Suganuma N. Pregnancy following placental abruption. Arch Gynecol Obstet. 2002;267:11-3.

42. Rasmussen S, Irgens LM, Albrechtsen S, Dalaker K. Women with a history of placental abruption: when in a subsequent pregnancy should special surveillance for a recurrent placental abruption be initiated? Acta Obstet Gynecol Scand. 2001;80:708-12.

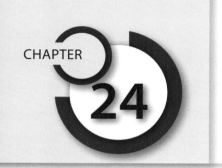

Rh Alloimmunization

Nitin S Kshirsagar

INTRODUCTION

Rh alloimmunization has an important place in the history of obstetrics. It is one of the first genotypic diseases affecting fetus that can be detected and treated before birth. It exemplifies the achievements of systematic scientific and clinical research. In just over 40 years, it has been possible to unravel the pathophysiology, devise useful treatments, and introduce an effective means to prevent a condition which had previously caused extensive fetal morbidity and mortality.

TERMINOLOGY

Exposure to foreign red cell antigens results in the production of anti-red-cell antibodies in a process known as red cell alloimmunization (formerly known as isoimmunization). The term sensitization can be used synonymously. The active transport of these antibodies across the placenta accounts for hemolysis in the fetus resulting in anemia, hyperbilirubinemia, and ultimately hydrops fetalis. These effects were detected only after birth. Hence, the term used was hemolytic disease of the newborn (HDN). Because the peripheral smear of these infants demonstrated a large number of immature red cells (erythroblasts), it was called erythroblastosis fetalis. Some authors use the term hemolytic disease of the fetus and newborn (HDFN) which appears to be an appropriate term. Milestones in the history of Rh alloimmunization:

- *1609:* First case of HDFN described by a midwife in French literature
- *1932:* Diamond proposed that erythroblastosis fetalis, icterus gravis, neonatorum, and hydrops fetalis represented different manifestations of the same disease.
- *1939:* Levin described an antibody in a woman who delivered a still birth.
  She developed a severe hemolytic transfusion reaction after receiving her husband's compatible blood.
- *1940:* Landsteiner and Wiener discovered the "Rhesus antigen".
- *1941:* Levin demonstrated a causal relationship between RhD antibody in Rh negative women and HDFN in baby.

- *1945:* Wallerstein described the technique of neonatal exchange transfusion.
- *1956:* Bevis performed spectrophotometric analysis of amniotic fluid to diagnose Rh hemolytic disease.
- *1957:* Kleihauer described acid elution test to detect fetomaternal hemorrhage.
- *1961:* Liley designed his charts based on the work of Bevis.
- *1961-62:* Finn in Liverpool and Gorman in New York reported prevention of disease by passive immunization. These experiments were done using male volunteers.
- *1963:* Liley performed first intrauterine transfusion.
- *1964:* Dr Gorman's sister-in-law was the first at-risk woman to receive injection
  Anti-D on January 31, 1964.
- *1966:* Several investigators made futile attempts to transfuse blood to fetus via hysterotomy (Freda 1964; Asensio, 1966).
- *1965:* Freda reported successful clinical trials using postpartum passive immunization in Rh-negative mothers.
- *1968:* The Food and Drug Administration (FDA) approved use of injection Anti-D from postpartum prophylaxis.
- *1971:* Qeenan demonstrated isoimmunization following first- and second-trimester abortions and strongly recommended injection Anti-D.
- *1981:* Rodeck and coworkers are credited with the first intravascular fetal transfusion using a fetoscope.
- *1982:* Bang et al. performed the first ultrasound-guided intravascular transfusion through the umbilical vein.
- *1993:* Bennett and colleagues utilized genetic techniques on amniotic fluid to determine fetal Rh type.
- *2000:* Mari et al. proposed peak systolic velocity of fetal middle cerebral artery to diagnose fetal anemia.
- *2002:* Finning and coworkers detected fetal D status by examining maternal plasma.

RHESUS BLOOD GROUP SYSTEM

There are various classification systems:

- *Fisher–Race system:* Fisher and Race proposed the concept of three genes that encode for the three major antigens—D, C/c, and E/e.[1,2] An Rh gene complex is described by three letters—Cde, cde, cDE, cDe, Cde, CDE, and CdE (the first three being the most common). These genes are located on the short arm of chromosome.

- *Weiner system:* Weiner put forth the concept of one gene instead of three.[3] He postulated that a gene gives rise to an agglutinogen on the red cell surface and this in turn possesses a number of blood factors. The eight genotypes are R1, R2, R0, R2, r', r'', ry, and r. For example, gene R1 gives rise to the agglutinogen Rh1 which possesses the three blood factors Rh0, rh', and hr''.

- *Rosenfield system:* It is based on the belief that other systems do not explain the quantitative differences in the expression of Rh antigen.[4]

  Rosenfield suggested a numerical nomenclature for Rh system. For example, D or Rho became Rh_1, C or rh' become Rh_2, and Rh antigens were numbered from Rh_1 to Rh_{48}.

- *ISBT (International Society of Blood Transfusion) numeric terminology:* The ISBT working committee proposed assigning numbers to specificities as standard alternatives to current alphabetical names mainly for some computer systems.[5] For example, D, C, and E are 004001, 004002, and 004003, respectively.

PATHOGENESIS OF MATERNAL ALLOIMMUNIZATION

For Rh alloimmunization to occur:
- The woman must be Rh negative and the fetus Rh positive.
- Fetal erythrocytes must enter maternal circulation in sufficient quantity.
- The mother must be immune-competent.

TRANSPLACENTAL HEMORRHAGE

Seventy-five percent of women have transplacental hemorrhage (TPH) during pregnancy or at delivery. The volume of hemorrhage is usually small. The prevalence and volume of TPH rise with advancing gestation, e.g., 3% in the first trimester (0.03 mL) to 12% in the second trimester (<0.1 mL) and 45% in the third trimester.

MATERNAL RESPONSE

Initial exposure to Rh-positive cells leads to weak primary response in the form of production of immunoglobulin M (IgM) antibodies. It does not cross the placenta and fetus is unaffected. It takes about 5–16 weeks. With further exposure, IgG antibodies are produced which can readily cross the placenta. In one-third of the cases, only subclasses IgG_1 and IgG_3 are found.[6] B lymphocytes differentiate into plasma cells that can rapidly produce IgG.

SENSITIZATION PHENOMENON

Sensitization phenomenon describes how some women can become sensitized but their immune response remains occult until revealed by a subsequent exposure to Rh antigen. It was reported by Nevanlinna.[7]

FETAL RESPONSE

Maternal IgG antibodies cross the placenta and enter the fetal circulation. They are attached to fetal red blood cells (RBCs). These cells are sequestered by macrophages in the spleen where they undergo hemolysis. It results in fetal anemia. The higher the antibody response, the more the hemolysis and anemia.

Male fetuses are 13 times more likely than their female counterparts to become hydropic.[8]

Clinical manifestations depend upon the severity of anemia and hemolysis, namely, neonatal anemia, neonatal jaundice, hydrops fetalis, and intrauterine death (IUD).

To compensate for anemia, extramedullary hematopoiesis is initiated in liver and spleen. There is hepatosplenomegaly. Tissue hypoxia ensues as anemia progresses and ultimately there is hydrops fetalis.

Causes of Hydrops Fetalis

- Severe anemia [hemoglobin (Hb) < 4 g%] resulting in cardiac failure
- Lowering of serum albumin due to hepatic dysfunction[9]
- Portal hypertension
- Decrease in colloid osmotic pressure
- Tissue hypoxia enhancing capillary permeability
- Endothelial cell dysfunction
- Blockage of lymphatic system due to raised central venous pressure (CVP)
- Myocardial dysfunction

DEGREES OF ALLOIMMUNIZATION

It is estimated that about 10–15% of Rh-negative women bearing Rh-positive fetus become sensitized after delivery. The incidence of primary antenatal sensitization is 1%.

This low index of sensitization is due to the following factors:

- *Size of inoculum:* Obviously, the greater the number of fetal cells entering the maternal circulation, the more the risk of alloimmunization **(Table 1)**.
- *ABO incompatibility:* If the mother is group O and baby group A, B or AB, the chances of sensitization are decreased by 50–75% due to the following mechanisms:

TABLE 1: Volume of fetal red cells and risk of alloimmunization.

Volume of fetal red cells	Risk of alloimmunization
0.1 mL	3%
0.25–1 mL	25%
>5 mL	65%

– Maternal anti-A or anti-B antibodies destroy the fetal red cells carrying Rh antigen.
– These antibodies deviate the fetal cells away from immune apparatus.

- *Nonresponders:* About 30–35% Rh-negative women do not produce antibodies. It is probably genetically controlled.

Mild Disease

About 50% fetuses will have mild disease and they do not require treatment of their umbilical cord. Their Hb is about 12 g% and cord bilirubin is <4 mg%.

Intermediate Disease

Some 25–30% of affected babies have intermediate disease. The characteristics are as follows:

- *Cord Hb:* 9–12 g%
- Modest extramedullary hematopoiesis
- Normal liver functions
  Some of these infants develop severe hyperbilirubinemia by day 3 to 5 which results in kernicterus.

Severe Disease

Around 20–25% fetuses have severe disease; half of these fetuses develop hydrops fetalis between 18 and 34 weeks and the other half between 34 weeks and term.

■ MANAGEMENT

In the management of Rh alloimmunization, one of the following circumstances is encountered:

- Pregnant Rh-negative nonimmunized women
- Pregnant Rh-negative immunized women

Management of the Pregnant Rh-negative Nonimmunized Women

In an Rh-negative pregnant lady, the first step is to detect the blood group of the husband. If he is Rh negative, nothing further is required as the baby will also be Rh negative.

If the husband is Rh positive, indirect Coombs test (IDCT) is done to know if the mother has already developed antibodies to Rh-positive cells.

If IDCT is negative, the problems for the obstetrician are

- To assess the chances for the patient to become alloimmunized

- To detect alloimmunization at the earliest
- Antenatal and if required postnatal injection Anti-D

Indirect Coombs test is done at every 4 weeks from 24 to 40 weeks provided it remains negative. The aim is not to miss an occasional patient who becomes immunized antepartum. If at any time, IDCT becomes positive, the patient is managed as per protocol for the immunized patient.

Fetal Blood Typing

Fetal blood typing can be determined by:

- Amniocentesis
- Cordocentesis
- Free DNA in maternal plasma
- Trophoblasts recovered from endocervix
- Chorion villus biopsy

Amniocentesis was reported to be a reliable method for assessing fetal blood type through DNA testing.[10]

Free DNA in maternal plasma is a noninvasive method. It can be done after 8 weeks. Its accuracy has been reported to be 99.5-100%.[11] At present, it is expensive.

Antenatal Injection Anti-D

There is evidence that administration of injection Anti-D at 28 weeks decreases the incidence of alloimmunization from 18-20 per 1,000 to 2 per 1,000.

The dose used is 300 µg.

In some countries, it is given in two doses of 100 µg at 28 and 34 weeks, respectively.

The efficacy of both regimes is same.

There is a flip side of antenatal Anti-D also:"

- 40% women bear Rh-negative babies who will unnecessarily receive it
- It is estimated that 278 women will have to receive it to prevent one case of alloimmunization.
- Cost-benefit ratio has to be considered.
- Cochrane review 2015 [also quoted by the World Health Organization (WHO)] stated that routine antenatal anti-D prophylaxis has no substantial benefits in preventing Rh alloimmunization and neonatal jaundice.

After antepartum administration of injection Anti-D, IDCT becomes positive. But the titer should not be greater than a trace. If it is 1:2 or greater, alloimmunization should be suspected.

It is not necessary to perform further Coombs testing after giving injection Anti-D. It provides protection for 12 weeks or 84 days. If pregnancy extends beyond 40 weeks, one more dose of injection Anti-D should be administered. In the Rh-negative nonimmunized gravida or who receives injection Anti-D antepartum, the eligibility for postpartum injection Anti-D is determined by the following factors:

- Rh typing of infant
- Direct Coombs test

Investigations to be done on cord blood at the time of delivery are:

- Rh typing
- Direct Coombs test
- Hb, total leukocyte count (TLC), differential leukocyte count (DLC), reticulocytes
- Serum bilirubin

Injection Anti-D, 300 µg, is administered within 72 hours after delivery provided the baby is Rh positive and direct Coombs test is negative. However, it can be given up to 4 weeks after delivery.

Injection Anti-D Immunoglobulin

The development of Rh immunization prophylaxis was a major advance in the management of the Rh-negative pregnant women. In 1900, Van Dungern showed that administration to rabbits of antibody from ox red cells along with ox red cells prevented the development of rabbit anti ox red cells antigen, in sufficient amount, and suppresses active immunization to the antigen. This information was used 60 years later by Freda, Clarke, Bowman, and Pollock to develop injection Anti-D immunoglobulin.

Initial experiments were done on male prisoners: The jail authorities allowed follow-up of prisoners only after 72 hours. Hence, the arbitrary limit of 72 hours for injection Anti-D after delivery came into existence!

Mechanism of Action: The precise mechanism of action of injection Anti-D immunoglobulin is unknown. There are theories which are as follows:

Antigen deviation: It was proposed by Race and Sanger. Rh-positive cells bound by RhJG succumb to intravascular hemolysis that destroys or alters the Rh antigen so as to prevent anti-D antibody production. It is now known that injection Anti-D does not cause intravascular hemolysis.

Antigen blocking: Competitive inhibition: It is also an unlikely mechanism that antibody preparations that lack the Fc portion also avidly bind the antigen but do not suppress the immune response. It was also shown that approximately 20% of D antigen sites were occupied by anti-D.

Central inhibition: It appears to be the most likely mechanism. It was put forth by Gorman and elaborated by Pollack. Erythrocytes coated with anti-D are filtered out of circulation to spleen and lymph nodes. The increase in the local concentration of anti-D bound to D-antigen affects the suppression of immune response. Specialized T lymphocytes bind the Rh immunoglobulin-D antigen complexes. The binding stimulates the production of a soluble immune suppressor substance that acts locally to inhibit the elaboration of helper factors by T helper lymphocytes or macrophages. This inhibition of helper factors' production limits the recruitment of B lymphocytes for the synthesis of anti-D antibody.

Antibody-mediated immune suppression (AMIS): It accounts for downregulation of maternal immature dendritic cells or anti-D-specific B cells before development of anti-D response.

Passive anti-D: It causes rapid clearance of anti-D-coated RBCs which prevents the destruction of fetal red cells.

Experimentally 300 µg of Rh Ig prevents Rh immunization after an exposure of up to 30 mL of Rh-positive blood (15 mL of red cells).

In the presence of massive TPH, the doses that are recommended are given in **Table 2**.

The following clinical conditions are likely to be associated with large TPH:

- Traumatic deliveries including cesarean section
- M.R.P
- Still births and IUDs
- Twin pregnancy at delivery
- Abdominal trauma in the third trimester
- Abruptio placenta
- Induced abortions

TABLE 2: Transplacental hemorrhage and doses.

Transplacental hemorrhage	Dose of injection Anti-D
25–50 mL	600 µg
50–75 mL	900 µg
75–100 mL	1,200 µg

Anti-D Preparations

There are two types of injection Anti-D preparations available in the market: polyclonal and monoclonal.

Polyclonal injection Anti-D: Traditionally, this preparation was used for prevention of alloimmunization. These antibodies are obtained from carefully screened human plasma of sensitized Rh-negative blood donors.

Advantages:

- Proved efficacy
- Antibody-dependent cell-mediated cytotoxicity (ADCC) is better than with monoclonal preparation. This is because polyclonal antibodies interact better with Fc receptors on splenic cells.
- Has both IgG_1 and IgG_3 activity which is essential for reliable immunoprophylaxis
- There are about 30 epitopes of Rh antigen, and polyclonal antibody is effective against them including week D antigen.

Disadvantages
- Limited supply
- High cost
- Rare possibility of transmitting viral infections

Monoclonal injection Anti-D: Monoclonal Anti-D is obtained from heterohybridoma lymphoblastoid cell lines which have been transformed by using Epstein-Barr virus.

Advantages
- Unlimited supply
- Less expensive
- No fear of transmission of diseases

Disadvantages
- Still requires extensive trials
- Has less ADCC activity
- Has only IgG_1 activity
- As there are about 30 epitopes of Rh antigen, monoclonal antibody may not be effective in all patients.

It is recommended that polyclonal injection Anti-D should be preferred to monoclonal injection Anti-D which requires further trials.

Other Indications for Injection Anti-D

- First-trimester spontaneous or induced abortions (50 µg)
- First-trimester ectopic pregnancy (50 µg)
- Full dose of 300 µg in the following conditions—second-trimester abortions and ectopic pregnancy, chorion villous biopsy, amniocentesis, cordocentesis, external cephalic version, threatened abortion, antepartum hemorrhage (APH), abdominal trauma, and IUD

There is controversy in case of molar pregnancy. Those who advocate injection Anti-D maintain that (1) there is possibility of partial mole and (2) trophoblast contains D antigen.

The opponents say that if the diagnosis of complete vesicular mole is certain, there is no need of injection Anti-D.

Injection Anti-D is available for intramuscular or for intravenous use. Although it is administered intramuscularly in almost all cases, the following conditions may warrant IV injection:
- Thrombocytopenia
- Other bleeding disorders
- Massive fetomaternal hemorrhage (FMH) requiring higher dose of Anti-D

Precautions while giving Injection Anti-D

- Informed consent of the woman (as we are injecting blood product) is required.
- Inject it in deltoid muscle and not in the buttock (as absorption is quick).
- Be prepared to treat anaphylactic reaction in an occasional patient.
- Never give intramuscular preparation intravenously.
  ACOG Practice Bulletin (August 2017)[13]

Some selected recommendations:
- The median half-life of Anti-D is 23 days. If the patient delivers within 3 weeks after antenatal injection Anti-D, there is no need of postnatal injection if there is no significant FMH.
- If the patient does not deliver in 12 weeks of antenatal Anti-D injection, there is no need of one more injection before delivery.
- Injection Anti-D is recommended after tubectomy as there can be tubectomy failure. Further alloimmunization can complicate cross matching of blood (Author' comment: Some patients may remarry or some may demand tubal recanalization following death of a child).
- If the patient has weak D type 1, 2, and 3, there is no need of Anti-D injection.

But there can be partial or variant D that can cause alloimmunization; hence, administer Anti-D injection.

Determination of Fetomaternal Hemorrhage

Various tests have been used to assess the FMH:
- *Rosetting test:* It is a qualitative screening test.
  Principle: Rh-positive fetal cells coated with Anti-D form rosettes with Rh-positive indicator cells, thus making them distinguishable from Rh-negative maternal cells.
  Disadvantage: Not reliable when the mother or baby is weak D positive
- *Kleihauer-Betke test:* It is based upon the principle that fetal Hb (Hbf) is more resistant than HbA to acid.
  A thin blood smear is prepared from maternal hemoglobin. The smear is stained by erythrocin to stain fetal red cells. Maternal cells appear as ghost cells against the stained fetal cells. Under the light microscope, the number of fetal cells per 100,000 ghost cells is counted (**Table 3**).

Quantitating the volume of fetal bleed is done by the following formulae:

TABLE 3: Relationship between the number of fetal cells and amount of blood.

Fetal cells/100,000 maternal cells	Amount of fetomaternal hemorrhage (mL)
1–4	0.15
5–8	0.25
9–13	0.5
14–24	0.75
25–32	1
33–64	2
65–96	3
97–157	5

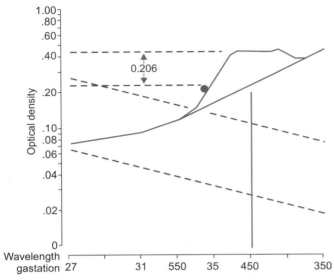

Fig. 1: Relationship between optical density and wavelength.

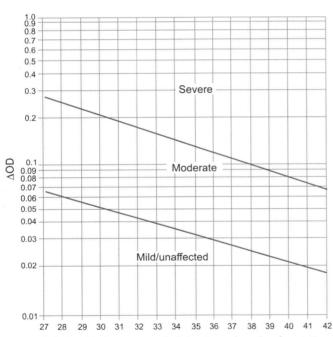

Fig. 2: Relationship between optical density and weeks of gestation.

- 1) $\text{mL of fetal bleed} = \dfrac{\text{No. of fetal cells}}{\text{No. of adult cells}} \times 5{,}000$

- *Mollison formula:*

  $$\text{FMH in mL} = \dfrac{\text{Ratio of fetal}}{\text{Adult}}\ \text{Cells} \times 2{,}400$$

  Fallacies of the test:
  - Variable maternal blood volume
  - Maternal HbF-containing cells are increased during pregnancy
  - Some conditions with high HbF give wrong results, e.g. sickle cell anemia, thalassemia, aplastic anemia

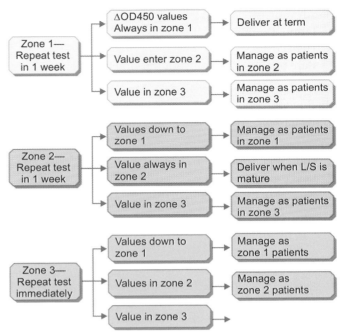

Fig. 3: Liley's method.

- *Flow cytometry:* The estimation of FMH depends upon the identification of D-positive red cells in the presence of D-negative red cells.

  The limit of sensitivity is 2 mL of FMH.

  Accuracy is false below 2 mL of FMH but is better than Kleihauer-Betke test in large FMH.

  It is more useful in assessing the need for additional injection Anti-D in large FMH, where the D status of the body is unknown, and in conditions where maternal HbF is high.

Management of an Rh-negative Immunized Patient

Immunized patients are divided into two subgroups depending upon past obstetric history:
- Past history of babies requiring intensive care or who had hydrops fetalis or IUD. They are managed by amniotic fluid analysis, fetal middle cerebral artery peak systolic velocity (MCA-PSV) and cordocentesis.
- *No significant past history:* They are managed by maternal antibody titers.

Indirect Coombs Test

The critical titer may vary in different laboratories (e.g., 1:6 or 1:32).
- The titer may be above the critical level at the first visit.
- The titer exceeds the critical level during follow-up.
- Significant rise in titer between two consecutive samples even if the critical level is not crossed.

If any of these three conditions is fulfilled, there is no further use of antibody titers in the management. Further management is based on examination of amniotic fluid.

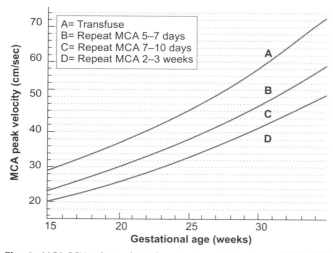

A = Transfuse
B = Repeat MCA 5–7 days
C = Repeat MCA 7–10 days
D = Repeat MCA 2–3 weeks

Fig. 4: MCA-PSV values plotted against gestational age. (MCA-PSV: middle cerebral artery peak systolic flow velocity)
Source: Modified from Mari et. al. Ultrasound Obstet Gynecol. 1995;5:400.

Amniotic Fluid Analysis

When there is fetal hemolysis due to Rh alloimmunization, the bilirubin content of the amniotic fluid is raised. When normal amniotic fluid is examined in a spectrophotometer, optical density (OD) readings between 350 and 650 nm form almost a straight line. If the amniotic fluid contains bilirubin, the OD readings will show a peak at 450 nm and the size of the peak will be proportional to the bilirubin content. Majority of the laboratories measure OD at 375, 450, and 525 nm. The results are plotted on a semilogarithmic paper, and a straight line is drawn between 375 and 525 nm. The difference is noted between the point where the line crosses the 450-nm mark [expected value and actual reading is the delta OD at 450 (ΔOD)].

Management Based on ΔOD450 Values

Liley's method: Liley plotted gestational age on the X-axis and OD450 on the Y-axis and divided the group into three zones:

- *Zone l:* Mildly affected or nonaffected fetus
- *Zone 2:* Includes mild or severely affected fetus
- *Zone 3:* Severely affected fetus

If values are persistently in zone 3, consider the following factors: neonatal intensive care unit (NICU) facilities, experienced clinician, malpresentation, anterior placenta, obese mother, gestational age around 30 weeks, fetal weight near 1 kg, hydrops fetalis, etc.

Depending upon these factors, either intrauterine transfusion is given or baby is delivered.

Robertson's method: Robertson proposed zones such as A, B, B_2, C_1, C_2, D_1, D_2, E, F_1, F_2, G_1, and G_2. Robertson's method has the advantage of greater individualization of care.

Freda's method: Freda's method uses net values of OD at 450. Freda correlated these absolute values with bilirubin concentration in fluid.

Disadvantages of methods using amniocentesis:
- Requires several invasive procedures and their complications
- Indirect test of fetal anemia
- Advent of MCA-PSV has rendered it outdated.

Estimation of Anti-D Levels

- Maternal anti-D levels <4 IU/mL—the fetus is likely to be minimally affected with <5% requiring neonatal exchange transfusion.
- Levels between 4 and 8 IU/mL—may lead to moderate disease and warrant delivery by 38 weeks.
- Levels > 15 IU/mL—baby will be severely affected. The fetus has 29% chance of becoming anemic.

■ MIDDLE CEREBRAL ARTERY PEAK SYSTOLIC FLOW VELOCITY

This technique to assess fetal anemia was proposed by Mari et al.[14] It is a noninvasive and practical way to predict the fetus at risk of moderate and severe anemia. MCA-PSV closely correlates with the degrees of fetal anemia and has reduced the need for invasive testing by 70%. It is done during 18–35 weeks of gestation Practically, it has replaced amniocentesis and Liley's method.

Principle

As the fetus becomes anemic, it tries to compensate hypoxia by pumping more blood to the brain by MCA which is estimated as PSV.

MCA-PSV values are expressed in multiples of median (MoM) for that gestational age. If it is >1.5 MoM, it is abnormal. There are tables of gestational age and MCA-PSV but roughly if MCA-PSV is more than gestational age in weeks multiplied by 2, it is >1.5 MoM and hence abnormal.

The MCA-PSV values are plotted against gestational age. The following patients are selected for MCA-PSV:
- Anti-D titer above 15 IU/mL or IDCT 1:128 or more
- Significant past history, namely, fetal loss, hydrops fetalis, fetal transfusion

Management based on MCA-PSV is shown in **Flowchart 1**.

■ FETAL BLOOD SAMPLING

Indications

- All hydropic cases
- ΔOD450 values in high zone 2
- Rapid rise in ΔOD450 values
- Fetal blood typing

Flowchart 1: Management based on MCA-PSV.

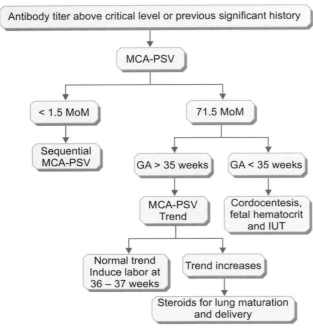

(IUT: intrauterine transfusion; GA: gestational age)

Flowchart 2: Management protocol for Rh alloimmunized patient.

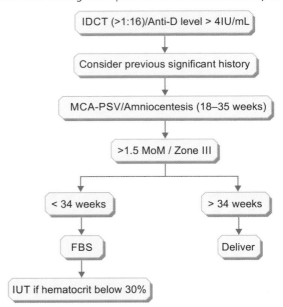

(FBS: fetal blood sampling; IDCT: indirect Coombs test; IUT: intrauterine transfusion; MoM: multiples of median)

- Risk of severe anemia in early to mid-second trimester
- MCA-PSV values > 1.5 MoM

Fetal blood is obtained by cordocentesis under ultrasound guidance. The blood is examined for hematocrit, direct Coombs test, bilirubin, reticulocyte count, and blood type.

Intrauterine Transfusion

The primary objective of IUT is to allow pregnancy to complete 34 weeks so that the baby is reasonably mature. The decision of IUT is based upon:

- Amniocentesis
- OD 450 values
- *Cordocentesis:* Fetal hematocrit
- *Doppler flow studies:* MCA-PSV values

If amniocentesis and Liley's charts are utilized, IUT is performed once OD 450 values reach zone 3.

The fetal hematocrit values at which IUT is given vary. It is not required for values above 40%.

By and large, it is necessary below 30% hematocrit.

IUT may be:

- Intravascular umbilical vein
- Interperitoneal only if vascular access is not available
- Intracardiac only if urgent transfusion is required and other routes are unavailable

Fresh O-negative double-packed cells with a hematocrit of 60–70% are used based on the following formula:

$$\text{Volume to be transfused} = \frac{(\text{Desired hematocrit} - \text{fetal Hct})}{(\text{Donor Hct} - \text{Desired Hct})} \times \text{Fetal blood volume}$$

Complications

- Umbilical cord hematoma
- Bradycardia (8%)
- Fetal demise (0.6-4%)
- Thrombocytopenia
- Chorioamnionitis
- Preterm labor

■ MANAGEMENT PROTOCOL FOR Rh ALLOIMMUNIZED PATIENT (FLOWCHART 2)

■ REFERENCES

1. Fisher RA, Race RR. Rh gene frequencies in Britain. Nature (London). 1946;15-48.
2. Race RR. The Rh genotype and Fisher's theory. Blood. 1948;32t.
3. Weiner AS. Genetic theory of the Rh blood types. Proc Soc Exp Biol. 1943;54:316-9.
4. Rosenfield RE, Allen Jr FH, Swisher SN, Kochwa S. A review of Rh serology and presentation of a new terminology. Transfusion. 1962;2:287-312.

5. Daniels GL, Anstee DJ, Cartron JP, Dahr W, Garratty G, Henry S. Terminology for red cell surface antigens. ISBT Working Party Oslo Report. International Society of Blood Transfusion. Vox Sang. 1999;77(1):52-7.

6. Pollock JM, Bowmen JM. Anti-Rh(D) IgG subclasses and severity of Rh hemolytic disease of the newborn. Vox Sang. 1990;59(3):176.

7. Nevanlinna HR. Factors affecting maternal Rh immunisation. Ann Med Exp Biol Fenn. 1953;31(2):1-80.

8. Ulm B, Svolba G, Ulm MR, Bernaschek G, Panzer S. Male fetuses are particularly affected by maternal alloimmunization to D antigen. Transfusion. 1999;39:169-73.

9. Nicolaides KH, Warenski JC, Rodeck CH. The relationship of fetal plasma protein concentration and hemoglobin level to the development of hydrops in rhesus isoimmunization. Am J Obstet Gynecol. 1985;152:341-4.

10. Bennet PR, Le Van Kim C, Colin Y, Warwick RM, Cherif-Zahar B, Fisk NM, et al. Prenatal determination of fetal RhD type by DNA amplification. N Engl J Med. 1993;329;607-10.

11. Finning KM, Martin PG, Soothill PW, Avent ND. Prediction of fetal D status from maternal plasma: introduction of a new noninvasive fetal RHD genotyping service. Transfusion. 2002;42:1079-85.

12. Bowman JM. Antenatal suppression of Rh alloimmunization. Clin Obstet Gynecol. 1991;34(2):296-303.

13. Committee on Practice Bulletins—Obstetric. Practice Bulletin No. 181: Prevention of RhD alloimmunization. Obstet Gynecol. 2017;130(2):e57-70.

14. Mari G, Deter RL, Carpenter RL, Rahman F, Zimmerman R, Moise Jr KJ, et al. Noninvasive diagnosis by Doppler ultrasonography of fetal anemia due to maternal red-cell alloimmunization. N Engl J Med. 2000;342:9-14.

CHAPTER 25

Intrauterine Growth Restriction

Vandana Kanumury

INTRODUCTION

The term intrauterine growth restriction (IUGR) or fetal growth restriction (FGR) is used for a fetus when it has note reached its complete genetic growth potential due to various environmental factors. The underlying cause of the problem may be fetal, placental, or maternal or a combination of these.

A major concern of antenatal care is to ascertain if a fetus is at risk for growth restriction and to diagnose the growth-restricted fetus. Not only are those fetuses at risk of poor perinatal outcome, but they are also prone to some adult-onset problems such as diabetes mellitus, hypertension, hyperlipidemia, and coronary heart diseases.

Fetal growth restriction and small for gestational age (SGA) are not synonymous. Often when a small fetus is identified, it is difficult to identify a constitutionally small fetus from a growth-restricted one. It also remains a challenge to identify a fetus that may not be small but maybe growth restricted relative to its genetic potential. Majority of FGR fetuses are SGA, while 50–70% of SGA fetuses have grown appropriately but are constitutionally small.

Diagnosing antenatally may be difficult but helps in prognostication and to estimate future recurrence risk.

DEFINITION

The commonly accepted definition of FGR (based on sonography) is an estimated fetal weight below the 10th percentile for gestational age [American College of Obstetricians and Gynecologists (ACOG)]. However, this definition fails to distinguish a fetus that is:

- Constitutionally small or
- Small due to a pathological process or
- Not small but short of achieving its genetic growth potential.

Structurally, normal SGA fetuses are at an increased risk for perinatal mortality and morbidity. Majority of the adverse effects are encountered in the growth-restricted group.

Fetal growth restriction is sometimes defined as SGA with abnormal Doppler indices such as umbilical artery pulsatility index above the 95th percentile or mean uterine artery pulsatility index above the 95th percentile.

Small for Gestational Age

Small for gestational age are term newborns with a birth weight of less than 10th percentile for their gestational age in weeks. These fetuses need to be distinguished from preterm neonates. While preterm neonates have problems related to organ immaturity, SGA neonates have mostly metabolic and nutritional problems.

Low Birth Weight

Low birth weight (LBW) is commonly used for a fetus that weighs <2,500 g irrespective of gestational age. The term very low birth weight (VLBW) is used for a fetus <1,500 g and extremely low birth weight (ELBW) for a fetus <1,000 g.

Low birth weight newborns who are SGA are often designated as having FGR. These infants are at an increased risk for neonatal death. The mortality rate of SGA neonates born at 38 weeks was 1% compared to 0.2% in those with appropriate birth weights.

Restricted Growth

Restricted growth means when hyperplasia and hypertrophy occur in a suboptimal manner in second and third trimesters leading to deficiency in fetal growth (weight, size, metabolism).

Retarded Growth

Retarded growth means when there is a central nervous system (CNS) involvement in additional to deficient growth in terms of fetal weight, size, and maturation.

CLASSIFICATION

Fetal growth restriction may be classified as symmetric or asymmetric **(Table 1)**.

PONDERAL INDEX

Ponderal index (PI) is a useful tool to detect FGR, particularly in infants with asymmetric IUGR.

Ratio of body weight to length: Weight (g) × 100/Length (cm³)

PI < 10th percentile reflects malnutrition and <3rd percentile indicates severe wasting.

RISK FACTORS AND ETIOLOGY

Risk factors for impaired fetal growth potential include abnormalities in the mother, fetus, and placenta. These three compartments and some of these factors are known causes of FGR and may affect more than one compartment.

- *Maternal (80%):* Maternal risk factors, medical diseases, and obstetric factors are given in **Table 2**.
- Fetal (20%)
- Placenta and Cord Factors

Cord abnormalities and placental factors are given in **Table 3**.

OTHER ETIOLOGIES

Assisted Reproductive Technologies

Singleton pregnancies conceived via assisted reproductive technologies (ARTs) have a higher prevalence for SGA than naturally occurring pregnancies.

TABLE 1: Classification of fetal growth restriction.

	Symmetric	Asymmetric
Incidence	20–30%	70–80%
Growth pattern	All fetal organs decreased proportionately	A relatively greater decrease in abdominal size (e.g., liver and subcutaneous fat) than in head circumference
Cause	Global impairment of cellular hyperplasia	Adaptation of fetus to a pathologic environment by redistribution of blood flow to vital organs at the cost of nonvital organs
Timing	Early gestation	Late gestation

Residing at High Altitude

Studies performed in Denver, Colorado, Tibet, and Peru demonstrated a direct relationship between birth weight and altitude. Birth weight declined at an average of 65 g for every additional 500 m in altitude above 2,000 m.

Placental Insufficiency

Defects in early placentation are associated with FGR. Implantation site disorders such as incomplete/abnormal trophoblastic invasion may be both a cause and a consequence of hypoperfusion at the placental site leading to FGR with or without hypertension. Mechanisms leading to abnormal trophoblastic invasion are multifactorial.

Interactions between fetal and maternal circulations in the placenta are crucial for adequate exchange of oxygen and nutrients **(Fig. 1)**. This adaptation occurs by a continuous physiological process referred to as "waves of trophoblast migration." Trophoblastic tissue invades the muscular layer of maternal arteries, thereby converting them from high- to low-resistance vessels.

The absence of destruction of the muscle and elastic portion of spiral arteries by trophoblastic migration leads to inadequate placentation. This leads to high resistance to blood flow and decreased nutrition to intervillous space. This is associated with a greater frequency of preeclampsia and SGA.

Booking Assessment (First Trimester)

All women at booking should be assessed for risk factors for an SGA fetus/neonate to identify those who require increased surveillance.

Women with *one or more major risk factors* need to have serial ultrasound measurements of fetal size along with umbilical artery Doppler from 26 to 28 weeks of pregnancy.

Women with *three or more minor risk factors* must have uterine artery Doppler done at 20–24 weeks of gestation.

TABLE 2: Maternal risk factors, medical diseases, and obstetric factors contributing to FGR.

Maternal risk factors	Maternal medical diseases	Obstetric factors

Age: Teenage
  Age > 35 years
Parity: Nulliparity
Weight: BMI < 20 mg/m²
  BMI > 30 mg/m²
Exercise:
Intense daily exercise
Substance abuse: Smoking, alcohol, and drugs
	Anemia
	Cardiovascular disease
	Hypertension
	Diabetes with vascular disease
	Chronic renal insufficiency
	Sickle cell disease
	Chronic pulmonary disease
	Antiphospholipid syndrome
		Previous obstetric history:
		• Previous SGA
		• Previous stillbirth
		• Preeclampsia
		• Pregnancy interval < 6 months or >60 months
		Present obstetric factors:
		• Heavy bleeding in the first trimester
		• PIH and preeclampsia
		• Unexplained APH
		• Low maternal weight gain
		• Echogenic bowel

(APH: antepartum hemorrhage; BMI: body mass index; PIH: pregnancy-induced hypertension; SGA: small for gestational age)

- If normal—assessment of the fetal size and uterine artery Doppler in the third trimester
- If abnormal [defined as a pulsatility index (PI) > 95th percentile] and/or notching)—serial assessment of fetal size and uterine artery Doppler from 26 to 28 weeks.

For women who are not suitable for monitoring of growth by symphysial fundal height (SFH) measurements (e.g., large fibroids), serial assessment of the fetal size and uterine artery Doppler from 26 to 28 weeks is recommended.

Measurement of fetal size by serial ultrasound and in cases of fetal echogenic bowel, assessment of fetal well-being with umbilical artery Doppler should be offered.

However, when a woman has a normal uterine artery Doppler, there is no need for either a serial measurement of fetal size or serial assessment of well-being with umbilical artery Doppler unless she develops specific pregnancy complications such as antepartum hemorrhage or hypertension.

However, these women should have a scan for fetal size and umbilical artery Doppler in the third trimester.

■ SCREENING

Rationale

Prenatal detection of FGR will provide an opportunity to employ interventions to reduce the morbidity and mortality associated with this problem. Adverse outcomes include prematurity, perinatal asphyxia, poor thermoregulation, hypoglycemia, polycythemia resulting in hyperviscosity, impaired immune function, stillbirth, neonatal death, neurodevelopmental delay, and some adult-onset disorders **(Table 4)**.

Symphysis Fundal Height Measurement with Selective Ultrasonography

Measurement of distance between the upper edge of the pubic symphysis and the top of the uterine fundus using a tape is an easy, simple and widely used method to identify FGR during an antenatal examination.

Discordancy is defined in many ways. The common criteria are:
- Fundal height in cm is at least 3 cm less than the gestational age in weeks.
- Fundal height measurement below the 3rd or 10th percentile can be used.

Serial measurement of SFH is recommended at each antenatal visit from 24 weeks of pregnancy as it improves the prediction of an SGA neonate.

Women should be referred for ultrasound measurement for fetal size who have single SFH which plots below 10th percentile or serial measurements which demonstrate slow or static growth by crossing percentiles.

Factors that affect sensitivity include maternal body mass index (BMI) > 35 kg/m², bladder fullness, parity, large fibroid, and hydramnios.

Biochemical Markers

For an SGA fetus, several biochemical markers have been investigated as screening tests due to their placental origin.

For delivery of an SGA neonate, second-trimester Down screening markers have limited predictive accuracy.

TABLE 3: Cord abnormalities and placental factors.	
Cord abnormalities	*Placental factors*
• Single umbilical artery • Velamentous cord insertion • Marginal cord insertion • Vasa previa • Umbilical cord knots • Umbilical cord cysts	• Chronic placental separation • Abruptio placentae • Infarction • Placenta previa • Circumvallate placenta • Placenta hemangioma • Placental mesenchymal dysplasia

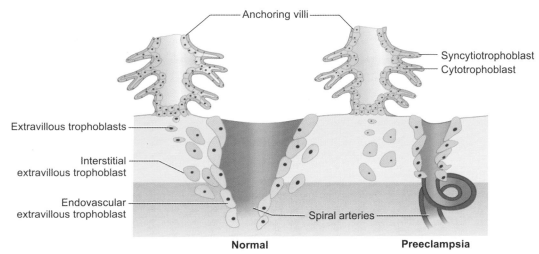

Fig. 1: Normal placental implantation.

TABLE 4: Causes of symmetric FGR.

Genetic	Infection	Metabolic
Trisomy 13,18,21	Cytomegalovirus	Phenylketonuria
Single-gene mutations	Toxoplasma gondii	
Partial deletions or duplications	Plasmodium malariae	
Aberrant genomic	Treponema pallidum	
	Rubella	
	Herpes simplex	
	Varicella-zoster	

TABLE 5: Booking assessment of first trimester.

Minor risk factors	Major risk factors
Maternal age ≥ 35	Maternal age ≥ 40
Nulliparity	Smoker ≥ 11/day
BMI < 20 kg/m²	Previous SGA
BMI 25–29.9 kg/m²	Previous stillbirth
Smoker 1–10/day	Maternal SGA
Mild PIH	Cocaine
Pregnancy interval < 6 months	Diabetes with vasculopathy
Pregnancy interval > 60 months	Renal impairment
Paternal SGA	Chronic HTN
	Antiphospholipid syndrome
	Heavy bleeding in the first trimester
	Echogenic bowel
	Severe PIH
	Preeclampsia
	Unexplained APH
	Low maternal weight gain
	PAPP-A < 0.4 MoM

(APH: antepartum hemorrhage; BMI: body mass index; HTN: hypertension; MoM: multiple of median; PAPP-A: pregnancy-associated plasma protein-A; PIH: pregnancy-induced hypertension; SGA: small for gestational age)

A low level [<0.4 multiple of median (MoM)] of the first-trimester marker pregnancy-associated plasma protein-A (PAPP-A) should be considered a major risk factor for delivery of an SGA neonate.

A low beta human chorionic gonadotropin (hCG; <0.5 MoM) is also a risk factor for an SGA neonate.

Universal Ultrasonography

An alternate method of screening for FGR is routine universal ultrasound. Two screening examinations can be done after TIFFA (Targeted Imaging for Fetal Anomalies) scan at 32 and 36 weeks of gestation, respectively. If only one ultrasound is to be performed, it is done between 32 and 36 weeks.

Choice of Test

Most countries recommend screening for FGR using risk assessment for impaired fetal growth **(Table 5)** and serial SFH measurements at each antenatal visit.

In women with high risk for FGR or with a lag in fundal height, a detailed ultrasound assessment is done. Universal ultrasound in late pregnancy is not routinely recommended as there is no clear, proven benefit.

■ DIAGNOSIS

The single best test for diagnosing FGR is an ultrasound estimation of fetal weight <10th percentile. Maternal history, information from a customized growth curve, and amniotic fluid volume can add to the diagnostic performance and help differentiate the following:

- Constitutionally small fetus
- Growth-restricted fetus
- The fetus not small but has not reached its growth potential.

Ultrasound Findings

Estimated Fetal Weight

Estimated fetal weight (EFW) is the most common method to identify a growth-restricted fetus. However, using a universal standard for fetal growth can lead to overdiagnosing either large for gestational age (LGA) or SGA

fetuses. This can have a negative impact on clinical care. EFW, when performed 1–2 weeks before delivery, is more predictive than performed earlier in gestation.

Customized Growth Charts

It is a fact that fetal weight is affected by various factors, such as fetal sex, and maternal factors, such as parity, ethnicity, age, height, and weight. The fetus is more influenced by maternal than paternal characteristics. It is best to interpret EFW using local population-based birthweight percentiles.

Biometry

Abdominal Circumference

Abdominal circumference (AC) is the most sensitive single biometric indicator of FGR. During fetal growth compromise, depletion of abdominal adipose tissue and a reduction in hepatic size (depleted glycogen) lead to a decreased AC. There is increased morbidity when AC decreases.

The optimal time to screen for FGR with AC was at approximately 34 weeks of gestation. The sensitivity of AC is more in detecting asymmetric FGR and more when it is taken near or at term.

Measurement of AC was more predictive of FGR than measurement of either head circumference (HC) or biparietal diameter (BPD) or the combination of AC with either one of these two parameters.

Biometric Ratios

The HC/AC and femur length (FL)/AC have been used to identify the growth-restricted fetus and are *most sensitive in detecting asymmetric FGR*.

HC/AC ratio: In the case of asymmetric FGR, the liver is smaller when compared to HC and FL for that gestational age.

Since the HC/AC ratio decreases linearly throughout pregnancy, a ratio of >2 SDs above the mean for that gestational age is taken as abnormal.

FL/AC ratio: The FL/AC ratio uses biometric parameters that relate to both weight and length in the prediction of FGR and is independent of gestational age in normally grown fetuses in the last half of pregnancy.

Amniotic Fluid Measurement

An association between pathological FGR and oligo-hydramnios has long been recognized. Oligohydramnios is one of the sequelae of FGR.

Although some fetuses with FGR may have normal amniotic fluid volume, presence of oligohydramnios without a history of ruptured membranes, prolonged pregnancy or presence of genitourinary anomalies, FGR is the most likely possibility.

A decreased amniotic fluid volume between 24 and 34 weeks' gestation was significantly associated with malformations.

Hypoxia-induced redistribution of blood flow to vital organs and diminished renal blood flow have been hypothesized as an explanation for oligohydramnios.

Amniotic fluid volume interpretation should be *based on the single deepest vertical pocket*. Using the oligohydramnios definition of deep pocket <1 cm, Manning reported specificity and positive predictive values for prediction of FGR as 97 and 90%, respectively.

Changing the definition of oligohydramnios to a vertical amniotic fluid pocket of <2 cm resulted in poor sensitivity (16 %), with specificity and positive predictive value of 98 and 78%, respectively.

Either cardiotocography (*CTG*) *or amniotic fluid index (AFI) alone* should *not* be used as the only form of surveillance in SGA fetuses.

Doppler Velocimetry

Uterine Artery

The systolic/diastolic (S/D) ratio of the uterine artery in normal pregnancies should be <2.7 after the 26th week of gestation. If the end-diastolic flow does not increase throughout pregnancy or a small uterine artery notch is detected at the end of systole, the fetus is at high risk for developing FGR.

Diastolic blood flow may be absent or even reversed with extreme degrees of placental dysfunction. Such findings are ominous and may precede fetal death or signal high risk for an abnormal fetal neurologic outcome.

Early changes in placenta-based growth restriction are detected in peripheral vessels such as the umbilical and middle cerebral arteries.

Late changes are characterized by abnormal flow in the ductus venosus and fetal aortic and pulmonary outflow tracts and by reversal of umbilical artery flow.

Umbilical Artery

Umbilical artery Doppler velocimetry is the main surveillance tool for monitoring cases of suspected FGR, and it is a valuable tool for predicting perinatal outcomes.

It is recommended by ACOG in the management of FGR as an adjunct to standard surveillance techniques such as nonstress testing (NST) and biophysical profile (BPP).

Increase in umbilical artery resistance occurs when 30% of villous vasculature ceases to function. When 60–70% of villous vasculature if obliterated, there is an absent/reversal of flow in umbilical artery with poor fetal prognosis. Persistently absent or reversed end-diastolic flow has been correlated with hypoxia, acidosis, and fetal death.

Umbilical artery Doppler flow indices if:

- Normal—repeat surveillance every 2 weeks
- Abnormal (decreased end diastolic velocities) and delivery is not indicated—repeat surveillance weekly in fetuses
- Absent/reversal end-diastolic velocities—daily surveillance

More frequent surveillance with Doppler may be appropriate in a severely SGA fetus.

Middle Cerebral Artery

When fetal hypoxemia is present in growth restriction, a phenomenon of blood flow redistribution occurs, known as the *brain-sparing reflex*, to compensate for the decrease in available oxygen. Blood is preferentially redistributed to the brain, heart, and adrenal glands at the expense of the peripheral circulation. Asymmetric FGR occurs likely.

In predicting acidemia and adverse outcome, middle cerebral artery (MCA) Doppler has limited accuracy in the preterm SGA fetus and should not be used to time delivery.

However, an abnormal MCA Doppler (PI < 5th percentile) has a moderate predictive value for acidosis at birth and must be used to time delivery in a term SGA fetus with normal umbilical artery Doppler.

Fetal Venous Doppler (Figs. 2 and 3)

Venous Doppler abnormalities are late, ominous circulatory findings in FGR.

In cases of preterm SGA with abnormal uterine artery Doppler, fetal well-being must be assessed with fetal ductus venosus Doppler to decide timing of delivery.

Cerebroplacental ratio (CPR): Ratio of MCA pulsatility index divided by uterine artery pulsatility index. A low CPR indicates fetal blood flow redistribution.

Sequence of Doppler changes: A fetus with severe growth restriction first demonstrates:

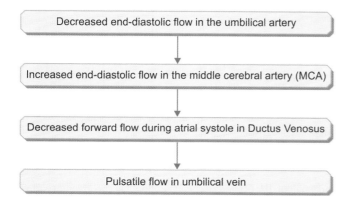

Decreased end-diastolic flow in the umbilical artery

↓

Increased end-diastolic flow in the middle cerebral artery (MCA)

↓

Decreased forward flow during atrial systole in Ductus Venosus

↓

Pulsatile flow in umbilical vein

Karyotyping should be offered in severely SGA fetuses with structural anomalies and in those detected before 23 weeks of gestation, especially if uterine artery Doppler is normal.

Serological screening for congenital cytomegalovirus (CMV) and toxoplasmosis infection should be offered in severely SGA fetuses.

Testing for syphilis and malaria should be considered in high-risk populations.

■ PREDICTION OF INTRAUTERINE GROWTH RESTRICTION

A scoring system developed by the Radiological Society of North America uses a combination of the following parameters:
- USG estimated fetal weight
- Amniotic fluid volume
- Maternal blood pressure

The scoring system has a range of 0–100.

IUGR score: Amniotic fluid volume score + fetal weight score + maternal blood pressure + 39.2
- Score < 50 rules out possibility of IUGR.
- Score > 75 means confident diagnosis of IUGR.
- Score of 50–75 means likelihood of IUGR.

The IUGR score is a practical tool that can be easily used in an ultrasound facility.

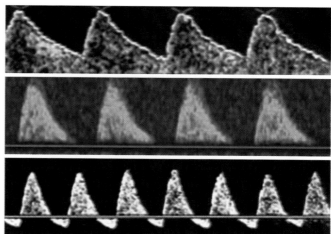

Fig. 2: Umbilical artery—normal, absent, and reversal of blood flow.

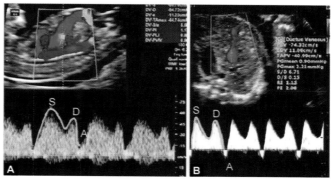

Figs. 3A and B: Ductus venosus. (A) Normal; (B) Abnormal waveforms.

■ MANAGEMENT

Early onset growth restriction is easier to recognize but presents challenging issues in management.

In pregnancies in which there is a strong suspicion of fetal anomalies, patient counseling and prenatal diagnostic testing are indicated.

Management of the Near-term Fetus

In cases of a suspected growth-restricted fetus having normal umbilical artery Doppler velocimetry, normal amniotic fluid volume, and reassuring fetal heart rate, delivery is recommended >37 weeks.

In case of clinically significant oligohydramnios, most clinicians recommend delivery at 34 weeks or beyond.

Summary of Management

Deliver immediately: If
- Abnormal ductus venosus Doppler
- Reversed diastolic flow ≥ 32 weeks
- Absent diastolic flow ≥ 34 weeks

Daily BPP regardless of the presence or absence of oligohydramnios in:

Flowchart 1: Management protocol for FGR according to Green-top guidelines.

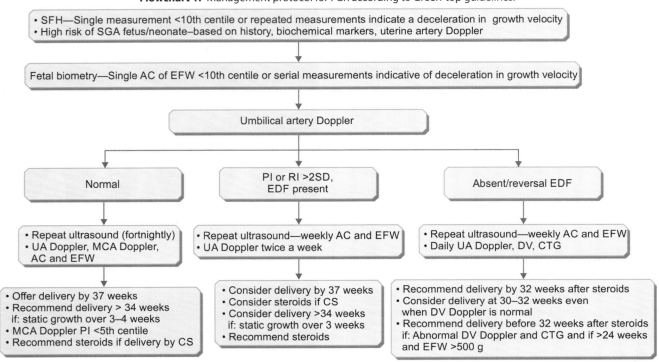

(EDF: end diastolic flow; SGA: small for gestational age; SFH: symphysial fundal height; UA: uterine artery; AC: abdominal circumference; EFW: estimated fetal weight; MCA: middle cerebral artery; CTG: Cardiotocography; PI: Ponderal index; CS: cesarean section)

- Reversed diastolic flow < 32 weeks
- Absent diastolic flow < 34 weeks

Deliver immediately: If BPP or ductus venosus Doppler becomes abnormal in the above situations.

Decrease diastolic flow: BPP twice weekly and *deliver at term* or when BPP becomes abnormal.

Management protocol for FGR according to Green-top guidelines is shown in **Flowchart 1**.

■ FETUS REMOTE FROM TERM (FLOWCHART 2)

In cases of growth-restricted fetuses (<34 weeks) having no anatomical abnormality and normal amniotic fluid volume and fetal surveillance findings, observation is recommended.

Some recommend screening for toxoplasmosis, cytomegalovirus infection, rubella, herpes, and other infections.

As long as interval fetal growth and fetal surveillance test results are normal, pregnancy is allowed to continue until fetal lung maturity is reached.

Fetal growth should be reassessed after an interval of 3–4 weeks. However, umbilical artery Doppler velocimetry and amniotic fluid volume along with NST must be done weekly.

Flowchart 2: Management of FGR fetus remote from term.

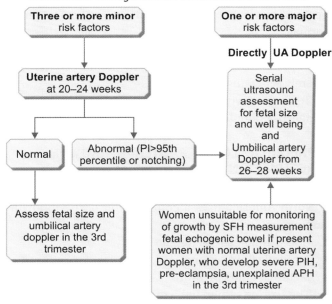

(PI: Ponderal index; PIH: pregnancy-induced hypertension; SFH: symphysial fundal height)

■ MODE OF DELIVERY

Cesarean section is advocated for SGA fetuses showing absent or reversed end-diastolic velocity (AREDV) in umbilical artery.

Induction of labor can be tried in cases with normal umbilical artery Doppler or in those having abnormal umbilical artery PI with end-diastolic velocities. However, continuous fetal heart rate monitoring is advocated from the onset of labor. However, some of these fetuses do not tolerate labor, necessitating cesarean delivery.

For fetuses < 32 weeks of gestation, magnesium sulfate is given before delivery for neuroprotection. A decrease in significant neurodevelopmental impairment and death was observed.

FETAL AND NEONATAL COMPLICATIONS

Fetal Hypoxia and Acidosis

Fetal hypoxia and acidosis are the most important and frequent complications of FGR, particularly if FGR is due to placental insufficiency.

Stillbirth

Approximately 20% stillbirths show signs of growth restriction. They are more common in infants whose birth weight is <1,500 g. Fetal death in FGR may occur at any time but is frequent at >35 weeks.

Oligohydramnios

Oligohydramnios is a common finding in FGR. This is due to decreased fetal urine output secondary to redistribution of fetal blood flow with decreased renal perfusion. The incidence of FGR when AFI is normal is 5% but in case of oligohydramnios it is approximately 40%.

Intrapartum Complications

Intrapartum complications include a high incidence of intrapartum hypoxia, increasing the rates of emergency cesarean section for a nonreassuring pattern of FHR.

Neonatal Complications

Diagnosis of FGR is easier after birth. An FGR infant shows signs of soft-tissue wasting, and skin is loose and thin with little subcutaneous fat. Abdomen is scaphoid, ribs are protuberant, muscle mass is reduced and HC is larger than AC.

Respiratory Distress Syndrome

Respiratory distress syndrome is the leading cause of comorbidity and mortality in a preterm growth-restricted infant.

Other Complications

Meconium aspiration syndrome, persistent fetal circulation, intraventricular hemorrhage, newborn encephalopathy, hypoglycemia, hypocalcemia, and hyperviscosity syndrome are some other complications.

Long-term Complications

As a result of partial resetting of fetal metabolic homeostasis and endocrine systems in response to in utero nutritional deprivation, an association starts between poor fetal growth, accelerated postnatal growth and development of obesity later, metabolic dysfunction, insulin sensitivity, type 2 diabetes, and cardiovascular and renal diseases.

The combination of severe FGR and prematurity increases risk of long-term neurodevelopmental abnormalities and decreased cognitive functions.

Maternal

Studies have shown that delivering a newborn with idiopathic growth restriction may be predictive of long-term maternal risk of ischemic heart diseases. A sevenfold increased risk of ischemic heart disease or death is observed with a combination of growth restriction, preterm birth, and preeclampsia.

Recurrence Risk

A prospective study on the risk of recurrence of birth of a nonanomalous SGA in second pregnancy whose first delivery was SGA and not SGA was 23 and 3%, respectively.

PREVENTION OF SMALL FOR GESTATIONAL AGE

Antiplatelet agents (low-dose aspirin) are recommended for patients at risk of preeclampsia. These must be started before 16 weeks to reduce the incidence of preeclampsia, SGA, and other complications.

Smoking cessation achieved <15 weeks has shown to reduce the incidence of LBW.

Dietary changes and supplements (calcium), bed rest, and progesterone do not prevent SGA.

KEY POINTS
- Ultrasonography-estimated fetal weight (EFW) of less than the 10th percentile for the specific gestational age (GA) is required for the diagnosis of FGR.
- Some fetuses are constitutionally small and at less than 10th percentile in weight for GA in accordance with their genetic growth potential. They are not growth restricted and may be appropriately characterized as small for gestational age fetuses.
- The severity of FGR is determined by the EFW.
  - EFW between 3rd and 9th percentile—moderate FGR
  - EFW less than the 3rd percentile—severe FGR
- Based on additional fetal biometric parameters, such as head circumference (HC), abdominal

circumference (AC), femur length (FL), and biparietal diameter (BD), FGR can be categorized as symmetrical and asymmetrical. In symmetrical FGR, all growth parameters are proportionally reduced, whereas, in asymmetrical FGR, classically, the abdominal circumference is reduced below 10 percentile, while other measurements are relatively preserved and may be within normal limits.

- ACOG) recommends performing serial fundal height during every prenatal visit. A serial ultrasonography study is warranted if the fundal height is less by 3 cm or more than the gestation in weeks. The ultrasound scan also serves to detect the presence of anatomical abnormalities in the fetus. An accurate assessment of the gestational age is of utmost importance for differentiating FGR from a misdated pregnancy.

- The guidelines also stress the need for early detection of high-risk pregnancies, such as those with a prior history of FGR, substance abuse (tobacco, alcohol, others), advanced maternal age, preeclampsia, or previous pregnancy complicated with preeclampsia among others.

- Serial ultrasonography is strongly indicated if risk factors are identified. If FGR is detected, amniotic fluid volume estimations and umbilical arterial Doppler blood flow velocimetry (UADV) studies should be performed. Routine screening with third-trimester ultrasound in low-risk pregnancy is not recommended.

- AC is the single most sensitive biometry for FGR and yields the best results when done at 34 weeks of gestation, or closer to term, especially in the cases of asymmetric FGR. Other useful biometric studies are HC/AC and FL/HC ratios, which can differentiate between symmetrical and asymmetrical FGR. An interval of 3–4 weeks between scans is recommended in pregnancies with suspected FGR.

- Uterine artery Doppler velocimetry (UADV) is commonly used for surveillance as well as to determine the timing of delivery. Delivery is indicated at ≥34 weeks if absent end-diastolic blood flow velocity (AEDV) and at ≥32 weeks of gestation if reversed end-diastolic velocity (REDV) are detected.

- Twice weekly CTG and/or BPP are indicated if the UADV study is abnormal. Abnormal CTG or BPP reports are indications for interruption of pregnancy by cesarean section (CS). FGR alone is not an indication for CS.

- Antenatal corticosteroids should be administered in pregnant mothers up to 34 weeks of gestation to improve fetal lung maturation. Magnesium sulfate is recommended for neuroprotection if a very preterm delivery (<32 weeks) is anticipated.

- FGR infants are susceptible to both short term and long-term complications.

■ SUGGESTED READING

1. Faraci M, Renda E, Monte S, Di Prima FA, Valenti O, De Domenico R, et al. Fetal growth restriction: current perspectives. J Prenat Med. 2011 Apr;5(2):31-3.

2. Longo S, Borghesi A, Tzialla C, Stronati M. IUGR and infections. Early Hum Dev. 2014;90 Suppl 1:S42-4.

3. Marsico C, Kimberlin DW. Congenital cytomegalovirus infection: advances and challenges in diagnosis, prevention and treatment. Ital J Pediatr. 2017;43(1):38.

4. Morse K, Williams A, Gardosi J. Fetal growth screening by fundal height measurement. Best Pract Res Clin Obstet Gynaecol. 2009;23(6):809-18.

5. Paul SP, Kirkham EN, Hawton KA, Mannix PA. Feeding growth restricted premature neonates: a challenging perspective. Sudan J Paediatr. 2018;18(2):5-14.

6. Rotshenker-Olshinka K, Michaeli J, Srebnik N, Terlezky S, Schreiber L, Farkash R, et al. Recurrent intrauterine growth restriction: characteristic placental histopathological features and association with prenatal vascular Doppler. Arch Gynecol Obstet. 2019;300(6):1583-9.

7. Shan HM, Cai W, Cao Y, Fang BH, Feng Y. Extrauterine growth retardation in premature infants in Shanghai: a multicenter retrospective review. Eur J Pediatr. 2009;168(9):1055-9.

8. Sharma D, Shastri S, Sharma P. Intrauterine Growth Restriction: Antenatal and Postnatal Aspects. Clin Med Insights Pediatr. 2016;10:67-83

9. Uzan J, Carbonnel M, Piconne O, Asmar R, Ayoubi JM. Preeclampsia: pathophysiology, diagnosis, and management. Vasc Health Risk Manag. 2011;7:467-74.

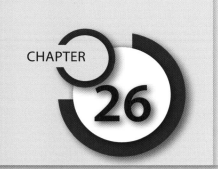

Intrauterine Fetal Demise

S Manikyarao

INTRODUCTION

Intrauterine fetal demise (IUFD) is a clinical and public health problem. However, very little attention is paid in the developed world.

Intrauterine fetal demise is a global issue which is historically misunderstood and underacknowledged, and awareness is growing with intention of good action. It is being used as an indicator for progress of women and child healthcare (WCHC).

DEFINITION

Fetal death refers to the demise of products of human conception before expulsion or extraction. It should not be a termination of pregnancy.

Antepartum death beyond the period of viability is termed as IUFD.

United States National Centre for Health Statistics definition: The United States National Centre for Health Statistics defines stillbirth as loss after 20 weeks of pregnancy, with further division into early stillbirth (<20 weeks), intermediate stillbirth (20–27 weeks), and late stillbirth (>28 weeks).[1]

Legal definition of stillbirth: Any child expelled or issued forth from its mother after the 24th week of pregnancy that did not breathe or showed any other signs of life is defined as stillbirth.

The current definition of fetal death adopted by the National Center for Health Statistics, part of the Centers for Disease Control and Prevention, is based on the definition recommended by the World Health Organization (MacDorman, 2015). It states that fetal death means death prior to complete expulsion or extraction from the mother of a product of human conception irrespective of the duration of pregnancy and which is not an induced termination of pregnancy. The death is indicated by the fact that after such expulsion or extraction, the fetus does not breathe or show any other evidence of life such as beating of the heart, pulsation of the umbilical cord, or definite movement of voluntary muscles. Heartbeats are to be distinguished from transient cardiac contractions and respirations are

to be distinguished from fleeting respiratory efforts or gasps.[1]

Green-top guidelines No. 55 deals extensively with IUFD. International coding for IUFD is 36.4A.

GLOBAL BURDEN

The impact of IUFD is significant and of wide range, costing around hundreds of millions throughout the globe for healthcare litigation, impact of psychological moods in family, and healthcare personnel.

In the UK, the mean health social care cost for IUFD is around 4191 pounds, i.e., approximately Rs. 3 lakhs; funeral charge is around 559 pounds, equivalent to Rs. 50,000; and workplace absence cost is 3829 pounds, equivalent to Rs. 3 lakhs. This costs a net total of approximately 7 lakhs of Indian rupees.

INCIDENCE

The incidence varies between 20 and 27 weeks at 25.2% and beyond 28 weeks it is 24.9%.

Global

Worldwide, the stillbirth rate has been falling from approximately 35/1,000 livebirths in 1980 to approximately 15/1,000 livebirths in 2015.[2] The reduction has been associated with improved access to and utilization of antenatal care and skilled birth attendants and attention to known maternal risks for stillbirth. At least half of the stillbirths in low-income countries occur during labor and birth, largely because of lack of skilled birth attendants and facilities for cesarean delivery.[3]

Prospective Rate of Fetal Death

In clinical studies, researchers are increasingly citing the prospective fetal mortality rate, which represents the number of fetal deaths at a given gestational age per 1,000 livebirths. In US in 2013, the prospective rate of fetal deaths at 20–22 weeks was high (0.52–0.56) and declined at 29–33 weeks to the lowest level (0.18–0.19), remained relatively low until approximately 37 weeks, then began to climb at 38 weeks, and increased to its highest level at 42 weeks (0.62).[4]

ETIOLOGY

The etiological factors can be categorized under subheadings given in the following text.

Fetal growth restriction constituted the highest risk factor. The risk increased fivefold if it was not recognized antenatally. In the next order of incidence are obstetric complications, fetal malformations, and consanguinity.

If the cause is known, estimation of the chance of recurrence, preconceptional counseling, pregnancy management, further diagnostic procedures, and neonatal management can minimize the incidence.

- *Maternal*
  - *Race:* African-Americans
  - Consanguinity of parents
  - Advanced maternal age > 35 years
  - Obesity
  - Low socioeconomic status
  - Smoking
  - Nulliparity
- *Fetal*
  - Congenital malformations (monosomy X, Trisomy 21, 18, 13)
  - Genetic anomalies
  - Male sex
  - Fetal infections: Parvovirus B19, cytomegalovirus (CMV), Listeria, hydrops fetalis
  - Iatrogenic causes such as external version
- *Pregnancy complications*
  - *IUGR:* It contributes as the highest risk factor and the risk increases fivefold if it is not recognized antenatally.
  - Maternal trauma
  - Uterine rupture
  - Pregnancy-induced hypertension (PIH)
  - Placental abruption
  - Rh isoimmunization
  - Multiple pregnancy
  - Post-term pregnancy > 42 weeks
  - Uterine anomalies
  - Infections
  - Antepartum asphyxia
  - Previous history of stillbirth
  - Prior history of preterm delivery, growth restriction, or preeclampsia which lead to increased risk of stillbirth in subsequent pregnancies
- *Placental causes* (one prospective study reported that 64.9% of IUFD contributed to placental causes)
  - Placental insufficiency
  - Antepartum hemorrhage
  - Cord accidents
  - Twin-to-twin transfusion syndrome
  - Vasa previa
- *Cord causes*
  - Cord prolapse
  - True knots
  - Cord entanglement
  - Tight nuchal cord
- *Medical disorders*
  - Diabetes
  - Hypertension
  - Chronic nephritis
  - Systemic lupus erythematosus (SLE)
  - Thrombophilias
  - Cholestasis of pregnancy
  - Antiphospholipid antibody syndrome
- *Unexplained:* An unexplained stillbirth is a fetal death that cannot be attributed to an identifiable fetal, placental, maternal, or obstetric etiology due to lack of sufficient information or because the cause cannot be determined at the current level of diagnostic ability.[5] It is reported to account for 25–60% of all fetal deaths.[6-9]

CLINICAL FEATURES

- *Symptoms*
  - Absence of perception of fetal movements
  - History of trauma and antepartum bleeding to be excluded.
  - Relevant maternal and obstetric factors must be reviewed.
  - Family history, particularly of pregnancy loss, congenital malformations, consanguinity, mental retardation, and diabetes, should not be forgotten.
- *Signs*
  - *Per abdomen*
    - Gradual retrogression of the fundal height
    - Uterine tone is diminished and the uterus feels flaccid; Braxton–Hicks contractions may not be easily felt.
    - Fetal movements are not felt on palpation.
    - Look for signs of bleeding diathesis and PIH.
    - Absent fetal heart sounds will confirm the diagnosis. Use of Doppler is a better choice if available.
    - Cardiotocography (CTG): Flat trace
    - Egg-shell crackling feel of the fetal head is a late feature.

INVESTIGATIONS

General Principles of Investigation

Clinical assessment and laboratory tests should be recommended to assess maternal well-being (including coagulopathy) and to determine the cause of death, the chance of recurrence, and the possible means of avoiding further pregnancy complications.

The basic investigations include:

- Hemoglobin
- Blood grouping and typing
- Glucose tolerance test (GTT) with 75 g of glucose
- Clotting time and bleeding time

Coagulation profile and all necessary investigations are mandatory because IUFD can sometimes cause disseminated intravascular coagulation (DIC) if it is delayed in diagnosis.

To enumerate, all special investigations are given in **Table 1**.

Major fetomaternal hemorrhage (FMH) is a silent cause of IUFD and a Kleihauer test is recommended for all women to diagnose the cause of death. Karyotyping is important as about 6% of stillborn babies will have a chromosomal abnormality.[30-32]

TABLE 1: Tests recommended for women with IUFD.

Test	Reason for test	Additional comments
Maternal standard hematology and biochemistry including CRPs and bile salt[10-12]	Preeclampsia and its complications Multiorgan failure in sepsis or hemorrhage Obstetric cholestasis	Platelet count to test for occult DIC (repeat twice weekly)
Maternal coagulation times and plasma fibrinogen[11]	DIC	Not a test to know cause of late IUFD Maternal sepsis, placental abruption, and preeclampsia increase the probability of DIC Especially important if the woman desires regional anesthesia
Kleihauer test[13,14]	Lethal fetomaternal hemorrhage To decide level of requirement for anti-D gammaglobulin	Fetomaternal hemorrhage is a cause of IUFD Kleihauer test should be recommended for all women, not simply those who are Rh D-negative (ensure that the laboratory is aware if a woman is Rh D positive) Tests should be undertaken before birth as red cells might clear quickly from maternal circulation In Rh-negative women, a second Kleihauer test also determines whether sufficient anti-Rh D has been given
Maternal bacteriology:[15-17] • Blood cultures • Midstream urine • Vaginal swabs • Cervical swabs	Suspected maternal bacterial infections including Listeria monocytogenes and Chlamydia spp.	Indicated in the presence of: • Maternal fever • Flu-like symptoms • Abnormal liquor (purulent appearance /offensive odor) • Prolonged ruptured membranes before late IUFD Abnormal bacteriology is of doubtful significance in the absence of clinical or histological evidence of chorioamnionitis. In one study, amniotic fluid culture was positive in only 1 of 44 women with IUFD despite evidence of chorioamnionitis in further 9 women Also used to direct maternal antibiotic therapy
Maternal serology:[18] • Viral screen • Syphilis • Tropical infections	Occult maternal–fetal infections	Stored serum from booking tests can provide baseline serology Parvovirus B-19, rubella (if nonimmune at booking), CMV, herpes simplex and Toxoplasma gondii (routinely) Hydrops not necessarily a feature of parvovirus-related; late IUFD treponemal serology—usually known already Others if presentation suggestive, e.g., travel to endemic areas
Maternal random blood glucose[19]	Occult maternal diabetes mellitus	Rarely a woman will have incidental type 1 diabetes mellitus, usually with severe ketosis Women with gestational diabetes mellitus return to normal glucose tolerance within a few hours after late IUFD has occurred
Maternal HbA1c[10]	Gestational diabetes mellitus	Most women with gestational DM have a normal HbA1c Need to test for gestational DM in future pregnancy Might also indicate occult types 1 and 2 DM
Maternal thyroid function[20]	Occult maternal thyroid disease	TSH, free T3 and T4
Maternal thrombophilia screen[21]	Maternal thrombophilia	Indicated if evidence of fetal growth restriction or placental disease The association between inherited thrombophilias and IUFD is weak, and management in future pregnancy is uncertain Most tests are not affected by pregnancy—if abnormal, repeated after 6 weeks; antiphospholipids screen is also repeated if abnormal

Contd...

Contd...

Test	Reason for test	Additional comments
Anti-red-cell antibody serology[22]	Immune hemolytic disease	Indicated if fetal hydrops evident clinically or on postmortem
Maternal anti-Ro and anti-La antibodies[23]	Occult maternal autoimmune disease	Indicated if evidence of hydrops endomyocardial fibroelastosis or AV node calcification at postmortem
Maternal alloimmune antiplatelet antibodies[24]	Alloimmune thrombocytopenia	Indicated if intracranial hemorrhage found on postmortem
Parental bloods for karyotype[25] Occult drug use maternal urine for cocaine metabolites[26]	Parental balanced translocation Parental mosaicism	Indicated if fetal unbalanced translocation Other fetal aneuploidy, e.g., 45X (Turner syndrome) Fetal genetic testing fails and history suggestive of aneuploidy With consent, if history and/or presentation are suggestive
Fetal and placental microbiology:[27] • Fetal blood • Fetal swabs • Placental swabs	Fetal infection	Cord or cardiac blood in heparin Written consent advisable for cardiac bloods Need to be obtained using clean technique
Fetal and placental tissues for karyotyping (and possible single gene testing):[28] • Deep fetal skin • Fetal cartilage • Placenta	Aneuploidy Single-gene disorders	Absolutely contraindicated if parents do not wish (written consent essential) Send several specimens—cell cultures might fail Culture bottles must be kept on labor ward stored separately from formalin preservation bottles Genetic material should be stored if a single gene syndrome is suspected
Postmortem examination:[29] • External • Autopsy • Microscopy • X-ray • Placenta and cord		Absolutely contraindicated if parents do not wish (written consent essential) External examination should include weight and length measurement FGR is a significant association for late IUFD

(CMV: *Cytomegalovirus*; CRP: C-reactive protein; DIC: disseminated intravascular coagulation; DM: diabetes mellitus; FGR: fetal growth restriction; IUFD: intrauterine fetal demise; T3: triiodothyronine; T4: thyroxine; TSH: thyroid stimulating hormone)

Perinatal specimens suitable for karyotyping include skin, cartilage, and placenta. Skin specimens are associated with a higher rate of culture failure (~60%), twice that of other tissues, including placenta. Placenta usually has the advantages of being the most viable tissue and of more rapid cell culture, but the disadvantages of maternal contamination and placental pseudomosaicism. The next best is cartilage, e.g., patella, but cartilage is harder to sample.[33]

Placental biopsy (approximately 1-cm diameter) should be taken from the fetal surface close to the cord insertion (to avoid tissue of maternal origin). Skin biopsy should be deep to include underlying muscle (about 1 cm in length from the upper fleshy part of the thigh). The skin can be closed with wound adhesive strips and tissue adhesives, but this is less successful when the baby is severely macerated.

Parents should be offered full postmortem examination to help explain the cause of an IUFD.

A written consent must be obtained for any invasive procedure on the baby including tissues taken for genetic analysis.

Postmortem examination should include external examination with birth weight, histology of relevant tissues, and skeletal X-rays.

TABLE 2: Radiological signs of intrauterine fetal death.

Sign	Interval (After Death)
Robert sign (gas in great vessels)	12 hours
Spalding sign (overlapping of skull bones)	1 week
Blair-Hartley/Ball sign (hyperflexion/hyperextension of spine with overcrowding of ribs **(Fig. 1)**	3–4 weeks

Pathological examination of the cord, membranes, and placenta should be recommended, whether or not postmortem examination of the baby is requested.

MRI can be a useful adjunct to conventional postmortem.

The role of X-ray and ultrasound are shown in **Table 2**.

Roberts sign refers to the presence of gas (N_2) in great vessels. It is the earliest radiological sign of IUFD.

Spalding sign denotes the collapse of fetal skull bones due to liquefaction of the brain matter. Spalding sign is named after *Alfred Baker Spalding*. A minimum of 2 cm of overlapping must be taken as a positive sign. It is most reliable between 28 and 36 weeks.

The third sign is overcrowding of the ribs. This is also called **Blair Hartley** or **Ball sign**.

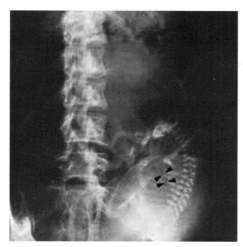

Fig. 1: Straight X-ray of abdomen showing a single fetus with hyperflexion of spine and gas in great vessels.

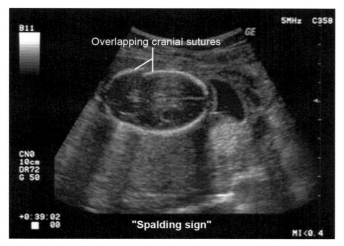

Fig. 2: Sonographic plate showing collapsed cranial bones, a late feature of intrauterine fetal demise.

TABLE 3: Changes in dead-born.	
>6 hours	Desquamation measuring at least 1 cm in diameter, brown-red discoloration of umbilical cord stump
>12 hours	Desquamation involving the face, abdomen, or back
>18 hours	Desquamation involving at least >5% of body surface area
>24 hours	Brown skin discoloration, moderate or severe extent of desquamation
>2 weeks	Mummification

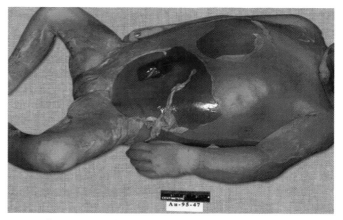

Fig. 3: Brownish skin discoloration with desquamation (moderate extent).

Sonography

The earliest diagnosis is possible with sonography.

- Lack of all fetal movements (including cardiac) during a 10-minute period of careful observation with a real-time sonar is a strong presumptive evidence of fetal death.
- Oligohydramnios and collapsed cranial bones are evident.

Spalding sign: Overlapping of skull bones as enumerated above can be diagnosed by ultrasound **(Fig. 2)**.

The extent of maceration depends on the time of fetal death in the newborn.[31]

Usually after 6 hours, desquamation will be at least 1 cm in diameter and brown-red discoloration of the umbilical cord stump will be seen. After 12 hours, the face, back, and abdomen will be involved. It takes 18 hours for covering the 5% of the body surface for desquamation. After 2 weeks,

the mummification sets in. **Table 3** shows changes in dead-born.

Figure 3 shows brownish skin discoloration with desquamation (moderate extent).

■ DEAD-BORN/STILLBORN EXAMINATION

Examination of the dead-born has impeccable values. This follows the examination of placenta. All the changes involving head, skin, chest, arms, ears, neck, and toes are given in **Box 1**.

■ MANAGEMENT

Management depends upon the mother's preferences as well as her medical condition and previous intrapartum history.

Immediate steps should be taken toward delivery if there is sepsis, preeclampsia, placental abruption, or membrane rupture.

Expectant Management

More than 85% of women with an IUFD labor occurs spontaneously within 3 weeks of diagnosis. If the woman is physically well, her membranes are intact and there is no evidence of preeclampsia, infection, or bleeding, and the risk of expectant management for 48 hours is low. There is a 10% chance of maternal DIC within 3–4 weeks from the date of fetal death and an increasing chance thereafter.

Vaginal birth can be achieved within 24 hours of induction of labor for IUFD in about 90% of women.

BOX 1: Changes observed in the body during the examination of the dead-born.

- *Date*
- *Weight*
- *Head circumference*
- *Crown–heel length (stretched)*
- *Gestational age*

Head
- Normal
- Hydrocephalic
- Scalp defects
- Anencephaly
- Abnormal skull shape
- Collapsed
- Others (describe)

Eyes
- Normal
- Close together
- Far apart
- Straight
- Upslanting
- Downslanting
- Abnormally small
- Abnormally large
- Epicanthus
- Others (describe)

Nose
- Normal
- Others (describe)

Mouth
- Normal
- Cleft lip
- Cleft palate
- Large tongue
- Small chin
- Others (describe)

Ears
- Normal
- Low set (top below eyes)
- Tags
- Pits
- Symmetric
- Others (describe)

Neck
- Normal
- Excess skin
- Cystic mass
- Others (describe)

Skin
- Intact
- Macerated
- Other (describe)

Chest
- Normal
- Asymmetric
- Small
- Others (describe)

Contd...

Contd...

Abdomen
- Normal
- Distension
- Omphalocele
- Gastroschisis
- Hernia
- Three-vessel cord
- Others (describe)

Back
- Normal
- Spina bifida (defect level)
- Scoliosis
- Kyphosis
- Others (describe)

Limbs
- Length: normal, short, long
- Form: normal, symmetric, missing parts
- Position: normal, abnormal

Arms: Length
Form Position
Right
Left

Legs: Length
Form Position
Right
Left

Hands:
- Right
  - Fingers
  - Webbing/syndactyly
  - Transverse crease
  - Others (describe)
- Left
  - Fingers
  - Webbing/syndactyly
  - Transverse crease
  - Others (describe)

Vaginal birth carries the potential advantages of immediate recovery and quicker return to home. Cesarean birth might occasionally be clinically indicated by virtue of maternal condition.

Induction of Labor in an Unscarred Uterus

A combination of mifepristone and prostaglandin preparation should usually be recommended as the first-line intervention for induction of labor. When compared with prostaglandin E_2 (PGE2) and PGF2α, the vaginal misoprostol is equally effective in achieving vaginal birth within 24 hours, with a similar induction to birth interval but less gastrointestinal side effects (nausea, vomiting, and diarrhea).[34]

Vaginal misoprostol is more effective orally but with fewer adverse effects.

We can also use Panicker's rapid cervical ripening device in patients with poor Bishop's score.

Mifepristone can also be useful as a single 200-mg dose for this indication.

TABLE 4: WHO guidelines.

Gestational age	Dosage
13–17 weeks	200 μg PV 6th hourly (max 4 doses)[35]
18–26 weeks	100 μg PV 6th hourly (max 4 doses)
27 weeks to term	25 μg PV 6th hourly (max 6 doses) or 20–25 μg PO 2 hourly (max 12 doses)[36]

TABLE 5: NICE guidelines.

Gestational age	Dosage
<27 weeks	100 μg 6th hourly
>27 weeks	25–50 μg 4th hourly

(NICE: National Institute for Health and Care Excellence)

TABLE 6: FIGO Misoprostol-only regimens 2017 chart.

Gestational age	Dosage
13–26 weeks	200 μg PV/sublingual/buccal every 4–6 hours
27–28 weeks	100 μg PV/sublingual/buccal every 4–6 hours
>28 weeks	25 μg PV 6th hourly 25 μg oral 2nd hourly

(FIGO: The International Federation of Gynecology and Obstetrics)

The recommended dose of Misoprost for induction in IUFD as per the different regimens is given in **Tables 4 to 6.**

Induction of Labor in a Scarred Uterus

A discussion of the safety and benefits of induction of labor should be undertaken by a consultant obstetrician.

Mifepristone can be used alone to increase the chance of labor significantly within 72 hours (avoiding the use of prostaglandin). Mechanical methods for induction of labor in women with an IUFD should be used only in the context of a clinical trial.

Women with a single lower segment scar should be advised that, in general, induction of labor with prostaglandin is safe but not without risk.

Misoprostol can be safely used for induction of labor in women with a single previous lower segment cesarean section (LSCS) and an IUFD but with lower doses than those marketed in the UK.

Women with two previous LSCS should be advised that in general, the absolute risk of induction of labor with prostaglandin is only a little higher than for women with a single previous LSCS.

Women with more than two LSCS deliveries or atypical scars should be advised that the safety of induction of labor is unknown.

Mechanical methods of induction might increase the risk of ascending infection in the presence of IUFD.[37]

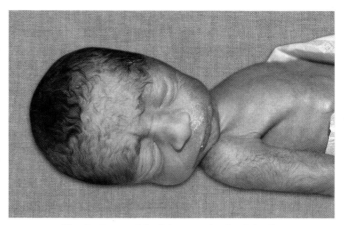

Fig. 4: A case of fresh intrauterine fetal death.

The Society of Obstetricians and Gynaecologists of Canada recommended that misoprostol is contraindicated in women with previous cesarean delivery because of a high rate of uterine rupture.[38] A more recent narrative review of induction of labor for late IUFD concluded that misoprostol can be used safely at lower doses for women with a previous cesarean (25–50 μg).[35]

Women undergoing vaginal birth after cesarean (VBAC) should be closely monitored for features of scar rupture.

Oxytocin augmentation can be used for VBAC but the decision should be made by a consultant obstetrician.

Fetal heart rate abnormality, usually the most common early sign of scar dehiscence, does not apply in this circumstance. Other clinical features include maternal tachycardia, atypical pain, vaginal bleeding, hematuria on catheter specimen, and maternal collapse.[39]

■ RECOMMENDATIONS FOR INTRAPARTUM ANTIMICROBIAL THERAPY

Women with sepsis should be treated with intravenous broad-spectrum antibiotic therapy (including antichlamydial agents).

Routine antibiotic prophylaxis should not be used.

■ OPTIONS FOR SUPPRESSION OF LACTATION

Dopamine agonist such as cabergoline is superior to bromocriptine. They should not be given to women with hypertension or preeclampsia. Dopamine agonists are contraindicated in women with hypertension or preeclampsia.[40] They increase blood pressure and have been associated with intracerebral hemorrhage.[41]

In such cases, Pyridoxine 10 mg tid for 5 days can be used.

Simple measures, such as support brassiere, ice packs, and analgesics,[42] can also be helpful.

PSYCHOLOGICAL AND SOCIAL ASPECTS OF INTRAUTERINE FETAL DEMISE

In stillbirths, particularly in recurrent stillbirth, most of the patients have depression because of paternal harassment and also occupying more beds for admission.[43]

Unresolved normal grief responses can evolve into post-traumatic stress disorder[44,45] as well.

COMPLICATIONS

- Psychological upset
- Infection—*Clostridium welchii*. It is a dreadful condition. Transplacental infections associated with IUFD include CMV, syphilis, Parvovirus B19, listeria, rubella, toxoplasmosis, herpes simplex coxsackievirus, *Leptospira*, Q fever, and Lyme disease. Malaria parasitemia has also been associated with stillbirth. Ascending infection, with or without membrane rupture, with *Escherichia coli*, *Klebsiella*, Group B Streptococcus, Enterococcus, mycoplasma/ureaplasma, *Haemophilus influenzae*, and *Chlamydia* are the more common infectious causes in developed countries.
- Blood coagulation disorders are rare. They are due to gradual absorption of thromboplastin liberated from dead placenta and decidua into the maternal circulation. There is also a moderate risk of maternal disseminated intravascular coagulation (DIC): 10% within 4 weeks after the date of late IUFD, rising to 30% thereafter. This can be tested for by clotting studies, blood platelet count, and fibrinogen measurement.
- *Social aspects:* Divorce and suicides are described in low socioeconomic and illiterate families.

LEGAL ASPECTS

International coding for IUFD is 36.4A.

The current law on stillbirth registration is set out in the Births and Deaths Registration Act 1953 amended by the Still-Birth Definition Act 1992 (Green-top guidelines).

The parents are responsible for registering the stillbirth, normally within 42 days (21 days in Scotland) but with a final limit of 3 months for exceptional circumstances. In unmarried women, she is solely responsible as per law.

STRATEGIES FOR PREVENTION OF STILLBIRTH

Basic Interventions

A 2011 systematic review identified the following 10 interventions as those with the best evidence for reducing the burden of stillbirth worldwide:

1. Periconceptional folic acid fortification
2. Prevention of malaria
3. Syphilis detection and treatment
4. Hypertensive disorders of pregnancy detection and management
5. Diabetes of pregnancy detection and management
6. Fetal growth restriction detection and management
7. Post-term pregnancy (≥41 weeks of gestation) identification and induction
8. Skilled birth attendant at birth
9. Availability of basic emergency obstetric care
10. Availability of comprehensive emergency obstetric care

Maternal Preventive Strategies

Weight reduction in obese women, avoidance of delayed childbearing (i.e., plan pregnancy before the age of 35 years), smoking cessation, and avoidance of alcohol and recreational use of drugs are some of the preventive strategies. Limiting the number of embryos transferred during in vitro fertilization or multifetal pregnancy reduction could reduce the number of stillbirths related to multiple gestation.

Antepartum Fetal Monitoring

Theoretically, antepartum fetal monitoring in the late second or the third trimester should reduce the risk of stillbirth by identifying fetuses in whom timely intervention will prevent death. The best evidence that antepartum fetal monitoring can play a role in reducing stillbirth rates involves the use of Doppler velocimetry for monitoring the growth-restricted fetus.

Patient Education for Fetal Movement

Patients who report decreased fetal movement are at an increased risk of having an adverse pregnancy outcome, including stillbirth, and approximately half of stillbirths are preceded by decreased fetal movement.

Perinatal Audit

Developing strategies for stillbirth reduction requires an ongoing audit process to evaluate the specific causes of stillbirth and the results of intervention programs. As an example, perinatal audits have identified stillbirths resulting from deficiencies in intrapartum care, and quality improvement processes have been initiated to prevent recurrence.

Elective Delivery at Term

Studies consistently report that the risk of stillbirth increases late in pregnancy, especially after 38 weeks of gestation. A strategy of selective induction appears to be useful in pregnancies at high risk of stillbirth, such as monoamniotic twin pregnancy, poor glycemic control in a pregnancy complicated by diabetes mellitus, post-term pregnancy, women with a previous stillbirth.

Preconception interventions include optimizing medical status; discussing cessation of illicit drug, tobacco, and alcohol use; and optimizing body mass index, as appropriate.

Antenatal Interventions

Assessment of the prior risk of stillbirth is important.

Decide on the appropriate type and frequency of antepartum monitoring and determine when the maternal/fetal risks of ongoing pregnancy warrant intervention for delivery.

The odds of gestational diabetes are fourfold higher after an unexplained stillbirth. If the previous stillbirth was unexplained or related to fetal anomalies, we suggest maternal assessment for diabetes early in pregnancy and, if normal, repeat at 24–28 weeks.

Early ultrasound examination for gestational age assessment and ongoing assessment of fetal growth are important, given the increased risk for fetal growth restriction. A fetal anatomic survey should be performed at 18–22 weeks of gestation.

Low-dose aspirin prophylaxis is indicated for women with a bad obstetric history.

In otherwise healthy women with a previous stillbirth, we agree with the American College of Obstetricians and Gynecologists' recommendation for initiation of antepartum fetal testing 1–2 weeks prior to the gestational age of the previous stillbirth and by 32–34 weeks of gestation.

We agree with an expert consensus guideline that suggested avoiding scheduled delivery before 39 weeks if the previous stillbirth was unexplained and the current pregnancy is uncomplicated.

■ FUTURE RESEARCH

Intrauterine fetal demise demands future research for the betterment of humankind. They are as follows:
- The optimal system for classification of stillbirth
- Safety and efficacy of methods for induction of labor with a previous cesarean section
- The optimal dose of misoprostol for induction of labor according to gestational age
- The diagnostic power and accuracy of MRI for postmortem investigation
- The optimal psychological care of women and their partners
- A comparison of hospital and home follow-up appointments

┌─ **KEY POINTS** ─────────────────────────────
- Real-time ultrasonography is essential for the accurate diagnosis of IUFD

- Clinical assessment and laboratory tests should be recommended to assess maternal wellbeing (including coagulopathy) and to determine the cause of death, the chance of recurrence and possible means of avoiding further pregnancy complications.
- Women who are rhesus D (RhD)-negative should be advised to have a Kleihauer test undertaken urgently to detect large feto-maternal hemorrhage (FMH) that might have occurred a few days earlier. Anti-RhD gammaglobulin should be administered as soon as possible after presentation.
- Parents should be offered full postmortem examination to help explain the cause of an IUFD.
- Women should be strongly advised for immediate delivery if there is sepsis, preeclampsia, placental abruption or membrane rupture, but a more flexible approach can be discussed if these factors are not present
- A combination of mifepristone and a prostaglandin preparation is usually recommended as the first-line intervention for induction of labor. Misoprostol can also be used in combination with prostaglandin.
- Assessment for DIC and sepsis should be undertaken.
- Counseling should be done for woman and her partner including family members.

■ REFFERENCES

1. MacDoman MF, Kirmeyer SE, Wilson EC. Fetal and perinatal mortality, United States, 2006. Natl Vital Stat Rep. 2012;60(8):1-22.
2. GBD 2015 Child Mortality Collaborators. Global, regional, national, and selected subnational levels of stillbirths, neonatal, infant, and under-5 mortality, 1980-2015: a systematic analysis for the Global Burden of Disease Study 2015. Lancet. 2016;388:1725.
3. Lawn JE, Blencowe H, Pattinson R, Cousens S, Kumar R, Ibiebele I, et al. Stillbirths: Where? When? Why? How to make the data count? Lancet. 2011;377:1448.
4. MacDorman MF, Gregory EC. Fetal and Perinatal Mortality: United States, 2013. Natl Vital Stat Rep. 2015;64:1.
5. Aminu M, Bar-Zeev S, van den Broek N. Cause of and factors associated with stillbirth: a systematic review of classification systems. Acta Obstet Gynecol Scand. 2017;96:519.
6. Huang DY, Usher RH, Kramer MS, Yang H, Morin L, Fretts RC. Determinants of unexplained antepartum fetal deaths. Obstet Gynecol. 2000;95:215.
7. Frøen JF, Arnestad M, Frey K, Vege A, Saugstad OD, Stray-Pedersen B. Risk factors for sudden intrauterine unexplained death: epidemiologic characteristics of singleton cases in Oslo, Norway, 1986-1995. Am J Obstet Gynecol. 2001;184:694.
8. Yudkin PL, Wood L, Redman CW. Risk of unexplained stillbirth at different gestational ages. Lancet. 1987; 1:1192.
9. Stillbirth Collaborative Research Network Writing Group. Causes of death among stillbirths. JAMA. 2011;306:2459.
10. Confidential Enquiry into Maternal and Child Health (CEMACH). Perinatal Mortality 2007: United Kingdom. CEMACH: London; 2009. [online] Available from http://www.cmace.org.uk/

getattachment/1d2c0ebc-d2aa-4131-98ed-56bf8269e529/Perinatal-Mortality-2007.aspx [Last accessed October, 2020]

11. Parasnis H, Raje B, Hinduja IN. Relevance of plasma fibrinogen estimation in obstetric complications. J Postgrad Med. 1992;38:183-5.

12. Glantz A, Marschall HU, Mattsson LA. Intrahepatic cholestasis of pregnancy: Relationships between bile acid levels and fetal complication rates. Hepatology. 2004;40:467-74.

13. Royal College of Obstetricians and Gynaecologists. Green-top Guideline No. 22. Anti-D immunoglobulin for Rh prophylaxis. London: RCOG; 2002. Available at https://www.rcog.org.uk/en/guidelines-research-services/guidelines/gtg22/

14. Biankin SA, Arbuckle SM, Graf NS. Autopsy findings in a series of five cases of fetomaternal haemorrhages. Pathology. 2003;35:319-24.

15. Osman NB, Folgosa E, Gonzales C, Bergström S. Genital infections in the aetiology of late fetal death: an incident case referent study. J Trop Pediatr. 1995;41:258-66.

16. Moyo SR, Hägerstrand I, Nyström L, Tswana SA, Blomberg J, Bergström S, et al. Stillbirths and intrauterine infection, histologic chorioamnionitis and microbiological findings. Int J Gynaecol Obstet. 1996;54:115-23.

17. Moyo SR, Tswana SA, Nyström L, Bergström S, Blomberg J, Ljungh A. Intrauterine death and infections during pregnancy. Int J Gynaecol Obstet. 1995;51:211-8.

18. Syridou G, Spanakis N, Konstantinidou A, Piperaki E, Kafetzis D, Patsouris E, et al. Detection of cytomegalovirus, parvovirus B19 and herpes simplex viruses in cases of intrauterine fetal death: association with pathological findings. J Med Virol. 2008;80:1776-82.

19. Aberg A, Rydhström H, Källen B, Källén K. Impaired glucose tolerance during pregnancy is associated with increased fetal mortality in preceding sibs. Acta Obstet Gynecol Scand. 1997;76:212-7.

20. Cove DH, Johnston P. Fetal hyperthyroidism: experience of treatment in four siblings. Lancet. 1985;1:430-2.

21. Kist WJ, Janssen NG, Kalk JJ, Hague WM, Dekker GA, de Vries JI. Thrombophilias and adverse pregnancy outcome – A confounded problem! Thromb Haemost. 2008;99:77-85.

22. Wikman A, Edner A, Gryfelt G, Jonsson B, Henter JI. Fetal hemolytic anemia and intrauterine death caused by anti-M immunization. Transfusion. 2007;47:911-7.

23. Nield LE, Silverman ED, Taylor GP, Smallhorn JF, Mullen JB, Silverman NH, et al. Maternal anti-Ro and anti-La antibody associated endocardial fibroelastosis. Circulation. 2002;105:843-8.

24. Kjeldsen-Kragh J, Killie MK, Tomter G, Golebiowska E, Randen I, Hauge R, et al. A screening and intervention program aimed to reduce mortality and serious morbidity associated with severe neonatal alloimmune thrombocytopenia. Blood. 2007;110:833-9.

25. Pauli RM, Reiser CA. Wisconsin Stillbirth Service Program: II. Analysis of diagnoses and diagnostic categories in the first 1,000 referrals. Am J Med Genet. 1994;50:135-3.

26. Lutiger B, Graham K, Einarson TR, Koren G. Relationship between gestational cocaine use and pregnancy outcome: a meta-analysis. Teratology. 1991;44:405-14.

27. Martinek IE, Vial Y, Hohlfeld P. [Management of in utero foetal death: Which assessment to undertake?] J Gynecol Obstet Biol Reprod (Paris). 2006;35:594-606. (Article in French.)

28. Thein AT, Abdel-Fattah SA, Kyle PM, Soothill PW. An assessment of the use of interphase FISH with chromosome specific probes as an alternative to cytogenetics in prenatal diagnosis. Prenat Diagn. 2000;20:275-80.

29. Kidron D, Bernheim J, Aviram R. Placental findings contributing to fetal death, a study of 120 stillbirths between 23 and 40 weeks gestation. Placenta. 2009;30:700-4.

30. Genest DR. Estimating the time of death in stillborn fetuses: II. Histologic evaluation of the placenta; a study of 71 stillborns. Obstet Gynecol. 1992;80:585-92.

31. Genest DR, Singer DB. Estimating the time of death in stillborn fetuses: III. External fetal examination; a study of 86 stillborns. Obstet Gynecol. 1992;80:593–600.

32. Genest DR, Williams MA, Greene MF. Estimating the time of death in stillborn fetuses: I. Histologic evaluation of fetal organs; an autopsy study of 150 stillborns. Obstet Gynecol 1992;80:575-84.

33. Gelman-Kohan Z, Rosensaft J, Ben-Hur H, Haber A, Chemke J. Cytogenetic analysis of fetal chondrocytes: a comparative study. Prenat Diagn. 1996;16:165-8.

34. Dodd JM, Crowther CA. Misoprostol for induction of labour to terminate pregnancy in the second or third trimester for women with anomaly or after intrauterine fetal death. Cochrane Database Syst Rev. 2010;(4):CD004901.

35. Gomez Ponce de Leon R, Wind D, Fiala C. Misoprostol for intrauterine fetal death. Int J Gynaecol Obstet. 2007;99(Suppl 2):S190-3.

36. WHO recommendations for induction of labour. Geneva: World Health Organization; 2011.

37. Boulvain M, Kelly A, Lohse C, Stan CM, Irion O. Mechanical methods for induction of labour. Cochrane Database Syst Rev 2001;(4):CD001233.

38. Society of Obstetricians and Gynaecologists of Canada. SOGC clinical practice guidelines. Guidelines for vaginal birth after previous caesarean birth. Number 155 (Replaces guideline number 147), February 2005. Int J Gynaecol Obstet. 2005;89:319-31.

39. Royal College of Obstetricians and Gynaecologists. Green-top Guideline No. 45: Birth after previous caesarean birth. London: RCOG; 2007 https://www.rcog.org.uk/en/guidelines-research-services/guidelines/gtg45/

40. British Medical Association and Royal Pharmaceutical Society of Great Britain. British National Formulary (BNF) 54. London: BMJ Publishing Group and RPS Publishing; 2007.

41. Iffy L, Zito GE, Jakobovits AA, Ganesh V, McArdle JJ. Postpartum intracranial haemorrhage in normotensive users of bromocriptine for ablactation. Pharmacoepidemiol Drug Saf 1998;7:167-71.

42. Spitz AM, Lee NC, Peterson HB. Treatment for lactation suppression: little progress in one hundred years. Am J Obstet Gynecol. 1998;179:1485-90.

43. National Institute for Health and Clinical Excellence. NICE clinical guideline 45: Antenatal and postnatal mental health. Clinical management and service guidance. London: NICE; 2007 https://www.nice.org.uk/guidance/cg192

44. Hughes P, Turton P, McGauley GA, Fonagy P. Factors that predict infant disorganization in mothers classified as U in pregnancy. Attach Hum Dev. 2006;8:113-22.

45. Turton P, Hughes P, Evans CD, Fainman D. Incidence, correlates and predictors of post-traumatic stress disorder in the pregnancy after stillbirth. Br J Psychiatry. 2001;178:556-60.

Multifetal Gestation

Vidya Thobbi

INTRODUCTION

Presence of more than one fetus in the gravid uterus is described as multifetal gestation. The number and rate of multifetal gestation have increased dramatically in the last two decades as a result of increased use of fertility drugs and various assisted reproductive techniques (ARTs). Multiple pregnancies have substantially high risks of perinatal morbidity and mortality as well as maternal morbidity. The epidemic of these high-risk multiple gestation which was on the rise is slowly decreasing because of advances in reproductive technology and guidelines. Almost 30–50% of twin pregnancies occur after infertility treatment.

The incidence of twin frequency is approximately 1 per 80 live births, but there is significant variation amongst different countries and different populations.

Hellin's law states the following incidences of multiple pregnancy:

- *Twins 1:* 80
- *Triplets 1:* 80²
- *Quadruplets 1:* 80³
- *Quintuplets 1:* 80⁴

The incidence of monozygotic (MZ) twinning is constant worldwide at 3.5 per 1,000 live births while dizygotic (DZ) twinning rates and higher order birth rates vary widely and are affected by various factors such as race, parity, age, use of ARTs, and ethnic differences.

With the use of ultrasound (USG), it is apparent that the incidence maybe more common than previously indicated and about half of these pregnancies fail to be recognized as twin gestation because one of the sacs spontaneously aborts or reabsorbs early in pregnancy.[1]

Multifetal pregnancies are responsible for:

- 17% of all preterm births before 37 weeks of gestation
- 23% of early preterm births before 32 weeks of gestation
- 24% of low birth weight births
- 25% of very low birth weight births (<1,500 g)[2]

ASSISTED REPRODUCTION TECHNOLOGY

Assisted reproduction technology is responsible for 14% of all multifetal gestations. The risk incidence of multifetal gestation with clomiphene citrate is between 6.8 and 17% and with gonadotrophins it is between 18 and 53%. The incidence is more in hypogonadotropic women, followed by normogonadotropic, oligomenorrheic, and then women with corpus luteum deficiency.[3]

The incidence is more when pregnancy occurs after cessation of oral contraception; if oral contraception is used for >6 consecutive months, then the possibility of twins gets doubled.

An incidence in the total number of follicles (>7) and serum estradiol level concentration (>1,385 pg/mL) correlates with an increase in high-order multifetal gestation (if the patient's age is younger). 20% multifetal gestation occur with double-embryo transfer and 25% with triple-embryo stransfer.[4]

MATERNAL AGE, RACE, PARITY, AND ETHNICITY

Twinning rates double as the woman's age advances. Due to delayed child bearing, there is use of ARTs and ovulation-inducing agents.

Women with a larger body mass index (BMI) have increased frequency of multiple gestations.[5] The increase was limited to DZ pregnancies.

The highest rate of twin births was in 45–49-year-old women (approximately 200 per 1,000 live births) compared with (the lowest rate of 20 per 1,000 live births) those between 15 and 24 years of age. Greater use of fertility services in this age group and the higher levels of follicle-stimulating hormone (FSH) with advancing age are responsible for a higher rate of multifetal gestation with increasing age.

Multifetal pregnancies are more common in multiparas, and heredity influences only DZ twins.

The frequency of twinning is highest amongst black race and low in Orientals.

CLASSIFICATION

By Zygosity

There are two types of twins:

1. Monozygotic, identical, uniovular, or single egg
2. Dizygotic, fraternal, biovular, nonidentical, or two eggs

Two-third of all twins are DZ.

a. MZ twins have identical genotypes and therefore have the same sex, because of early division of an ovum fertilized by one sperm cell into two cell masses containing identical genetic information.

b. DZ twins are the result of fertilization of two separate ova liberated during the same menstrual cycle by different sperms resulting in different maternal and paternal genetic contributions to each fetus.

The proportions of DZ and MZ twins are 69 and 31%, respectively.

Multifetal gestations of higher orders can result from any one or combination of these mechanisms:

■ *Superfecundation* refers to fertilization of two separate ova in the same menstrual cycle at two separate episodes of intercourse.

■ *Superfetation* occurs when two separate ovas are fertilized during separate menstrual cycles, i.e., second ovulation occurred after the first pregnancy has occurred.

■ *Chorionicity (Fig. 1)*
  – *Monochorionic:* Presence of one common placenta. These twins are always MZ. The septum dividing the two sacs has only two layers—an amnion from each fetus.
  – *Dichorionic:* Presence of two placentas. The twins may be MZ or DZ. The placentas may be separately located or they may be fused (lying in close proximity). The septum dividing the two sacs has four layers, one amnion and one chorion from each twin.

■ *Amnionicity:* Number of amniotic sacs within the uterus **(Figs. 2A to C)**
  – *Monoamniotic:* Presence of only one sac. Such twins are MZ. There is a potential risk of cord entanglement as there is no intervening septum.
  – *Diamniotic:* Presence of two sacs. These twins may be MZ or DZ.

Dizygotic twin pregnancies are dichorionic and diamniotic (di-di); they always have two placentas and two amniotic sacs.

Monozygotic twin placentation is complex and the number of chorions and amnions varies according to the timing of zygotic division.

If the splitting occurs before the eight-cell stage (within 3 days of fertilization) while the cells are still not specialized and retain their potentiality for differentiation, splitting results in differentiation of two separate blastocysts and if both blastocysts are implanted twin pregnancy results; both blastocysts may or may not be closely implanted. Each has its own placenta and amnion. Both are identical and are of the same sex and genetic constitution. This accounts for one-third of MZ twins (25–30%).

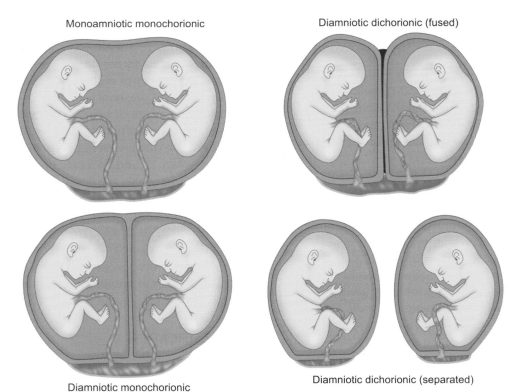

Monoamniotic monochorionic

Diamniotic dichorionic (fused)

Diamniotic monochorionic

Diamniotic dichorionic (separated)

Fig. 1: Chorionicity—monochorionic and dichorionic.

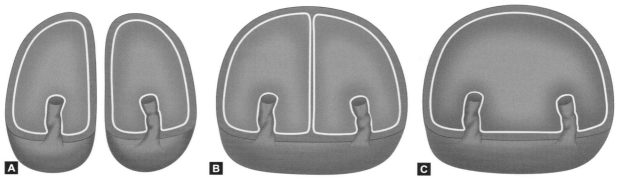

Figs. 2A to C: Number of amniotic sacs. (A) Dichorionic-diamniotic; (B) Monochorionic-diamniotic; (C) Monochorionic-monoamniotic.

If splitting is delayed (4–7 days) until after the inner cell mass starts forming, single blastocyst implantation occurs with single chorion. There are anastomoses between fetal circulations. Each embryo has its own amnion (monochorionic-diamniotic twins). Two-thirds of MZ twins are of such cases (65%).

If splitting of inner cell mass occurs after differentiation of the amnion but before the appearance of primitive streak (8–12 days), two identical twins are formed having single amnion, chorion, and placenta, and there is communication between the circulations (monochorionic-monoamniotic). Only 9% of MZ twins fall in the category.

After the appearance of primitive streak, 13 days later, incomplete splitting of germinal disc (rare cases) leads to formation of conjoined twins. The incidence is 1 in 60,000 live births.

Multifetal gestations of higher orders are the result of multizygosity and other combinations.

The factors responsible for the timing of division of fertilized ovum are not known.

Twins of opposite sex are always dizygotic.

ETIOLOGY OF MULTIPLE BIRTHS

The etiology of MZ twinning is not clear, but DZ twinning appears as a result of ovulation from multiple follicles.

Elevated Follicle-stimulating Hormone

The plasma concentration of FSH appears to correlate with rates of DZ multiple births and hence is the principal determinant of ovulation.

Plasma concentrations of FSH, luteinizing hormone, and estradiol are higher in women who have had at least one set of DZ twins.

Ovarian Stimulation

Assisted reproductive technologies use various drugs to stimulate ovaries and induce ovulation. Depending upon the used drug and its dosage, the frequency of twins is increased by 5–50%. Clomiphene citrate, the most widely used drug, exerts its major effects on the hypothalamus, pituitary, ovary, and uterus. It disrupts the normal feedback inhibition of gonadotropin-releasing hormone (GnRH) and gonadotropin secretion by circulating estrogen by binding to the hypothalamic estrogen receptors. The enhanced gonadotropin secretion thus induces ovulation.

In vitro Fertilization

The risk of multiple births from in vitro fertilization (IVF) varies inversely with maternal age and directly with the number of embryos transferred.

Placentation

DZ twins have di-di placentas, although these may fuse during pregnancy. In MZ twins, the timing of egg division determines placentation:

- Diamniotic, dichorionic placentation occurs with division prior to the morula stage (within 3 days post fertilization).
- Diamniotic, monochorionic placentation occurs with division between 4 and 8 days post fertilization.
- Monoamniotic, monochorionic placentation occurs with division between 8 and 12 days post fertilization.
- Division at or after day 13 results in conjoined twins.

The factors responsible for timing of egg division are not known.

Examination of Placenta (Fig. 3)

Placenta examination reveals zygosity in cases of like-sex twins. Determination is based on chorion/amnion status.

Histologic evaluation of the membrane as they join the body of the placenta at the T section (transverse section) may be needed to establish the presence of one or two chorions.

Demonstration of vascular anastomosis by injection of milk or dye through the vessels may reveal communications between the placentas and also indicates MZ twinning.

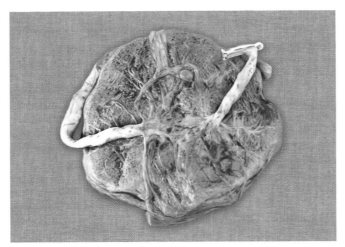

Fig. 3: Examination of placenta.

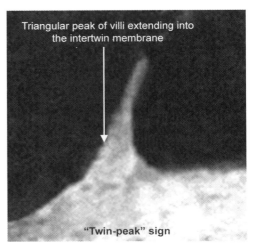

Fig. 4: Twin-peak sign seen in USG.

In indeterminate situations, zygosity can be established by blood types and chromosomal or DNA polymorphism.

The diagnosis of chorionicity is important and more specific than monozygosity as a risk factor for adverse perinatal outcome.

- *Dichorionic-diamniotic:*
  - Two layers of chorionic tissues in between two amnions
- *Monochorionic-diamniotic:*
  - One chorionic layer between two amniotic layers

Chorionicity may be determined antenatally and can be used for the management.

Monochorionic twins are at higher risk than dichorionic twins:

- Neurologic complications and morbidity
- Birth weight discordance
- Death

10–15% develop twin-to-twin transfusion syndrome (TTTS) and have poor obstetric and neonatal outcomes.[6]

■ AMNIONICITY AND ITS CLINICAL IMPORTANCE

Monoamniotic twins are always monochorionic, with an incidence of 1 in 10,000 live births and high perinatal mortality rate (PNMR) of 23%. Complications such as entanglement of cord are common, affecting about two third of cases, and leads to serious neurological morbidity and mortality; congenital anomalies are also common (25%) such as renal malformation and defects of abdominal wall. Birth weight discordance affects 20% of monoamniotic twins. High risk and poor outcome require intensive fetal surveillance and early delivery.

Diagnosis of Chorionicity and Amnionicity by Ultrasound Examination

Fetuses with opposite sex confirm di-di pregnancy; it is useful in advanced gestation, but when fetuses are of the same sex this method is not useful.

If two placentas are identified, then pregnancy is di-di. But it is difficult to identify when they are fused.

Visualization of membrane is utmost important in twins by USG. The membrane is thicker in dichorionic as it is formed by four layers of tissues (two amnions and two chorions).

In monochorionic, it is formed by two layers of amnion. To be accurate, it is to be performed in the first trimester of pregnancy. The mean thickness in mono-chorionic pregnancy is 1.4 ± 0.3 mm and in dichorionic is 2.4 ± 0.7 mm. The threshold to differentiate mono-to-di placentation is 2 mm. The accuracy for mono is 82% and for di is 95%.

In di-di twin pregnancy USG, lambda or twin-peak sign **(Fig. 4)** is seen that corresponds to triangular projection of chorionic tissue between the membrane layers in the areas of insertion of the membranes in the uterus.

Counting the layers of dividing membranes is another accurate method for the determination of chorionicity, 3.5 ± 5 MHz transducers to 7.5–20 MHz.[7]

Ultrasound and Chorionicity

The USG is best done in the first and second trimesters. The results are excellent if done before 14 weeks. It is difficult to interpret in advanced pregnancy and oligohydramnios.

Difficulty in localizing interfetal membrane can mislead to diagnosis of monoamniotic pregnancy.

Invasive Methods for Diagnosing Monoamniotic Pregnancy

- X-ray of abdomen is taken after injecting 30 mL of water-soluble contrast into the amniotic cavity. After 24 hours of injection, the X-ray will show contrast medium in the gastrointestinal tract (GIT) of both twins if it is monoamniotic pregnancy.
- Inject 0.1 mL of air and 5 mL of amniotic fluid after obtaining an amniotic fluid sample for genetic

evaluation. USG done following this injection will show microbubbles around one or both twins depending on amnionicity.

MATERNAL ADAPTATION

Maternal adaptation involves exaggeration of normal pregnancy response and all maternal organ systems.

Cardiovascular System

Diastolic blood pressure is lower in the second trimester and exhibits a greater increase near term. They are at a greater risk for postural hypotension. The increase in maternal heart rate is by 15%. Mean total peripheral resistance decreased by 30%. The incidence of pregnancy-induced hypertension (PIH) is increased in twins and increases with higher order multiple pregnancies. Cardiac output increases and peak is achieved at 9 L/min by 21–24 weeks. It is still higher during labor and when the patient is treated with beta mimetics.

Blood volume increases significantly and directly corelates with the size of the fetal mass. Plasma volume increases by 67% (6–7 L), maternal red cell volume by 24%, hematocrit drops, and dilutional anemia occurs. Iron and folic acid deficiency is more common in women with twins than singletons.

Levels of components of coagulation systems are also altered. Fibrinogen levels are increased by >50%. The coagulation factors VII, VIII, IX, and X all increase. The woman is in a hypercoagulable state. The plasma fibrinolytic activity decreases.

Endocrine Changes

There is an increase in maternal cortisol, aldosterone, and free thyroxin. The hormones made by placenta are increased in multiple pregnancies. Human chorionic gonadotropin (HCG) levels are 2.5 times higher than singleton pregnancy. The human placental lactogen levels are also higher. Serum progesterone levels are double. Serum estradiol is elevated. Levels of pregnancy-specific β1 glycoprotein (sp1) are higher in twin gestations than singletons. Urinary estriol excretion is increased and maternal estriol is higher in twin pregnancy.

The maternal serum α-fetoprotein (MSAFP) level is elevated in multiple pregnancy compared with singleton pregnancy.

The mean MSAFP value in twin pregnancy is 2.0–2.5 multiples of the median (MoM). The measurement should be done at 16–20 weeks. In twins without birth defects, the relative risk of perinatal death was 4.8 if the MSAFP value was at least 4 MoM compared with structurally normal twins where the MSAFP values were 2 and 3 MoM. If the values are >4 MoM, patients need more evaluation with further tests such as amniocentesis and acetylcholinesterase (AChE) levels.

Respiratory Functions

There is an increase in tidal volume than in singletons by 20%. The overall increase in ventilation is necessary to compensate the 20% increase in oxygen consumption in the normal pregnant woman.

Gastrointestinal System

Several physiological changes occur and are exaggerated. There is exaggerated morning sickness, increased gastric reflux due to lowered esophageal sphincter tone, increased intragastric pressure, and increased risk of aspiration during general anesthesia.

Renal Functions

Glomerular filtration rate (GFR) is higher than in singleton pregnancy. Obstructive uropathy is common because of pressure effects, especially in hydramnios.

Nutrition and Weight Gain

Mothers of multiple pregnancy gain more weight during pregnancy with improved intrauterine growth in twins, with good weight gain before 24 weeks. The birth weight of an infant is related to maternal weight gain.

Nutrition and calorie intake should be more and nutritional institutes have recommended 2,800 kcal/day for twins.

COMPLICATIONS

In multiple pregnancies, all pregnancy complications are aggravated. The incidence of complications is 83% in twins compared with 25% in singleton.[8]

Maternal Complications

- Spontaneous abortion
- Hyperemesis gravidarum
- Anemia
- Pregnancy-induced hypertension
- Diabetes mellitus
- Preterm labor
- Oligohydramnios
- Acute fatty liver of pregnancy
- Cholestasis of pregnancy
- Placenta previa
- Abruptio placenta
- Preterm premature rupture of the membranes (PPROM)
- Cord entanglement
- Cord prolapse
- Postpartum hemorrhage (PPH)
- Operative deliveries

- Puerperal infection/increased hospital stay
- Psychological stress

Fetal Complications

- Prematurity
- Fetal growth discordance
- Fetal growth restriction
- Fetal demise (one or both)
- Congenital anomalies
- Fetal malpresentation
- TTTS
- Acardiac twins

Spontaneous abortion: It is at least twice as often as singleton pregnancy. With increasing use of USG, early abortion or resorption of one twin (vanishing twin syndrome) can be observed in 21–63% of spontaneous twin pregnancies. It is estimated that only 50% of twins diagnosed by USG in the early first trimester continue as such until delivery.

Pregnancy-induced hypertension: The incidence of PIH as reported in various studies is around 12.9%. Early severe pre-eclampsia and HELLP (hemolysis, elevated liver enzymes, low platelet count) syndrome happen more frequently in multiple gestations. It occurs with equal frequency in monozygotic and dizygotic pregnancy and especially resulting from ART pregnancies. The frequency of recurrent pre-eclampsia is less with multiple gestations.[9]

Anemia: It is due to iron deficiency, increased fetomaternal demand, and additional physiological dilution from plasma volume expansion.

Polyhydramnios: In monozygotics, due to TTTS in one or both sacs, a greater or lesser degree of polyhydramnios occurs.

Gestational diabetes: It occurs more often in twins and triplets and may be due to a large placental mass producing human placental lactogen.

Fatty liver of pregnancy: It is a rare complication.

Placenta previa and abruptio placentae: Placenta is large so it approaches the lower segment. Due to PIH and sudden decompression, abruptio placentae is more common.

Postpartum hemorrhage: Its incidence is increased—27.8% in twins and 35% in triplet gestation. Overdistention, atony of uterus, and anemia are contributory factors.

Preterm labor: 50% of the twins deliver preterm before 37 weeks. The single largest factor for perinatal mortality is preterm and low-birth-weight babies.

Neonatal complications associated with preterm birth are hypothermia, hypoglycemia, respiratory problems, patent ductus arteriosus (PDA), intracranial bleeding, infections, retinopathy, and necrotizing enterocolitis, leading to neonatal morbidity and mortality.

Overdistension of uterus and intrauterine infection are two main causes for preterm deliveries.

Overall, all twins account for about 10% of all preterm babies. The mean length of gestation in twins is 35 weeks, in triplets 33 weeks, and in quadruplets 31 weeks.

■ FETAL COMPLICATIONS UNIQUE IN MULTIPLE GESTATIONS

Discordant Growth

The incidence of discordant growth is about 15–29% of all twin pregnancies. It causes differences in weight between the twins. A discrepancy of 20% or more is significant.
- *Grade I:* Difference of 15–25%
- *Grade II:* Difference of >25%

Smaller twins are at more risk of perinatal complications. They may also die due to congenital anomalies or prematurity. Neonatal morbidity along with physical and intellectual squeale is common, and prognosis is worst.

An ultrasonographic criterion, which is most commonly used, is a difference of 15–25% in estimated fetal weight.

Etiology

- *Unequal placental mass:* It occurs in monochorionic and dichorionic twins (more common). Asymmetrical growth is usually noticed after 24 weeks.
- *Genetic syndrome:* It occurs in monochorionic (more common) and dichorionic twins. It can be detected by 16–20 weeks. Neural tube defects, cardiac abnormalities, and chromosome defects are common underlying problems. USG shows symmetrical growth restriction.
- *Twin-to-twin transfusion syndrome:* It affects monochorionic pregnancies and is responsible for 15% of overall fetal mortality.

In addition, the neonatal mortality rate (per 1,000 live births) of the smaller twin increased with increasing discordance:
- No discordance—3.8
- 15–19% discordance—5.6
- 20–24% discordance—8.5
- 25–30%—18.4
- 30% or more—43.4

Management

Management of twin pregnancy with growth discordance differs depending on the etiology.

Intrauterine Fetal Demise of One Twin: The Vanishing Twin

Stoeckel (1945) (10 advances) described vanishing twin syndrome where multifetal gestation is identified followed by disappearance of one or more fetuses. The incidence is around 30% and increases with age; this may lead to a higher rate of incidence of multiple gestations. Intrauterine fetal demise (IUFD) occurs in 2–4% of twins.[10] When one twin dies in utero, the surviving twin gets affected and succumbs in about 25% cases.[11] The condition is diagnosed more frequently by USG.

In vanishing twin syndrome, there may be:

- Complete resorption of a fetus
- Formation of fetus papyraceous (mummified or compressed fetus)
- Development of abnormality on placenta like a cyst, or amorphous material

The timing of the above affects the outcome of the remaining live twin and other maternal complications.

Etiology

The etiology of the event is frequently unknown. Placental or fetal factors reveal chromosomal abnormalities and genetic factors.

It can cause spastic cerebral palsy or intrauterine fetal demise (IUFD) of the remaining twin. It could be due to a large amount of blood loss to low resistance system of the vanishing twin through placental anastomosis which causes intraventricular hemorrhages. It can also lead to skin necrosis. Disseminated intravascular coagulation (DIC) occurs due to release of thromboplastin proteins from the vanishing twin to the surviving twin. It takes 5 weeks for coagulopathy to develop. It has been observed that coagulation problems in mother are temporary and resolve spontaneously.[12]

Fetal Morbidity and Mortality

- In the first trimester, if death of one twin occurs no effect is observed on the surviving twin or mother.
- In the second half of pregnancy, the surviving fetus can be affected by cerebral palsy and cutis aplasia.
- Same sex twins are at a higher risk (2.6%).[13]
- Maternal complications include preterm labor, infection, consumption coagulopathy, and puerperal hemorrhage.
- The rates of fetal demise of the co-twin in monochorionic and dichorionic pregnancies were 15 and 3%, respectively.
- The rates of preterm birth in monochorionic and dichorionic pregnancies were 68 and 54%, respectively.
- The rates of abnormal postnatal cranial imaging in monochorionic and dichorionic pregnancies were 34 and 16%, respectively.
- The rates of neurodevelopmental impairment of the co-twin in monochorionic and dichorionic pregnancies were 26 and 2%, respectively.

Investigations

Ultrasonography: There should be follow-up USG for pregnancy loss and raised alpha fetoprotein levels are raised.

Management

Prognosis: Prognosis for surviving twin depends on:

- Gestational age at the time of demise
- Chorionicity
- Duration between demise and delivery
  Risk factors include monochorionicity and severe PIH.
  Placenta should be examined and sent for histology in suspicious cases.

In dichorionic pregnancies, the other twin is not affected. In dichorionic twins, the death of one twin is not an indication for delivery of the surviving twin, until and unless close surveillance is necessary in certain conditions (e.g., pre-eclampsia, chorioamnionitis), where timely delivery of the surviving twin is indicated to prevent a second fetal loss.

In monochorionic pregnancies, it is difficult to calculate the effect and to know the ischemic insult. Middle cerebral artery peak velocity is useful. Patients should be counseled regarding guarded prognosis, fetal morbidity, and outcome. When one twin dies prior to viability, one must discuss the option of pregnancy termination, although the risk to the co-twin is not clear when the death occurs in the first trimester. USG and magnetic resonance evaluation of the surviving co-twin can identify signs of brain injury, such as white matter lesions or intracranial hemorrhage, which develop over time. However, the ability of imaging studies to predict or exclude fetal brain injury in this setting is unknown. The risk of cerebral palsy greatly increases in such cases. The release of thromboplastin and emboli from the dead twin may cause injury to the surviving twin.

Structural defects related to ischemic disruption that typically occur in the surviving co-twin include:

- Porencephalic cyst, hydranencephaly, or microcephaly
- Intestinal atresia
- Gastroschisis
- Limb amputation
- Aplasia cutis

Twin-reversed Arterial Perfusion (TRAP) (Fig. 5)

- It is referred to as acardiac and is a rare event.
- It is a complication of MZ twins.
- Normal twin has a high risk of perinatal mortality and morbidity because of cardiac failure and preterm birth.
- It occurs in 1% monochorionic twins.
- The incidence is 1 in 35,000 pregnancies.

Driggers et al.[14] postulated that TRAP occurs during the period of organogenesis. Extensive anastomosis and

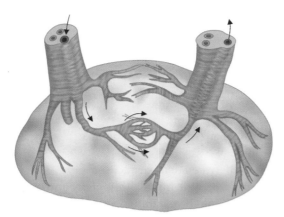

Fig. 5: Twin-reversed arterial perfusion. (TRAP sequence)

formation of shunts lead to dysfunction of twin A. Twin A (absent cardiac function) fails to transmit the pressure from heart to umbilical artery and because of loss of positive pressure in the umbilical artery which causes reversal of flow from twin A, which becomes dependent for its supply on its co-twin B (pump twin). Twin A gets majority of supply through the umbilical artery; inadequate deoxygenated perfusion leads to organ atrophy and absent or nondevelopment of various organs occurs during organogenesis.

Liver is most commonly affected.[15] The pump twin has its own complications due to hyperdynamic circulation and congestive cardiac failure leading to hydrops fetalis and death (12%). Mortality of 50–70% is observed in pump twin.[16,17]

Classification of Acardius[14]

- *Acardius acephalus:* Head and upper extremities absent; thorax, kidneys, intestines, lower extremities present
- *Acardiac amorphous:* Formless mass of bones, connective tissue. No head or extremities, cord is attached to the surface.
- *Acardius anceps:* Head is poorly developed and rudimentary.
- *Acardius acornus:* Very rare, only head is developed. Rest of the body is absent or rudimentary.

Diagnosis

USG is the mainstay of diagnosis showing an acardiac fetus in monochorionic twin pregnancy.[18]

- Absent cardiac motion
- Large cystic structures and soft-tissue echoes, skeletal echoes

It can be confused with IUFD but follow-up USG shows "growth of dead fetus" and reflex limb movements.

First-trimester discordance can be early manifestation in TRAP and color Doppler studies are of immense help. Color Doppler shows perfusion of acardiac fetus and

differentiates it from dead fetus which does not show any flow. In TRAP, reversal of flow in the umbilical artery of the perfused twin is diagnostic.

Management of TRAP (Flowchart 1)

It is challenging with two options:
1. Expectant
2. Interventional

Expectant management may be done in mild cases of TRAP when there is presence of a small acardiac twin and no signs of cardiac failure in the other twin.

Symptomatic interventions to control amniotic fluid volume by serial amniocentesis, digitalization of mother, and use of indomethacin are required.[19,20] Selective delivery of a nonviable twin was tried, but complications were more such as abruption, PROM, preterm birth, and maternal morbidity.[21]

Minimal invasive technique includes insertion of thrombogenic coil in the single umbilical artery of acardiac twin. Risk of embolization and death of normal twin may occur as complications. The endoscopic approach was first done by McCurdy as cord ligation, blocking the vessel by embolization under endoscopic and USG guidance.[22]

A new minimally invasive percutaneous technique for selective reduction of acardiac twin with radiofrequency (RFA) (3m – 14G). Radiofrequency needle under USG guidance has been reported. Though safe and effective, it is expensive and available in only few centers.[23]

Interruption of the vascular anastomosis between the donor and the recipient twin can be accomplished using endoscopic laser coagulation in pregnancies which are <24 weeks' gestation. In advanced gestational ages, ligation of the umbilical cord can be done using endoscopic or sonographic guidance. Another approach is to use radiofrequency ablation to obliterate the blood supply of the acardiac twin. In one series, 12 of 13 donor twins survived following this procedure and were neurodevelopmentally normal in the neonatal period.

In one report, 9 of 10 healthy donor twins survived when the acardiac twin pregnancy was managed expectantly. In four of these cases, flow to the acardiac twin stopped entirely or decreased, and the donor twin was born at >36 weeks' gestation.

Twin-to-twin Transfusion Syndrome (Fig. 6)

Twin-to-twin transfusion syndrome is a serious progressive disorder.

- Affects 15% monochorionic pregnancies and 15% of overall fetal mortality in twin pregnancies
- The recipient as a consequence of maximum increased intravascular volume develops cardiomegaly and congestive cardiac failure (CCF).

Flowchart 1: Management of twin-reversed arterial perfusion.

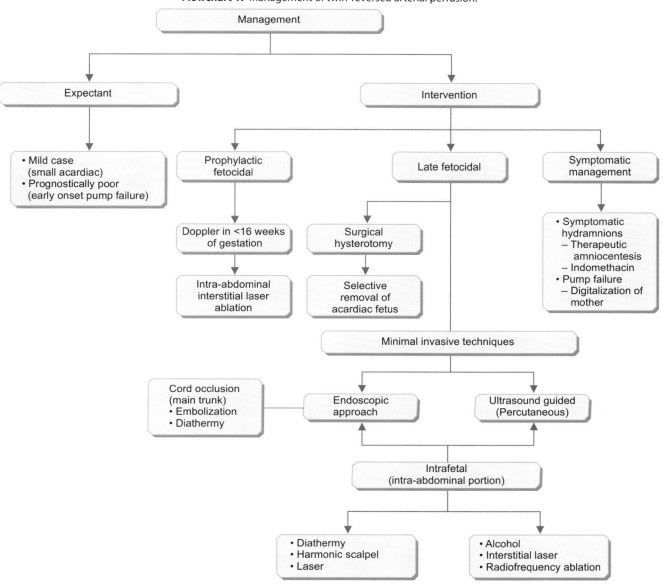

- Frequently dies in utero. If alive, it may develop respiratory distress and CCF in the early neonatal period.
- Hyperbilirubinemia is another complication. The recipient produces increased amount of natriuretic peptide to control intravascular volume and leads to excessive urination leading to polyhydramnios.
- Donor twin has retarded somatic growth and develops hydrops fetalis and high output heart failure if anemia is severe. Oliguria is common.
- Mechanisms of fetal death in TTTS are placental insufficiency and severe anemia in the donor twin, CCF in the recipient twin, and due to complications of preterm birth and congenital anomalies. The incidence

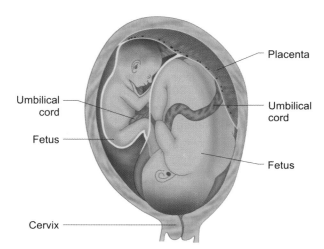

Fig. 6: Twin pregnancy: Twin-to-twin transfusion (TTTS).

of cerebral palsy and neurological abnormalities is greater in twin pregnancies complicated by TTTS.

- Although perinatal mortality was 100% earlier, improvements in outcome have resulted from better management options.

Mechanism

Twin-to-twin transfusion syndrome results from the presence of placental vascular communications that generate hemodynamic imbalance. Anastomosis may be (A-A)(A-V)(V-V) (A: artery, V: vein). A-A and V-V are localized on the fetal surface of chorion and as flow is in both directions it is balanced. A-V is unidirectional and deeply situated vascular anastomosis. If umbilical cord ligation is delayed after the delivery of the first twin in monochorionic placentation and the interval of the delivery of the second twin is delayed, acute fetoplacental circulation may occur and the second twin is endangered as it loses blood into placenta of the first twin.

Diagnosis

The following criteria are used for the neonatal diagnosis of TTTS:

- Difference of Hb% ≥ 5 g/dL
- Difference of birth weight > 20%

Antenatal diagnosis: It is a presumptive diagnosis. On USG, there is one placenta seen with twins of the same sex and diamniotic placentation with a thin membrane between the twins. Umbilical cords are of different sizes. There is discrepancy in amniotic fluid volume surrounding each twin and 20% or larger discrepancy in estimated fetal weight between the twins is significant. Fetal hydrops may be noticed in one or both twins.

The fundamental diagnostic criterion is oligo/poly sequence.

- *Oligohydramnios:* There is no fluid or a pocket fluid < 2 cm in its largest diameter.
- *Polyhydramnios:* Pocket of fluid 8 or more cm in its largest diameter

"Stuck" twin is an extreme variety of TTTS; the donor twin is so small that it gets stuck to the uterine wall. The mortality of stuck twin is 80%.

The use of Doppler in the diagnosis is not useful as its analysis varies with anemia, heart, and vascular pattern changes.

Classification

For the assessment of severity of the condition, Quintero's classification is used.

It is sonographic evaluation (it also detects the perinatal risks).

Prediction of TTTS

Twins presenting with severe TTTS in the mid trimester may have hemodynamic imbalance from the first trimester manifesting as discordant growth. Increased nuchal translucency (NT) is observed at 10–14 weeks. Another finding which can predict TTTS is folding of the intertwin membrane at 15–17 weeks.[24]

Doppler Studies of Placental Anastomosis

Twin-to-twin transfusion syndrome develops in 15% of patients with A-A versus 61% without an A-A. A-A anastomosis is associated with higher perinatal survival. A-A can be detected after 18 weeks with usual spectral and color Doppler with 85% sensitivity and 97% specificity. Presence of A-A is revealed by a bidirectional speckled pattern on color or power Doppler.

Quintero's Classification of the Severity of TTTS[25] (Modified)

- *Stage I:* Oligo/poly sequence and bladder seen in donor twin
- *Stage II:* Oligo/poly sequence donor bladder not seen. Normal Doppler studies
- *Stage III:* Oligo/poly sequence donor bladder not seen
    - *IIIa:* A-A anastomosis is present.
    - *IIIb:* A-A anastomosis is absent.

Doppler with one of the following factors:

- Absent or reversed diastolic flow in the umbilical artery of the donor twin
- Reversed flow in the ductus venosus of the donor twin
- Pulsatile flow in the umbilical vein of the recipient twin
- *Stage IV:* Fetal hydrops in any one of twins
- *Stage V:* Death of one or both twins

Differential Diagnosis

- Placental insufficiency
- Congenital abnormality
- Umbilical cord abnormality
- Fetal infection
- Preterm PROM in one of the twins

Treatment Modalities

- Serial amnioreduction
- Laser ablation of vascular anastomosis between the twins
- Amniotic septostomy
- Selective feticide

Serial amnioreduction: Removal of amniotic fluid decreases intraamniotic pressure and improves placental perfusion.

The rate of complications is 3–5% which include PROM, preterm labor, and chorioamnionitis.

For stages I and II, it is the best treatment option.

Laser photocoagulation of placental vascular anastomosis: Identify the A-V anastomosis between the twins endoscopically and then these anastomoses are photocoagulated with YAG lasers using microfiber of 400 m which is inserted through the operative channel of the fetoscope. Additionally, amnioreduction is performed.

- PROM is a common complication (10–12%).
- Serious complication is sudden reverse transfusion due to incomplete separation of placental circulation.
- Other complications are pulmonary edema, abruptio placenta, fetal ischemic lesions, and maternal deaths.

Fetal survival requires at least 18% of placental mass for nutrition of donor twin, following photocoagulation of vascular anastomosis.[25]

Laser photocoagulation is more effective than serial amnioreduction with respect to fetal survival and neurological complications and possibly more effective when cardiac dysfunction and growth discordance or Doppler abnormalities are found.[25]

Septostomy: It is intentional perforation of intertwin amniotic membrane to have equilibrium of both sacs amniotic fluid volume. The size should be small, to avoid monoamniotic pregnancy.

Selective feticide: Selective termination of one of the twins is performed after 20 weeks, indications being acardiac twin with TRAP sequence and fetal hydrops in TTTS.

The methods most commonly used are ligature or bipolar cauterization of the umbilical cord, under ultrasonic or fetoscopic guidance.

The survival rate of the other twin is 70–85%.

Complications occur in <15% of the cases.

Preterm delivery is necessary in majority of TTT patients. Use of steroids for accelerating lung maturity should be done.

Outcome

The prognosis of untreated severe TTTS is poor with high reported PNMRs (70–100%) and associated comorbidities such as neurologic, cardiac, and renal impairment in survivors. With advances in the obstetrical management of TTTS, the mortality has decreased, and survivors have improved long-term outcome.

■ MONOAMNIOTIC TWINS

- 1 in 12,500 births
- 50% perinatal mortality mostly due to umbilical cord entanglement, 42–60% which can be detected <24 weeks. In two-third of the cases both of the twins and one-third of the cases one of the twins die.

Complications

TTTS (less due to AA anastomosis), congenital anomaly, preterm birth, low birth weight, and birth weight discordance > 20% are some of the complications.

Fetal surveillance with Doppler is important.

In cord compression: High-velocity blood flow in vein and diastolic notching or absent diastolic flow is seen in umbilical artery.

Fetal heart rate variable deceleration is observed when cord entanglement is present.

Pharmacological treatment by sulindac 200 mg BD has been tried for reduction of amniotic fluid volume which limits fetal movements and cord entanglement.[26]

Monoamniotic twin pregnancy is terminated at 32 weeks by cesarean section to avoid further complications and managed at tertiary centers.

■ CONGENITAL ABNORMALITY

Congenital abnormality is more common in monozygotic.

Neural tube defects (33%), genitourinary system and abdominal wall defects (33%), cardiac defects (14%), VATER sequence (14%), and isolated limb deformity (8%) are seen.[27]

Conjoined twins and fetal acardia are uniquely seen in MZ twins.

Perinatal mortality is 43%.

■ CONJOINED TWINS (FIG. 7)

This is rare and affects 1 in 200 MZ twins, 1 in 900 twins, and 1 in 25,000 live births

Conjoined twins are mono-ovular. They have the same sex and karyotypes.

The female-to-male ratio is 3:1.

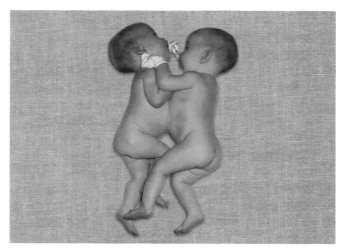

Fig. 7: Conjoined twins.

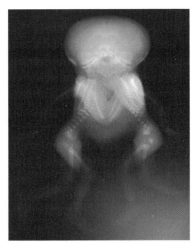

Fig. 8: Ultrasonography of conjoined twins.

Its cause is unknown, may be because of incomplete fission of the embryonic inner cell mass, and appears before the second week of fertilization.

According to the site of unions, it can be *ventral* or *dorsal*.[28]

Ventrally
- Thoracopagus (19%)—joined at chest
- Omphalopagus (18%)—joined at the anterior abdominal wall
- Ischiopagus (11%)—joined at ischium
- Craniopagus (11%)—joined at head

Dorsally
- Craniopagus (5%)—joined at head
- Pyopagus (6%)—joined at buttocks
- Rachipagus (2%)—joined at spine

Ultrasonography (Fig. 8)

Both fetuses
- Thorax and abdomen at same position
- Head at same level and plane and hyperextended
- Face each other
- No change in position on repeat USG

At 18–22 weeks, USG—anatomy of shared organs and other malformations

2D/3D/MRI/CT is done to know the connections.

Termination of pregnancy is done when the brain and heart are shared.

Cesarean section is the treatment option in advanced pregnancy.

Outcomes:
- 40% still born
- 35% die after 1 day

Surgical separation in very few is successful.

After birth, surgical separation can be performed. Nonoperative comfort care may be provided depending upon the extent of the abnormality. In cases of emergency (one of the twins is dead or threatens the survival of the other twin, or if a life-threatening condition exists in one of the twins), separation is performed. Preferably, elective separation should be performed, as it allows stabilization of the infants and extensive evaluation and planning. The survival rate is very low in emergency cases but fairly high for elective separation (80%).

Umbilical Cord Problems

- Single artery
- Velamentous insertion of cord is nine times more common.
- Cord prolapse/vasa previa and torsion of cord
- Cord entanglement in monoamniotic twins

Cerebral Palsy

Neurologic problems are seven times more common in monochorionic preterm fetuses, due to IUFD of co-twin, TTTS, intrauterine growth restriction (IUGR), and discordant twins. [29]

Complete Hydatidiform Mole and Coexisting Fetus

In this condition, there is normal placenta in one twin and complete molar pregnancy in the other; this condition is different from partial mode. Persistent trophoblastic tumors occur more commonly following complete mole. The management of complete mole with coexisting fetus is not certain. These frequently require preterm delivery because of bleeding complications or severe PIH. In some cases, they may require evacuation. Postnatal follow-up with HCG levels is advised.

■ DIAGNOSIS OF MULTIPLE GESTATIONS

Early diagnosis is important for successful outcome and to minimize perinatal losses.

History and Clinical Examination

History
- Maternal family history of twins
- Advanced maternal age and high parity
- History of ART procedure, use of fertility drugs
- Previous history of twins

Clinical Examination
- Clinical examination reveals the height of uterus larger than expected gestational age.
- Uterine palpation may reveal the palpation of three fetal poles.
- Fetal heart rate monitoring with Doppler ultrasonic equipment shows two fetal heart beats at rates distinct

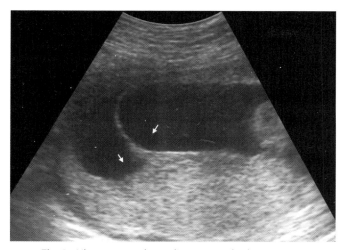

Fig. 9: Ultrasonography to diagnose multiple gestation.

from each other. Careful auscultations with a fetal stethoscope show that two fetal heart sounds are heard as early as 18–20 weeks.

Ultrasonography (Fig. 9)

Sonographical diagnosis of twins can be made as early as 6–7 weeks with the use of vaginal probe. Early in pregnancy, the membrane in between amniotic sacs is difficult to visualize if monochorionic diamniotic pregnancy is present. USG should include assessment of placentation

- Number of placentas and intertwin membranes for assessing amnionicity and chorionicity
- Gender of the baby if only one placenta is seen to confirm the chorionicity

▨ ANTEPARTUM MANAGEMENT

- To reduce perinatal mortality and morbidity in multiple pregnancy
- To predict and prevent preterm labor in multiple gestation
- To monitor fetal growth for early identification of discordant growth
- To monitor maternal and fetal complications common for multifetal gestation
- To counsel patient regarding nutrition and genetic counseling for screening for chromosomal anomalies

Gestational Weight Gain

The following are the recommendations by the Institute of Medicine regarding weight gain by term for women carrying twins:

- BMI < 18.5 kg/m^2 (underweight)—no recommendation due to insufficient data
- BMI 18.5–24.9 kg/m^2 (normal weight)—weight gain 16.8–24.5 kg
- BMI 25.0–29.9 kg/m^2 (overweight)—weight gain 14.1–22.7 kg
- BMI ≥ 30.0 kg/m^2 (obese)—weight gain 11.4–19.1 kg

Prediction and Prevention of Preterm Labor in Multiple Gestations

Multiple gestations have high rates of preterm birth and low birth weight. Majority of adverse perinatal outcomes are because of high rates of prematurity. Complications such as respiratory distress syndrome (RDS), intraventricular hemorrhage, and necrotizing enterocolitis might be present.[30]

Elevated fetal fibronectin level and short cervical length on USG examination may predict pregnancies at increased risk of preterm delivery, although their predictive value is low, and no intervention has been proven to be effective in reducing preterm birth rates.

Prediction of Preterm Labor

Cervical length: There is evidence that extremes of cervical length are useful predictors of preterm delivery in multiple gestations. Cervical length below 2.5 cm at 24 weeks of gestation is the most powerful predictor of preterm birth. Digital cervical assessment is subjective but has the advantage of being inexpensive, widely available, easy to perform and informative when performed by an experienced examiner. The cervical score is calculated as cervical length in centimeters minus internal os dilation in centimeters. A score of 0 or less has a positive predictive value of 69% for preterm labor in primies and 80% for multies.[31]

Ultrasonography: This is the best tool to assess the cervical length. Transvaginal is better.

Fetal fibronectin: Fetal fibronectin detected in cervicovaginal secretions after 21 weeks of gestation in patients of multifetal gestation is associated with an increased risk of preterm birth. The negative predictive value of the test is to reassure and to avoid unnecessary interventions. ELISA (enzyme-linked immunosorbent assay) test concentration > 50 mg/mL in cervicovaginal secretions of twin pregnancy and combined marker. Additionally, risk scoring systems and combined markers which include combinations, history, clinical data, and measurements are useful predictors.

Prevention of Preterm Birth in Multiple Gestations

It is a goal to prevent morbidity and mortality.

Early diagnosis of multiple gestations: Routine use of USG is associated with 98% detection rate of multiple gestations. The RADIUS (Routine Antenatal diagnostic Imaging with Ultrasound) trial did a prospective multicenter study which found USG as useful tool for detection of twins.[32]

Flowchart 2: Management of vaginal delivery with first cephalic twin.

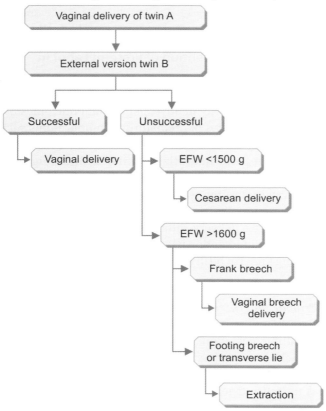

(EFW: estimated fetal weight)

Home uterine monitoring: It has been used to alert both patients and treating doctors to appreciate prelabor contractions. Home uterine monitoring for multiple gestations has been advocated based on observations that they have more frequent contractions. It may be useful in certain situations but is not cost effective and has not become standard treatment for multiple gestations.

Use of progesterone: Progesterone is useful as it encourages uterine quiescence through downregulation of oxytocin receptors, reduction in gap junctions, and direct relaxation of myometrial muscles.[33]

Prophylactic cervical encirclage: The majority of available evidence does not support the use of routine cerclage for multiple gestations. The Royal College of Obstetricians and Gynaecologists (RCOG) conducted trials that showed no difference in outcome with or without cerclage.[34] No benefit was associated. Moreover, complications such as PPROM and chorioamnionitis were increased. With potential harm and no proven benefit, prophylactic cerclage is not recommended for twin gestation. However, it can be used for usual indications such as extremely short cervix and incompetent os. There is no convincing evidence till date that encirclage is effective in preventing preterm births and reducing perinatal morbidity/mortality.

Prophylactic tocolysis: Routine prophylactic use of oral tocolytics cannot be recommended in multiple gestations according to current evidence. Administration of tocolytic drugs to asymptomatic women for prevention of preterm labor and birth does not significantly reduce preterm birth. Randomized controlled trials failed to show an increase in gestational age or improvement of perinatal morbidity and mortality with the use of prophylactic β mimetics in multiple gestations.[35]

Beta-adrenergic drugs should be used judiciously in women with multiple gestations, as they have a higher blood volume and lower colloid osmotic pressure than women with singleton pregnancies and hence are at a higher risk of pulmonary edema.

Hospitalized bed rest: The Cochrane database systematic reviews published a meta-analysis of six randomized prospective trials of routine hospitalized bed rest and multiple gestations.[36] In the analysis of 600 patients, no difference was seen in perinatal mortality, preterm delivery or very low birth weight babies, and significant statistical decrease in low birth weight infants. The other studies available and data do not support routine hospitalization for twin gestation. There is increase in cost care in patient management. There does not appear to be a benefit involving either gestational age at preterm delivery or perinatal morbidity. Prolonged bed rest (unrelated to delivery) was proven harmful in a population-based cohort study of pregnant women as it was found to be associated with an increased risk of venous thromboembolism.

Decreased maternal activity and bed rest: Bed rest is well accepted and inexpensive. There is evidence that maternal rest decreases the frequency of uterine contractions. It increases fetal weight and preterm birth. Decreased activity and outpatient bed rest are widely recommended by obstetricians, and evidence suggests that there is likely small benefit in terms of reducing the risk of preterm delivery and subsequent sequel but at what gestational age to initiate restrictions and how long to maintain are unknown.[37]

Steroids: Use of maternally administered steroids for fetal benefit is more widespread.[38] The benefits of use of steroids on various fetal organs include decrease in RDS, ICH, and necrotizing enterocolitis.

Two doses of betamethasone (12 mg, 12 hours apart) or four doses of dexamethasone (6 mg 12 hours) intramuscularly are given. Routine prophylactic administration of steroids in all multifetal gestations is not recommended and may have adverse effects.

Screening for Chromosomal Anomalies

Risk of aneuploidy is higher for twin pregnancy because there is more than one fetus at risk and with advanced maternal age, risk increases.[39]

First-trimester screening using NT and biochemical markers for detection of Down syndrome has a sensitivity of 80%. Using NT alone for aneuploidy screening for multifetal pregnancy, it is possible to know the individual twin affected. Increased NT thickness is a predictor of TTTS[40] and risk factor for congenital heart disease and other conditions.

Abnormal first-trimester screening requires further evaluation with chorionic villus sampling (CVS) or amniocentesis. Because of associated complications with these procedures, it is better to screen them in the second trimester with quad test. CVS and amniocentesis are indicated in high-risk twin pregnancy for aneuploidy. CVS is equally effective, but individual samples cannot be obtained unless placentas are separate.

Screening for Down Syndrome:
- *Combined test:* Screening with the first-trimester combined test can provide fetus-specific risk assessment. Increased NT is a marker for Down syndrome, other aneuploidies, development of TTTS, and congenital malformation.
- *Noninvasive screening (cell-free DNA):* Prenatal screening using cell-free DNA is challenging as the fetal cell-free DNA in the maternal circulation is derived from each fetus. Less validation data are available from twin gestations than from singletons because it is impossible to determine which twin is abnormal based on cell-free DNA analysis alone. The results are reported for the entire pregnancy, and further invasive testing is required to distinguish which twin is affected. Moreover, the amount of cell-free DNA contributed by each twin is lower than in a singleton pregnancy.

Second-trimester screening with triple or quad test has sensitivity of 60–70% and false-positive rate of 5%. Tests based on zygosity, maternal age, period of gestation, NT, and biochemical analysis give sensitivity up to 73%, but contribution of both fetuses to serum markers is criticized. Karyotyping is recommended when major structural anomalies are detected at the time of USG in the second trimester

■ GENETIC COUNSELING

Multifetal gestation presents special problems in prenatal testing, problems of genetic evaluation, and interpretation of results.[41]

Structural anomalies are more common in MZ twin and USG diagnosis may be difficult due to position, crowding, and transducer application. The risk of aneuploidy is increased in DZ twins. Biochemical screening procedures are affected due to different contributions from fetus and changes in maternal plasma volume. Interpretation of the results is complicated in the amniocentesis procedure due to diffusion of amniotic fluid across the membrane. Patients should be counseled regarding postprocedure pregnancy loss.

Chorionic villous sampling done in the first trimester of pregnancy in twin pregnancy has a high (5%) risk of twin-to-twin contamination. The ethical and practical management problems regarding one fetal demise or abnormality of one fetus should be discussed with the patients.

Selective fetal reduction leads to better survival of the other twin, and it is a safe procedure. Proper counseling should be done.

■ ANTENATAL CARE

Extra precautions and screening are required in multifetal gestation.
- Antenatal visits are required for every 2 weeks and more frequently if she develops complications.
- Special attention for checking blood pressure, weight gain, and uterine fundal growth. Routine lab investigations should include proteinuria and Hb frequently.
- Fetal surveillance should start earlier.
- *Counseling regarding nutrition and genetics:* The diet of the mother should include increased calorie intake to 300 kcal and optimal weight gain should be around 1.75 pounds/week after 20 weeks. The total weight gain should be at least 18–20 kg with an emphasis on adequate weight gain before 24 weeks. Inadequate early weight gain is associated with pre-eclampsia and poor intrauterine growth. Elemental iron 60 mg/day; folic acid 1 mg/day; and other minerals such as calcium, magnesium, and zinc; antioxidants; and vitamins E and C should be supplemented in diet.
- USG examination every 3–4 weeks to evaluate fetal growth
- Cervical length assessment from 18 weeks onward, effacement if seen early—rule out intrauterine infections and other causes
- Repeat USG at 24 weeks to know the cervical length and do fetal fibronectin level. USG also helps to rule out congenital abnormalities and chorionicity of placenta.
- Extra rest is required for mutifetal gestation.
- Hospital rest if complication ensues. Steroid in the form of betamethasone 12 mg IM 12 hourly should be given in all multifetal gestations.

Antepartum Fetal Surveillance to Evaluate Fetal Well-being

Antepartum fetal surveillance is indicated in high-risk situations such as:
- Fetal growth restriction in one or both fetuses
- Discordant growth

- Abnormal amniotic fluid distribution
- Monochorionic-monoamniotic twins, monochorionic-diamniotic twins
- Associated maternal conditions such as PIH and diabetes

Nonstress test (NST) and modified biophysical profile are useful tests. Amniotic fluid volume and index can be measured by various methods, and subjective valuation is the preferred method.

Among all tests, NST and Doppler velocimetry are more predictive of fetal well-being.[17]

The positive predictive value of abnormal Doppler outcome was 90% and negative predictive value was 95.6% in twin pregnancies.[18]

Doppler velocimetry may provide a measure of fetal well-being as in singleton.

Fetal Pulmonary Maturity

Pulmonary maturation done by determination of the lecithin-sphingomyelin (L:S) ratio is often required in multifetal gestation. It occurs simultaneously in both the sacs. But in twins with discordant growth, a growth-restricted baby has more advanced lung maturation so the testing should be done in the larger fetus.

Chorionicity-based Follow-up

Monochorionic Twins

Monitoring of monochorionic/diamniotic pregnancies should begin at 16–18 weeks by assessment of amniotic fluid volume and fetal bladder in both twins for early detection of TTTS. Middle cerebral artery peak systolic velocity (MCA-PSV) measurement must begin in both fetuses at 26–28 weeks for early detection of twin anemia-polycythemia sequence (TAPS). The diagnosis of TAPS is based on MCA-PSV > 1.5 MoM in one twin and <0.8 MoM in the other twin.

There are no guidelines to determine the optimal frequency of monitoring, but measurement every 2–3 weeks is reasonable. Monitoring may be more frequent if abnormalities are detected. The sonographic finding of oligohydramnios (maximal vertical pocket < 2 cm) and polyhydramnios (maximal vertical pocket > 8 cm before 20 weeks and >10 cm after 20 weeks) can detect TTTS.

Monochorionic placentation results in unequal sharing of the placenta and hence is a significant risk factor for discordant growth and TTTS. Every 2–4-weekly ultrasonographic evaluation for fetal growth is required to monitor for TTTS and TAPS.

Dichorionic Twins

It is unnecessary to do close fetal monitoring for TTTS and TAPS in dichorionic twins. An USG examination may be performed every 4–6 weeks after the fifth month of gestation to monitor fetal growth (as fetal growth deceleration leading to discordancy is optimally detected between 20 and 28 weeks). Continue serial USG assessment until delivery unless some anomaly is detected.

■ PRETERM PREMATURE RUPTURE OF MEMBRANES

An ideal approach to PPROM in multiple pregnancies involves balance between maternal and fetal risks.

The incidence is two times higher than in singleton pregnancy.[42]

It is common in the presenting sac and clinical evaluation of vaginal pooling, ferning, and nitrazine testing confirms the diagnosis.

Premature rupture of membranes typically occurs in the presenting sac but can develop in the nonpresenting twin too (e.g., after amniocentesis).

The diagnosis is more difficult in PPROM of nonpresenting sac as leakage is intermittent.

The exact incidence and clinical course of PPROM in nonpresenting sac are unknown.

The rupture of dividing membranes in monochorionic-diamniotic twins is a unique complication, and complications are similar to monoamniotic twins. It can be iatrogenic following amniocentesis or due to infections or developmental disturbances or actions. It carries a perinatal mortality of 44%.

The latency period between rupture of membranes and delivery of conservatively managed twins is the same as singletons. The length of latency is related to gestation at the time of rupture of membranes and is prolonged when PPROM occurs prior to 30 weeks and shorter before 30 weeks. Neonatal outcome is the same for singletons and multiple gestations. Median latency is of 1.1 days.

Chorioamnionitis and funisitis in the nonpresenting twin are less common in dichorionic than in monochorionic twins.

Management of PPROM in Multiple Pregnancy[43]

PPROM in multifetal gestation is associated with an increased risk of:

- Infection
- Abruptio placenta
- Cord accidents

In twins, if PPROM is in a nonpresenting twin, there is an increased risk of RDS and prolonged neonatal intensive care unit (NICU) stay because of relative immaturity. The patient should be counseled that the nonpresenting fetus has a higher risk of respiratory complications. Gestational age at which PPROM occurs is critical for the management, in the point of view of prematurity infection and oligohydramnios.

Infections can affect mother and fetus from ruptured sac and adjacent fetus with intact sac.

Oligohydramnios can lead to pulmonary hypoplasia, skeletal deformities, and amniotic band syndrome. PPROM is classified as follows:

- *Previable:* <23 completed weeks of gestation
- *Remote from term:* 23–31 weeks
- *Near term:* 32–36 weeks

Once the diagnosis is confirmed:

- Avoid digital examination
- Visualize with sterile speculum and send culture
- Watch for labor, infection, abruption, fetal status

In PPROM after 34 weeks, the risk of chorioamnionitis and cord complications, such as cord compression, is more likely so delivery is recommended. Antibiotic prophylaxis should be given.

In PPROM between 32 and 34 weeks, conservative management with close monitoring is recommended; adjunctive antibiotic therapy and antenatal corticosteroids are given.

In PPROM at remote from term, conservative management is given as above with tocolytics for steroids and antibiotics to act to prolong the pregnancy till 34 weeks.

In PPROM at <23 weeks, patients are counseled about fetal and maternal risks and benefits of expectant versus termination. Assessment of maternal and fetal status is done carefully till viability is reached. Exclude any infections. Tocolysis antibiotics and cerclage can be tried. Selective reduction of a previable fetus in a ruptured sac is a reasonable option in carefully selected cases or termination of the entire pregnancy may be the best approach as there are increased chances of infections and related complications.

■ INTRAPARTUM MANAGEMENT OF TWINS

Timing of the Delivery

The gestational age that is considered term is earlier in twin gestation.

Various population data shows increased perinatal morbidity, and mortality increases as gestational age is advanced beyond 38 weeks. It is recommended that delivery of uncomplicated twin pregnancy should be electively done at 38 weeks and not later than 39 weeks. In complicated twin pregnancies by IUGR, growth discordance, or maternal complications such as PIH, delivery should be at earlier gestation (36–37 weeks). Fetal lung maturity should be seen in twins complicated with maternal diabetes before undertaking elective delivery.[44]

Careful assessment of amniotic fluid volume, fetal growth, and complete biophysical profile must be undertaken and should be completely reassuring.

Intrapartum management of multiple gestation is a multidisciplinary approach, and a team to handle obstetric emergencies and neonatal problems should be available.

- Obstetrician experienced with operative vaginal deliveries
- Anesthetist
- Neonatologist
- Additional staff sisters

Apart from routine management as in singletons, special precautions are needed to handle twin delivery.

- Delivery should be conducted in a well-equipped operative labor room with all facilities.
- Upon admission complete blood count, including blood grouping and Rh typing, should be sent.
- Intravenous access with a large-bore indwelling catheter should be obtained and maintained during labor.
- The American College of Obstetricians and Gynecologists (ACOG) practice bulletin on obstetric analgesia and anesthesia recommends placement of an epidural catheter in cases of twin gestation in high risk and is ideal for analgesia during labor.[45]
- A bedside USG is done after admission to verify the fetal weight of each fetus.
- USG examination is repeated after the delivery of the first fetus to ascertain the position and presentation of the second twin.
- Electronic fetal monitoring should include both twins simultaneously.
- Oxytocin drip can be used if there is an abnormal pattern of uterine contractions.
- Active management of the third stage prevents PPH and its complications.

Even though there are 10 possible combinations of fetal positions for twins, they can be simplified and categorized in three groups:[46]

1. *Both fetuses in vertex position (vertex–vertex):* 40–50%
2. *Twin A vertex twin B nonvertex:* 25–35%
3. *Twin A nonvertex twin B any other:* 20–25%

Intrapartum assessment of fetal positions and assessment of fetal positions and fetal weight are very important in decisions and management.

It is necessary to counsel the patients about the potential morbidity and mortality of preterm births, discordant growth babies, and deciding the route of delivery of vertex nonvertex twins. Kiely reported that the overall intrapartum death rate with twins is about three times higher (6.1/1,000 live births) than for singletons.[47]

If birth weight is below 2,500 g, twins have a lower likelihood of intrapartum death. The prediction of fetal weight based on the measurement of abdominal circumference and femur length is as reliable as derived from the measurement of three or more biometric parameters.[48]

Both the fetuses may be delivered vaginally or by cesarean section. Additionally after the birth of the first fetus a breech extraction, external cephalic version (ECV), internal podalic version (IPV), with assisted or total breech extraction, cesarean or combination of operative interventions may be necessary to deliver the second fetus.[49]

Understanding of alternative options and proper expertise are needed to reduce the rising rates of cesarean section births in twin delivery.

■ ROUTES OF DELIVERY

Twin A Vertex–Twin B Vertex

This combination is seen in 40%. It is the most common presentation.

In majority of them, vaginal delivery is anticipated. Presentation of the second fetus is assessed after the delivery of the first fetus. Cesarean may be necessary for twin B vertex in 5% of cases with cord prolapse, fetal distress, abruptio placenta, and malpresentation.

The time interval between the deliveries of the two fetuses should be optimally <30 minutes and shorter intervals may correlate with decreased incidence of fetal acidosis in the second twin, as was observed earlier has undergone change. The interval between the births is no longer considered critical; close monitoring of the second twin by continuous electronic fetal monitoring and sonography is recommended.[50] Oxytocin drip and augmentation help to achieve satisfactory vaginal delivery.

Delivery should be hastened in cases of cord prolapsed, premature separation of placenta, or fetal distress.

Twin A Vertex–Twin B Nonvertex

It occurs in about one-third of the cases.
Controversial issues exist regarding management.
Decisions are based on:
- Gestational age
- Expected fetal weight
- Associated complications
- Clinical expertise to perform ECV, IPV, and breech extraction as well as availability of the facilities for neonatal care

Options available:
- Cesarean delivery
  - Vaginal delivery of both twins by successful ECV[46] of twin B or breech extraction of twin B

The ACOG in its bulletin has acknowledged the conflicting data on the management of twins—vertex breech or vertex transverse positions.[8]

Success of ECV depends on five factors:[51]
1. Parity
2. Cervical dilatation
3. EFW
4. Location of placenta
5. Station of the vertex

Another option is breech extraction, and various studies indicate that breech extraction is safer than ECV of malpresenting twin B. IPV and breech extraction are other treatment options available and need expertise.

Before undertaking breech extraction, attempts should be made so that the actual weight of the second baby is at least ≥1,500 g for better outcome.[48]

The third option for vertex–nonvertex twins is cesarean delivery. The published research "term breech collaborative trial over two singletons to breech extractions versus cesarean sections" concluded that for every 14 abdominal deliveries one newborn will avoid death or serious morbidity.[51]

The ACOG and RCOG issued statement encouraging clinicians to undertake breech extraction for nonvertex second twin.[52]

Recommendations were based on the randomized trial of Rabinovici et al. involving vaginal or cesarean section for the second nonvertex twin which showed the same neonatal outcome and more febrile morbidity with the cesarean delivery group.[53]

Twin A Nonvertex–Twin B Others

It occurs in 20% of cases and is the least common presentation (twin A in nonvertex position). The intrapartum management is dictated by the presentation of twin A. The twins are at risk of fetal entanglement and perinatal mortality if vaginal delivery is attempted. The risk factors for entanglement include twin A breech–twin B vertex, IUGR, fetal weight below 2 kg, and demise of one twin.

According to ACOG recommendation, cesarean delivery is the best route of delivery for this twin.[8]

There are reports in the literature where ECV was performed of twin A successfully and breech delivery of twin A in various centers of Europe.[54,55] Due to lack of larger studies and expertise and complications, the ACOG recommends cesarean delivery for twin A/nonvertex twin B as the best option.

Monoamniotic Twins

They occur in 1% of MZ twins. Once monoamniotic twins are diagnosed, the possible complications such as congenital abnormalities, TTTS, cord entanglement or accidents, preterm births or IUFD can occur. Patients should be counseled. Cesarean delivery is the best option to deliver these patients. Conjoined twins are to be delivered by cesarean section.

Indications of Elective Cesarean Section in Twins

- *Malpresentation:* First twin nonvertex
- Dystocia
- Conjoined twins at term
- Monoamniotic twins
- Previous cesarean scar
- Obstetric factors

Cesarean section

- Epidural anesthesia is preferred as it avoids fetal hypoxia or depression.
- Transverse incision is preferred (abdominal and over the uterus).
- Conjoined twins may need classical uterine incision.

Summary of Recommendations[56]

- *Level A (consistent scientific evidence)*
  - Upon admission, a sonographic examination should be completed to evaluate fetal position.
  - If vaginal delivery is planned, an estimate of fetal weight should be assessed unless this has been recently documented (within 2–4 weeks).
  - For twins in vertex–vertex position, lower segment cesarean section LSCS delivery should be reserved for obstetric indications.
- *Level B (limited evidence)*
  - ECV of malpresenting twin B is associated with a higher rate of complications than breech extraction.
  - For vertex–nonvertex vaginal delivery

▤ INTERLOCKING TWINS

It is a rare complication (1 in 1,000 twins; 1: 50,000 births).

The PNMR is 62–80%; it is possible with breech–vertex combination and cesarean section will save twin B.

Interlocking of various body parts may also happen in vertex–vertex, VX-Tr, Br-Br may present as abnormal labor pattern and arrest disorders.

▤ MANAGEMENT OF GESTATION WITH HIGH FETAL NUMBER

Triplets occur in 6,000–9,000 deliveries. They have a five-fold increase in adverse perinatal outcome, mainly because of PROM and TTTS. Fetal and neonatal morbidity and mortality are high in patients with high fetal numbers. Preterm delivery affects >85% and is an important hazard with high fetal numbers. The mean gestational age at delivery for triplets is 32–33 weeks and for quadruplets it is 30–32 weeks. The incidences of other complications

are greater such as anemia, pre-eclampsia, and PPH. Cesarean section is common because of the difficulties in monitoring and has more mortality and morbidity. Multiple pregnancies with high fetal numbers require tertiary care centers and NICU setup. With proper modern perinatal management, the survival rates are improving.

Consensus expert views relating to clinical practice[57]

- The risk of multiple pregnancies should be reduced by conservative use of ovarian stimulation with careful monitoring according to published guidelines (RCOG, 1999; NICE, 2004; Grade A).
- In view of the risks associated with multiple pregnancies, consideration should be given to transferring only a single embryo in women undergoing IVF (Grade A).
- In view of the changing effects of maternal age and fertility treatment on multiple pregnancy rates, there needs to be a mechanism for recording their impact on the rates of multiple pregnancies.
- Prepregnancy counseling regarding the risks of multiple pregnancies should be given to a woman undergoing fertility treatment (Grade C).
- Parents of high-order multiple pregnancies (≥3) should be counseled and offered multifetal pregnancy reduction (MFPR) to twins in specialist centers (Grade B).
- Long-term neurodevelopmental follow-up studies are needed for survivors of multiple pregnancies who have undergone MFPR (Grade C).
- All women with a multiple pregnancy should be offered an USG examination at 10–13 weeks of gestation (Grade B) to assess:
  - Viability
  - Chorionicity
  - Major congenital malformation
  - NT for designation of risk of aneuploidy and TTTS
- All monochorionic twins should have a detailed USG scan which includes extended views of the fetal heart (Grade B).
- Monochorionic twins require increased USG surveillance from 16 weeks of gestation onward to detect TTTS and growth discordance. This should be offered at an interval of 2 weeks (Grade C).
- NT-based screening should be offered as the preferred method of aneuploidy screening in women with multiple pregnancy (Grade B).
- Monochorionic twins that are discordant for fetal anomaly must be referred at an early gestation for assessment and counseling in a regional fetal medicine center (Grade B).
- Twins that are discordant for fetal anomaly should be managed in fetal medicine centers with specific expertise (Grade C).

- Hospitals should organize antenatal and postnatal care around specialist-led, multidisciplinary multiple pregnancy clinics (Grade C).
- The organization of antenatal twin clinics should be facilitated by care pathways and allow referral to regional fetal medicine centers when appropriate (Grade C).
- The lead clinician for multiple pregnancy clinics should have expertise in USG and in the intrapartum care of multiple pregnancies (Grade C).
- TTTS should be managed in conjunction with regional fetal medicine centers with recourse to specialist expertise (Grade C).
- Fetoscopic laser ablation is the treatment of choice in severe TTTS presenting prior to 26 weeks of gestation (Grade A).
- Single-twin demise in a monochorionic twin pregnancy should be referred and assessed in a regional fetal medicine center (Grade B).
- The survivor after single-twin demise in monochorionic twins should have follow-up USG and, if normal, an MRI examination of the fetal brain 2–3 weeks after the co-twin death. Counseling should include the long-term morbidity in this condition (Grade C).
- Vaginal delivery of twins should be performed in a setting with continuous intrapartum monitoring, immediate recourse to cesarean section, appropriate analgesia, and an obstetrician experienced in twin delivery (Grade B).
- In view of the increased risk of stillbirth in twin pregnancy, elective delivery is recommended between 37 and 38 weeks of gestation (Grade C).
- Mothers with a multiple pregnancy have a need for specific information, including discussion of delivery and postnatal well-being, including breastfeeding (Grade C).
- The role of midwives and other healthcare specialists is integral to the management of multiple pregnancies within specialist clinics (Grade C).
- Additional support to women is available from TAMBA (Twins and Multiple Birth Association) and the Multiple Births Foundation, and this should be encouraged (Grade C).
- There is a need to support women emotionally with multiple pregnancies (Grade A).
- There is a need to recognize early signs of perinatal psychological disturbance, which is increased after multiple births, and to offer treatment (Grade A).

■ KEY PRE- AND POSTNATAL EVENTS TO BE OFFERED IN PREGNANCY

Dichorionic Twins

- *Multiples clinic:* Lead clinician with multidisciplinary team

- *USG at 10–13 weeks:* (1) viability, (2) chorionicity, (3) NT: aneuploidy
- Structural anomaly scan at 20–22 weeks
- Serial fetal growth scans, e.g., 24, 28, 32 and then 2–4-weekly
- BP monitoring and urinalysis at 20, 24, 28 and then 2-weekly
- Discussion of a woman's/family needs relating to twins
- *34–36 weeks:* Discussion of the mode of delivery and intrapartum care
- Elective delivery at 37–38 completed weeks

Monochorionic Twins

- *Multiples clinic:* Lead clinician with multidisciplinary team
- *USG at 10–13 weeks:* (1) viability, (2) chorionicity, (c) NT: aneuploidy/TTTS
- *USG surveillance for TTTS and discordant growth:* At 16 weeks and then 2-weekly
- Structural anomalies scan at 20–22 weeks (including fetal ECHO)
- Fetal growth scans at 2-weekly intervals until delivery
- BP monitoring and urinalysis at 20, 24, 28 and then 2-weekly
- Discussion of a woman's/family needs relating to twins
- *32–34 weeks:* Discussion of the mode of delivery and intrapartum care
- Elective delivery at 36–37 completed weeks (if uncomplicated)
- Postnatal advice and support (hospital- and community-based) to include breastfeeding and contraceptive advice

Postnatal Issues

Breast-feeding is ideal for twin gestation as in singletons. The rate of successful breast-feeding of both is dependent on proper counseling, motivation, and support. The success rate also depends on proper training of specific techniques such as double football and double cradle positions. One must also realize that partial breast-feeding may also be helpful. Counseling should start in the antenatal period which usually yields satisfactory results

Perinatal Mortality

Averaging five times higher than singletons, the risk is higher for MZ twins and twins displaying discordant growth.[47]

The largest single cause of perinatal death however is prematurity (cerebral palsy, microcephaly, porencephaly, multicystic encephalomalacia). Twins are responsible for 25% of preterm perinatal deaths and 10% of all perinatal mortality. In addition to prematurity, etiologies include congenital malformations, TTTS, uteroplacental insufficiency, birth trauma or hypoxia, infection, and growth retardation.

Neonatal mortality (51 per 100) rather than fetal (28 per 100) PNMR, it varies with birth order and type of placentation. The second twin is at risk. Monoamniotic-monochorionic has poor prognosis. Monoamniotic-dizygotic has 26% PNMR.

Twins or higher order multiple order pregnancy may at a later age demonstrate increased rates of neonatal morbidity.

■ PREVENTIVE INTERVENTIONS FOR MULTIPLE PREGNANCIES

The American Society for Reproductive Medicine has initiated effort to reduce the incidence of multifetal gestation by optimizing ARTs. It is observed that the fewer the numbers of embryos transferred after IVF, the lower the risk of multiple pregnancies.[58]

Recent practice is to offer only two embryos to optimize the chance of pregnancy without significantly increasing the risks of multiple pregnancies.

Gonadotropin stimulation which is less intensive reduces the incidence of multiple gestation.

■ MULTIFETAL PREGNANCY REDUCTION

To reduce the risk and avoid complications of high-order pregnancy, MFPR is done.

It can be done by various methods—transcervical, transvaginal, transabdominal. The preferred method is transabdominal at 10–13 weeks. This gestational age was chosen because any spontaneous abortions have already occurred, the remaining fetuses are large enough to be evaluated ultrasonographically, the amount of devitalized fetal tissue remaining after the procedure is small, and the risk of aborting the entire pregnancy as a result of the procedure is low. Smallest or anomalous fetus is chosen and potassium chloride is injected into the heart or thorax of the selected fetus under ultrasonic guidance. Postprocedure loss is 11.7% and the incidence of fetal growth restriction in the remaining fetus is increased.[59]

■ SELECTIVE TERMINATION

A structurally or genetically anomalous fetus which can affect the other fetus can be terminated selectively. With the identification of multiple fetuses discordant for structural or genetic abnormalities, two options are available—either abortion of all fetuses or selective termination of the abnormal fetus, and continuation of the pregnancy. Selective termination is performed later in gestation (unless the anomaly is severe but not lethal) than selective reduction as the anomalies are typically not discovered until the second trimester.

Before selective termination, a precise diagnosis for the anomalous fetus and its location is a mandate. The same holds true while performing a genetic amniocentesis on a multifetal gestation. Selective termination is usually done using potassium chloride and results in the delivery of a viable neonate in >90% of cases. The pregnancy loss rates are 7.1% (pregnancies reduced to singletons) and 13% (those reduced to twins). The gestational age at the time of the procedure does not appear to affect the rate of pregnancy loss.

KEY POINTS

- The chorionicity and amnionicity should be determined in the first trimester. The chorionicity is determined by examining the membrane thickness at the site of their insertion into the placenta; a T sign indicates monochorionicity, while a lambda (λ) sign is diagnostic of dichorionicity

- Twins conceived by in-vitro fertilization should be dated using the date of fertilization. In all other cases, the pregnancy should be dated according to the crown–rump length of the larger twin. Dating should take place when the crown–rump length is between 45 mm and 84 mm (equivalent to 11+0 to 13+6 weeks of gestation). Twin pregnancies presenting later than 14 weeks' gestation should be dated according to the head circumference of the larger twin.

- In uncomplicated dichorionic twin pregnancies, following the first trimester scan, subsequent scans should be performed around the following gestations: weeks 20 (the second trimester anomaly scan), 24, 28, 32, and 36.

- In uncomplicated monochorionic twin pregnancies, following the first trimester scan, further scans should be performed at least every 2 weeks from 16 weeks' gestation in order to detect twin-to-twin transfusion syndrome

- Mode of delivery is recommended as following:
  - Vaginal delivery on labor ward if twin one is cephalic
  - Cesarean section if both twins or twin one are non-cephalic
  - Cesarean section if monochorionic monoamniotic twins

- Continuous cardiotocography of both twins throughout labor. It is recommended that twin one should be monitored using fetal scalp electrode, unless it is contraindicated. Twin two should be monitored using an external transducer

- Delivery should take place in a setting where ready recourse to operative delivery, if necessary, is available

- The anesthetist and neonatologist should be alerted at delivery

- Delivery of twin two should not be rushed if there is no cord prolapse or bleeding, and if the fetal heart rate remains normal. The interval between delivery of twin one and twin two should generally be less than 30 minutes, but may be prolonged if the fetal heart rate is normal
- Twin two may need stabilization of lie, internal podalic version, breech extraction, or immediate cesarean section
- Active management of the third stage of labor is indicated.

■ REFERENCES

1. Dickey RP, Taylor SN, Lu PY, Pelletier WD, Zender JL, Matulich EM, et al. Spontaneous reduction of multiple pregnancy: Incidence and effect on outcome. Am J Obstet Gynecol. 2002;186:77.
2. American College of Obstetricians and Gynecologists (ACOG). Multiple gestation: Complicated twin, triplet, and high order multifetal pregnancy. Practice Bulletin No. 56. Washington, DC: ACOG; 2004.
3. Blondel B, Kogan MD, Alexander GR, Dattani N, Kramer MS, Macfarlane A, et al. The impact of the increasing number of multiple births on the rates of preterm births and low birth weight: an international study. Am J Public Health. 2002;92:1323.
4. Umstad MP, Gronow MJ. Multiple pregnancy; a modern epidemic? Med J Aust. 2003;178(12):613-5.
5. Basso O, Nohr E. Risk of twinning as a function of material height and body mass index. J Am Med Assoc. 2004;291:1564-6.
6. Leduc L, Tasker L, Rinfret D. Persistence of adverse obstetric and neonatal outcomes in monochorionic placentation. Am J Obstet Gynecol. 2005;193:1670-5.
7. Vyssiere C, Heim N, Campus EP, Hilton YE, Nisand YF. Determination of chorionicity in twin gestation by high frequency abdominal ultrasonography; counting the layers of the dividing membranes. Am J Obstet Gynecol 1996; 175:1529-33.
8. American College of Obstetricians and Gynecologists (ACOG). Special problems of multiple gestations. Educational Bulletin No. 253. Washington, DC: ACOG; 1998.
9. Trogstad L, Krondal AS, Stoltenberg C, Magnus P, Nesheim BI, Eskild A. Recurrent risk of preeclampsia in twin and singleton pregnancies. Am J Med Genet. 2004;126A:41-5.
10. Rydhstroem H, Heraib F. Gestational duration, and fetal and infant mortality for twins vs singletons. Twin Res. 2001;4(4):227-31.
11. Riley M, Halliday J. Births in Victoria 1999-2000. Melbourne: Department of Human Services; 2001.
12. Pharoah PO, Adi Y. Consequences in utero death in a twin pregnancy. Lancet. 2000;355:1594-602.
13. Rydhstroem H. Discordant birth weight and late fetal death in like sexed and unliked sexed twin pairs; A population based study. Br. J Obstet Gynecol. 1994;101:765-9.
14. Driggers R W, Blakemore KJ, Bird C, Ackerman KE, Hutchins GM. A pathogenesis of acardiac twinning; clues from an almost acardiac twin. Fetal Diagn. Ther. 2002;17(3):185-7.
15. Gimmenez-Scherer JA, Davies BR. Malformations in acardiac twins are consistent with reversed blood flow: liver as a clue to their pathogenesis. Ped Develop Pathol. 2003. [online] Available from https://doi.org/10.1007/s10024-002-1002-0 [Last accessed October, 2020]
16. Van Allen MI, Smith DW, Sheppard TH. Twin reversed arterial perfusion (TRAP) sequence: A study of 14 twin pregnancy with acardius. Semin Perinatal. 1983;7:285-93.
17. Hanafy A, Peterson CM. Twin reversed arterial perfusion (TRAP) sequence: Case reports and review of literature. Aust NZ J Obstet Gynecol. 1997;37:187-91.
18. Billah KL Shah K, Odwin C. Ultrasonographic diagnosis and management of acardiac acephalus twin pregnancy. Med Ultrasound. 1984;8:108-10.
19. Ash K, Harman CR, Gritter H. TRAP sequence a successful outcome with indomethacin treatment. Obstet Gynecol. 1990;76:960-2.
20. Simpson PD, Trudinger BJ, Walker A, Baird PJ. The intrauterine treatment fetal cardiac failure in a twin pregnancy with an acardiac, acephalic monster. Am J Obstet Gynecol. 1983;147:842-4.
21. Robie GF, Payne GG, Morgan MA. Selective delivery of an acardiac acephalic twin. N Engl Med. 1989;320:512-3.
22. McCurdy CM, Childers JM, Seeds JW. Ligation of the umbilical cord of an acardiac acephalus with an endoscopic intrauterine technique. Obstet Gynecol. 1993;82:708-11.
23. Tsao K, Feldstein VA, Albanase CT, Sandberg PL, Lee H, Harrison MR, et al. Selective reduction of acardiac twin by radiofrequency ablation. Am J Obstet Gynecol. 2002;187(3):635-40.
24. Taylor MJ, Denbow ML, Duncan KR, Overton TG, Fisk NM. Antenatal factors at diagnosis that predict outcome in twin-twin transfusion syndrome. Am J Obstet Gynecol. 2000;183:1023-8.
25. Quintero RA, Morales WJ, Allen MH. Staging of twin-twin transfusion syndrome. J Perinatal. 1997;19:550.
26. Pasquin PL, Wimmalesundera RC, Fichera A, Barigye O, Chappell L, Fisk NM. High perinatal survival in monoamniotic twins managed by prophylactic sulindac, intestine ultrasound surveillance and cesarean delivery at 32 weeks gestation. Ultrasound Obstet Gynecol. 2006;28:681-7.
27. Cameron AH, Edwards JH, Derom R, Thiery M, Boelaert R. The value of twin surveys in the study of malformations. Eur J Obstet Gynecol Reprod Biol. 1983;14:347.
28. Spencer K. Anatomic description of conjoined twins: A plea for standardized terminology. J Pediatr Surg. 1996;31:941.
29. Adegbite AL, Castille S, Ward S, Bajoria R. Neuromorbidity in preterm twins in relation to chorionicity and discordant birth weight. Am J Obstet Gynecol. 2004;190:156-63.
30. Goldernberg RL, Iams JD. the preterm prediction study: the risk factors in twin gestations. Am J Obstet Gynecol. 1996;175:1047-53.
31. Houston MC, Marivate M, Philpott RH. Factors associated with preterm labor and changes in the cervix before labour in twin pregnancy. Br J Obstet Gynecol. 1982;89:190.
32. Ewingman BG, Crane JP. Effect of prenatal ultrasound scanning for on perinatal outcome. N Engl J Med. 1993;329:821-37.
33. Keirse MJ. Progesterone administration in pregnancy may prevent preterm delivery. Br J Obstet Gynecol. 1990;97:149-154.
34. Medical Research Council/Royal College of Obstetricians and Gynecologists working party on cervical cerclage. Multicenter trial of cervical cerclage. Br J Obstet and Gynecol. 1988;95:437-45.
35. Keirse MJ. Prophylactic oral betamimetics in twin pregnancies. Cochrane Pregnancy and Child Database (March 24, 1993) Cochrane Collaboration, Issue 2. 1995.
36. Jeffrey RL, Bowes WA, Delaney JJ. Role of bed rest in twin gestation. Obstet Gynecol. 1974;6:822-6.
37. Crowther CA. Hospitalisation and bed rest for multiple pregnancy. Cochrane Database Syst Rev. 2001;(1):CD000110.

38. National Institute of Health (NIH). Consensus development confidence. Effect of corticosteroids for fetal maturation on perinatal outcomes. Am J Obstet Gynecol. 1995;173:246.

39. Meyers C, Adam R, Dungan J, Prenger V. Aneuploidy in twin gestations: when is maternal age advanced. Obstet Gynecol. 1997;89(2):248-51.

40. Sebire NJ, Dercolec, Hughes K, Carvalho M, Nicolaides NH. Increased nuchal translucency thickness at 10-14 weeks of gestation as a predictor of severe TTTS. Ultrasound Obstet Gynecol. 1997;10:86-9.

41. Drugan A, Johnson MP, Krivchenia EL, Evans MI. Genetics and genetic counseling in multiple pregnancy and delivery. In: Gall SA (Ed). Multiple Pregnancy and Delivery. St Louis, MI: Mosby; 1996.

42. Mercer BM, Crocker LG, Pierce WF, Sibai BM. Clinical characteristics and outcome of twin gestation complicated by preterm premature rupture of the membranes. Am J Obstet Gynecol. 1993;168:1467-73.

43. Mercer BM. Preterm premature rupture of membranes. Obstet Gynecol. 2003;101:178-93.

44. Lluke B. Reducing fetal deaths in multiple births; optimal birth weights and gestational age for infants of twin and triplet births. Acta Genet Med Gemellol (Roma). 1996;45:333-48.

45. American College of Obstetricians and Gynecologists. Obstetric analgesia and anesthesia. ACOG Practice Bulletin No. 36. Washington, DC: ACOG; 2002.

46. Chervenak FA, Johnson RE, Youcha S, Hobbins JC, Berkowitz RL. Intrapartum management of twin gestation. Obstet Gynecol. 1985;65:119-24.

47. Keily JL. The epidemiology of perinatal mortality in multiple births. Bull N Y Acad Med. 1990;66:618-37.

48. Chervenak FA, Johnson RE, Berkowitz RL, Hobbins JC. Intrapartum external version of the second twin. Obstet Gynecol. 1983;62:160-5.

49. Chauhan SP, Roberts WE. Intrapartum management of twin. In: Gall SA (Ed). Multiple Pregnancy and Delivery. St. Louis, MI: Mosby-Year Book; 1996. pp. 243-80.

50. Rayburn WF, Lavin JP, Miodovnik M, Varner MW. Multiple gestation: time interval between delivery of first and second twin. Obstet Gynecol. 1984;63:502-6.

51. Hannah ME, Hannah WJ, Hewson SA, Hodnett ED, Saigal S, Willan AR. Planned caesarean section versus planned vaginal birth for breech presentation at term: A randomized multicenter trial. Term Breech Trial Collaborative Group. Lancet. 2000;356:1375-83.

52. Royal College of Obstetricians and Gynecologists. The management of breech presentation. London: RCOG Press; 2001. Guideline number 20.

53. Rabinovici J, Barkai G, Reichman B, Serr DM, Mashiach S. Randomized management of the second non vertex twin; Vaginal delivery or cesarean section. Am J Obstet Gynecol. 1987;156:52-6.

54. Bloomfield MM, Philipson EH. External cephalic version of twin A. Obstet Gynecol. 1997;89:814-5.

55. Blickstein I, Goldman RD, Kupfermine M. Delivery of breach of first twins: A multicentre retrospective study. Obstet Gynecol. 2000;95:37-42.

56. Robinson C, Chauhan S. Intrapartum management of twins. Clin Obstetr Gynecol. 2004;47(I):248-62.

57. Kilby M, Baker P, Critchley H, Field D. Consensus views arising from the 50th Study Group: Multiple Pregnancy. UK: RCOG Press; 2009.

58. Adashi EY, Ekins MN, Lacoueries Y. On the discharge of Hippocratic obligations challenges and opportunities. Am J Obstet Gynecol. 2004;190:885-93.

59. Evans MI, Berkowitz RL, Wapner RJ, Carpenter RJ, Goldberg JD, Ayoub MA, et al. Improvement in outcome of multifetal pregnancy reduction with increased experience. Am J Obstet Gynecol. 2001;184:97-103.

■ SUGGESTED READINGS

1. Bejar R, Vigliocco G, Gramajo H, Solana C, Benirschke K, Berry C, et al. Antenatal origin of neurologic damage in newborn infants. II. Multiple gestations. Am J Obstet Gynecol. 1990;162:1230.

2. Blondel B, Kaminski M. Trends in the occurrence, determinants, and consequences of multiple births. Semin Perinatol. 2002; 26:239.

3. Conde-Agudelo A, Romero R, Hassan SS, Yeo L. Transvaginal sonographic cervical length for the prediction of spontaneous preterm birth in twin pregnancies: a systematic review and metaanalysis. Am J Obstet Gynecol. 2010; 203:128.e1.

4. Lambalk CB, De Koning CH, Braat DD. The endocrinology of dizygotic twinning in the human. Mol Cell Endocrinol. 1998;145:97.

5. Landy HJ, Weiner S, Corson SL, Batzer FR, Bolognese RJ. The "vanishing twin": ultrasonographic assessment of fetal disappearance in the first trimester. Am J Obstet Gynecol. 1986;155:14.

6. Martin NG, Olsen ME, Theile H, El Beaini JL, Handelsman D, Bhatnagar AS. Pituitary-ovarian function in mothers who have had two sets of dizygotic twins. Fertil Steril. 1984;41: 878.

7. Petterson B, Nelson KB, Watson L, Stanley F. Twins, triplets, and cerebral palsy in births in Western Australia in the 1980s. BMJ. 1993;307:1239.

8. Pharoah PO. Twins and cerebral palsy. Acta Paediatr Suppl. 2001;90:6.

9. Schieve LA, Peterson HB, Meikle SF, Jeng G, Danel I, Burnett NM, et al. Live-birth rates and multiple-birth risk using in vitro fertilization. JAMA. 1999;282:1832.

10. Singer E, Pilpel S, Bsat F, Plevyak M, Healy A, Markenson G. Accuracy of fetal fibronectin to predict preterm birth in twin gestations with symptoms of labor. Obstet Gynecol. 2007;109:1083.

11. Sullivan AE, Varner MW, Ball RH, Jackson M, Silver RM. The management of acardiac twins: a conservative approach. Am J Obstet Gynecol. 2003;189:1310.

12. Vermesh M, Kletzky OA. Follicle-stimulating hormone is the main determinant of follicular recruitment and development in ovulation induction with human menopausal gonadotropin. Am J Obstet Gynecol. 1987;157:1397.

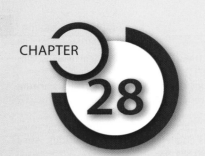

Induction of Labor

Jayanti Reddy

INTRODUCTION

Stimulation of uterine contractions before the spontaneous onset of labor, with or without ruptured membranes, is referred to as induction of labor (IOL). Initially, the cervix is closed and uneffaced. Labor often commences with cervical ripening, which involves gradual softening and opening of cervix due to prostaglandins. The term augmentation of labor refers to enhancement of spontaneous contractions that are considered inadequate because of failed cervical dilation and fetal descent.

The pinnacle of normal pregnancy involves three stages: (1) prelabor, (2) cervical ripening, and (3) labor occurring as a continuous process rather than as isolated events.[1]

INCIDENCE

The incidence of IOL varies from 20 to 30%. Unpublished data from the World Health Organization (WHO) Global Survey on Maternal and Perinatal Health, which included 373 healthcare facilities in 24 countries and nearly 3 lakh deliveries, showed that 9.6% of the deliveries involved labor induction. On the whole, the survey also found that African countries tended to have lower rates of IOL (lowest: Niger, 1.4%) compared to Asian and Latin American countries (highest: Sri Lanka, 35.5%).[2]

IMPORTANT POINTS TO EVALUATE BEFORE INDUCTION

- *Maternal considerations*
  - Confirm the indication for induction.
  - Review if there are any contraindications to labor and/or vaginal delivery.
  - Perform clinical pelvimetry to assess pelvic shape and adequacy of bony pelvis.
  - Assess the cervical condition (assign Bishop score).
  - Review risks, benefits, and alternatives of IOL with the patient along with a written informed consent.
- *Fetal considerations*
  - Confirm the gestational age [by last menstrual period (LMP)/ultrasonography (USG) dating].
  - Assess the fetal lung maturity status.
  - Estimate fetal weight (either by clinical or by ultrasound examination).
  - Determine fetal presentation and lie.
  - Confirm fetal well-being.

INDICATIONS FOR INDUCTION OF LABOR[3,4]

Induction is often employed in situations where the risks associated with shortening of the duration of pregnancy by induction outweigh waiting for the onset of spontaneous labor.

The benefits of induction typically outweigh the risks in the following situations:
- *Maternal indications*
  - Hypertensive disorders
  - Medical disorders
  - Prolonged pregnancy
  - Premature rupture of membranes
  - Chorioamnionitis
  - Antepartum hemorrhage
  - Rhesus sensitization
  - Oligohydramnios
- *Fetal indications*
  - Compromised fetus, e.g., growth restriction
  - Fetal abnormality or death: The main reason for intervention is to alleviate distress in the mother.
- *Social indication*: This means where IOL is done at the request of the pregnant woman to shorten the duration of pregnancy or to time the birth of the baby according to the convenience of the mother and/or healthcare workers although currently, no guidelines recommend this.

Centuries ago, the only indication used to be fetal demise but since the last 50–60 years prolonged pregnancy and maternal hypertensive disorders have become the major indications.

CONTRAINDICATIONS

- *Maternal*
  - Contracted pelvis
  - Prior uterine incision (classical/inverted-T)

- Prior uterine surgery
- Active genital herpes/cervical cancer
- Abnormal placentation
- Previous vesicovaginal fistula repair
- *Fetal*
  - Appreciable fetal macrosomia
  - Severe hydrocephalus
  - Malpresentation
  - Nonreassuring fetal status

■ PREINDUCTION CERVICAL RIPENING

Cervical ripening is the most important event involved in the outcome of successful IOL **(Fig. 1)**.

In the beginning during the first trimester, the composition of cervix is: 50% tightly aligned collagen, 20% smooth muscle, and the rest is ground substance composed of elastin and glycosaminoglycans (chondroitin dermatan sulfate and hyaluronidase). The proportion of muscle cells varies from 30% in the internal os to 6% in the external os.

During labor, collagenase, elastase enzymes along with vascularity, and water content increase and hyaluronidase increases from 6 to 33%, whereas dermatan and chondroitin decrease.

There is increased production of interleukin-1-beta (IL-1β), tumor necrosis factor-alpha and interleukin-8 along with rise in prostaglandin E_2 (PGE_2), relaxin, and progesterone antagonists.

Remodeling of Cervix

Degradative enzymes → Collagenases, matrix metalloproteinase-1 (MMP-1) and -8, and elastases:
- *Source:* Stromal cells, neutrophils, and macrophages
- Activity enhanced by cytokines such as IL-1β and IL-8
  Inhibitors → Tissue inhibitors of MMPs, alpha-2 macroglobulin.

Affecting Elements

Cytokines
For example, IL-1β
and IL-8
} Enhance the activity of collagenases

Platelet-activating factor
Monocyte chemotactic factor-1

Hormonal influences: Estrogens increase collagenases. Progesterones inhibit collagenases, hyaluronic acid, and IL-8.

Nitric oxide stimulates leukocytes' infiltration and induces prostaglandin secretion.

The ideal agent for cervical ripening should be:
- Noninvasive
- Physiological (effectively induce labor and convert an unfavorable cervix to one receptive to delivery)

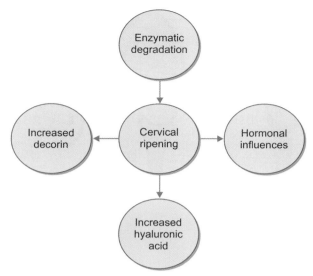

Fig. 1: Cervical ripening.

TABLE 1: Modified Bishop's score or Calder's score (where effacement has been replaced with cervical length to avoid subjective variations).

Score	0	1	2	3
Cervical dilation (cm)	0	1–2	3–4	5+
Cervical length (cm)	3	2	1	<1
Station of the presenting part or more	–3	–2	–1, 0	+1
Consistency	Firm	Moderate	Soft	
Position	Posterior	Midposition	Anterior	

Total score: 13; Favorable score: 6–13; Unfavorable score: 1–5
Bishop Score Modifiers
Add 1 point for: Preeclampsia, each previous vaginal delivery
Subtract 1 point for: Postdate pregnancy, nulliparity, PPROM (preterm premature rupture of the membranes)

- Safe
- Easy to administer
- Acceptable to the patient
  (Technically, it is difficult to differentiate between cervical ripening and labor induction.)

Cervical ripening typically refers to the preparation of unfavorable cervix, i.e., softening of the cervix that typically begins prior to the onset of labor.

Predictors for the Success of Induction of Labor

Bishop Score

Bishop score is a globally accepted method of recording the degree of ripeness of cervix before the onset of labor **(Table 1)**.

Other predictors are as follows:
- *Maternal:* Age, parity, body mass index (BMI)
- *Fetal:* Gestational age, fetal weight > 3.5 kg, fetal fibronectin in cervical secretions, insulin-like growth factor (IGF) binding protein.

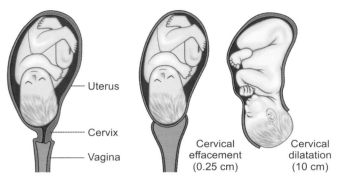

Fig. 2: Depicting formation of lower uterine segment.

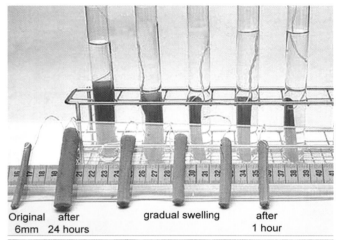

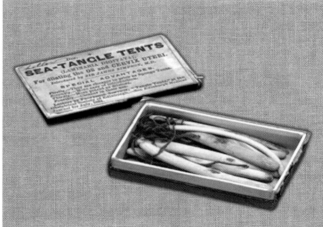

Fig. 3: Expanding capability of laminaria tents immersed in water.

Other Scoring Systems

- Field's system
- Burnett modification of Bishop's score
- Weighted Bishop's score by Friedman
- Pelvic score by Lange
  However, despite this, none of the modifications has shown improved predictability.
  Both Bishop's score and transvaginal ultrasound (TVUS) predicted successful induction.

- Bishop's score predicted delivery within 24 hours and TVUS within 48 hours.
- Cervical length has been related to the latent phase of labor whereas funneling is related to both latent and active phases of labor.[5]

Methods of Cervical Ripening

1. Nonpharmacological

- *Herbal supplements:* Evening primrose oil, blue and black cohosh
- Raspberry leaves, wild ginger, pineapple (contains enzyme bromelain)
- *Breast stimulation:* Causes oxytocin release
  - *Advantages: Noninvasive, inexpensive, simple*
  - *Disadvantage: Fetal heart rate (FHR) abnormalities*
- Castor oil, hot baths, enemas
- *Miscellaneous:* Acupuncture, transcutaneous electrical nerve stimulation (TENS), sexual intercourse, music therapy.
  There is insufficient evidence either of effectiveness or of benefits over the pharmacological methods.

2. Mechanical Methods

Osmotic dilators:

- Natural osmotic dilators **(Fig. 3)**:
  - Laminaria japonicum
  - Laminaria digitata
  - Isaphgol
- Synthetic osmotic dilators:
  - Lamicel
  - Dilapan
  They absorb endocervical and local tissue fluids, swell up to four to five times, causing the device to expand within the endocervix, and provide mechanical pressure thereby causing mechanical dilation and release of prostaglandins.

Advantages:

- Cheap
- Outpatient placement
- Easy for placement
- No need for fetal monitoring
- Rapid improvement of cervical status

Disadvantages:

- Need of skill for proper placement in internal os
- Delay in obtaining maximum effect
- Patient discomfort
- Inability of tents to be molded without compromising mechanical integrity
- Lack of manufacturer specifications for natural dilators
- Potential for incomplete sterility. Ethylene oxide (ETO) gas does not eradicate spores in the interstices of the seaweed stem.

Sweeping of membranes:
- Separating the membranes from the lower uterine segment by a circular motion of a finger inserted through the cervix is a common procedure used to curtail pregnancy.
- It is associated with an increase in circulating prostaglandins *(Ferguson's reflex)* and reduces formal labor inductions but is uncomfortable and not possible when the cervix is closed or very posterior.

Extra-amniotic Foley's catheter:
- Extra-amniotic Foley's catheter acts by physical stretching of the cervix and release of endogenous prostaglandins as a result of stimulation of the cervix and lower uterine segment.
- Although the effect is slower than PGE_2 analogs, it causes less uterine hyperstimulation and FHR changes.

Extra-amniotic saline infusion: The stimulatory effect of the extra-amniotic balloon catheter may be enhanced by infusion of normal saline into the extra-amniotic space at a rate of 50 mL/h. It is much more effective and safer than methods using exogenous uterine stimulants.

Technique of balloon placement **(Fig. 4)**:
- Taking all aseptic precautions, the catheter is introduced into the endocervix either by direct visualization or blindly by sliding it over fingers through the endocervix into the potential space between the amniotic membrane and the lower uterine segment.
- The balloon is then inflated with 30–50 mL of normal saline and is retracted so that it rests on the internal os.
- *Constant pressure* may be applied over the catheter. For example, a bag filled with 1 L of fluid may be attached to the catheter end or an intermittent pressure may also be exerted on the catheter end two to four times per hour.
- The catheter may be expelled spontaneously or is removed at the time of rupture of membranes.

3. Pharmacological Agents
- Prostaglandins
  - PGE_2: Dinoprostone
  - PGE_1: Misoprostol
  - $PGF_{2\alpha}$
- Oxytocin
- *Others:* Estrogen, relaxin, hyaluronic acid, progesterone receptor antagonist.

Prostaglandins: Prostaglandins are endogenous compounds found in the myometrium, deciduas, and fetal membranes during pregnancy. Their chemical precursor is arachidonic acid.

Cervical production of PGE_2, PGI_2, and PGF increases at term.

These modulate the fibroblast activity and increase hyaluronic acid production.

Acting as chemotactic agents, inflammatory cells further release degradative enzymes, causing cervical ripening.

Unlike oxytocin, the response to prostaglandins does not change throughout gestation.

PGE_1 analog (misoprostol), which was initially used for peptic ulcer prevention, is now used as an off-label drug for cervical ripening.

Pharmacokinetics:
- *Route of administration:* Oral, vaginal, and sublingual routes for induction
- *Bioavailability:* Extensively absorbed from the gastrointestinal tract
- *Metabolism:* De-esterified to prostaglandin F analogs
- *Half-life:* 20–40 minutes
- *Excretion:* Mainly renal (80%), remainder is fecal (15%)
- Maximum plasma concentration with 400 μg misoprostol—34 minutes after oral and 80 minutes after vaginal administration

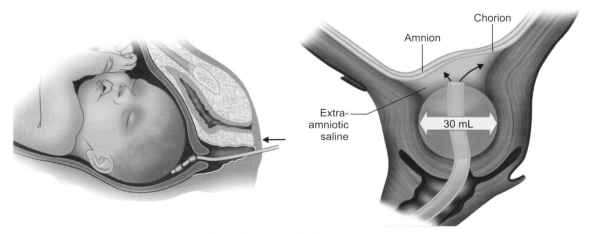

Fig. 4: Technique of balloon placement.

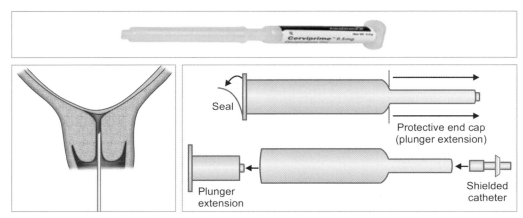

Fig. 5: Cerviprime gel.

■ Rapid onset of action along with greater peak is evidenced with the oral route of administration whereas longer duration of action is attained with the vaginal route.

Recommendations:
■ Oral misoprostol (25 µg, 2-hourly) is recommended for IOL.
■ Vaginal low-dose misoprostol (25 µg, 6-hourly) is recommended for IOL.
■ Misoprostol is not recommended in women with a previous cesarean section.

The American College of Obstetricians and Gynecologists reaffirmed its recommendation for use of the drug because of proven safety and efficacy.

PGE_2 analogs:
■ Vaginal gel: *Prepidil, Cerviprime*
■ Removable tampon: *Cervidil*
■ Vaginal pessary: *Prostin E2*

Dinoprostone gel (Cerviprime) **(Fig. 5)***:* It is available in a 2.5-mL prefilled syringe for an intracervical application of *0.5 mg of dinoprostone.* The tip of the syringe is placed intracervically and the gel is deposited just below the internal cervical os and the patient is asked to lie in lying-down position for at least 30 minutes.

The dose may be repeated every 6 hours, with a maximum of three doses recommended in 24 hours.

One must be cautious not to initiate oxytocin until 6–12 hours after the last dose of PGE_2 gel because of high risk for uterine hyperstimulation with concurrent oxytocin and prostaglandin administration.

Dinoprostone vaginal insert (Cervidil) **(Fig. 6)***:* The vaginal dinoprostone insert has 10 mg of drug embedded in a mesh, which is placed in the posterior fornix of the vagina for 24 hours. It releases the medication at a rate of 0.3 mg/h and may be left in place for up to 24 hours.

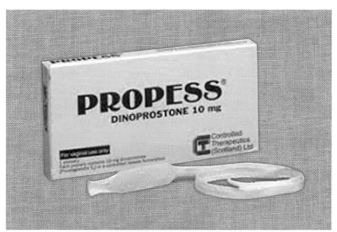

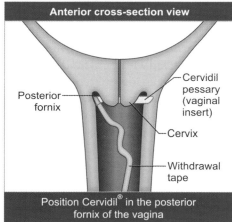

Fig. 6: Cervidil.

Advantage: The insert may be removed with the onset of active labor, with the rupture of membranes, or with the development of uterine hyperstimulation.

Complications include hyperstimulation, meconium-stained liquor, precipitate labor, and rupture of uterus. *Vaginal pessary (Prostin;* **Fig. 7)**

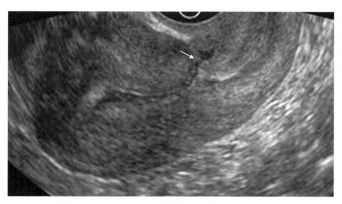

Fig. 4: Cesarean scar defect in ultrasonography.

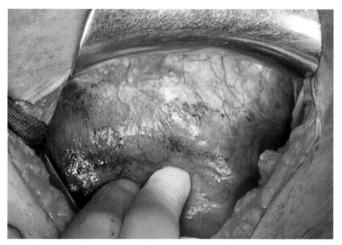

Fig. 5: Intraoperative finding of scar dehiscence.

- Previous uterine rupture
- The presence of a contraindication to labor, such as placenta previa, malpresentation, cephalopelvic disproportion (CPD), or contracted pelvis.
- Presence of any obstetric factor which makes this pregnancy precious, i.e., elderly patient, long-standing secondary infertility, previous perinatal death, severe preeclampsia, uncontrolled diabetes mellitus (DM), and obesity are also contraindications to VBAC.

■ MATERNAL RISKS OF VAGINAL BIRTH AFTER CESAREAN

Uterine Scar Rupture

Even though the absolute risk is very low, uterine scar rupture is the major cause of short-term morbidity. The risk of rupture with planned VBAC varies from 39 to 74/10,000.

Two Previous Cesarean Sections

Women with a prior history of two uncomplicated lower transverse CSs in an otherwise uncomplicated pregnancy at term, with no contraindication for vaginal birth, may be considered suitable for planned VBAC.

In these women, the rate of uterine rupture and VBAC success is similar to women with one previous uncomplicated lower transverse segment CS. These women do however have higher rates of hysterectomy and transfusion compared to women with one previous uncomplicated lower transverse CS. These women need to be reviewed at booking, 28, 36, and 38 weeks.

Factors Affecting Uterine Scar Rupture

The risk of rupture depends upon the type of previous scar, number of previous CS, and factors concerned with healing of the uterine scar.

- *Type of previous scar: Risk of rupture*
    - *Low transverse scar:* 0.2–1.5%
    - *Classical CS scar:* 2–9%
    - *Previous ruptured uterus scar:* Much increased
- *Number of previous LSCS*
    - *One LSCS:* 1%
    - *Two LSCSs:* 3.7%
- *Healing of uterine scar:* Uterus heals by formation of smooth muscle and without any fibrous tissue when suturing of the uterine incision is done well with perfect cooptation of incised tissue. Incision heals by complete muscular regeneration in 80–90% of the cases. At the end of 3 weeks, it has 30% of its final strength, and at 3 months and beyond, it has approximately 80% of its final strength.

Histologically, the scar tissue shows fibrin formation, fibroblast proliferation, smooth muscle regeneration, and hypertrophy of myometrial muscles.

In the presence of sepsis, more fibrous tissue is formed with fewer regenerated muscle fibers resulting in a weak scar. This can occur in the whole thickness of the wound (serosal to mucosal) or to a part of it.

Factors Concerned with Healing and Integrity of Scar

Operative technique: A large amount of tissue included in each suture, poor hemostasis, edges of unequal thickness, ragged margins, eversion of the endometrium or inclusion of decidua in scar, and increased levels of corticosteroids all are responsible for weak scar.

Systemic factors: Age, nutrition, general condition of patient, anemia, diabetes, obesity ambulation, involution, and lochia drainage affect the healing of scar.

Local factors: Many local factors play a role in scar healing such as location of placenta over the previous incision, devitalized uterine muscle, greatly stretched lower uterine segment (LUS), poorly formed thick LUS (prematurity, transverse lie), number of previous sections, overdistension (healing occurs by fibroblast proliferation), adequacy of blood supply (continuous interlocking technique causes weak scar by tissue ischemia), and suture material (thick suture causes more tissue reaction). Since the introduction of synthetic suture, one could also reasonably argue that chromic gut is obsolete due to its marked tissue reactivity, inconsistent tensile strength absorption, and knotting trouble. Chromic catgut has tensile strength for 7–10 days while polyglactin and polyglycolic acid sutures have tensile strength for 30 days.

Polyglycolic acid suture material causes less tissue trauma and induces less intense inflammatory response than catgut. Other important properties such as tensile strength, knot security, thickness or caliber, rate of absorption, and coating are better with delayed absorbable sutures.

Layered Closure of Prior Incision

Whether the risk of subsequent uterine rupture is related to the number of layers in which closure is done is controversial. While a study by Durnwald and Mercer[2] (2003) showed that single-layer closure has no increased risk of rupture and uterine dehiscence, studies by Chapman[3] (1997) and Tucker (1993) showed no relationship between one- and two-layered closure and risk of subsequent uterine rupture.

Maternal Mortality

The absolute risk of maternal death is 1–2/100,000 with an attempt at VBAC and 5–10/100,000 with ERCS. However, the mortality risk is increased when the emergency section is undertaken following a failed VBAC.

■ FETAL RISKS

The incidence of intrapartum hypoxic ischemic encephalopathy, TTN, and other perinatal morbidities is increased in cases of planned VBAC as compared to ERCS.

■ PREDICTORS OF VAGINAL BIRTH AFTER CESAREAN SUCCESS

- *Indication of previous CS*: In cases where indications for previous cesarean have been CPD, the success rate of VBAC (60–65%) is the lowest, followed by indication such as fetal distress (69–73%). Nonrecurring indications such as breech and placenta previa have the highest success rate (77–89%).
- *Prior vaginal delivery*: Patients who have had a successful VBAC following a CS have a very good chance of another successful and shorter duration of VBAC (93%).
- *Induction of labor*: Patients with a history of CS when induced for labor have a two- to three-fold increased risk of another cesarean delivery compared to spontaneous labor.

- *Condition of cervix on admission*: The more favorable the Bishop score (>6), the higher the rate of successful VBAC. Patients presenting in active labor with dilatation of 5 cm or more have an 86% rate of successful VBAC.
- An *interdelivery interval* of 24 months or less is associated with a two- to three-fold increase in the risk of uterine rupture compared to an interval of >24 months.
- *Previous scar thickness*: Many studies boast of the ultrasonographic assessment of the scar in LUS between 36 and 38 weeks' gestation as a successful predictor of uterine rupture. The scar thickness can be measured transabdominally or through the transvaginal route. Transvaginal sonography with high-frequency transducers offers better delineation of structures. If the lower segment thickness was <2.5 mm, the risk of uterine rupture or dehiscence was 11.8% whereas the risk of uterine rupture was minimal with measurement >3.5 mm. For patients with scar thickness between 2.5 and 3.5 mm, labor should be carefully monitored.

Thinning of the LUS is seen in patients with previous CS after 28 weeks of gestation. 74% of women with lower segment thickness of <2 mm [detected by transvaginal ultrasonography (USG)] developed incomplete uterine rupture 1 week before ERCS. Women with a history of previous CS, abdominal pain, and sonographic finding of thinning of LUS with ballooning of membranes into the scar should suggest a diagnosis of uterine dehiscence and be offered ERCS.

Hysterosalpingography (HSG) is not routinely used for evaluation of a CS scar; however, if done, HSG should be done at least 4 months after the CS. Accumulation of blood or secretions in the scar leads to unreliable HSG results.

Assessment of Uterine Scar

Baker in 1955, for the first time, reported imaging for the uterine scar by HSG.

Poidevin and Bockner (1958)[4]: Large wedge defects or sacculations in the anterior wall of size > 5 mm in depth were indicative of weak scars, and women with these findings were advised to undergo repeat CS in subsequent pregnancy.

Uterine Scar Classification (in Nonpregnant Uterus-based on HSG Findings)

Poidevin's classification

- Spicule
- Saccule < 6 mm in depth
- Saccule > 6 mm in depth
- Moth-eaten appearance

Oblonsky's classification:

- Defect < 2 mm
- Defect 2–6 mm
- Defect > 6 mm

Ultrasonography Monitoring of Lower Uterine Segment Scar

Donald in 1974 advocated use of ultrasonography during pregnancy to diagnose abnormal LSCS scars. USG scar evaluation is done first around 32–34 weeks and a scan is repeated at term. Monitoring before 28 weeks of pregnancy will not be very useful because the length of the LUS is:

- 0.5 cm at 20 weeks
- 1 cm at 28 weeks
- 4 cm at 34 weeks
- 5 cm at 38 weeks

An isolated scan in labor is not recommended but is useful for diagnosis of asymptomatic or symptomatic dehiscence. The irregular and puckered appearance of the posterior wall of the bladder suggests a bad scar. Results of many studies clearly prove that a sonographic LUS wall thickness of <3 mm is abnormally thin.

Fukuda et al. (1988)[5] showed:

- *LUS wall thickness of <2 mm:* Associated with poor healing
- *LUS wall thickness of >3 mm:* Associated with good healing

Lower uterine segment is measured (in millimeters) from interphase of amniotic fluid and deciduas to interphase of bladder and urine. A maximum of four measurements are taken and average recorded. Further LUS is studied for any areas of defects (thinnest area) or any discontinuation of LUS. For scar integrity, a transabdominal ultrasound with full bladder helps in finding out a thinned-out scar, notching in the region of scar and ultrasonic window in the lower segment. Windows are more dangerous than thinned-out lower segment. A study conducted at the University of Bosnia showed that a scar thickness of 3.5 mm or more, homogeneity of the scar, triangular scar shape, qualitatively richer perfusion, and scar volume verified by a 3D technique up to 10 cm are attributes of a quality scar. A study by Lebedev et al.[6](1991) analyzed the uterine myometrium by sonography and determined that the myometrium adequate for vaginal delivery should have a V shape of the LUS, a minimum thickness of 3–4 mm, continuous contour of the LUS, homogeneous echo structure, or structures with small areas of increased echogenicity. A balloon-like shape of the LUS, thickness <3 mm, discontinuity of uterine structures, and predominance of areas of increased echogenicity in the scar area determine a myometrium inadequate for vaginal delivery. The sensitivity and specificity of the transvaginal ultrasound for scar assessment were 77.8 and 88.6%, respectively. At the same time, the positive predictive value of ultrasound was 25.9% and negative predictive value was 98.7% (Asakura et al., 2000)[7]. A study by Flamma et al. (1988)[8] concluded that the thickness of the LUS from 3.0 to 3.5 mm is associated with a very low risk of uterine scar separation from previous CS and hence higher chances of successful VBAC. Multidimensional color Doppler is now the "gold standard" in assessing the quality of the scar after a previous CS. Measurement of scar thickness in both late second trimester and third trimester can be done, but the latter has better correlation with the mode of delivery.[9] This association is explained by the fact that thinner scars have more chances of fetal bradycardia and meconium staining of liquor.

Flamm Geiger Scoring System (Table 1)

Flamm score is useful to predict the outcome of previous one cesarean patient who has undergone TOL. With >5 score, the chances of vaginal birth are >90% while with <2 score, the chances of CS rate are 80–90%. Application of Flamm scoring gives fare judgment of successful vaginal birth in TOLAC. It was proposed by Flamm et al.[10] (1997) after a prospective study on 5,022 patients with previous LSCS.

The score is calculated based on the age of the patient, prior successful vaginal delivery, history of CPD, and cervical dilatation and effacement. So the practice of protocol of applying Flamm score and monitoring by partogram will reduce the rate of CS and morbidity in previous one LSCS patient. It enables the obstetricians to predict the chances for success of TOLAC in the individual patient and to evaluate the risks and benefits, thus improving outcome.

TABLE 1: Flamm score for prediction of VBAC success.

Parameter	Finding	Points
Woman's age	<40 years	2
	>40 years	0
Vaginal birth history	Before and after first cesarean section (CS)	4
	After first CS	2
	Before first CS	1
	None	0
Reason for first CS	Failure to progress	0
	Other reason	1
Cervical effacement on admission	>75%	2
	25–75%	1
	<25%	0
Cervical dilatation on admission	>4 cm	1
	≤4 cm	0

(VBAC: vaginal birth after cesarean)

TABLE 2: Modified Dhall–Mittal scoring system.

	Clinical features	Score		
		0	1	2
I	Indication for previous LSCS	• Cervix dystocia • Failed induction • Labor arrest • CPD	• Fetal distress • APH, PIH • Cord prolapse	• Malpresentation • Multiple pregnancy with BOH/DM
II	H/O intermittent vaginal delivery	Nil	1	2 or more
III	EBW	>3.3 kg	3–3.3 kg	2.5–2.9 kg
IV	Period of gestation	Post date	Up to 40 completed weeks	<37 weeks
V	Type of labor	Oxy/PG induction	Artificial rupture of membranes	Spontaneous

Note: Score ≥ 6: High percentage of successful vaginal deliveries
(APH: antepartum hemorrhage; BOH: bad obstetric history; CPD: cephalopelvic disproportion; DM: diabetes mellitus; EBW: estimated birth weight; H/O: history of; LSCS: lower segment cesarean section; PG: prostaglandin; PIH: pregnancy-induced hypertension)

The highest score is 10. The 0–2 range had a 49% VBAC success rate, while the 8–10 group had a 95% VBAC rate.

Modified Dhall–Mittal Scoring System

The modified Dhall–Mittal scoring system is given in **Table 2**.

Weinstein Scoring System

The Weinstein scoring system is shown in **Table 3**.

■ MANAGEMENT

Antenatal Management

- It is a high-risk pregnancy requiring special antenatal care.
- Correct dating of pregnancy from history, examination, and ultrasonography is essential.
- Early detection of complications such as anemia, hypertension, and adequate treatment is indicated.
  All routine antenatal investigations are carried out.
  If VBAC is to be considered, malpresentations, multiple pregnancy, and macrosomia should be ruled out.
  USG is a must as it helps in:
- Establishing fetal maturity, particularly in cases of unknown last menstrual period (LMP)
- Estimating approximate fetal weight
- Placental localization
- Scar integrity assessment
  Based on various clinical research results, it was concluded that the ultrasonic measurement of the thickness of the LUS has a practical application in the decision on the mode of delivery in women who had previously given birth by CS.

In the last trimester at every visit, the patient is asked for any suprapubic pain and palpation for detecting scar tenderness is carried out.

For trial of vaginal delivery, the pelvis is assessed clinically for adequacy after 37 weeks.

TABLE 3: Weinstein scoring system.

Factor	Nil	Yes
Bishop > 4	0	4
Vaginal delivery before CS	0	2
Indications:		
Grade A: Malpresentation, twins, PIH	0	6
Grade B: APH, preterm, PROM	0	6
Grade C: Distress, CPD, cord prolapse	0	5
Grade D: Macrosomia, IUGR		3

Note: More score means higher chances of VBAC.
(APH: antepartum hemorrhage; CPD: cephalopelvic disproportion; CS: cesarean section; IUGR: intrauterine growth restriction; PIH: pregnancy-induced hypertension; PROM: prelabor rupture of membranes; VBAC: vaginal birth after cesarean)

CT pelvimetry gives better detailed information with no risk of radiation.

Conduct of VBAC: Intrapartum Management

Admission

A woman planned for a TOL should be admitted at 37–38 weeks and assessed early in labor. As with all women in labor, the members of the care team should be notified in a timely manner of the admission of such a patient with relevant clinical details. Spontaneous labor has high success for vaginal delivery. The emergency CS rate is more in the induction group rather than spontaneous labor.

Continuous Fetal Surveillance

A uterine scar is an indication for continuous electronic fetal surveillance in labor. Studies by Ayres et al.[11] and Ridgeway et al.[12] have evaluated the use of cardiotocography (CTG) during a TOLAC, and the results are conflicting. The CTG tracings are interpreted according to international guidelines, but specific guidelines regarding the interpretation of fetal heart tracings during a VBAC do not exist. However, recommendations in guidelines for TOLAC imply that changes in the fetal heart tracings are the most frequent and sometimes the only indicator. Severe bradycardia is strongly correlated with a rupturing uterus.

Analgesia

There appears little evidence that regional anesthesia is harmful in a TOL, and this should be freely accessible in the absence of other contraindications. Epidural anesthesia is a good technique for adequate pain relief during TOLAC with few contraindications. It has not been found to mask the signs and symptoms of uterine rupture, and success rates for VBAC are similar to those experienced by women who receive other types of pain relief **(Table 4)**.

Intravenous Fluids, Blood Sampling, and Oral Intake

Placement of an intravenous line is advisable in a TOL. At that time, blood can be taken for blood grouping and cross matching, keeping adequate blood ready. Oral intake should be restricted to clear fluids because of a greater than normal probability of needing an immediate CS under general anesthesia. Solid foods are best avoided.

Induction and Augmentation of Labor

The most favorable intrapartum factor associated with successful VBAC is the onset of spontaneous labor with advanced cervical dilatation. But when the patient presents with spontaneous ruptured membranes or is at term or post-term with an unfavorable cervix and not in labor, induction of labor becomes an important issue. These should only be undertaken with caution. Whilst good evidence is lacking, mechanical methods of cervical ripening might be preferred to pharmacological methods and an infusion of oxytocin is not contraindicated but should be used with caution. However, great care needs to be exercised if a decision is taken to augment spontaneous labor with prostaglandins. Oxytocin has also been used for both induction and augmentation. Its doses exceeding 20 mU/min increase the risk of uterine rupture at least fourfold.

■ ASSESSMENT OF PROGRESS IN LABOR AND MANAGEMENT OF FAILURE TO PROGRESS

A TOL mandates vigilant assessment of progress in labor with vaginal examinations at least 4-hourly in the active phase of labor and more frequently as full dilatation approaches. The cervix should dilate at least at 1 cm/h in the active phase of labor and the second stage should not exceed an hour in duration.

The pattern of cervical dilatation in women with a previous CS showed that initial dilatation rate (IDR) > 0.5 cm/h and average dilatation rate (ADR) ≥ 1.0 cm/h have 95 and 97% positive predictive values, respectively, for

TABLE 4: Guidelines and level of evidence for VBAC-TOL.

	Level of evidence
Antenatal counseling	
In the absence of relevant complications, VBAC should be offered to every woman who has had one previous transverse lower segment cesarean section	II-2B
Multiple pregnancy, post-dates pregnancy, diabetes mellitus and suspected fetal macrosomia are not contraindications to VBAC	II-2B
VBAC within 18–24 months of a previous cesarean section may be associated with an increased risk of scar rupture	II-2B
Every effort should be made to confirm that a transverse lower segment incision was used for previous cesarean section	II-2B
Document planned mode of delivery in the woman's notes and record the type of previous uterine scar	II-2B
VBAC may be considered after more than one previous cesarean section but is associated with an increased risk of scar rupture	II-2A
Plan delivery in hospitals equipped and staffed for urgent cesarean section and with a documented VBAC policy	II-2A
Induction of labor	
Misoprostol should be avoided for induction of labor but a Foley catheter can be considered for cervical ripening	II-2A
Prostaglandin E2 is associated with an increased risk of scar rupture and should be used rarely and with caution	II-2B
Oxytocin infusion for induction is not contraindicated but should be used with care	II-2B
Intrapartum care	
Continuous electronic fetal monitoring is recommended in VBAC to detect early signs of impending rupture	II-2A
Judicious use of oxytocin augmentation is not contraindicated	II-2A
Suspected uterine rupture requires urgent laparotomy to reduce associated maternal and fetal complications	II-2A
Practitioners should be aware that single layer uterine closure may be associated with an increased risk of subsequent scar rupture	Good practice
Routine digital assessment of the uterine scar post-delivery is not beneficial	Good practice

success of VBAC. There is some evidence that prolonged labor is associated with an increased risk of failure and uterine rupture.

A partogram should be maintained in all cases because an arrest of active phases is associated with a higher incidence of scar rupture. Abnormal progress of labor must be taken seriously. CS should be done in all those cases in which labor extends 2 hours or more beyond the alert line in partogram.

Preparation for emergency LSCS is kept ready including an anesthetist and a neonatologist on call.

Monitoring of maternal pulse, blood pressure, and uterine contractions is done every half hourly along with continuous electronic fetal monitoring. Scar tenderness is assessed at the suprapubic area. Intrauterine pressure catheters have not been found to be superior to external monitoring in preventing or detecting uterine rupture.

Scar Rupture/Dehiscence

Theoretically, dehiscence means amniotic sac should be intact, incomplete rupture means visceral peritoneum should be intact, and complete rupture means all layers have given way.

However, practically, the following meanings are more appropriate: Scar dehiscence means disruption of part of the scar and not the entire length and fetal membranes remain intact. Usually, the visceral peritoneum is also intact, bleeding is minimal, and a small hematoma on the scar line may be present. Scar rupture means that disruption of the entire thickness of the scar may be along the entire length of the scar or partial. Usually, it is called complete rupture. This is associated with varying amounts of internal and external hemorrhage.

Site of Rupture

The uterus is dextrorotated in >85% cases and the uterine contraction pressure is centrally directed; thus, the left end of the scar is at potential risk.

The most reliable first sign of uterine rupture is a nonreassuring fetal heart tracing. CTG heralds uterine rupture in 50–70% of cases. Studies confirm that the occurrence of pathological CTG tracings and severe variable decelerations may be predictors for uterine rupture but alone they cannot provide the sole evidence of threatening uterine rupture, and other risk factors or signs should also be carefully evaluated.

Other clinical signs include:
- Scar tenderness
- Tachycardia
- Cessation of contractions (even decrease in uterine activity)
- Vaginal bleeding
- Hematuria
- Superficial palpation of fetal parts
- Loss of the presenting part on vaginal examination
- Hypotension

First Stage

When any of the features suggesting scar dehiscence develops, immediate CS is carried out. In case of frank rupture, hypotension and tachycardia are always present, the fetus is usually dead, and uterine contractions have

stopped. Immediate resuscitation of the mother is done alongside the preparations for urgent laparotomy.

Second Stage

Liberal episiotomy is a must. The second stage should be cut short by prophylactic forceps or vacuum and is not allowed to go beyond 1 hour.

Third Stage

Active management of the third stage of labor (AMTSL) is done. A careful watch for vitals and bleeding per vaginum after delivery of the placenta is a must. Routine examination of the scar after successful vaginal delivery is not done. It is unnecessary and dangerous as finger exploration might increase the silent defect and cause bleeding. Laparotomy and surgical correction of scar dehiscence is only necessary if significant bleeding occurs.

▇ IMPORTANT

- In spite of the risks of uterine rupture, VBAC remains an option for many patients with a success rate of 60–75%. Increasing recourse of VBAC, after careful selection of cases, can potentially reduce the prevailing high cesarean incidence.
- The decision to undergo a TOL for CS should be individualized. Counseling and informed consent are of paramount importance. The choice between ERCS and VBAC, like every other medical decision, involves a fine balance between risk and benefits.
- The ACOG defines the term trial of labor as a trial of labor in women who have had a previous cesarean delivery, regardless of the outcome, i.e., TOLAC. Also, the term vaginal birth after cesarean delivery is used to denote a vaginal delivery after a TOL.
- The ACOG guidelines now consider most women with two previous low transverse cesarean incisions, women with twin pregnancy, and women with an unknown type of uterine scar to be appropriate candidates for TOLAC.
- Even for nonrecurrent indications, in case of previous two LSCS, a trial of vaginal delivery can be given. Many cases of previous two LSCS are reported with success rate up to 75%. This is not practiced normally.
- Induction and augmentation of labor by appropriate means are now permitted in VBAC. But one should be vigilant in such a situation as there is a slightly increased risk of rupture as compared to spontaneous labor.
- About 90% of those who have had previous cesarean are candidates for VBAC. Those with previous indications such as CPD and dystocia can also be included. Still, TOL with a previous CS or uterine scar has inherent risks for the mother and the baby. So, our aim should be to prevent the primary (first) CS.

- Acute bradycardia of <80 minutes lasting for >10 minutes suggests that the fetus has severe acidosis and whatever may be the cause, immediate LSCS is required.
- If the interval between the last cesarean and this pregnancy (conception) is <9 months, a three-times increase in scar rupture is reported.
- History of prior vaginal delivery is protective against uterine rupture lowering the risk to 1/5th.
- ACOG recommendations:[13-15] The following recommendations and conclusions are based on good and consistent scientific evidence (Level A):
  - Most women with one previous cesarean delivery with a low-transverse incision are candidates for and should be counseled about and offered TOLAC.
  - Misoprostol should not be used for cervical ripening or labor induction in patients at term who have had a cesarean delivery or major uterine surgery.
  - Epidural analgesia for labor may be used as part of TOLAC.

SPECIAL POINTS

History

- Detailed history of previous CS
- Why it was done? Indication
- When was it done? Elective or emergency after TOL—what duration of trial?
- History and duration of PROM
- Baby weight and whether alive or dead?
- History of blood transfusion after cesarean
- History of abnormal puerperium: (1) Febrile illness, (2) wound gap, (3) wound discharge, and (4) poor wound healing
- Type of cesarean incision—LSCS or extended incision, T-shaped incision from earlier operative notes
- Whether the patient was advised about the next pregnancy and mode of delivery (check the discharge card if available)
- Time since the last cesarean
- History of vaginal delivery before or after cesarean
- Complaint of pain at the scar region

SUMMARY

Women with a uterine scar should be counseled as to the risks and benefits involved with both TOL and ERCS. They should be given all pertinent information free of bias, in order to make an appropriately informed decision.

Successful VBAC is a desirable outcome for the mother and newborn. VBAC failure, resulting in emergency CS and, rarely, in uterine rupture, can be minimized with appropriate patient selection, good antenatal counseling, careful review of the case notes, and adherence to guidelines. Senior obstetricians' backup in the labor ward is needed in rare cases of uterine rupture and catastrophic maternal and fetal consequences. These cases are tackled by prompt diagnosis and rapid resort to emergency CS.

KEY POINTS

- Cesarean delivery emerged as a life-saving surgical procedure when vaginal delivery not possible due to either maternal or fetal factors.
- Parenteral antibiotic prophylaxis (ampicillin or first-generation cephalosporins) 30–60 minutes before the skin incision reduces the risk of postpartum endometritis.
- Most preferred anesthesia for cesarean section is regional anesthesia.
- Intestinal obstruction and the adhesions are more common after classical cesarean section usually occur in the second or third week.
- Gynecological complications that can occur are menstrual irregularities, pelvic pain, dysmenorrhea, fistulae, infertility, urinary infection, scar endo-metriosis, and adenomyosis.
- Of these dysmenorrhea is the most important compli-cation.
- Women with a uterine scar should be counseled as to the risks and benefits involved with both TOL and ERCS.
- VBAC is successful in 60–75% cases selected for trial.
- Most reliable first sign of uterine rupture is a non-reassuring fetal heart tracing. In spite of the risks of uterine rupture, VBAC remains an option for many patients with a success rate of 60–75%.
- To decrease the pandemic of increased LSCS rates, steps must be taken to reduce primary cesarean sections.
- There is a need to universally follow a particular system of classification for LSCS . This will help in the audit of LSCS.

REFERENCES

1. National Institutes of Health. (2010). National Institutes of Health Consensus Development Conference Statement on Vaginal Birth After Cesarean: New Insights, Vol. 27, No. 3. [online] Available from https://consensus.nih.gov/2010/images/vbac/vbac_statement.pdf [Last accessed October, 2020].
2. Durnwald C, Mercer B. Uterine rupture, perioperative and perinatal morbidity after single-layer and double-layer closure at cesarean delivery. Am J Obstet Gynecol. 2003;189(4):925-9
3. Chapman SJ, Owen J, Hauth JC. One- versus two-layer closure of a low transverse cesarean: the next pregnancy. Obstet Gynecol. 1997;89(1):16-8.
4. Poidevin Lo. Caesarean section scar safety. Br Med J. 1959;2(5159):1058-61.

5. Fukuda M, Fukuda K, Mochizuki, M. Examination of previous caesarean section scars by ultrasound. Arch Gynecol Obstet. 1988;243:221-4.

6. Lebedev VA, Strizhakov AN, Zhelnezov BI. Echographic and morphological parallels in the evaluation of the condition of the uterine scar. Akush Ginekol. 1991;8:44-9.

7. Asakura H, Nakai A, Ishikawa G, Suzuki S, Araki T. Prediction of uterine dehiscence by measuring lower uterine segment thickness prior to the onset of labor: evaluation by transvaginal ultrasonography. J Nippon Med Sch. 2000;67(5):352-6.

8. Flamm BL, Lim OW, Jones C, Fallon D, Newman LA, Mantis JK. Vaginal birth after cesarean section: results of a multicenter study. Am J Obstet Gynecol. 1998;158:1079-84.

9. Royal College of Obstetricians and Gynaecologists. (2007). Birth after previous caesarean birth (Green-top Guideline No. 45). [online] Available from https://www.rcog.org.uk/en/guidelines-

10. Bruce L Flamm, Ann M Geiger. Vaginal birth after cesarean delivery: an admission scoring system. Obstetrics & Gynecology. 1997;90(6):907-10.

11. Ayres AW, Johnson TR, Hayashi R. Characteristics of fetal heart rate tracings prior to uterine rupture. Int J Gynaecol Obstet. 2001;74(3):235-40.

12. Jeffrey R, Darin W, Thomas B. Fetal heart rate changes associated with uterine rupture. Obstetrics and Gynecology. 2004;103:506-12.

13. ACOG Practice Bulletin No. 54: vaginal birth after previous cesarean. Obstet Gynecol. 2004;104:203-12.

14. Gonen R, Nisenblat V, Barak S, Tamir A, Ohel G. Results of a well defined protocol for a trial of labor after prior Cesarean delivery. Obstet Gynecol. 2006;107(2):240-5.

15. American College of Obstetricians and Gynecologists. ACOG Practice bulletin no. 115: Vaginal birth after previous cesarean delivery. Obstet Gynecol. 2010;116(2 Pt 1):450-63.

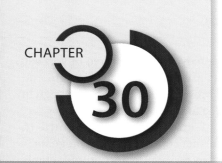

Ectopic Pregnancy

Amrita Chaurasia

DEFINITION

The word "ectopic" means "out of place." An ectopic pregnancy is defined when the embryo implants and grows outside of the uterus.

INCIDENCE

The rate of ectopic pregnancy is about 1%–2% of all live births in developed countries but may be as high as 4% among those using assisted reproductive technology.[1] The associated risk of death in the developing world is 1–3% and it is the leading cause of maternal deaths in the first trimester, being responsible for 6% of all first-trimester maternal deaths.[2]

CLASSIFICATION

- *Tubal ectopic pregnancy:* More than 90% of all ectopic pregnancies are tubal ectopic pregnancies, out of which maximum occur in the ampullary section (80%), followed by isthmus (12%), the fimbrial end (5%), and the cornual and interstitial parts of the tube (2%).[3] Here, interstitial and cornual pregnancies need special mention as these parts are more muscular; hence, pregnancygrows longer before rupture resulting in major internal hemorrhage and greater morbidities and mortalities.
- *Nontubal ectopic pregnancies:* These include pregnancies implanted in the abdomen (1%), cervix (1%), ovary (1–3%), and cesarean scar (1–3%). They often result in greater morbidity because of delayed diagnosis and treatment.[4]
- *Heterotopic pregnancy:* This is defined as co-existence of intrauterine pregnancy along with the ectopic pregnancy. The documented incidence is very low, ranging from 1 in 4,000 to 1 in 30,000, whereas the risk among women who have undergone in vitro fertilization is estimated to be as high as 1 in 100. The patient usually presents as ectopic pregnancy and intrauterine pregnancy is discovered while we are trying to locate the ectopic one.[5]

- *Pregnancy of unknown location:* Pregnancy of unknown location (PUL) is defined as a positive pregnancy test but no visualization of pregnancy in transvaginal ultrasonography.[4] PUL should not be considered a diagnosis; rather every effort should be made to establish a definitive diagnosis by repeating transvaginal ultrasound or serial measurement of serum β-human chorionic gonadotropin (β-hCG) or both.[6] The true nature of PUL may be an ongoing viable intrauterine pregnancy, a failed pregnancy, an ectopic pregnancy, or rarely a persisting PUL.[4]

RISK FACTORS

To understand the risk factors for ectopic pregnancy, it is important to understand the physiology of occurrence of intrauterine pregnancy, which requires an anatomically and physiologically normal fallopian tube so as to transfer the sperm and ovum, allowing them a favorable surrounding to get fertilized and finally transporting the embryo to the uterine cavity to get hatched out of nonadhesive zona pellucida and get implanted in the uterine cavity on day 6 of fertilization. Hair-like fallopian cilia located on the internal surface of the fallopian tubes carry the fertilized egg to the uterus. Thus, tubal ectopic pregnancy is caused by a combination of retention of the embryo within the fallopian tube due to impaired embryo-tubal transport and alterations in the tubal environment allowing early implantation to occur.[7]

The risk factors for ectopic pregnancy include all the conditions adversely affecting fallopian cilia or tubal mobility. *Previous ectopic pregnancy, prior fallopian tube surgery, certain sexually transmitted infections (STIs) such as chlamydia, pelvic inflammatory diseases, and genital tuberculosis, Asherman syndrome, and cigarette smoking* cause tubal adhesions and damage the fallopian cilia predisposing women to tubal pregnancies. *Previous pelvic surgery and endometriosis* cause peritubal adhesions, again affecting tubal mobility and predisposition to ectopic pregnancy. The chance of a *repeat ectopic* pregnancy after one ectopic is approximately 10% and after two or more ectopic pregnancies 25%.[8]

Other less-described predisposing factors include *age older than 35 years, infertility treatment, use of assisted reproductive technology, and use of birth control measures.* The chance of getting pregnant while using an intrauterine device (IUD) is rare. However, if failure occurs, there are 53% chances of ectopic pregnancy.[9] In spite of all these explanations, about a third to one half of all women do not have known risk factors.[10]

■ CLINICAL FEATURES

The symptomatology varies with the unruptured and ruptured ectopic pregnancy. Up to 10% of women with ectopic pregnancy have no symptoms, and one third have no signs.[1] *Unruptured tubal pregnancy* may feel like a typical pregnancy with few suggesting symptoms of abdominal pain, vaginal spotting, tender cervix, an adnexal mass, and/or tenderness. The typical triad of amenorrhea, abnormal vaginal bleeding, and pain, either low back pain or mild pain on one side of the abdomen or pelvis, is present in only 50% of the patients.

Acutely ruptured ectopic pregnancies have more dramatic presentation with suggestive history followed by sudden, severe abdominopelvic pain, weakness, dizziness, or fainting attacks with features of shock and sometimes associated with shoulder pain that may occur due to diaphragmatic irritation. Signs include abdominal distension, tenderness, and signs of peritonitis.[1]

■ DIAGNOSIS

A high index of suspicion aids in early diagnoses. Every woman of reproductive age with suggestive symptoms regardless of their contraceptive uses should be screened for ectopic pregnancy.[11]

Clinical features along with ultrasonography have high yield for diagnosing ectopic; however, inconclusive results may need serial estimation of serum β-hCG levels.

Diagnosis of Tubal Pregnancy

Transvaginal Ultrasonography

This has reported sensitivity of 87.0–99.0% and specificity of 94.0–99.9% for diagnosis of tubal pregnancies.[12-14]

The typical finding is an inhomogeneous or noncystic adnexal mass with or without yolk sac/embryo with or without cardiac activity moving separately from the ovary. There is no typical endometrial appearance to support the diagnosis of tubal pregnancy; however, 20% cases may show a pseudogestational sac inside the cavity due to collection of fluid giving rise to suspicion of heterotopic pregnancy.[15] The differentiating features of true intrauterine gestation sac and pseudosac are a regular margin and eccentric placement of true gestation sac that may contain embryo or yolk sac while the pseudosac has usually an irregular margin and is centrally placed.[4] The presence of the double-sac sign in true gestational sac is also to be sought for.

A small amount of anechogenic-free fluid in the rectouterine pouch further confirms ectopic pregnancy. The amount of this fluid may be small in unruptured ectopic pregnancies or slow leakage from fimbrial end as a result of slow-going tubal abortion. The presence of significant fluid along with collections in different abdominal potential spaces such as pouch of Douglas, paracolic gutters, hepatorenal recess, and subhepatic spaces strongly suggest ruptured ectopic.[1] Currently, Doppler ultrasonography is not considered to contribute significantly to the diagnosis of ectopic pregnancy.[1]

In patients with a laterally implanted pregnancy in an arcuate uterus and tubal pregnancy implanted in proximal parts, diagnosing ectopic pregnancy needs high expertise.[4]

Serum β-hCG Measurement

This is not primarily used to make diagnosis; rather it aids in diagnosis where there is strong suspicion of ectopic pregnancy but ultrasonography is inconclusive.[16] Normally, an intrauterine gestation sac with the yolk sac becomes visible by 5 weeks and with the embryo by 6 weeks.[17,18]

Nonvisualization of the gestation sac with low levels may interpret too early pregnancy to be visible on ultrasonography or early pregnancy failure or ectopic pregnancy. As has been described, the discriminatory level above which an intrauterine pregnancy becomes visible on transvaginal ultrasound is around 1,500 IU/mL of serum β-hCG. An empty uterus with levels higher than 1,500 IU/mL may not only be an evidence of an ectopic pregnancy, but also be consistent with an intrauterine pregnancy which is simply too small to be seen on ultrasound. However, the utility of β-hCG discriminatory level has been challenged and relatively high discriminatory levels up to 3,500 IU/mL have been suggested to avoid misdiagnosis and potential harm to intrauterine pregnancy that women might want to continue.[15,19]

Obtaining a repeat level of β-hCG after 48 hours is another tool to solve the dilemma. If the β-hCG doubles, it suggests normal intrauterine pregnancy because 99% of normal pregnancies have a faster rate of rise of β-hCG. If the levels rise but not up to the doubling point, it suggests either failed intrauterine pregnancy or ectopic pregnancy. Declining levels strongly suggest a spontaneous abortion or ruptured ectopic.

If the levels are falling, follow-up till the β-hCG levels have reached a nonpregnant level is suggested as even though low, the possibility of rupture is there with a resolving ectopic pregnancy too. However, at the same time we should keep in mind that though the majority of cases of

hemorrhage in the form of uterine artery ligation or uterine artery embolization.[45] However, rates of excessive bleeding necessitating hysterectomy were high and therefore, its use should be restricted to those women for whom alternative measures are unsuitable.

Treatment Options for Cesarean Scar Pregnancy
(RCOG Green-top Guideline No. 21, 2016)

These pregnancies are associated with severe maternal morbidity and mortality.

There is insufficient evidence to recommend any one specific intervention over another, but the current literature supports a surgical rather than medical approach as the most effective.

Medical treatment consisting of intramuscular methotrexate or ultrasound-guided local injection into the gestational sac or surgical interventions in the form of suction evacuation or surgical excision with scar repair with or without additional hemostatic measures should be considered.

Expectant management may be suitable for women with small, nonviable scar pregnancies provided they have given a written informed consent.[46]

Treatment Options for Interstitial Pregnancy
(RCOG Green-top Guideline No. 21, 2016)

Nonsurgical management is an acceptable option for stable interstitial pregnancies. A pharmacological approach using methotrexate has been shown to be effective, although there is insufficient evidence to recommend a local or systemic approach.

Surgical management by laparoscopic cornual resection or salpingotomy is an effective option.

Treatment Options for Cornual Pregnancy
(RCOG Green-top Guideline No. 21, 2016)

Cornual pregnancies should be managed by excision of the rudimentary horn via laparoscopy or laparotomy.

Treatment Options for Ovarian Pregnancy
(RCOG Green-top Guideline No. 21, 2016)

Minimal access surgery with removal of the gestational products by enucleation or wedge resection with preservation of normal ovarian tissue is indicated. Oophorectomy is occasionally required when there is coexisting ipsilateral ovarian pathology or excessive bleeding.[47]

Treatment Options for Abdominal Pregnancy
(RCOG Green-top Guideline No. 21, 2016)

Early abdominal pregnancy: Laparoscopic removal is an option with possible alternative treatment with systemic methotrexate in combination with intrasaccular injection with methotrexate or with ultrasound-guided fetocide.[48]

Advanced abdominal pregnancy: This is associated with significant maternal and fetal morbidity and mortality and should be managed by laparotomy promptly. The rule is to avoid incision of the placenta. The placenta may be removed along with its attached structure if that is a less vital structure and removal is possible but it will have to be left in situ for spontaneous resorption if the attachment involves major vessels or vital structures. Though leaving placenta is associated with significant morbidity (ileus, bowel obstruction, fistula formation, hemorrhage, peritonitis), the mortality is lower than with its removal.[49,50]

Treatment Options for Heterotopic Pregnancy
(RCOG Green-top Guideline No. 21, 2016)

The intrauterine pregnancy must be considered in the management plan. Methotrexate should only be considered in eligible candidates for tubal ectopic if the intrauterine pregnancy is nonviable or if the woman is not desirous to continue the pregnancy. Local injection of potassium chloride or hyperosmolar glucose with aspiration of the sac content of ectopic gestation is also an option for clinically stable women who want to continue with the intrauterine pregnancy. Surgical removal of the ectopic pregnancy is always an option both in hemodynamically stable and in unstable women. The fate of intrauterine pregnancy may be sometimes favorable with reported survival rates of 70% when tubal ones are removed early in the pregnancy.

▓ RHESUS D (RHD)-NEGATIVE WOMEN WITH AN ECTOPIC PREGNANCY (RCOG GREEN-TOP GUIDELINE NO. 21, 2016)

Anti-D prophylaxis is recommended for all RhD-negative women having surgical removal of an ectopic pregnancy or where bleeding is repeated, heavy, or associated with abdominal pain. There is a paucity of evidence regarding the risk of alloimmunization associated with medical and expectant management of ectopic pregnancy, but viewing the serious adverse effects on future pregnancy outcome in cases with alloimmunization even with the slightest possibility of fetomaternal blood mixing in women treated with medical/expectant management protocol, it will be wiser to offer anti-D prophylaxis to these women too.

KEY POINTS

- Ectopic pregnancy is usually a diagnosis of exclusion with high index of suspicion It may be tubal, non-tubal, heterotopic or PUL.

- Any woman of reproductive age group presenting with H/O overdue cycle with acute abdomen, signs of shock, abdominal distension and tenderness, cervical motion tenderness with or without adnexa mass is an acute ectopic pregnancy unless proved otherwise.
- In a chronic ectopic pregnancy, cassic picture is missing and examination is inconclusive. H/O amenorrhoea with on and off abdominal pain along with USG findings and mild anemia may help.
- Clinical findings along with ultrasonography is highly conclusive of ectopic pregnancy. Incolclusive findings may need serial βhCG estimation.
- Strong suggestive points for ectopic pregnancy:
  - No visible intrauterine pregnancy on transvaginal ultrasonography with a serum β-hCG of >2,000 IU/mL,
  - An abnormal rise in β-hCG level. A rise of 35% over 48 hours is proposed as the minimal rise consistent with a viable intrauterine pregnancy.
  - An abnormal fall in β-hCG level, as <20% in 2 days
- Management may be conservative, pharmacological or surgical.
- Pharmacological management is contraindicated in a hemodynamically unstable patient, ruptured ectopic, breast feeding, immunodeficiency, chronic liver disease, active pulmonary disease, hematological dysfunction and ectopic mass >4cm or with fetal cardiac activity.
- Single dose (currently treatment of choice), two- dose or multiple dose regimen of methotrextae may be followed.
- Anti-D should be offered to Rh negative women.

■ REFERENCES

1. Kirk E, Bottomley C, Bourne T. Diagnosing ectopic pregnancy and current concepts in the management of pregnancy of unknown location. Human Reprod Update. 2014;20(2):250-61.
2. The WHO Reproductive Health Library; Mignini L. (2008). Interventions for tubal ectopic pregnancy. [online] Available from Interventions for tubal ectopic pregnancy. The WHO Reproductive Health Library [Last accessed October, 2020]
3. Speroff L, Glass RH, Kase NG. Clinical Gynecological Endocrinology and Infertility, 6th edition. Philadelphia; Lippincott Williams & Wilkins; 1999. p. 1149ff.
4. Bouyer J, Coste J, Fernandez H, Pouly JL, Job-Spira N. Sites of ectopic pregnancy: a 10 year population-based study of 1800 cases. Hum Reprod. 2002;17:3224-30.
5. Barrenetxea G, Barinaga-Rementeria L, Lopez de Larruzea A, Agirregoikoa JA, Mandiola M, Carbonero K. Heterotopic pregnancy: two cases and a comparative review. Fertil Steril. 2007;87:417.e9-15.
6. Barnhart KT. Early pregnancy failure: beware of the pitfalls of modern management. Fertil Steril. 2012;98:1061-5.
7. Lyons RA, Saridogan E, Djahanbakhch O. The reproductive significance of human Fallopian tube cilia. Human Reprod Update. 2006;12(4):363-72.
8. Barnhart KT, Sammel MD, Gracia CR, Chittams J, Hummel AC, Shaunik A. Risk factors for ectopic pregnancy in women with symptomatic first-trimester pregnancies. Fertil Steril. 2006;86:36-43 (Level II-2)
9. Backman T, Rauramo I, Huhtala S, Koskenvuo M. Pregnancy during the use of levonorgestrel intrauterine system. Am J Obstet Gynecol. 2004;190:50-4. (Level II-3)
10. Farquhar CM. Ectopic pregnancy. Lancet. 2005;366(9485):583-91 (ACOG, 2017)
11. van Mello NM, Mol F, Opmeer BC, Ankum WM, Barnhart K, Coomarasamy A, et al. Diagnostic value of serum β-hCG on the outcome of pregnancy of unknown location: a systematic review and meta-analysis. Hum Reprod Update. 2012;18:603-17.
12. Kirk E, Papageorghiou AT, Condous G, Tan L, Bora S, Bourne T. The diagnostic effectiveness of an initial transvaginal scan in detecting ectopic pregnancy. Hum Reprod. 2007;22(11): 2824-8.
13. Condous G, Okaro E, Khalid A, Lu C, Van Huffel S, Timmerman D. The accuracy of transvaginal ultrasonography for the diagnosis of ectopic pregnancy prior to surgery. Hum Reprod, 2005;20(5):1404-9.
14. Atri M, Valenti DA, Bret PM, Gillett PJ. Effect of transvaginal sonography on the use of invasive procedures for evaluating patients with a clinical diagnosis of ectopic pregnancy. Clin Ultrasound. 2003;31(1):1-8.
15. Connolly A, Ryan DH, Stuebe AM, Wolfe HM. Reevaluation of discriminatory and threshold levels for serum beta-β-hCG in early pregnancy. Obstet Gynecol. 2013;121:65-70. (ACOG).
16. Morse CB, Sammel MD, Shaunik A, Allen-Taylor L, Oberfoell NL, Takacs P, et al. Performance of human chorionic gonadotropin curves in women at risk for ectopic pregnancy: exceptions to the rules. Fertil Steril. 2012;97:101-6.e2. (ACOG)
17. Goldstein I, Zimmer EA, Tamir A, Peretz BA, Paldi E. Evaluation of normal gestational sac growth: appearance of embryonic heartbeat and embryo body movements using the transvaginal technique. Obstet Gynecol. 1991;77:885-8. (Level II-3)
18. Rossavik IK, Torjusen GO, Gibbons WE. Conceptual age and ultrasound measurements of gestational sac and crown-rump length in in vitro fertilization pregnancies. Fertil Steril. 1988;49:1012-7.
19. Doubilet PM, Benson CB, Bourne T, Blaivas M, Barnhart KT, Benacerraf BR, et al. Diagnostic criteria for nonviable pregnancy early in the first trimester. Society of Radiologists in Ultrasound Multispecialty Panel on Early First Trimester Diagnosis of Miscarriage and Exclusion of a Viable Intrauterine Pregnancy. N Engl J Med. 2013;369:1443-51.
20. Silva C, Sammel MD, Zhou L, Gracia C, Hummel AC, Barnhart K. Human chorionic gonadotropin profile for women with ectopic pregnancy. Obstet Gynecol. 2006;107(3):605-10.
21. Godin PA, Bassil S, Donnez J. An ectopic pregnancy developing in a previous caesarian section scar. Fertil Steril. 1997;67: 398-400.
22. Jurkovic D, Hillaby K, Woelfer B, Lawrence A, Salim R, Elson CJ. First-trimester diagnosis and management of pregnancies implanted into the lower uterine segment cesarean section scar. Ultrasound Obstet Gynecol. 2003;21:220-7.40.
23. Timor-Tritsch IE, Monteagudo A, Santos R, Tsymbal T, Pineda G, Arslan AA. The diagnosis, treatment, and follow-up of cesarean scar pregnancy. Am J Obstet Gynecol. 2012;207:44.e1-13.41.
24. Seow KM, Hwang JL, Tsai YL. Ultrasound diagnosis of a pregnancy in a cesarean section scar. Ultrasound Obstet Gynecol. 2001;18:547-9.
25. Osborn DA, Williams TR, Craig BM. Cesarean scar pregnancy: sonographic and magnetic resonance imaging findings, complications, and treatment. J Ultrasound Med. 2012;31: 1449-56.

26. Ackerman TE, Levi CS, Dashefsky SM, Holt SC, Lindsay DJ. Interstitial line: sonographic finding in interstitial (cornual) ectopic pregnancy. Radiology. 1993;189:83-7.

27. Whonamedit; Spiegelberg O. Spiegelberg's criteria. [online] Available from http://www.whonamedit.com/synd.cfm/2274. html [Last accessed October, 2020].

28. Aliyu LD, Ashimi AO. A multicentre study of advanced abdominal pregnancy: a review of six cases in low resource settings. Eur J Obstet Gynecol Reprod Biol. 2013;170:33-8.

29. Lipscomb GH, Meyer NL, Flynn DE, Peterson M, Ling FW. Oral methotrexate for treatment of ectopic pregnancy. Am J Obstet Gynecol. 2002;186:1192-5.

30. Menon S, Colins J, Barnhart KT. Establishing a human chorionic gonadotropin cutoff to guide methotrexate treatment of ectopic pregnancy: a systematic review. Fertil Steril. 2007;87:481-4.

31. Methotrexate—injection. In: Drug Facts and Comparisons. St. Louis (MO): Wolters Kluwer; 2017. pp. 3883-90.

32. Pisarska MD, Carson SA, Buster JE. Ectopic pregnancy. Lancet. 1998;351:1115-20.

33. Dasari P, Sagili H. Life-threatening complications following multidose methotrexate for medical management of ectopic pregnancy. BMJ Case Rep. 2012;2012:bcr0320126023.

34. Stovall TG, Ling FW. Single-dose methotrexate: an expanded clinical trial. Am J Obstet Gynecol. 1993;168:1759-62; discussion 1762–5.

35. Barnhart K, Hummel AC, Sammel MD, Menon S, Jain J, Chakhtoura N. Use of "2-dose" regimen of methotrexate to treat ectopic pregnancy. Fertil Steril. 2007;87:250-6.

36. Rodi IA, Sauer MV, Gorrill MJ, Bustillo M, Gunning JE, Marshall JR, et al. The medical treatment of unrupted ectopic pregnancy with methotrexate and citrovorum rescue: preliminary experience. Fertil Steril. 1986;46:811-3.

37. Lipscomb GH, Givens VM, Meyer NL, Bran D. Comparison of multidose and single-dose methotrexate protocols for the treatment of ectopic pregnancy. Am J Obstet Gynecol. 2005;192:1844-7; discussion 1847–8.

38. Barnhart KT, Gosman G, Ashby R, Sammel M. The medical management of ectopic pregnancy: a meta-analysis comparing "single dose" and "multidose" regimens. Obstet Gynecol. 2003;101:778-84.

39. Yang C, Cai J, Geng Y, Gao Y. Multiple-dose and double-dose versus single-dose administration of methotrexate for the treatment of ectopic pregnancy: a systematic review and meta-analysis. Reprod Biomed Online. 2017;34:383-91.

40. Oriol B, Barrio A, Pacheco A, Serna J, Zuzuarregui JL, Garcia-Velasco JA. Systemic methotrexate to treat ectopic pregnancy does not affect ovarian reserve. Fertil Steril. 2008;90:1579-82.

41. Svirsky R, Rozovski U, Vaknin Z, Pansky M, Schneider D, Halperin R. The safety of conception occurring shortly after methotrexate treatment of an ectopic pregnancy. Reprod Toxicol. 2009;27:85-7.

42. Hackmon R, Sakaguchi S, Koren G. Effect of methotrexate treatment of ectopic pregnancy on subsequent pregnancy. Can Fam Physician. 2011;57:37-9.

43. Practice Committee of American Society for Reproductive Medicine. Medical treatment of ectopic pregnancy: a committee opinion. Fertil Steril. 2013;100:638-44.

44. Craig LB, Khan S. Expectant management of ectopic pregnancy. Clin Obstet Gynecol. 2012;55:461-70

45. Benson CB, Doubilet PM. Strategies for conservative treatment of cervical ectopic pregnancy. Ultrasound Obstet Gynecol. 1996;8:371-2.

46. Michaels AY, Washburn EE, Pocius KD, Benson CB, Doubilet PM, Carusi DA. Outcome of cesarean scar pregnancies diagnosed sonographically in the first trimester. J Ultrasound Med. 2015;34:595-9.

47. Joseph RJ, Irvine LM. Ovarian ectopic pregnancy: aetiology, diagnosis, and challenges in surgical management. J Obstet Gynaecol. 2012;32:472-4.

48. Andres MP, Campillos JM, Lapresta M, Lahoz I, Crespo R, Tobajas J. Management of ectopic pregnancies with poor prognosis through ultrasound guided intrasacular injection of methotrexate, series of 14 cases. Arch Gynecol Obstet. 2012;285:529-33.

49. Opare-Addo HS, Deganus S. Advanced abdominal pregnancy: a study of 13 consecutive cases seen in 1993 and 1994 at Komfo Anokye Teaching Hospital, Kumasi, Ghana. Afr J Reprod Health. 2000;4:28-39.

50. Nkusu Nunyalulendho D, Einterz EM. Advanced abdominal pregnancy: case report and review of 163 cases reported since1946. Rural Remote Health. 2008;8:1087.

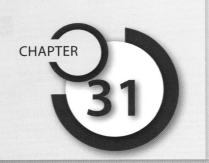

Hyperemesis Gravidarum

Shubharanjan Smantarai

INTRODUCTION

Nausea and vomiting of pregnancy (NVP) is a minor disorder observed during the first trimester of pregnancy with occasional persistence until delivery.[1] Approximately 70–80% of women during pregnancy experience some type of NVP.[2] Hyperemesis gravidarum is considered as a severe form of NVP. Till now, there is no single accepted definition of hyperemesis gravidarum. The Royal College of Obstetricians and Gynaecologists (RCOG) published the first national guideline for NVP and hyperemesis gravidarum in 2016 which defines hyperemesis gravidarum as protracted NVP with a triad of >5% prepregnancy weight loss, dehydration, and electrolyte imbalance.[3] Other potential causes of severe vomiting must be excluded before diagnosis of hyperemesis gravidarum. Other criteria included are signs of acute starvation and patient requiring hospitalization.[4]

EPIDEMIOLOGY

The incidence of hyperemesis gravidarum is approximately 0.3–3% of pregnancy.[5] The estimated incidence varies across the globe because of the lack of uniform diagnostic criteria of hyperemesis gravidarum. A higher incidence is observed in low-income countries (4.5–10.8%) and a low incidence (0.3–1.5%) is observed in high-income countries.[6] Hyperemesis gravidarum is the most common cause of hospital admissions in the first half of pregnancy and is overall the second common cause of hospitalization throughout pregnancy (first being preterm labor).[7,8] The risk of recurrence in subsequent pregnancy ranges from 15 to 80%.[9]

ETIOLOGY

The exact mechanism of parthenogenesis has not yet been established, but a number of proposed associations suggest that the etiology of hyperemesis gravidarum is multifactorial. Various theories have been postulated regarding the probable cause of hyperemesis gravidarum including hormonal stimulus, evolutionary adaptation, and psychological predisposition.[10,11] Hyperemesis gravidarum

is clearly related to the product of placental metabolites, since it does not require the presence of fetus as seen in molar pregnancy and multiple pregnancy. None of the hormones are validated scientifically. Since hyperemesis gravidarum occurs in early pregnancy when there is a sudden change in hormonal milieu, various hormones are being postulated as the cause. Majority of the studies support the role of human chorionic gonadotropin (hCG) and estrogen. Limited studies show the association of other hormones such as progesterone, growth hormone, leptin, and prolactin.

Human Chorionic Gonadotropin

Direct correlation between hCG levels and severity of hyperemesis gravidarum is not established, but there is a strong temporal association observed between hCG concentrations and the time course of NVP.[12,13] Hyperemesis is observed in conditions where the hCG concentrations are higher like molar pregnancy and multiple pregnancy. Additionally in almost all studies of thyroid hormone and pregnancy, there is an association between transient biochemical hyperthyroidism and NVP. As because hyperthyroidism itself seldom causes nausea and vomiting, the focus changed back to hCG for its role in NVP.[14] hCG is thought to be the thyroid stimulator in pregnancy.[15] This thyroid stimulation can be due to the fact that hCG is a family of uniform isoforms that differ in potency and half-life at luteinizing hormone (LH)/hCG receptor. It is seen that the isoforms lacking carboxylic terminal are more potent stimulator of LH/hCG and thyroid-stimulating hormone (TSH) receptors but have a shorter half-life. In contrast, hyperglycosylated isoforms have a longer half-life and longer duration of action.[16]

Estrogen

Estrogen is also thought to influence NVP. NVP is more common when the estradiol level is increased and less common when the estradiol level is decreased. Cigarette smoking is associated with a decreased level of hCG and estradiol. Many studies have shown that smokers are less likely to have hyperemesis gravidarum.[14] Estrogen in combined oral contraceptive pills has shown to induce nausea and vomiting in a dose-related manner. Women who develop nausea and vomiting after estrogen exposure are more likely to develop NVP than the women who did not have that sensitivity to estrogen.[17]

Evolutionary Adaptation

It is thought that NVP is an evolutionary adaptation developed to protect the woman and her fetus from the food that might be potentially dangerous.[18] It is evidenced by the fact that women with NVP are less likely to have spontaneous abortion and conversely the pregnancy destined to end in spontaneous abortion has deficient production of placental factors responsible for NVP. Clinical application of this theory may lead to undertreatment of women suffering from NVP and is potentially dangerous.[14]

Psychologic Predisposition

A number of current studies postulated the association of NVP with certain personality type or with some psychological disorders. There is no controlled study to support this. *Simpson* observed the association between NVP and conversion disorders.[19] However, if these changes are due to stress of being ill or due to reflection of a preexisting personality disorder is debatable.

Role of Cytokines

Recent studies depict the role of cytokines in the development of hyperemesis gravidarum. Increased concentration of tumor necrosis factor α (TNFα) and interleukin 4 (IL4) is observed in women with hyperemesis gravidarum. Both TNFα and IL4 favor production of hCG and development of hyperemesis gravidarum. Normal shift in pregnancy to TH2 over TH1 dominance has been reported to be more exaggerated in women with hyperemesis gravidarum and hence increased production of TNFα and IL4.[20,21]

Genetic Predisposition

Supporting evidence in favor of genetic predisposition includes (1) concordance in frequency of NVP observed in monozygotic twins,[22] (2) significant family history among siblings and mother of woman affected with NVP, (3) variation in frequency of NVP observed among different ethnic groups,[23] and (4) association of NVP in women with inherited glycoprotein hormone receptor defects.[24]

Helicobacter pylori

Helicobacter pylori has been suggested in the pathogenesis of hyperemesis gravidarum, but the available data are inconclusive. The American College of Obstetricians and Gynecologists (ACOG) 2015 guideline advocates that the treatment of *H. pylori* is safe in pregnancy and found to be beneficial in refractory cases of hyperemesis gravidarum.[25]

To summarize, NVP and hyperemesis gravidarum may be considered as a syndrome with primary emitogenic stimulus arising from the placenta or its metabolism. The response of the mother to this stimulus is determined in part by her susceptibility to such stimulus and may be mediated through vestibular, gastrointestinal, behavioral, and central nervous system (CNS) pathways. The genetic component may influence more than one of these pathways.[26]

■ RISK FACTORS

Common risk factors associated with hyperemesis gravidarum are (1) increased placental mass as seen in multiple pregnancy and molar pregnancy, (2) family history of hyperemesis gravidarum, (3) female gender of fetus, and (4) history of migraine. An interesting finding observed that smoking decreases the risk of hyperemesis gravidarum and it is associated with decreased concentration of hCG and estradiol, while the female gender of fetus is associated with increased concentration of hCG and increased risk of hyperemesis gravidarum.[27]

■ CLINICAL PRESENTATION AND DIAGNOSIS

The onset of NVP is typically observed in the first trimester. Almost all women who develop NVP will have some symptoms by 9 weeks, and onset of symptoms after that virtually excludes the diagnosis of hyperemesis gravidarum and may be due to some other cause. It is observed that 7% of women are symptomatic before the first missed period and 60% are symptomatic by 6 weeks.[26] Usually, it starts between the 4th and 7th weeks of gestation, peaks approximately by 9 weeks, and resolves by 20 weeks in 90% of women.[28] About 35% of women suffer severe enough to miss work or are unable to perform daily activity. Apart from nausea and vomiting, other symptoms observed include ptyalism and increased olfactory and gustatory aversion. There is no single accepted definition of hyperemesis gravidarum. According to the RCOG guideline 2016, hyperemesis gravidarum can be diagnosed when there is a protracted vomiting not related to other cause with the triad of 5% prepregnancy weight loss, dehydration, and electrolyte imbalance. Other criteria which may be included are the presence of features of acute starvation (ketonuria) and requirement of hospitalization. The symptoms and signs of dehydration include orthostatic hypotension, tachycardia, dry mouth and skin, mood changes, and lethargy. Electrolyte imbalance includes hypochloremic alkalosis, hyponatremia, hypokalemia, etc. Other abnormalities associated with hyperemesis gravidarum are mild elevation of amylase, lipase, and liver enzymes; raised hematocrit;

TABLE 1: Pregnancy Unique Quantification of Emesis (PUQE) index.[33]

PUQE scoring system					
In last 24 hours, for how long have you felt nauseated or sick of your stomach?	Not at all (1)	1 hour or less (2)	2–3 hours (3)	4–6 hours (4)	More than 6 hours (5)
In last 24 hours, have you vomited or thrown up?	7 or more times (5)	5–6 times (4)	3–4 times (3)	1–2 times (2)	I did not throw up (1)
In last 24 hours, how many times have you had retching or dry heaves without bringing anything up?	No time (1)	1–2 times (2)	3–4 times (3)	5–6 times (4)	7 or more times (5)

PUQE 24 score: Mild ≤ 6; Moderate = 7–12, Severe = 13–15
How many hours have you slept out of 24 hours? _____ why_____
On a scale of 0 to 10, how would you rate your well-being? _____
                                    0 (worst possible) →10 (best you felt before pregnancy)
Can you tell me what causes you to feel that way? _____

and low serum urea. In severe cases, metabolic acidosis may develop. Abnormal thyroid function test is observed in two-thirds of patients with hyperemesis gravidarum, with biochemical thyrotoxicosis and raised free thyroxine levels with or without suppressed TSH level. These patients are euthyroid clinically and rarely have thyroid antibodies. This gestational transient biochemical thyrotoxicosis resolves as hyperemesis gravidarum improves. So, routine thyroid test and treatment with antithyroid drug are not needed.[29,30] It may be distinguished from intrinsic thyroid disease by (1) no history of thyroid disease before pregnancy, (2) lack of systemic sign of hyperthyroidism (except tachycardia), (3) absence of thyroid autoantibodies, and (4) absence of goiter.[31] Liver function test is abnormal in up to 40% women with hyperemesis gravidarum.[32] Common abnormalities include rise in transaminase and slight rise of bilirubin without clinical jaundice. These abnormalities are self-limiting and usually resolve as hyperemesis gravidarum improves. An ultrasound scan should also be done to check viability and number of fetus and rule out trophoblastic disease.

The severity of NVP can be assessed by a recently published classification system called Pregnancy Unique Quantification of Emesis (PUQE) scoring, which is calculated by using the number of hours of nausea per day, number of episodes of vomiting per day, and number of episodes of retching per day[33] (**Table 1**).

■ DIFFERENTIAL DIAGNOSIS

Nausea and vomiting of pregnancy typically appear before 9 weeks of gestation. When a patient experiences vomiting for the first time after 9 weeks, other conditions should be considered in differential diagnosis. **Box 1** shows the list of different conditions in pregnancy that may create confusion with NVP. These conditions should be excluded by detailed clinical history, focused examination, and investigation.

Important negative history should also be asked to exclude other causes of nausea and vomiting; e.g.,

BOX 1: Differential diagnosis of nausea and vomiting of pregnancy.

Pregnancy related:
- Acute fatty liver of pregnancy
- Preeclampsia

Gastrointestinal disorders:
- Gastroenteritis
- GERD
- Peptic ulcer disease
- Intestinal obstruction
- Hepatitis
- Biliary disorders
- Appendicitis
- Pancreatitis

Genitourinary disorders:
- Nephrolithiasis
- Pyelonephritis
- Uremia
- Ovarian torsion

Metabolic disorders:
- Hyperthyroidism
- Hyperparathyroidism
- Addison's disease
- Diabetic ketoacidosis

Neurologic disorders:
- Migraine
- CNS tumors
- Pseudotumor cerebri
- Vestibular abnormalities

(CNS: central nervous system; GERD: gastroesophageal reflux disease)

abdominal pain and tenderness, fever, and headache are not observed in women with NVP. Abnormal neurological examination is not seen in most of the cases until unless complicated with Wernicke's encephalopathy or central pontine myelinolysis (observed during correction of hyponatremia). Palpable goiter is also not seen with NVP. **Table 2** depicts the method of assessment of women with hyperemesis gravidarum.[3]

■ MATERNAL EFFECTS OF NAUSEA AND VOMITING OF PREGNANCY

Mortality with NVP is not reported nowadays because of better access to health care with early detection

TABLE 2: Evaluation of patient with hyperemesis.

History	• Previous history NVP/HG
	• *Quantify severity using PUQE score:* Nausea, vomiting, hypersalivation, spitting, loss of weight, inability to tolerate food and fluids, effect on quality of life
	• History to exclude other causes:
	  – Abdominal pain
	  – Urinary symptoms
	  – Drug history
	  – Chronic *Helicobacter pylori* infections

Examination	• Temperature • Pulse • Blood pressure • Respiratory rate • Oxygen saturation • Abdominal examination • Weight • Signs of dehydration • Signs of muscle wasting • Other examination as guided by history

Investigations	• *Urine dipstick:* Quantify ketonuria
	• Electrolyte and urea:
	  – Hypokalemia/hyperkalemia
	  – Hyponatremia
	  – Dehydration
	  – Renal disease
	• Complete blood count:
	  – Hematocrit
	  – Infection
	  – Anemia
	• Blood glucose monitoring: Exclude diabetic ketoacidosis if diabetic
	• Ultrasound scan:
	  – Confirm viable intrauterine pregnancy
	  – Excludes multiple pregnancy and trophoblastic disease
	• In refractory cases or history of previous admission, check:
	  – *TFTs:* Hypothyroid/hyperthyroid
	  – *LFTs:* Exclude other liver diseases such as hepatitis or gall stone
	  – Calcium and phosphate
	  – *Amylase:* To exclude pancreatitis
	  – *ABG:* To exclude metabolic disturbances/to monitor severity

(ABG: arterial blood gas; HG: hyperemesis gravidarum; LFT: liver function test; NVP: nausea and vomiting of pregnancy; PUQE: Pregnancy Unique Quantification of Emesis; TFT: thyroid function test)
Source: Royal College of Obstetricians and Gynaecologists. The management of nausea and vomiting of pregnancy and hyperemesis gravidarum. Green-top Guideline No. 69. London: RCOG; 2016. 1-27 pp.

and treatment. Untreated or refractory cases may be associated with significant morbidity such as Wernicke's encephalopathy, esophageal injury (Mallory–Weiss tear and sometimes rupture of esophagus), pneumomediastinum, retinal hemorrhage, splenic avulsion, acute tubular necrosis, central pontine myelinolysis, and peripheral neuropathy. Severe nausea and vomiting increase the hospital admission rate, increase psychological morbidity significantly, and increase the chance of termination of pregnancy.

Wernicke's Encephalopathy

Wernicke's encephalopathy is considered as one of the dreaded complications of hyperemesis gravidarum. This is due to loss of water-soluble vitamin B_1 (thiamine), leading to CNS dysfunction. Initially, the patient may present with symptoms such as lethargy and confusion. Other classical signs of Wernicke's encephalopathy described are hyporeflexia, ataxia, and oculomotor symptoms such as nystagmus and ophthalmoplegia. Blindness and cardiac dysfunction have also been reported. Permanent residual dysfunction and death are observed in severe cases. Thus, early diagnosis and treatment are necessary to avoid such complications. This condition may be precipitated by carbohydrate infusion prior to thiamine replacement, as a small amount of thiamine remaining in the body is consumed during metabolism of carbohydrate load. MRI is useful for diagnosis. Wernicke's encephalopathy can be avoided by preventive measures. All women with hyperemesis gravidarum must receive the recommended daily amount of thiamine 3 mg along with other vitamins. When intravenous hydration is required specifically before administering dextrose-containing fluids, a bolus dose of thiamine (100 mg) should be given by the parenteral route at least for the initial 3 days.

▪ FETAL EFFECTS OF NAUSEA AND VOMITING OF PREGNANCY

Mild-to-moderate NVP has a better outcome of pregnancy as compared to women who do not have NVP. This result is thought to be due to robust placental production of factors essential for a healthy pregnancy rather than the protective effect of vomiting.[34] In a study, it has been observed that women who had lost >5% of prepregnancy weight due to hyperemesis are associated with preterm delivery and low birth weight.[35] Major congenital anomalies are found to be less prevalent in women with hyperemesis gravidarum. Data are conflicting. Various congenital anomalies linked to hyperemesis gravidarum included Down syndrome, hip dysplasia, skeletal malformations, CNS defects, undescended testes, and skin abnormalities.[36] Vitamin K deficiency in women with hyperemesis gravidarum may lead to development of intracranial hemorrhage. Data are conflicting regarding the association of hyperemesis gravidarum and several childhood cancers such as testicular cancer and leukemia. Another association is found between hyperemesis gravidarum and the increased prevalence of psychiatric disorders in adulthood such as anxiety, depression, and bipolar disorders but there is limited data to support this.[37]

■ MANAGEMENT (FLOWCHART 1: TREATMENT ALGORITHM)

Prevention

Prevention is considered as the best approach for management of hyperemesis gravidarum. Studies found that women who were taking multivitamins preconceptionally or early in pregnancy are less likely to need medical attention for vomiting.[38,39] Therefore, preconceptional supplementation of multivitamins may reduce the incidence and severity of NVP.[40]

Dietary and Lifestyle Modifications

There is a little data regarding the efficacy of dietary changes for management of hyperemesis gravidarum. The possible dietary modifications that have been found to be helpful include (1) frequent and small meals every 1–2 hours to avoid full stomach, (2) avoidance of spicy and fatty foods, (3) eating bland and dry foods, (4) high-protein snacks, (5) toast or cracker in morning before raising from bed, and (6) discontinuation of iron supplementation. Other general measures found helpful are rest and avoidance of sensory stimulus that provoke the symptoms such as odor, noise, heat, humidity, and flickering light. In some cases behavioral therapy, deconditioning, and relaxation are found to improve the symptoms of NVP.

Alternate Medicine

Acupressure/Acupuncture/Stimulation

Acupressure, acupuncture, and electrical nerve stimulation at pericardium 6 (P6) or Neiguan point which is situated three finger-breadth below wrist between the tendon of palmaris longus and flexor carpi radialis have been studied with conflicting results.[41]

Ginger

Ginger has shown some beneficial effect in reducing the symptoms of nausea, but none of the studies showed any benefit in reducing vomiting.[5,41,42] Ginger is believed to stimulate gastrointestinal motility and flow of saliva, bile, and gastric secretion.

Supportive Measures

Adequate rehydration and electrolyte replacement are considered as mainstays of supportive measures. The initial recommended management includes keeping the patient nil per oral and immediate fluid resuscitation with normal saline and Ringer's lactate. Considering the fact that women with hyperemesis gravidarum are hyponatremic, hypokalemic, hypochloremic and ketotic, it is appropriate to use normal saline with addition of potassium chloride in each bag. Serum electrolyte monitoring and replacement should be considered as required with special attention to sodium, potassium, and magnesium. Dextrose-containing fluid is then included for maintenance. To prevent Wernicke's encephalopathy, 100 mg of parenteral thiamine should be administered before initiation of dextrose-containing fluid replacement. Studies have shown the beneficial effect of dextrose-containing fluid in faster improvement of nausea and vomiting.[43]

Pharmacologic Treatment

Early and prompt treatment of NVP should be initiated to improve the quality of life and progression of disease. Common drugs studied for use in NVP include pyridoxine, H_1 antihistamines [doxylamine, dimenhydrinate, diphenhydramine, phenothiazines (promethazine, prochlorperazine, and chlorpromazine)], benzamides (metoclopramide and trimethobenzamide), serotonin ($5HT_3$) antagonists (ondansetron), corticosteroids, and butyrophenones (droperidol).

Table 3 shows the list of drugs used for hyperemesis gravidarum.

All these medications have their potential benefits, risks, and adverse effects; thus, care must be taken before prescribing. With available efficacy and safety data, both antihistamines and phenothiazines are safe in pregnancy and are considered first-line medication in hyperemesis gravidarum. Metoclopramide and ondansetron are considered second-line medication and corticosteroids are considered third-line medication. A combination of antiemetics should be used for the patients who do not respond to a single agent, but care must be exercised for possible adverse effects. For example, simultaneous use of dopamine antagonists such as phenothiazines and metoclopramide may result in increased risk of extrapyramidal syndrome (Tardive dyskinesia) and rarely malignant neuroleptic syndrome (high fever, confusion, muscle rigidity, autonomic nervous system instability). Simultaneous use of serotonin inhibitors and phenothiazines may result in QT interval prolongation and arrhythmia.

Pyridoxine with or without Doxylamine

No relationship is found between the pyridoxine level and the degree of NVP.[44] Several studies have shown the improvement of NVP with use of pyridoxine.[45,46] A placebo-controlled trial demonstrates its benefit in hyperemesis gravidarum.[47] But a recent Cochrane review concluded lack

Flowchart 1: Algorithm of therapeutic treatment of nausea and vomiting of pregnancy (if no improvement, proceed to next step in algorithm). This algorithm assumes that other causes of nausea and vomiting have been ruled out. At any step, consider enteral nutrition if dehydration or persistent weight loss is noted.

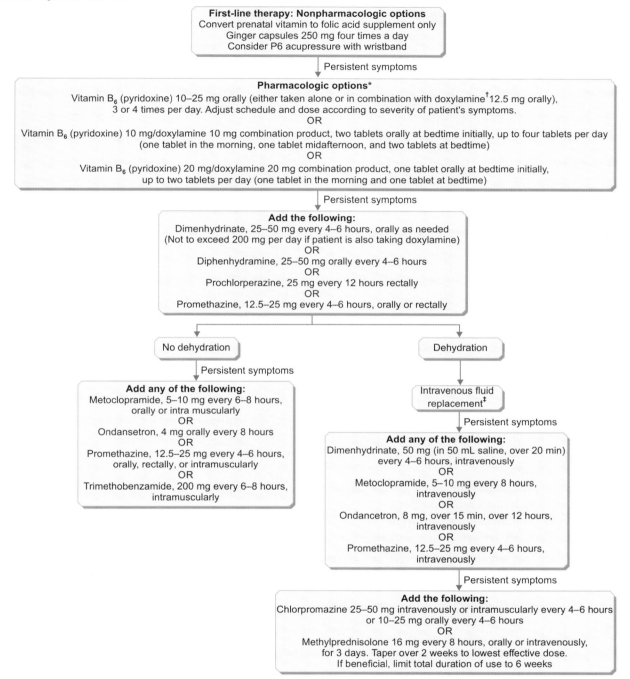

Notes:
*Some antiemetic medication have only been approved by the U.S. Food and Drug Administration for use in nonpregnant patients; however, off-label use is common. Obstetrician and other obstetric care providers should counsel patients and document such discussion accordingly. Care should be exercised if multiple antiemetic medications are used simultaneously. Parallel use of some medications may result in an increased risk of adverse effects.
†In the United States, doxylamine is available as the active ingredient in some over-the-counter sleep aid; one half of a scored 25-mg tablet can be used to provide a 12.5-mg dose of doxylamine.
‡Thiamine, recommended for women who require intravenous hydration and have vomited for more than 3 weeks to prevent a rare but serious maternal complication, Wernicke encephalopathy.
Source: Reprinted from American College of Obstetricians and Gynecologists. ACOG Practice Bulletin. Clinical management guidelines for obstetrician-gynecologists: nausea and vomiting of pregnancy. Obstet Gynecol. 2018;131:e15-e29.

TABLE 3: Antiemetic drugs for nausea and vomiting of pregnancy and hyperemesis gravidarum.[36]

Drug name/category	Pregnancy category	Recommended dose	Mechanism of action	Efficacy in HG	Side effects
Pyridoxine Pyridoxine 10 mg + Doxylamine 10 mg	• A • A/B	• 25 mg po q8h • 2–4 tabs daily	• May treat underlying pyridoxine deficiency • Treats pyridoxine deficiency and H_1 antagonist	± ±	• Paresthesia, nausea, fatigue • Drowsiness
Antihistamine: • Dimenhydrinate • Diphenhydramine	B	25–50 mg po q4–8h 50–100 mg po q3–6h	Peripheral H_1 antagonists	+	Drowsiness, dizziness, dry mouth, urinary retention
Phenothiazines: • Promethazine • Prochlorperazine	C	12.5–25 mg po q6–8h 10 mg po q6–8h	Central/peripheral dopamine antagonism	+	Drowsiness, decrease seizure threshold, extrapyramidal reaction
Benzamides: • Metoclopramide • Trimethobenzamide	B	10 mg po/IV q8h 200 mg PRq6–8h	Central/peripheral dopamine antagonism	+	Dystonia, restlessness, somnolence *FDA black box warning: Tardive dyskinesia
Serotonin (5HT3) receptor antagonists: Ondansetron	B	8 mg PO/IV q8–12h	Peripheral and central selective 5HT3 receptor antagonists	±	Constipation, fatigue, headache, arrhythmias (rare)
Corticosteroids: Methylprednisolone	C	16 mg po q8h × 3d, then taper	May treat relative ACTH deficiency, inhibit central PG synthesis, or decrease central 5HT turnover	±	Hyperglycemia, possible increase risk of oral facial cleft with first-trimester use
Butyrophenones: Droperidol	C	0.25–2.5 mg IV loading with 1 mg IV/hour	Dopamine antagonism in chemoreceptor trigger zone	±	Drowsiness, dizziness, cardiac arrhythmias, FDA black box warning for QT prolongation

(ACTH: adrenocorticotropic hormone; FDA: Food and Drug Administration; HG: hyperemesis gravidarum; PG: prostaglandin)

of considerable evidence to use pyridoxine as an effective agent for NVP.[5] The RCOG guideline 2016 concluded that pyridoxine is not recommended for use in NVP and hyperemesis gravidarum.

Combination of pyridoxine (pregnancy category A) and doxylamine (category B) was removed from the market in 1983 in the United States due to reported congenital malformation with early trimester of use. Later, it was reapproved by the US Food and Drug Administration (FDA) in 2013 for treatment of NVP in women who failed to respond to diet and lifestyle modification.[48] A randomized placebo-controlled trial attested the efficacy of the combination as compared to placebo.[49] Fetal safety for pyridoxine and doxylamine combination has been demonstrated in various epidemiological studies.[50] Pyridoxine is thought to have benefit in a patient with depleted nutritional status, and doxylamine is an H_1 antihistaminic (antiemetic).

Antiemetics

Antihistamines (doxylamine, dimenhydrinate, diphenhydramine): The effectiveness and efficacy of antihistamine for NVP has been demonstrated in a meta-analysis.[51] Studies have shown that their use in pregnancy is not associated with any birth defects.[52] Because of their effectiveness and safety profile, they are considered as one of the first-line agents for treatment of NVP. Common adverse effects observed are dry mouth, sedation, urinary retention, blurred vision, etc.

Phenothiazines (promethazine, prochlorperazine, chlorpromazine): Studies have demonstrated significant relief of nausea and vomiting with the use of phenothiazines.[53] They have a central and peripheral dopamine antagonism property. Majority of studies validated their safety in pregnancy.[51] Because of their safety and efficacy, they is also considered as a first-line drug for treatment of NVP. Common adverse effects seen with their use are sedation, drowsiness, dry mouth, and extrapyramidal reactions.

Metoclopramide: It is a dopamine receptor antagonist and has both central and peripheral actions. It is known to modulate the signal at the chemoreceptor trigger zone (CTZ). Peripherally, its actions are increased lower esophageal sphincter testing tone, accelerated gastrointestinal transit, and correction of gastric dysrhythmia. A recent double-blind randomized controlled trial of promethazine versus metoclopramide for treatment of hyperemesis found that both the drugs have similar efficacy, but the rate of side effects such as drowsiness, dizziness, and dystonia is less with metoclopramide.[53] In pregnancy, it is a category B drug.

Its safety is established in several studies and it is found that metoclopramide has no increased risk of major congenital malformations, low birth weight, preterm labor, and perinatal death.[36,54] The adverse effects of metoclopramide are dry mouth, drowsiness, dizziness, and extrapyramidal symptoms such as dystonia, akathesia, Parkinsonism, and Tardive dyskinesia. Due to the risk of extrapyramidal effects, it is used as a second-line agent for treatment of NVP.[3] The FDA in 2009 added a black box warning to metoclopramide due to the risk of Tardive dyskinesia with long-term use.

Ondansetron: It is a serotonin (5HT3) receptor antagonist and acts by blocking serotonin receptors centrally at the medullary vomiting center and peripherally in the small intestine. Ondansetron use in NVP is increasing because of its proven superiority in management of chemotherapy-related nausea and vomiting. The efficacy of ondansetron has shown mixed result. A double-blind randomized controlled trial and a Cochrane systematic review of intravenous metoclopramide and ondansetron found no clear difference in the management of severity of nausea and vomiting.[55,56] Another randomized controlled trial proved its superiority in controlling vomiting and nausea as compared to metoclopramide.[57] Ondansetron is found superior to doxylamine and pyridoxine combination in controlling nausea and vomiting in a small double-blind randomized controlled trial of 36 women.[58] The safety of ondansetron in pregnancy showed a mixed result from the available studies. A retrospective analysis by Posterna KB et al. revealed no increase in risk of major birth defects with ondansetron use in pregnancy.[59] Some studies have shown an association between ondansetron and some birth defects such as cleft palate and cardiac septal defects.[60,61] For these reasons, ondansetron is considered as second line of therapy and preferably used after the first trimester.[3] Adverse effects associated with ondansetron use include headache, drowsiness, fatigue, constipation, and prolongation of QT interval leading to arrhythmia (torse de pointes).

Corticosteroids: The effectiveness of corticosteroids was observed in a case series of women with refractory hyperemesis gravidarum.[62] Its antiemetic property is believed to be due to its effect at the CTZ located in brainstem and also thought to correct the relative adrenal insufficiency, induced by hyperemesis gravidarum (because of increased demand of cortisol during early pregnancy). A randomized controlled trial of 40 women with hyperemesis gravidarum treated with methylprednisolone versus promethazine found a lower rate of rehospitalization in the steroid treatment group.[63] Another randomized controlled trial by Yost et al. found no significant decrease in the rate of rehospitalization with addition of methylprednisolone.[64]

A recent systematic review of randomized controlled trial observed that corticosteroids' use in hyperemesis gravidarum reduced the hospital readmission rate, but no difference is observed in the days of hospitalization.[56] Regarding the safety of corticosteroids for use in hyperemesis gravidarum, a meta-analysis observed increase in the risk of major congenital malformations such as cleft palate.[65] It is considered as category "C" drug in pregnancy. Because of association of corticosteroids with congenital malformations, it should not be used as a first-line agent for treatment of hyperemesis gravidarum. The most commonly used regimen of methylprednisolone is 48 mg orally or intravenously in three divided doses for 3 days. Patients who will not respond within 3 days are less likely to respond after that, and the treatment should be discontinued. For patients who respond to the treatment, methylprednisolone may be continued and tapering of dose should be done over a period of 2 weeks.

Other Preventive Management Strategies

H_2 receptor blockers and proton-pump inhibitors: Prolonged vomiting may lead to development of gastroesophageal reflux disease, esophagitis, and gastritis. Treatment with H_2 receptor blockers and proton-pump inhibitors is safe in pregnancy and their use may be considered in such a situation.[66,67] The safety of esophageal-gastroduodenoscopy is proven safe in pregnancy and indicated if hyperemesis is associated with hematemesis and epigastric pain.[68]

Thromboprophylaxis: Different studies found increased risk of venous thromboembolism in women with hyperemesis.[69,70] This increased risk is specifically observed in patients with persistent vomiting.[71] Thus, thromboprophylaxis with low-molecular-weight heparin must be considered for women with hyperemesis gravidarum unless there is a specific contraindication such as active bleeding, and the treatment may be discontinued upon discharge.[3]

Avoiding iron-containing preparation: Oral iron is thought to cause nausea and vomiting. In a cohort study, it was observed that discontinuation of iron supplementation improves the severity of NVP.[72]

Nutrition

In women with severe hyperemesis gravidarum who are not responsive to medical therapy and cannot maintain their weight, nutrition support in the form of enteral or parenteral feeding should be considered as the last resort.

Enteral feeding: Enteral feeding options are nasogastric, nasoduodenal, nasojejunal, percutaneous endoscopic gastrectomy (PEG), and jejunostomy. Intragastric feeding is found to be associated with increased risk of nausea and vomiting, so the postpyloric tube (such as nasojejunal, PEG, and surgical jejunostomy) is described as the alternative to avoid the disadvantage of intragastric feeding.[73-75] The common problem with postpyloric feeding is dislodgement of the tube due to ongoing vomiting, retching, and gastric cooling.[76] Percutaneous endoscopic gastrojejunostomy is found to be safe, effective, and well tolerated for treatment of hyperemesis gravidarum. Dislodgement is minimal as compared to nasogastric tube placement. Possible complications observed are dislodgement, obstruction, migration of tube, cutaneous or intra-abdominal abscess, fistula formation, pneumatosis, intestinal occlusion, and ischemia.[77]

Total parenteral nutrition (TPN): TPN may be useful in refractory cases to provide adequate nutrition, but it is considered as a high-risk intervention as it is associated with serious complications such as thrombosis, infection, metabolic acidosis, and cardiac tamponade. Peripherally inserted central catheter (PICC) was thought to be associated with less complications, but studies show significant morbidity.[78,79] Because of the cost, inconvenience and complications, parenteral nutrition should be reserved as the last resort for management of hyperemesis gravidarum.

■ NEED OF HOSPITALIZATION

Women with mild NVP can be managed at home with antiemetic. Ambulatory day care management may be considered for patients in whom primary care measures failed and where PUQE score is <13.[3]

In the patient, management may be considered if there is at least one of the following: (1) Continued nausea and vomiting and inability to keep down oral antiemetic, (2) continued nausea and vomiting associated with ketonuria and/or weight loss (>5% of body weight) despite oral antiemetic, and (3) confirmed or suspected comorbidities (such as urinary tract infection and inability to tolerate oral antibiotics).

■ TERMINATION OF PREGNANCY

Termination may be offered only if all available therapeutic measures failed to control hyperemesis. A psychiatric opinion has also to be considered and the decision of termination needs to be multidisciplinary with documentations of therapeutic failure.[3]

CONCLUSION

Hyperemesis gravidarum is a complex syndrome. Little is known about its pathogenesis and if not timely treated may lead to serious maternal and fetal morbidity. Early diagnosis and aggressive treatment and support are essential to improve the outcome and quality of life.

KEY POINTS

- Hyperemesis gravidarum is protracted NVP with a triad of >5% prepregnancy weight loss, dehydration, and electrolyte imbalance
- Incidence of hyperemesis gravidarum is approximately 0.3–3%
- Etiology of the condition is multifactorial
- Untreated or refractory cases may be associated with significant morbidity such as Wernicke's encephalopathy, Mallory–Weiss tear, pneumomediastinum
- Early diagnosis and aggressive treatment and support are essential to improve the outcome and quality of life.
- Preconception supplementation of multivitamins may reduce the incidence and severity of NVP
- When intravenous hydration is required specifically before administering dextrose-containing fluids, a bolus dose of thiamine (100 mg) should be given by the parenteral route at least for the initial 3 days
- Management of severe hyperemesis needs a multidisciplinary approach with involvement of obstetrician, endocrinologists, gastroenterologists and psychiatrists.

■ REFERENCES

1. O'Brien B, Evans M, White-McDonald E. Isolation from "being alive": coping with severe nausea and vomiting of pregnancy. Nurs Res. 2002;51:302-8.
2. Gadsby R, Barnie-Adshead T. Severe nausea and vomiting of pregnancy: should it be treated with appropriate pharmacotherapy? Obstet Gynecol. 2011;13:107-11.
3. Royal College of Obstetricians and Gynaecologists. The management of nausea and vomiting of pregnancy and hyperemesis gravidarum. Green-top Guideline No. 69. London; 2016. 1-27 pp.
4. Grooten I, Roseboom T, Painter R. Barriers and challenges in hyperemesis gravidarum research. Nutr Metab Insights. 2015;8(Suppl 1):33-9.
5. Matthews A, Haas DM, O'Mathúna DP, Dowswell T. Interventions for nausea and vomiting in early pregnancy. Cochrane Database Syst Rev. 2015;9:CD007575.
6. Dinberu MT, Mohammed MA, Takelab T, Yimer NB, Desta M, Habtewold TD. Burden, risk factors and outcome of hyperemesis gravidarum in low-income and middle-income countries (LMICs): systematic review and meta-analysis protocol. BMJ Open. 2019;9:e025841.
7. Adams MM, Harlass FE, Sarno AP, Read JA, Rawlings JS. Antenatal hospitalization among enlisted servicewomen, 1987–1990. Obstet Gynecol. 1994;84:35-9.
8. Gazmarian JA, Petersen R, Jamieson CJ, Schild L, Adams MA, Deshpande AD, et al. Hospitalizations during pregnancy among managed care enrollees. Obstet Gynecol. 2002;100:94-100.
9. Dean C, Bannigan K, O'Hara M, Painter R, Marsden J. Recurrence rate of hyperemesis gravidarum in pregnancy: a systematic review protocol. JBI Database Rev Implement Rep. 2017;15(11):2659-65.
10. Simpson SW, Goodwin TM, Robins SB, Rizzo AA, Howes RA, Buckwalter DK, et al. Psychological factors and hyperemesis gravidarum. J Womens Health Gend Based Med. 2001;10:471-7.

11. Flaxman SM, Sherman PW. Morning sickness: a mechanism for protecting mother and embryo. Q Rev Biol. 2000;75:113-48.

12. Braunstein GD, Hershman JM. Comparison of serum pituitary thyrotropin and chorionic gonadotropin throughout pregnancy. J Clin Endocronol Metab. 1976;42:1123-6.

13. Godsby R, Barnie-Adshead AM, Jagger C. A prospective study of nausea and vomiting during pregnancy. Br J Gen Pract. 1993;43:245-8.

14. American College of Obstetricians and Gynecologists. ACOG Practice Bulletin. Clinical management guidelines for obstetrician-gynecologists: nausea and vomiting of pregnancy. Obstet Gynecol. 2018;131:e15-e29.

15. Yashimura M, Hershman JM. Thyrotrophic action of human chorionic gonadotropin. Thyroid. 1995;5:425-34.

16. Jordon V, Grebe SK, Cooke RR, Ford HC, Larsen PD, Stone PR, et al. Acidic isoform of chorionic gonadotropin in European and Samoan women are associated with hyperemesis gravidarum and may be thyrotrophic. Clin Endocrinol. 1999;50: 619-27.

17. Whitehead SA, Andrews PL, Chamberlain GV. Characterisation of nausea and vomiting in early pregnancy: a survey of 1000 women. J Obstet Gynaecol. 1992;12:364-9.

18. Sherman PW, Flaxman SM. Nausea and vomiting of pregnancy in an evolutionary perspective. Am J Obstet Gynecol. 2002;186:S190-7.

19. Buckwalter JG, Simpson SW. Psychological factors in the etiology and treatment of severe nausea and vomiting in pregnancy. Am J Obstet Gynecol. 2002;186:S210-4.

20. Kaplan PB, Gucer F, Sayin NC, Yüksel M, Ali Yüce M, Yardim T. Maternal serum cytokine levels in women with hyperemesis gravidarum in the first trimester of pregnancy. Fertil Steril. 2003;79(3):498-502.

21. Yoneyama Y, Suzuki S, Sawa R, Yoneyama K, Doi D, Araki T. The T-helper 1/T-helper 2 balance in peripheral blood of women with hyperemesis gravidarum. Am J Obstet Gynecol. 2002;187:1631-5.

22. Corey LA, Berg K, Solaas MH, Nance WE. The epidemiology of pregnancy complications and outcome in Norwegian twin population. Obstet Gynecol. 1992;80:989-94.

23. Vallacott I, Cooke E, James CE. Nausea and vomiting in early pregnancy. Int J Gynaecol Obstet. 1988;27(1):57-62.

24. Minturn L, Weiher AW. The influence of diet on morning sickness: a cross-cultural study. Med Antropol. Winter. 1984;8(1):71-5.

25. London V, Grube S, Sherer DM, Abulafia O. Hyperemesis gravidarum: A review of recent literature. Pharmacology. 2017;100:161-71.

26. Goodwin TM. Hyperemesis gravidarum. Progr Obstet Gynaecol. 2007;17:49-64.

27. James WH. The associated offspring sex ratios and cause(s) of hyperemesis gravidarum. Acta Obstet Gynecol Scand. 2001;80:378-9.

28. Einarson A, Maltepe C, Boskovic R, Koren G. Treatment of nausea and vomiting in pregnancy: an updated algorithm. Can Fam Physician. 2007;53:2109-11.

29. Malek NZ, Kalok A, Hanafiah ZA, Shah SA, Ismail NA. Association of transient hyperthyroidism and severity of hyperemesis gravidarum. Horm Mol Biol Clin Investig. 2017;30(3).

30. Alexander EK, Pearce EN, Brent GA, Brown RS, Chen H, Dosiou C, et al. 2017 Guidelines of the American Thyroid Association for the diagnosis and management of thyroid disease during pregnancy and the postpartum. Thyroid. 2017;27:315-89.

31. Goodwin TM, Montoro M, Mestman JH. Transient hyperthyroidism and hyperemesis gravidarum: clinical aspects. Am J Obstet Gynecol. 1992;167:648-52.

32. Rotman P, Hassin D, Mouallem M, Barkai G, Farfel Z. Wernicke's encephalopathy in hyperemesis gravidarum: association with abnormal liver function. Isr J Med Sci. 1994;30:225-8.

33. Ebrahimi N, Maltepe C, Bournissen FG, Koren G. Nausea and vomiting of pregnancy: using the 24-hour Pregnancy-Unique Quantification of Emesis (PUQE-24) scale. J Obstet Gynaecol Can. 2009;31:803-7.

34. Hinkle SN, Mumford SL, Grantz KL, Silver RM, Mitchell EM, Sjaarda LA, et al. Association of nausea and vomiting during pregnancy with pregnancy loss: a secondary analysis of a randomized clinical trial. JAMA Intern Med. 2016;176:1621-7.

35. Gross S, Librach C, Cecutti A. Maternal weight loss associate with hyperemesis gravidarum: a predictor of fetal outcome. Am J Obstet Gynecol. 1989;160:906.

36. Lee NM, Saha S. Nausea and vomiting of pregnancy. Gastroenterol Clin North Am. 2011;40:309-34, vii.

37. Mullin PM, Bray A, Schoenberg F, MacGibbon KW, Romero R, Goodwin TM, et al. Prenatal exposure to hyperemesis gravidarum linked to increased risk of psychological and behavioral disorders in adulthood. J Dev Orig Health Dis. 2011;2:200-4.

38. Czeizel AE, Dudas I, Fritz G, Tecsoi A, Hanck A, Kunovits G. The effect of periconceptional multivitamin mineral supplementation on vertigo, nausea and vomiting in the first trimester of pregnancy. Arch Gynecol Obstet. 1992;251:181-5.

39. Emelianova S, Mazzotta P, Einarson A, Koren G. Prevalence and severity of nausea and vomiting of pregnancy and effect of vitamin supplementation. Clin Invest Med. 1999;22:106-10.

40. American College of Obstetricians and Gynecologists. Practice Bulletin No. 187: Neural tube defects. ACOG Practice Bulletin No. 187. Obstet Gynecol. 2017;130:e279-90.

41. Viljoen E, Visser J, Koen N, Musekiwa A. A systematic review and meta-analysis of the effect and safety of ginger in the treatment of pregnancy-associated nausea and vomiting. Nutr J. 2014;13:20.

42. McParlin C, O'Donnell A, Robson SC, Beyer F, Moloney E, Bryant A, et al. Treatments for hyperemesis gravidarum and nausea and vomiting in pregnancy: a systematic review. JAMA. 2016;316:1392-401.

43. Tan P, Norazilah MJ, Omar SW. Dextrose saline compared with normal saline rehydration of hyperemesis gravidarum: a randomized control trial. Obstet Gynecol. 2013;121(2 pt 1):291-8.

44. Schuster K, Bailey LB, Dimperio D, Mahan CS. Morning sickness and vitamin B6 status of pregnant women. Hum Nutr Clin Nutr. 1985;39:75-9.

45. Sahakian V, Rouse D, Sipes S, Rose N, Niebyl J. Vitamin B6 is effective therapy for nausea and vomiting of pregnancy: a randomized, double-blind placebo-controlled study. Obstet Gynecol. 1991;78:33-6.

46. Niebyl J, Goodwin T. Overview of nausea and vomiting of pregnancy with an emphasis on vitamins and ginger. Am J Obstet Gynecol. 2002;186:S253-5.

47. Tan PC, Yow CM, Omar SZ. A placebo-controlled trial of oral pyridoxine in hyperemesis gravidarum. Gynecol Obstet Invest. 2009;67:151-7.

48. Slaughter SR, Hearns-Stokes R, van der Vlugt T, Joffe HV. FDA approval of doxylamine-pyridoxine therapy for use in pregnancy. N Engl J Med. 2014;370:1081-3.

49. Koren G, Clark S, Hankins GD, Caritis SN, Miodovnik M, Umans JG, et al. Effectiveness of delayed release doxylamine and pyridoxine for nausea and vomiting of pregnancy: a randomized placebo controlled trial. Am J Obstet Gynecol. 2010;203:571.e1-7.

50. Madjunkova S, Maltepe C, Koren G. The delayed release combination of doxylamine and pyridoxine (Diclegis(R)/

Diclectin (R)) for the treatment of nausea and vomiting of pregnancy. Paediatr Drugs. 2014;16:199-211.

51. Magee LA, Mazzotta P, Koren G. Evidence-based view of safety and effectiveness of pharmacologic therapy for nausea and vomiting of pregnancy (NVP). Am J Obstet Gynecol. 2002;186:S256-61.

52. Bustos M, Venkataramanan R, Caritis S. Nausea and vomiting of pregnancy—what's new? Auton Neurosci. 2017;202:62-72.

53. Tan PC, Khine PP, Vallikkannu N, Omar SZ. Promethazine compared with metoclopramide for hyperemesis gravidarum: a randomized controlled trial. Obstet Gynecol. 2010;115:975-81.

54. Matok I, Gorodischer R, Koren G, Sheiner E, Wiznitzer A, Levy A. Safety of metoclopramide use in first trimester of pregnancy. N Engl J Med. 2009;360(24):2528-35.

55. Abas MN, Tan PC, Azmi N, Omar SZ. Ondansetron compared with metoclopramide for hyperemesis gravidarum: a randomized controlled trial. Obstet Gynecol. 2014;123:1272-9.

56. Boelig RC, Barton SJ, Saccone G, Kelly AJ, Edwards SJ, Berghella V. Interventions for treating hyperemesis gravidarum. Cochrane Database of Systematic Reviews and Meta-analysis. J Matern Fetal Neonatal Med. 2018;31(18):2492-505.

57. Kashifard M, Basirat Z, Kashifard M, Golsorkhtabar-Amiri M, Moghaddamnia A. Ondansetrone or metoclopromide? Which is more effective in severe nausea and vomiting of pregnancy? A randomized trial double-blind study. Clin Exp Obstet Gynecol. 2013;40:127-30.

58. Oliveira LG, Capp SM, You WB, Riffenburgh RH, Carstairs SD. Ondansetron compared with doxylamine and pyridoxine for treatment of nausea in pregnancy: a randomized controlled trial. Obstet Gynecol. 2014;124:735-42.

59. Pasternak B, Svanstrom H, Hviid A. Ondansetron in pregnancy and risk of adverse fetal outcomes. N Engl J Med. 2013;368:814-23.

60. Anderka M, Mitchell AA, Louik C, Werler MM, Hernández-Diaz S, Rasmussen SA; National Birth Defects Prevention Study. Medications used to treat nausea and vomiting of pregnancy and the risk of selected birth defects. Birth Defects Res A Clin Mol Teratol. 2012;94:22-30.

61. Danielsson B, Wikner BN, Källén B. Use of ondansetron during pregnancy and congenital malformations in the infant. Reprod Toxicol. 2014;50:134-7.

62. Taylor R. Successful management of hyperemesis gravidarum using steroid therapy. QJM 1996;89:103-7.

63. Safari HR, Alsulyman OM, Gherman RB, Goodwin TM. Experience with oral methylprednisolone in the treatment of refractory hyperemesis gravidarum. Am J Obstet Gynecol. 1998;178:1054-8.

64. Yost NP, McIntire DD, Wians FH, Ramin SM, Balko JA, Leveno KJ. A randomized, placebo-controlled trial of corticosteroids for hyperemesis due to pregnancy. Obstet Gynecol. 2003;102:1250-4.

65. Park-Wyllie L, Mazzotta P, Pastuszak A, Moretti ME, Beique L, Hunnisett L, et al. Birth defects after maternal exposure to corticosteroids: prospective cohort study and meta-analysis of epidemiological studies. Teratology. 2000;62:385-92.

66. Gill SK, O'Brien L, Koren G. The safety of histamine 2 (H2) blockers in pregnancy: a metaanalysis. Dig Dis Sci. 2009;54:1835-8.

67. Gill SK, O'Brien L, Einarson TR, Koren G. The safety of proton pump inhibitors (PPIs) in pregnancy: a meta-analysis. Am J Gastroenterol. 2009;104:1541-5.

68. Debby A, Golan A, Sadan O, Glezerman M, Shirin H. Clinical utility of esophagogastroduodenoscopy in the management of recurrent and intractable vomiting in pregnancy. J Reprod Med. 2008;53:347-51.

69. Sanghvi U, Thankappan KR, Sarma PS, Sali N. Assessing potential risk factors for child malnutrition in rural Kerala, India. J Trop Pediatr. 2001;47:350-5.

70. Liu S, Rouleau J, Joseph KS, Sauve R, Liston RM, Young D, et al.; Maternal Health Study Group of the Canadian Perinatal Surveillance System. Epidemiology of pregnancy-associated venous thromboembolism: a population-based study in Canada. J Obstet Gynaecol Can. 2009;31:611-20.

71. Royal College of Obstetricians and Gynaecologists. Reducing the risk of thrombosis and embolism during pregnancy and the puerperium. Green-top Guideline No. 37a. London: RCOG; 2009.

72. Gill SK, Maltepe C, Koren G. The effectiveness of discontinuing iron-containing prenatal multivitamins on reducing the severity of nausea and vomiting of pregnancy. J Obstet Gynaecol. 2009;29:13-6.

73. Godil A, Chen YK. Percutaneous endoscopic gastrostomy for nutrition support in pregnancy associated hyperemesis gravidarum and anorexia nervosa. J Parenteral Enteral Nutr. 1998;22:238-41.

74. Vaisman N, Kaidar R, Levin I, Lessing JB. Nasojejunal feeding in hyperemesis gravidarum:a preliminary study. Clin Nutr. 2004;23:53-7.

75. Serrano P, Velloso A, Garcia-Luna PP, Pereira JL, Fernádez Z, Ductor MJ, et al. Enteral nutrition by percutaneous endoscopic gastrojejunostomy in severe hyperemesis gravidarum: a report of two cases. Clin Nutr. 1998;17:135-9.

76. Barclay BA. Experience with enteral nutrition in the treatment of hyperemesis gravidarum. Nutr Clin Pract. 1990;5:153-5.

77. Saha S, Loranger D, Pricolo V, Degli-Esposti S. Feeding jejunostomy for the treatment of severe hyperemesis gravidarum: a case series. J Parenter Enteral Nutr. 2009;33:529-34.

78. Ogura JM, Francois KE, Perlow JH, Elliott JP. Complications associated with peripherally inserted central catheter use during pregnancy. Am J Obstet Gynecol. 2003;188:1223-5.

79. Cape AV, Mogensen KM, Robinson MK, Carusi DA. Peripherally inserted central catheter (PICC) complications during pregnancy. J Parenter Enteral Nutr. 2014;38:595-601.

32

Gestational Trophoblastic Disease

Priya Ballal

■ INTRODUCTION

Gestational trophoblastic disease (GTD) is a group of trophoblastic disorders that arise from pregnancy. Some of them remain benign while others have the propensity for metastasis and malignancy. The most benign of them also have the capacity for spontaneous resolution.

The World Health Organization (WHO) classifies GTD into complete mole and partial mole and gestational trophoblastic neoplasia (GTN) or gestational trophoblastic tumors. Gestational trophoblastic tumors may be local invasive like the invasive mole, placental site trophoblastic disease, and choriocarcinoma **(Table 1)**. A rare and aggressive variety termed epithelioid trophoblastic tumor has also been described.

Benign trophoblastic lesions, termed exaggerated placental site and placental site nodule, are not included with GTD.[1]

■ MOLAR PREGNANCY

Two forms of molar pregnancy have been classified: complete mole and partial mole **(Table 2)**. Differentiation of complete and partial moles is of importance in management as partial mole is seldom followed by persistent trophoblastic disease (PTD).

Complete Mole

Complete mole is characteristically an abnormal proliferation of trophoblastic tissue, with dilated and edematous chorionic villi—hydropic degeneration, giving the characteristic appearance of grape-like vesicles filling the uterine cavity. No fetal tissue is seen within the cavity of uterus. The uterine size would have grown larger than the period of gestation in some cases due to excessive proliferation **(Fig. 1)**. Microscopically, the appearance of fluid-filled cisterns are seen within the villi. The vesicular pattern of villi and its translucent thin-walled nature earn it the terms vesicular mole or hydatidiform mole. Excessive and dilated villi on sonography appear as a "snowstorm" pattern. This typical pattern may not be seen in early gestation of 8 weeks or earlier where vesicles are not formed in abundance. An abortus at this gestation may show hydropic changes in the placenta that needs to be differentiated from a molar pregnancy. Hydropic changes in placenta are seen after a spontaneous abortion; they show typically absent circumferential proliferation of trophoblast and only occasional central cistern patterns **(Fig. 2)**. Immunohistochemistry (p57 (kip2)) helps to differentiate between the hydropic change of an abortus and a complete mole. When the fetal tissue is identified along with the trophoblasts, it is important to keep in mind a twin

TABLE 1: Placental tumors.[1]

Malformation of villi	Complete mole Partial mole	Premalignant	Cytotropho-blast and syncytiotro-phoblast
Malignant tumors	Invasive mole Choriocarcinoma Placental site trophoblastic tumor	Malignant	Intermediary trophoblast
	Epithelioid trophoblastic tumor		Intermediary trophoblast
Benign trophoblastic lesions	Exaggerated Placental site Placental site nodule	Benign	

TABLE 2: Comparison between complete and partial mole.

Features	Complete mole	Partial mole
Hydropic changes	Diffuse and placenta not present	Focal
Hyperplasia of trophoblasts	Marked	Mild to moderate
Fetal tissue	Absence of fetus	Present, malformed, or FGR
Fetal vessels	Absent	Present
Karyotype	46XX mostly and paternally derived	69XXY
Malignant potential	15–20%	Rare
β-hCG	Very high	Comparatively low

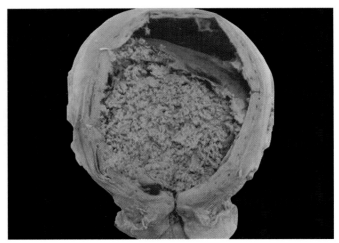

Fig. 1: Complete mole
Courtesy: Department of Pathology, KMC Mangalore

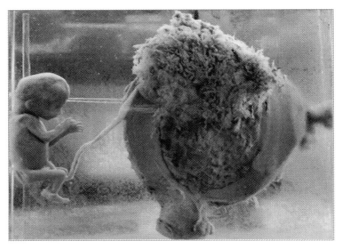

Fig. 3: Partial mole.
Courtesy: Department of Pathology, KMC Mangalore

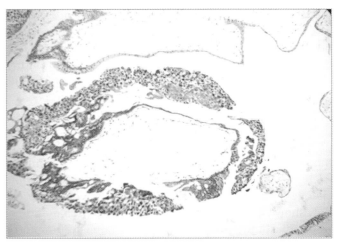

Fig. 2: Microscopic picture of complete mole.
Courtesy: Department of Pathology, KMC Mangalore.

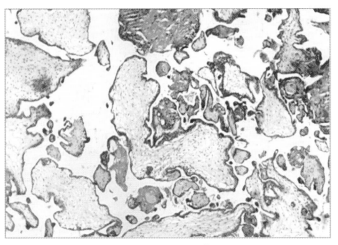

Fig. 4: Microscopic picture of partial mole.
Courtesy: Department of Pathology, KMC Mangalore.

pregnancy where one is molar and the other a normal fetus. Associated normal population of villi may be the clue along with clinical cytogenetic correlation.[2,3]

Partial Mole

Partial mole has few enlarged villi along with normal placenta and hence not as voluminous as a complete mole. Fetal tissue is present along with vesicular placental tissue; however, the fetus most often shows malformations **(Fig. 3)**. Microscopy reveals two types of villi: one large and edematous with central cisterns and the other small with stromal fibrosis. Circumferential fibrosis is typically focal giving a scalloped outline to the villi (Fjord-like) **(Fig. 4)**. Fetal tissue or RBC can be identified.[2,3]

A partial mole needs to be differentiated from a complete mole as a part of twin pregnancy as well as from abortus with hydropic change in placental tissue. Ploidy studies help differentiate a complete mole from partial moles which are triploid.

Complete moles are 46XX and arise by diandric diploidy (94%) or diandric dispermy (4%). Fertilization of an empty pronucleus by a haploid sperm that undergoes duplication is diandric diploidy **(Fig. 5)**. Fertilization of an empty egg by two sperms is diandric dispermy **(Fig. 5)**. Those women with abnormal events during meiosis are at a higher probability of inducing empty/inactive eggs. A biparental complete mole can arise in women who are carriers for mutation of NLRP7 or KHDC3L **(Fig. 5)**. Partial moles are triploid in nature with 69 chromosomes—diandric triploidy **(Fig. 5)**. They arise from fertilization of an oocyte by two sperms.[2,3]

of uterine perforation. The incidence is higher (8%) among women undergoing a secondary curettage, which is no more a part of protocol for managing molar pregnancy or PTD.

Theca Lutein Cysts

Theca lutein cysts are seen in 25–35% of molar pregnancy. They correlate with markedly elevated hCG levels above 1,00,000 mIU. They are physiologically and histologically similar to iatrogenic hyperstimulation caused by ovulation induction. They may cause symptoms of pain/pressure/torsion/rupture or bleeding. Although pain and pressure may be treated by aspiration, the latter will require surgical treatment.

Respiratory Distress

Impaired left ventricular function as a consequence of trophoblastic embolization may be contributory along with coexisting conditions of anemia, hyperthyroidism, hypertension, and iatrogenic fluid overload. Anticipation of central venous pressure monitoring and careful attention to fluid volume are required post evacuation, especially where the uterus volume is large (>14 weeks). It usually resolves in 48 hours with adequate care.

Thyroid Storm

It is suggested that patients who have been diagnosed with features of thyrotoxicosis (elevated thyroxin levels and with symptoms of tachycardia and tremors) prior to evacuation may be benefited from administration of beta-blockers to prevent a thyroid storm during the postevacuation period.

Persistent Trophoblastic Disease

Persistent trophoblastic disease is a complication following a molar pregnancy; its incidence ranges from 3 to 25%. 70–90% are likely to develop invasive mole whereas 10–30% are likely to develop choriocarcinoma. The risk of metastatic disease when PTD is diagnosed is 6–25%.[12] Diagnosis is based on rising/plateauing or persistently elevated hCG post evacuation of mole or an ectopic pregnancy or even in a term pregnancy. The condition can also be diagnosed based on the histological evidence of choriocarcinoma, PSTT, or metastatic disease.

Patients with PTD present with vaginal bleeding resulting from persistent or recurrent trophoblastic proliferation in the uterine cavity. Patients with vaginal bleeding should be subjected to chemotherapy. Performing a dilatation and evacuation increases the risk of perforation and hemorrhage requiring hysterectomy; such a procedure is recommended only in cases of life-threatening hemorrhage.

The risk of developing PTD is associated with advanced age and amount of trophoblastic proliferation which is reflected by factors given in **Box 2**.

BOX 2: Parameters that reflect trophoblastic proliferation.
- Uterine size larger than period of gestation
- Bilateral theca lutein cyst
- β-hCG >1,00,000 mIU/mL
- Hyperthyroidism
- Postevacuation hemorrhage, respiratory distress, and subinvolution

Attempts at predicting PTD have been tried; histological criteria from postevacuation tissue have remained unsuccessful. Studies on hCG assays have been done to identify predictors of PTD. Invasive trophoblastic antigen (ITA) has been found to have 100% sensitivity and specificity for identifying invasive trophoblastic tumors. Women with low levels of hCG (<50 mIU/L) are termed "quiescent gestational trophoblastic disease." Such of those in this category may be subjected to monitoring and surveillance without therapy until β-hCG is positive or ITA is positive.

PROPHYLACTIC CHEMOTHERAPY

Methotrexate used in the treatment of GTD has also been used for the prevention of postmolar GTD. Difficulty in specifically identifying patients who will develop postmolar GTD as well as the toxicity of the drug has made its use controversial. It has been estimated by a randomized controlled trial (RCT) that methotrexate and folinic acid used at the time of evacuation of molar pregnancy reduced the incidence of postmolar disease from 47 to 14% among patients with high-risk criteria but not among the low risk. These prophylactic regimens also involved the risk of developing drug resistance. Postprophylactic chemotherapy does not completely eliminate the risk to develop postmolar GTD, and hence surveillance with hCG cannot be done away with. Thus, it may be concluded that women with high risk for postmolar GTD benefit from chemoprophylaxis. Excellent cure rates in women with postmolar GTD have led to most centers forgoing the use of prophylactic chemotherapy.

POSTMOLAR SURVEILLANCE

The first hCG testing postmolar evacuation should be done after 48 hours. Weekly testing of hCG levels are recommended until three normal values are obtained. This is followed by once-a-fortnight evaluation for 3 months and thereafter monthly hCG monitoring up to 12 months. A pelvic assessment to ensure uterine involution is done when hCG values normalize. A chest X-ray at the time of evacuation is recommended as reference/baseline. Prevention of pregnancy during the surveillance period of 12 months is recommended. Use of OC pills may be advised for such. With low risk for developing postmolar GTD among cases of partial mole, surveillance in these women may be for a shorter period of up to 6 months.

The risk of recurrent mole ranges from 1 to 2%.[13] A third molar pregnancy in such cases has been 15–28%. Patients with a history of molar pregnancy do have a subsequent normal reproductive function and uneventful successful pregnancy with no greater risk for spontaneous miscarriages, preterm labor, intrauterine demise, or congenital anomalies than the general population. Extra care should be taken in these women to diagnose a normal pregnancy early. Postdelivery, it becomes important to rule out occult trophoblastic disease in placenta or products of conception. A chest X-ray to rule out occult metastasis masked by hCG rise in pregnancy should be obtained. hCG levels should be obtained 6 weeks post evacuation or delivery to confirm normalization.

STAGING AND EVALUATION OF GESTATIONAL TROPHOBLASTIC DISEASE

Patients diagnosed with GTD are either identified during surveillance of postmolar evacuation or by the signs and symptoms that occur following any pregnancy event. It is mandatory to send products obtained from MTP or check curettage following incomplete abortions for histopathological examination to rule out GTD. Most often, symptoms may be nongynecological such as hemoptysis, gastrointestinal (GI) bleed, cerebral hemorrhage, and hematuria. Abnormal uterine bleeding that is acyclical or amenorrhea following a pregnancy event also warrants investigations. A β-hCG evaluation in such patients and exclusion of concurrent pregnancy are important in diagnosis. Diagnosis of postmolar GTD is made by International Federation of Obstetrics and Gynecology (FIGO) criteria as already mentioned in **Box 3**.

Phantom hCG

Some women with persistent elevated levels of hCG are found to have false-positive hCG assays, most ranging as high as 200–300 mIU/mL. Even during postchemo or postevacuation surveillance, this false positive is caused by nonspecific heterophile antibodies in a patient's sera. If hCG values persist at low levels and do not respond to methotrexate, then "phantom hCG" is suspected.

BOX 3: Current FIGO criteria to diagnose postmolar GTD/PTD.

- 4 or more values of hCG documenting a plateau for at least 3 weeks (days 1, 7, 14, and 21)
- Rise of hCG of 10% or more for 3 values or longer over the last 2 weeks (days 1, 7, and 14)
- Presence of histologic choriocarcinoma
- Persistence of hCG 6 months after evacuation of mole

(FIGO: International Federation of Obstetrics and Gynecology; GTD: gestational trophoblastic disease; PTD: persistent trophoblastic disease)

Identification of this condition will need evaluation with different immunoassay techniques at different dilutions of serum combined with urinary hCG levels if serum levels are >60 mIU/mL. False-positive hCG assays are not affected by serial dilution. Heterophile antibodies are not excreted in urine and hence will not be detectable in such samples of false-positive hCG levels. It is important to rule out phantom hCG before subjecting patients to second-line chemotherapy or surgery.

EVALUATION

Gestational trophoblastic disease can spread by local invasion or by the hematogenous route. Venous metastasis into subvaginal plexus results in vaginal metastasis and through the uterine venous system into the parametrium and lungs. Disseminated metastasis usually arises once pulmonary metastasis is established, through the systemic circulation to brain, liver, GI tract, and kidneys. Lymphatic spread is uncommon.

Vaginal metastasis can be diagnosed by a clinical examination usually seen as darkened or bluish nodules in the anterior vagina; ulceration or bleeding from the nodule may be present. Due to the high vascularity, a biopsy is not recommended. A solitary vaginal metastasis responds well to chemotherapy. Vaginal packing or embolization may be resorted to in case of active bleeding from vaginal metastasis.

For the purpose of staging, imaging studies such as chest X-ray or CT scan (>30–40% of cases treated as nonmetastatic disease are identified with pulmonary metastasis on CT scan that were undetected by chest X-ray), CT of abdomen and pelvis, and MRI of brain are warranted to identify metastasis. USG of pelvis to rule out concurrent pregnancy should be the initial step in evaluation. It is also helpful in identifying intrauterine tumors and local myometrium invasion.

Secondary dilatation and curettage (D&C) for establishing diagnosis or debulking is not recommended. Basic work-up of the general condition along with routine hematological and clinical chemistry is warranted before chemotherapy is initiated.

CLASSIFICATION AND STAGING OF MALIGNANT GESTATIONAL TROPHOBLASTIC DISEASE

Search for a better classification system in GTD has a history of almost 40 years. The classification systems so evolved are on the basis of risk factors that affect prognosis. It is important to know at least three classification systems that have evolved over the years.

1. *Clinical Classification System:*[14] In this classification, the risk factors are those primarily used to detect

resistance to single-agent chemotherapy. It was found that patients in the poor prognosis group responded well to multiagent chemotherapy. Nonmetastatic disease is not classified on the assumption that this group usually has a good outcome **(Table 5)**.

2. *WHO classification system:* This system was based on analysis of retrospectively identified prognostic factors among patients mainly treated with single-agent chemotherapy. This scoring system applies weightage to each of the factors assumed to act independently. The total of scores was used to stratify risk into low-, medium-, and high-risk categories **(Table 6)**. Certain known risk factors are not included as information

regarding them may not be uniformly available, e.g., blood group. Weightage of scoring has been modified by others to 6, therefore requiring fewer risk factors to identify the highest and lowest risk categories. The lack of recommendations in radiographic studies used to identify the number and site of metastasis may impair uniformity in categorization. Despite the above drawbacks, the modified WHO scoring system has proven useful in identifying those patients with GTD who are at low or high risk for treatment failure.

The clinical classification identifies those patients at risk for treatment failure and death with better sensitivity and specificity whereas WHO prognostic indexed score stratified patients better into low-, medium-, and high-risk population. The clinical classification being relatively simple to use finds its place in the day-to-day practice of a generalist who needs to identify patients who require referral to specialist care for treatment of high-risk disease.[15]

3. *FIGO staging and scoring system:* The initially developed staging system by FIGO was anatomic and recognized progress of disease stepwise. This system did not take into account any of the risk factors **(Table 6)**.[16]

To stage and allot a risk factor score, a patient's diagnosis is allocated to a stage as represented by Roman numerals I, II, III, and IV. This is then separated by a colon from the sum of all the actual risk factor scores expressed in Arabic numerals, i.e., stage II:4, stage IV:9. This stage and score will be allotted for each patient. Those with a score of <6 consolidative score were considered to be low risk

TABLE 5: Clinical classification system for patients with malignant GTD.

Category	Criteria
Nonmetastatic GTD	No evidence of metastases; not assigned to prognostic category
Metastatic GTD	Any extrauterine metastases
Good prognosis metastatic GTD	No risk factors: • Short duration (<4 months) • Pretherapy hCG < 40,000 mIU/mL • No brain or liver metastases • No antecedent term pregnancy • No prior chemotherapy
Poor prognosis metastatic GTD	Any risk factor: • Long duration (>4 months) • Pretherapy hCG > 40,000 mIU/mL • Brain or liver metastases • Antecedent term pregnancy • Prior chemotherapy

(GTD: gestational trophoblastic disease)

TABLE 6: FIGO staging and scoring system.[16]

FIGO anatomical staging	Stages
	I. Disease confined to uterus
	II. GTN spread outside the uterus, limited to genital structures
	III. Lung metastases with or without genital tract involvement
	IV. Other metastases

Modified WHO prognostic scoring system as adapted by FIGO[16]

Scores	0	1	2	4
Age	<40 years	≥40 years	–	–
Antecedent pregnancy	Mole	Abortion	Term	–
Interval months from index pregnancy	<4	4–6	7–12	>12
Pretreatment serum hCG (IU/L)	$<10^3$	$10^3–10^4$	$10^4–10^5$	$>10^5$
Largest tumor size (including uterus)	<3 cm	3–4 cm	≥5 cm	–
Site of metastases	Lung	Spleen, kidney	Gastrointestinal	Liver, brain
Number of metastases	–	1–4	5–8	>8
Previous failed chemotherapy	–	–	Single drug	≥2 drugs
	Risk status • Low • High		*Total score* ≤6 ≥7	

(FIGO: International Federation of Obstetrics and Gynecology; GTN: gestational trophoblastic neoplasia; WHO: World Health Organization)

TABLE 7: Low-risk gestational trophoblastic disease.

Clinical classification	Low-risk metastatic disease
FIGO	Stage III or less
WHO	<6
Charing cross	<8

(FIGO: International Federation of Obstetrics and Gynecology; WHO: World Health Organization)

whereas those with a consolidative score of 7 or greater were considered as high risk.

The revised staging system in 1992 included two risk factors, that of hCG levels and of time from an antecedent pregnancy. In 2000, it was further revised to incorporate the modified WHO prognostic index score.

This new system of scoring intends for uniformity in scoring and helps to accumulate enough data globally for any further research and management plans.

■ TREATMENT OF LOW-RISK GESTATIONAL TROPHOBLASTIC DISEASE (TABLE 7 AND FLOWCHART 1)

Eighty per cent of patients with complete mole and 95% of patients with partial mole are completely cured by evacuation of uterus. For the small fraction of patients who develop persistent disease, management with methotrexate chemotherapy has completely changed the prognosis. Low-risk patients will require less aggressive chemotherapy. Therefore, patients with no metastasis or metastatic disease with low risk are together considered as low-risk malignant GTD. PSTT are considered as high-risk hysterectomy is suggested in such cases. Choriocarcinoma is considered as high risk and metastasis has to be looked for.

■ CHEMOTHERAPY FOR LOW-RISK GESTATIONAL TROPHOBLASTIC NEOPLASIA

All patients with malignant trophoblastic disease will require chemotherapy. The low-risk category will achieve 100% cure rates following chemotherapy if elevated. Those patients with failure of first-line chemotherapy among the low-risk category also have a chance for 100% cure after the next line of chemotherapy regimens. Chemotherapeutic agents such as methotrexate, actinomycin D, 5-fluorouracil, and etoposide are used in low-risk GTN protocols. Chemotherapeutic doses and regimens of administration are described in **Table 8**.

Comparison of various chemotherapeutic regimes identifies methotrexate and actinomycin D regimes to have excellent response with minimum side effects and better cost effectiveness, making them the choice for initial treatment **(Flowchart 2)**. Etoposide was found to have the highest remission rate of 90% compared to others (60–80%). Failure of first-line chemotherapy is likely to occur in a good number of patients, and such cases are subjected to second-line chemotherapy with a different agent from the list given in **Table 8**. Multidrug chemotherapy is reserved for cases who fail second-line chemotherapy. Treatment cycles are to be monitored by hCG measurement weekly. Remission is considered when 3 consecutive weekly hCG levels have normalized. Chemotherapy for low-risk malignant GTD is continued until hCG normalizes and one extra cycle is given thereafter.

Hysterectomy is suggested only in a few select situations of past GTD as mentioned in **Box 4**.

Ovarian preservation may be offered as ovarian metastasis from GTD is very rare. A rare possibility of germ cell tumor with clinical features similar to GTD must be kept in mind. Suspicion of such during hysterectomy warrants removal of ovaries. Posthysterectomy surveillance with hCG is mandatory and any elevated hCG levels warrant chemotherapy as per low-risk treatment protocol. Single-agent chemotherapy at the time of hysterectomy for the purpose of preventing hematogenous spread during surgery has not demonstrated any change in outcome and is not recommended.

Postchemotherapy surveillance begins with the three consecutive normal weekly hCG titers; thereafter, hCG values are evaluated every fortnight (2 weekly) for 3 months followed by monthly hCG estimation for 3 months. This is followed by 2-monthly hCG check for 6 months (total of 1 year). Contraception must be advised during this 1 year of surveillance preferably with OC pills. No detrimental effect was noted on pregnancy after successful completion of chemotherapy and surveillance. Although some studies reported fertility issues, there were no higher risks for fetal malformations. If the patient is desirous of pregnancy, she may be advised attempting pregnancy 6 months after completing treatment.

A rise of 10% or more hCG titer in 2 consecutive months or evidence of new metastasis indicates *resistance*. Recurrence is likely seen within 6 months of normalization of hCG. The incidence ranges from 2.5 to 3.5% among low-risk GTD and nonmetastatic GTD.

■ HIGH-RISK GESTATIONAL TROPHOBLASTIC DISEASE

In women classified as high-risk GTD, treatment is initiated with multidrug chemotherapy. One of the first multidrug combinations to be extensively studied for high-risk GTD was MAC[17] (methotrexate, actinomycin D, and chlorambucil). Bagshawe and co-workers then proposed the CHAMOCA (cyclophosphamide, hydroxyurea, actinomycin D,

Flowchart 1: Protocol for diagnosis and evaluation of low-risk gestational trophoblastic disease.

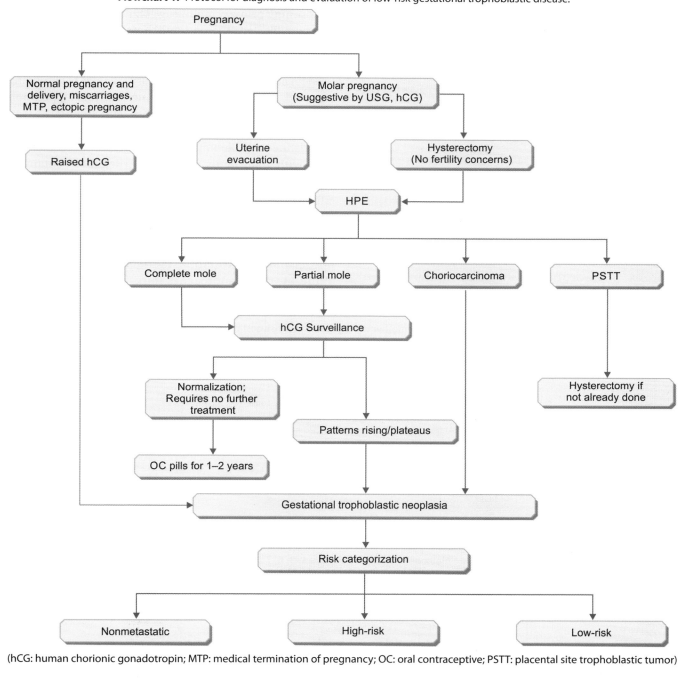

(hCG: human chorionic gonadotropin; MTP: medical termination of pregnancy; OC: oral contraceptive; PSTT: placental site trophoblastic tumor)

methotrexate, vincristine, and doxorubicin) regime.[18] Efficacy was no better than MAC regime, with higher overall toxicity rates. A new drug regime including etoposide was tried in the form of EMA-CO regime (etoposide, methotrexate, actinomycin D, cyclophosphamide, and vincristine) with better success rates of 80–82%. The regime also proved to be effective in those patients who had received prior chemotherapy.[19,20] This regime is now the treatment of choice for high-risk GTD, although several modifications

have been made to the original regime including addition of cisplatin. EMA-CO[16] has been described in **Table 9**.[16]

Although EMA-CO is well tolerated, acute and chronic adverse effects have been identified. Nausea, vomiting, and alopecia are common complaints. Neutropenia and thrombocytopenia are dose-limiting toxicities. Patients who receive EMA-CO regime have the propensity to develop a second cancer with a risk of >50%. Myeloid leukemia, colon cancer, and breast cancer have been known to occur.[21]

TABLE 8: Chemotherapy options for low-risk malignant gestational trophoblastic disease.

Methotrexate	• 20–25 mg (0.4 mg/kg) IM Q day × 5 days (repeat in 7–14 days) • 30–50 mg/m² IM (repeat weekly)
Methotrexate and folinic acid	• Methotrexate 1 mg/kg IM/PO days 1, 3, 5, 7 alternating with folinic acid 0.1 mg/kg IM/PO days 2, 4, 6, 8 (repeat every 14 days) • Methotrexate 300–500 mg/m² IV followed by folinic acid 15 mg PO Q 6° × 4 doses (repeat every 14 days)
Actinomycin D	• 9–13 µg/kg IV Q day × 5 days (repeat every 14 days) • 1.25 mg/m² IV bolus (repeat every 14 days)
Methotrexate and actinomycin D	Methotrexate 20–25 mg (0.4 mg/kg) IM Q day × 5 days in week 1 alternating with actinomycin D 9–13 µg/kg IV Q day × 5 days in week 2 (repeat every 14 days)
5-FU	28–30 mg/kg/day (continuous 10-day infusion)
Etoposide	200 mg/m² for 5 days orally (repeat every 2 weeks)

As about 15–30% of women with high-risk GTD may relapse after primary multidrug chemotherapy. Such cases may be subjected to second-line chemotherapy and surgical resection of persistent disease/metastatic sites. The EMA-EP regime **(Table 10)** containing cisplatin and etoposide are used for such cases, with overall survival rates of 88% being reported. This regime is also prone to myelosuppression requiring treatment delays and dose reductions.[22]

BVP and BEP regimes containing Etoposide or Vincristine with Bleomycin and Cisplatin have also been used with good remission rates.[23-25] Regimes containing VIP (etoposide, ifosfamide, and cisplatin) with cisplatin and vincristine have been tried.

Refractory and resistant patients have been found to tolerate taxane-based regimes better than EMA-EP regime, with equally efficient response. A combination of paclitaxel and cisplatin with etoposide has been described in **Table 11**. Other approaches to resistant and refractory

Flowchart 2: Representation of chemotherapy regimes in low-risk gestational trophoblastic disease.

(GTD: gestational trophoblastic disease; hCG: human chorionic gonadotropin)

BOX 4: Indications for hysterectomy.

- Molar pregnancy in patients not desirous of fertility and advanced maternal age
- Placental site trophoblastic tumor
- Nonmetastatic gestational trophoblastic tumors

TABLE 9: EMA-CO regime.

Regimens	Drug	Dose
Regimen 1		
Day 1	Etoposide	100 mg/m², IV infusion over 30 minutes
	Actinomycin D	0.5 mg, IV bolus
	Methotrexate	100 mg/m², IV bolus
		200 mg/m², IV infusion over 12 hours
Day 2	Etoposide	100 mg/m², IV infusion over 30 minutes
	Actinomycin D	0.5 mg, IV bolus
	Folinic acid rescue	15 mg, PO or IM every 12 hours × 4 doses, beginning 24 hours after methotrexate bolus infusion
Regimen 2		
Day 8	Cyclophosphamide	600 mg/m², IV infusion over 30 minutes
	Vincristine	1 mg/m², IV bolus (maximum 2 mg)

The two regimens alternate each week.

TABLE 10: EMA-EP regime.

Day	Drug	Dose
1	Etoposide	150 mg/m², IV infusion over 30 minutes
	Cisplatin	25 mg/m², IV in 1 L NS and 20 mmol KCL over 4 hours
	Cisplatin	25 mg/m², IV in 1 L NS and 20 mmol KCL over 4 hours
	Cisplatin	25 mg/m², IV in 1 L NS and 20 mmol KCL over 4 hours
8	Etoposide	100 mg/m², IV infusion over 30 minutes
	Methotrexate	300 mg/m², IV over 12 hours
	Actinomycin D	0.5 mg/m², IV bolus
9	Folinic acid	15 mg PO/IM every 12 hours × 4 doses, beginning 24 hours after methotrexate bolus infusion
15	Begin next cycle	

patients would be high-dose chemotherapy with peripheral stem cell transplantation.

Multidrug chemotherapy regimes are given for two to three cycles after three consecutive hCG are normal and there is no clinical evidence of metastasis.

■ MANAGEMENT OF METASTATIC SITES

Lung metastasis is the most common site. These pulmonary nodules may not resolve radiographically until completion

TABLE 11: TP/TE schedule for relapsed GTD[26]

Regimen	Schedule
Day 1	
Dexamethasone	20 mg oral (12 hours pre-paclitaxel)
Dexamethasone	20 mg oral (6 hours pre-paclitaxel)
Cimetidine	30 mg in 100 mL NS over 30 minutes IV
Chlorphenamine	10 mg bolus IV
Paclitaxel	135 mg/m² in 250-mL NS over 3 hours IV
Mannitol	10% in 500 mL over 1 hour IV
Cisplatin	60 mg/m² in 1-L NS over 3 hours IV
Posthydration	1-L NS + KCl mmol + 1 g MgSO₄ over 2 hours IV
Day 15	
Dexamethasone	20 mg oral (12 hours pre-paclitaxel)
Dexamethasone	20 mg oral (6 hours pre-paclitaxel)
Cimetidine	30 mg in 100 mL NS over 30 minutes IV
Chlorphenamine	10 mg bolus IV
Paclitaxel	135 mg/m² in 250 mL NS over 3 hours IV
Etoposide	150 mg/m² in 1 L NS over 1 hours IV

of treatment. Those with resistant disease may be subjected to thoracotomy and lung resection.

Hepatic metastasis is a poor prognosticator for GTD. Uncontrollable hepatic hemorrhage is often fatal to patients with hepatic metastasis. Liver irradiation, hepatic artery embolization, or partial hepatectomy has been used to prevent such hemorrhage. Hepatic chemoembolization has also been tried.

Brain metastasis occurs in 10–15% of patients with metastatic GTD most often seen on frontal and parietal bones. These patients present with symptoms of headache, vomiting, convulsions, and neurological deficit. Whole-brain irradiation along with multidrug chemotherapy is the treatment for such metastasis. Intrathecal administration has also been used for the treatment of brain metastasis. Craniotomy and tumor excision are reserved for select cases only.

Patients are likely to require resection and anastomosis of bowel in cases where *GI metastasis* has been found in resistant disease.

Pelvic metastasis: Vaginal nodules are highly vascular and require resection only if they are the sole focus of resistant disease. A hysterectomy in women with high-risk GTD is considered in a woman with recurrent neoplasia or in patients who have only a small extrauterine tumor burden.

Surveillance After Treatment of High-risk Gestational Trophoblastic Disease

Surveillance is required with serial hCG monitoring monthly for the first 2 years after remission. Recommendation for follow-up to 5 years is as per **Table 12**.[26]

Pregnancy should be discouraged for at least 1 year after completion of treatment. 5-year survival for patients with high-risk GTN after treatment is 86%.[27] New imaging

TABLE 12: UK follow-up protocol of gestational trophoblastic neoplasia patients who have been treated with chemotherapy

	Low-/high-risk postchemotherapy patients, hCG concentration sampling	
	Urine	Blood
Year 1 Week 1–6 after chemotherapy Months 2–6 Months 7–12	Weekly 2 weekly 2 weekly	Weekly 2 weekly –
Year 2	4 weekly	–
Year 3	8 weekly	–
Year 4	3 monthly	–
Year 5	4 monthly	–
After year 5	6 monthly	–

modalities and sensitive investigative tools have improved the diagnosis and follow-up such that prompt diagnosis and treatment can cure even those patients with metastatic disease.

KEY POINTS

- βhCG is a reliable tumor marker used for diagnosis and follow up of H mole patients.
- Complete moles are derived from paternal genome (46XX, diploid) whereas, partial moles are composed of both paternal and maternal genomes (triploid, 69XXX).
- Suction evacuation irrespective of size of uterus is the preferred method of evacuation.
- Pregnancy should be avoided for atleast 6 months following evacuation.
- Regular follow-up is essential for timely diagnosis of gestational trophoblastic neoplasia.
- GTN can be suspected by plateau, rising or prolonged persistence of elevated hCG values after molar evacuation.
- Low risk GTN is treated with Actinomycin D or Methotrexate.
- High risk GTN is treated with EMA/CO chemotherapy.

REFERENCES

1. Alteri A, Franceshchi S, Ferlay J, Smith J, La Vecchia C. Epidemiology and aetiology of gestational trophoblastic diseases. Lancet Oncol. 2003;4(11):670-8.
2. Hammond C, Soper J. Gestational trophoblastic diseases. Glob Libr Women's Med. [online] Available from 10.3843/GLOWM.10263. [Last accessed October, 2020]
3. Hawkins JL. Obstetric anesthesia. Clin Obstet Gynecol. 2003;46(3):614-5.
4. Union for International Cancer Control, 2014 Review of Cancer Medicines on the WHO List of Essential Medicines. Gestational trophoblastic neoplasia. [online] Available from https://www.who.int/selection_medicines/committees/expert/20/applications/GestationalTrophoblasticNeoplasia.pdf?ua=1 [Last accessed October, 2020]
5. Palmer JR. Advances in the epidemiology of gestational trophoblastic disease. J Reprod Med. 1994; 39:155.
6. Sekharan PK, Sreedevi NS, Radhadevi VP, et al. Hydatidiform mole in Calicut, India. Proceedings of XII World Congress on Gestational Trophoblastic Disease, Boston; 2003.
7. Ballal Priya K, Pralhad K, Shetty N, Polnaya R. Variation in prevalence of gestational trophoblastic disease in India. Indian J Gynecol Oncolog. 2016;14:1-4.
8. Takeuchi S. Incidence of gestational trophoblastic disease by regional registration in Japan. Hum Reprod. 1987;2:729.
9. Lorigan PC, Sharma S, Bright N, Coleman RE, Hancock BW. Characteristics of women with recurrent molar pregnancies. Gynecol Oncol. 2000;78:288-92.
10. Berkowitz RS, Cramer DW, Bernstein MR, Cassells S, Driscoll SG, Goldstein DP. Risk factors for complete molar pregnancy, case control study. Am J Obstet Gynecol. 1985;152:1016-20.
11. Royal College of Obstetricians and Gynaecologists. Gestational Trophoblastic Disease (Green-top Guideline No. 38). London: RCOG; 2010.
12. Lurain JR, Brewer JI, Torok EE, Halpern B. Natural history of hydatidiform mole after primary evacuation. Am J Obstet Gynecol. 1983;145:591.
13. Lurain JR, Sand PK, Carson SA, Brewer JI. Pregnancy outcome subsequent to consecutive hydatidiform moles. Am J Obstet Gynecol. 1982;142:1060.
14. Soper JT, Lewis JL, Hammond CB. Gestational trophoblastic disease. In: Hoskins WJ, Perez CA, Young RC (Eds). Principles and Practice of Gynecologic Oncology, 2nd edition. Philadelphia, Lippincott-Raven, 1996; pp. 1039-77.
15. Soper JT, Evans AC, Conaway MR, Clarke-Pearson DL, Berchuck A, Hammond CB. Evaluation of prognostic factors and staging in gestational trophoblastic tumor. Obstet Gynecol. 1994;84:969-73.
16. Ngan HYS, Seckl MJ, Berkowitz RS, Xiang Y, Golfier F, Sekharan PK, et al. Update on the diagnosis and management of gestational trophoblastic disease. Int J Gynecol Obstet. 2018;143(2):79-85.
17. Hammond CB, Borchert LG, Tyrey L, Creasman WT, Parker RT. Treatment of metastatic trophoblastic disease: good and poor prognosis. Am J Obstet Gynecol. 1973;115:451-7.
18. Bagshawe KD. Treatment of high risk choriocarcinoma. J Reprod Med. 1984;29: 813-20.
19. Newlands ES, Bagshawe KD, Begent RH, Rustin GJ, Holden L, Dent J. Developments in chemotherapy for medium and high risk patients with gestational trophoblastic tumors. (1979 – 1984). Br J Obstet Gynaecol. 1986;93:63-9.
20. Newlands ES, Bagshawe KD, Begent RH, Rustin GJ, Holden L. Results with EMA/CO (etoposide, methotrexate, actinomycin D, cyclophosphamide, vincristine) regimen in high risk gestational trophoblastic tumors, 1979 to 1989. Br J Obstet Gynaecol. 1991;98:550-7.
21. Rustin GJ, Newlands ES, Lutz JM, Holden L, Bagshawe KD, Hiscox JG, et al. Combination but not single agent methotrexate chemotherapy for gestational trophoblastic tumors increases the incidence of second tumors. J Clin Oncol. 1996;14:2769-73.

22. Newlands ES, Mulholland PJ, Holden L, Seckl MJ, Rustin GJ. Etoposide and cisplatin/etoposide, methotrexate, and actinomycin D (EMA) chemotherapy for patients with high-risk gestational trophoblastic tumors refractory to EMA/Cyclophosphamide and vincristine chemotherapy and patients presenting with metastatic placental site trophoblastic tumors. J Clin Oncol. 2000;18:854-9.

23. Gordon AN, Kavanagh JJ, Gerhenson DM, Saul PB, Copeland LJ, Allen Stringer G. Cisplatin, vinblastine, and bleomycin combination therapy in resistant gestational trophoblastic disease. Cancer. 1986;58:1407-10.

24. DuBeshter B, Berkowitz RS, Goldstein DP, Bernstein M. Vinblastine, cisplatin and bleomycin as salvage therapy for refractory high-risk metastatic gestational trophoblastic disease. J Reprod Med. 1989;34:189-92.

25. Azab M, Droz JP, Theodore C, Wolff JP, Amiel JL. Cisplatin, vinblastine, and bleomycin combination in the treatment of resistant high risk gestational trophoblastic tumors. Cancer. 1989;69:1829-32.

26. Secakl MJ, Sebire NJ, Fisher RA, Golfier F, Massuger L, Sessa C. Gestational trophoblastic disease: ESMO clinical practice guidelines for diagnosis, treatment and follow up. Ann Oncol. 2013;24(suppl 6): vi39-vi50.

27. Bower M, Newlands ES, Holden L, Short D, Brock C, Rustin GJ, et al. EMA/CO for high risk gestational trophoblastic tumors: results from a cohort of 272 patients. J Clin Oncol. 1997;15:2636-43.

Cesarean Section

Virendra Kumar CM

INTRODUCTION

Motherhood is the greatest and the hardest thing in the world. Pregnancy makes us realize how fragile and important life is as well as giving birth to life and why it must be protected at all cost. Obstructed labor and postpartum hemorrhage were the most dreaded complications faced by the women in labor. The latter was often secondary to prolonged labor. Cesarean delivery emerged as a life-saving surgical procedure when such or other complications arise during pregnancy or delivery. The dramatic and medically unjustified indications have transformed this surgery into one of the most performed surgeries in modern obstetric practice. 18.5 million cases were performed annually.[1]

New knowledge of human anatomy in the eighteenth century led to the first modern cesarean section by Henry Thomson and John Hunter in London in 1769. Further improvement in anesthesiology and transfusion medicine made cesarean section a more safer procedure.[1]

In 1985, the World Health Organization (WHO) in Fortaleza, Brazil, concluded, "there is no justification for any region to have a cesarean delivery rate higher than 10–15%." But this statement was subjected to maximum criticism. Both very high and very low cesarean section rates are dangerous for any region as they depict excessive unnecessary surgical interventions or resource-poor settings.[1]

HISTORY

Historically, cesarean sections were done to extract the baby from the mother in a deceased or in a moribund state just for the purpose of separate burial ceremonies as per the customs. They were rarely done to save the mother or the baby.[1]

The most prevailing myth on cesarean section is the birth of Gaius Julius Caesar (13 July 100 BC–15 March 44 BC), the Roman general and statesman, who was delivered abdominally. But such a delivery was certainly unlikely at that period of time. The term "cesarean" derived from "Julius Caesar" is still controversial.[1]

The Roman law "Lex Regia" forbids the burial of a pregnant woman before the young has been excised: who does otherwise clearly causes the promise of life to perish with the mother. This law Lex Regia became part of the "*Lex Caesaris or Lex Caesarea*." This would have led to the origin of the term "cesarean."

In Latin, verb "*caedere*" means "to cut."

The term cesarean section (la section cesarienne) was first used by the French obstetrician Jacques Guillimeau in his 1609 book on midwifery, *De l'heureux accouchement desfemmes*.

In the 16th century, obstetricians opposed performing surgery on live patients because maternal mortality was incredibly high. As well, during most of the 19th century (1787–1876), no successful cesarean operation had been performed in Paris. This was attributed to the wrong belief that the natural rhythmic contraction and relaxation of the uterus prevented the use of sutures. Therefore, after the baby was removed, incisions in the uterus were left open. Due to this, women died from hemorrhage and infection. As well, in those days, sutures had to be removed, and it was impossible to remove them from the uterine wall after the abdomen had been closed.[1]

The first man to close a uterine incision with sutures was Lebas, a French surgeon in 1769. However, the usage of sutures did not become popular until his method resulted in reduced mortality rates.

Important milestones in cesarean section since Renaissance are given in **Table 1**.[2]

CLINICAL ANATOMY

The nerve supply of the abdominal wall is provided by thoracic nerves T6–T12, including the subcostal nerve, and the cutaneous branches of the iliohypogastric nerve and the ilioinguinal nerve, both of which derive from the lumbar nerve L1. So, regional anesthesia for a cesarean section must extend up to the T6 level.

Langer's lines—also known as cleavage lines—are natural lines of cleavage of the skin, where the skin is least flexible and are determined by the direction of alignment of collagen fibers. There is minimal scarring when incision is over it.

TABLE 1: Important milestones in cesarean section since Renaissance.[2]

Year	Name and Country	Description
1543	A Vesalius, Belgium	First human anatomy book, De humani corporis fabrica
1581	F Rousset, France	Describes cesarean sections performed on living women in Hysterotomotokia
1596	S Mercurio, Italy	First detailed cesarean section indications in La Commare o raccoglitrice
1610	J Trautmann, Germany	First authenticated cesarean section with survival of the mother
1769	J Lebas, France	First closure of the uterus after cesarean section
1786	S Johnson, United Kingdom	First description of lower segment uterine incision
1876	E Porro, Italy	Cesarean section followed by supracervical partial hysterectomy and salpingo-oophorectomy
1882	F Kehrer and M Sanger, Germany	Transverse incision of lower uterine segment and uterine closure using sutures made of silver wire
1900	H Pfannenstiel, Germany	Described transverse suprapubic skin incisions
1908	M Munro Kerr, United Kingdom	First series of suprapubic skin incision and transperitoneal lower segment cesarean sections

The layers of the abdominal wall below the umbilicus are as follows: skin, superficial (Camper's) fascia, membranous (Scarpa's) fascia, rectus sheath, muscle, and parietal peritoneum which are all passed through in transverse incision.

The rectus sheath is formed from the medial aponeurotic extensions of the lateral abdominal wall muscles (from anterior to posterior, the external oblique muscle, the internal oblique muscle, and the transversus muscle).

In vertical incision, it passes through the linea alba, which is an almost bloodless line allowing rapid entry to the abdomen.

It is important to have in mind the mapping of the vascularity for a successful surgery with minimal blood loss. Superficially, the inferior part of the abdominal wall is supplied medially by the superficial epigastric artery and laterally by the superficial circumflex artery. Both are branches of the femoral artery. Below the superficial level, the inferior epigastric artery supplies the medial part of the lower abdomen, and the deep circumflex iliac artery supplies the lateral part. Both of these arteries are branches of the external iliac artery. The veins run in the plane between the superficial and the deep fascia.

The superficial inferior epigastric veins are approximately 4 cm lateral to the midline of the Pfannenstiel incision, on either side. They are superior to the rectus sheath. The inferior epigastric arteries are posterior to the rectus muscles. The branches of the superior epigastric artery and vein pierce the rectus at each intersection.

The uterus and fallopian tubes are supplied by the uterine arteries, with collateral supply from the ovarian arteries. The uterine arteries are branches of the internal iliac arteries. The internal iliac arteries arise from the common iliac arteries at the level of the fourth lumbar vertebra. The uterine artery passes medially from the pelvic side wall to the level of the junction between the uterus and the vagina. As it passes medially, it crosses the ureter at a point 1.5 cm lateral to the lateral fornices of the vagina. The ureters pass below the uterine arteries at this point.

The uterine arteries then divide into ascending and descending branches, with the former passing along the lateral margin of the uterus and the latter forming a vaginal branch. The ovarian arteries are branches of the abdominal aorta. They descend along the posterior abdominal wall and then cross over the external iliac arteries at the pelvic brim, at which point they enter the suspensory ligaments to supply the ovaries. Tubal branches then anastomose with tubal branches of the uterine arteries to supply the fallopian tubes.

The venous drainage of the uterus, the cervix, the upper vagina, and the ovaries is via a plexus of veins running within the parametrium. The plexus forms veins that run alongside the arterial blood supply. With the exception of the left ovarian vein, which drains into the left renal vein, these veins drain into the inferior vena cava.[3]

■ INDICATIONS FOR CESAREAN SECTIONS[4]

Rising cesarean section rates are a major public health concern and cause worldwide debates. To propose and implement effective measures to reduce or increase CS rates where necessary require an appropriate classification. Seven domains (ease, clarity, mutually exclusive categories, totally inclusive classification, prospective identification of categories, reproducibility, and implement ability) were assessed and graded. 27 classifications were identified. They were categorized as indication-based classifications, urgency-based classifications, woman-based classifications, and other types of classifications.

Two classifications, Althabe and Anderson's, respectively, obtained the best overall grade for *indication-based classification*. Althabe's classification was considered clear in its definition of categories. Anderson's classification provided clear hierarchical rules on how to classify a woman with more than one indication for cesarean section. Van Dillen's classification obtained the best overall grade among *urgency-based classifications*.

The 10-group (Robson's) classification received the maximum grade in *women-based classification*; the 8-group

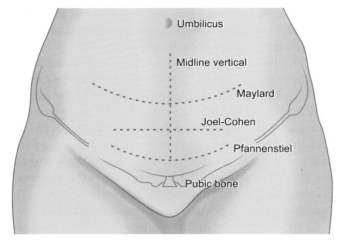

Labels: Umbilicus, Midline vertical, Maylard, Joel-Cohen, Pfannenstiel, Pubic bone

Fig. 1: Various incisions for cesarean section.

(Denk) and the case-mix (Cleary) classifications also obtained high grades.

The WHO recommends the 10-group (Robson) classification as the global standard for comparing varying cesarean section rates across facilities:

1. Nulliparous with single cephalic pregnancy, ≥37 weeks' gestation in spontaneous labor
2. Nulliparous with single cephalic pregnancy, ≥37 weeks' gestation who either had labor induced or were delivered by cesarean delivery before labor
3. Multiparous without a previous uterine scar, with single cephalic pregnancy, ≥37 weeks' gestation in spontaneous labor
4. Multiparous without a previous uterine scar, with single cephalic pregnancy, ≥37 weeks' gestation who either had labor induced or were delivered by cesarean delivery before labor
5. All multiparous with at least one previous uterine scar, with single cephalic pregnancy, ≥37 weeks' gestation
6. All nulliparous women with a single breech pregnancy
7. All multiparous women with a single breech pregnancy including women with previous uterine scars
8. All women with multiple pregnancies including women with previous uterine scars
9. All women with a single pregnancy with a transverse or oblique lie, including women with previous uterine scars
10. All women with a single cephalic pregnancy, <37 weeks' gestation, including women with previous scars

The 2008 WHO Surgical Safety Checklist (http://www.who.int/patientsafety/safesurgery/checklist/en/) was introduced to improve the safety of surgical procedures.

Modified versions of the checklist for obstetrics have been recently proposed (see http://www.nrls.npsa.nhs.uk/resources/type/guidance and http://sogc.org/wp-content/uploads/2013/04/JOGC-Jan2013-CPG286-ENG-Online.pdf). The most important modification of the checklist seems to be adoption of classification of the level of urgency of cesarean section (cesarean section grades).

PREOPERATIVE PREPARATION FOR CESAREAN SECTION

Pubic hair in the region of the proposed skin incision may be clipped.

The reason for hair removal is mainly to prevent interference with wound approximation, as there is no evidence that reduces the risks of wound infection.

The operating table should have a lateral tilt of 15°, or a pillow or folded linen should be placed under the woman's right lower back to avoid vena caval compression and supine hypotension syndrome.

It is now well established that parenteral antibiotic prophylaxis (ampicillin or first-generation cephalosporins) 30–60 minutes before the skin incision reduces the risk of postpartum endometritis.

Fixing an indwelling urethral catheter (Foley catheter) is to be done routinely and it is left in situ for 12–24 hours until the patient is able to be mobile. Painting with 0.5% chlorhexidine in methylated spirits was associated with lower rates of site infection than preparation with alcohol-based povidone-iodine.[1]

SURGICAL TECHNIQUE

In the last four decades, the main cesarean section procedure has been the so-called Pfannenstiel cesarean section (also known as the Pfannenstiel–Kehrer–Kerr cesarean section or the Monro Kerr cesarean section). This procedure is based on a technique described by Hermann Johannes Pfannenstiel (1862–1909) in 1900 to open the abdomen horizontally and is also described by Ferdinand Adolf Kehrer (1837–1914) in 1881 to open the lower segment of the uterus transversely.[1,5]

It became widespread following strong support by John Martin Munro Kerr (1868–1960), who combined the suprapubic transverse incision described by Pfannenstiel and the low transverse uterine opening described by Kehrer.

The traditional Pfannenstiel incision involves the transverse cutting of the skin and subcutaneous tissue along a straight or slightly curved cut approximately 15-cm long in the Malgaigne triangle area. This region has the approximate shape of an isosceles triangle that points down to the pubic symphysis and with its base at the top; along the top it is defined by the Bumm pelvic fold and on the sides and bottom by the two groin-femoral folds.

An alternative to the traditional Pfannenstiel abdomen opening is the Joel–Cohen transverse incision. With clear understanding of the anatomy of the anterior abdominal wall and by stretching technique instead of sharp dissection, it reduces surgical duration and improves healing.

In the Misgav Ladach method, two innovative principles followed are the Joel-Cohen's laparotomy and the nonclosure of the peritoneum, respectively.

The uterine incision type has not been studied separately in a trial. The transverse incision in the lower uterine segment (LUS) is recommended by most experts. Some experts advocate the classic vertical or at least low-vertical incision if the LUS is not large enough to allow a transverse incision [e.g., for the very preterm (<28 weeks of gestation) uterus, fibroids], but this has been associated with increased blood loss compared with low transverse incision (recommendation: B; quality: fair). Expansion of uterine incision either bluntly or by scissors was evaluated in two randomized trials. Sharp expansion significantly increases blood loss and the need for transfusion and is associated with more extensions. Because it is also quicker and is associated with less risk of inadvertently cutting the neonate or cord, blunt expansion should be preferred to sharp expansion of the uterine incision (recommendation: A; quality: good).

The baby is delivered by placing one hand inside the uterine cavity between the uterus and the baby's head.

The head is grasped, flexed, and gently lifted through the incision, taking care not to extend the incision. During manipulations to take out jammed head thinned segment can have tears in the lower portion. It is a good idea to apply a stay suture on the segment and then incise the uterus. Fetal extraction is difficult in 1–2% of cesarean deliveries.[1]

For a deeply engaged head:

- *Abdomino-vaginal delivery ("push method"):* The assistant places his/her gloved, cupped hand into the vagina to gently disengage and push the impacted fetal head up into the uterus for extraction via cesarean delivery.[6]
- *Patwardhan technique ("shoulder first method"):* The anterior shoulder is delivered out by hooking the arm first. With gentle traction on this shoulder, the posterior shoulder is then delivered. Next, the surgeon holds the trunk of the baby gently with both thumbs parallel to spine and with fundal pressure given by the assistant the buttocks are delivered, followed by legs. Finally, the baby's head, which is the only part still inside the uterus, is gently lifted out of the uterus.[7]
- *Fetal head elevators:* They take up less space than the obstetrician's hand; they are easier to get around a tightly impacted head.
- *Obstetric spoons:* Several variations of these instruments are available, including the Coyne spoon, the Sellheim spoon, and the Murless head extractor. For each instrument, the smooth, rounded edge is carefully slipped into the uterus, between the fetal head and the anterior LUS, and gently positioned below the fetal head. Using the handle, the instrument and fetal head are then carefully elevated out of the pelvis, and the delivery is completed in the usual manner.

For delivery of the floating fetal head, internal podalic version and extraction as breech are easier. Use of vacuum, Coyne spoon, or forceps are reasonable alternatives, depending on the operator's skill set and comfort with each technique.

- *Fetal pillow:* The fetal disimpacting system (fetal pillow) is another variation on the fetal elevator. The device has a balloon that is inserted into the vagina just below the fetal scalp when the patient is being prepared for cesarean delivery. A short time before the hysterotomy incision is made, the balloon is inflated with 60–120 mL saline, which is supposed to gently lift the fetal head 2–3 cm from its original position. After the newborn is delivered, the device is deflated and removed.
- *C-Snorkel:* The C-Snorkel is a disposable device consisting of a molded, polymer tube and a flat, curved polymer tip with multiple ventilation ports.

For hemostatic purposes, the Green-Armytage compressor clamps are best suited and tissue friendly to grasp the angles of the uterine incision.

Uterine incision closure is done with delayed absorbable suture material, preferably in two layers, where continuous interlocking first layer and imbricated second layer suturing are done. When a single layer is used, it is continuous locking or interlocking. A newer technique, Babu and Magon's uterine closure technique, is where delayed absorbable suture polyglactin 910(0) or PGA (0) is used by the continuous modified mattress suture technique in a single layer excluding the decidual layer. Deciduas to deciduas, myometrium to myometrium, and serosa to serosa layers' anatomical approximation is achieved here. But long-term studies are needed yet to establish the benefits of this technique.[8]

Regarding the uterine exteriorization, there are different schools of thought; various randomized controlled trials (RCTs) were done to study the outcome and benefits. Some are of the opinion that *"Exteriorization of uterus for repair following Cesarean delivery is not associated with significant problems and it is associated with less blood loss, shorter operative time, decreased hospital stay and less febrile morbidity."* While some say *"uterine exteriorization and **in situ** repair have similar effects on peri-operative cesarean section morbidity. No clinically significant differences between uterine exteriorization and **in situ** repair were found in pulse rate, mean arterial pressure, oxygen saturation and hemoglobin changes."* Uterine exteriorization can be done as and when the situation warrants for better visualization of the angles and as per the surgeon's comfort.

Randomized controlled trials have shown that nonclosure of parietal peritoneum is associated with shorter operative time, lesser incidence of febrile mortality, lesser antibiotic and analgesic use, and overall reduced cost of hospital stay.

Cesarean Section Surgical Techniques

CORONIS

CORONIS is a fractional, factorial, multicenter, unmasked, RCT at 19 sites in Argentina, Chile, Ghana, India, Kenya, Pakistan, and Sudan to assess two surgical techniques (intervention pairs) for five elements of the cesarean section operation. The five intervention pairs were as follows: (1) blunt versus sharp abdominal entry, (2) exteriorization of the uterus for repair versus intra-abdominal repair, (3) single-layer versus double-layer closure of the uterus, (4) closure versus nonclosure of the peritoneum (pelvic and parietal), and (5) chromic catgut versus polyglactin-910 for uterine repair.[9]

The findings of CORONIS, when combined with the existing evidence, suggest that clinicians are free to carry on with their existing practices, at least with respect to their effect on short-term postoperative morbidity. However, particularly for interventions that involve closure of the uterine incision (single-layer vs. double-layer closure or use of different suture materials) as well as closure or nonclosure of the peritoneum, longer term outcomes are needed to enable clinicians to make fully informed decisions about what surgical approaches to take.[9]

CAESAR

The CAESAR[10] study is a RCT was conducted to find whether the following alternative surgical techniques affect the risk of adverse outcomes : single-versus double-layer closure of the uterine incision, closure versus nonclosure of the pelvic peritoneum, and liberal versus restricted use of a subrectus sheath drain.

Results do have implications for clinical practice, particularly in relation to current guidance about closure of the peritoneum, which suggests that nonclosure is preferable.

■ ANESTHESIA FOR CESAREAN SECTION

The most preferred anesthesia for cesarean section is regional anesthesia. Spinal anesthesia is the most routinely opted option. The default fall-back technique when regional anesthesia not possible or contraindicated is general anesthesia where intubation with rapid-sequence induction is expected. It is indicated for sick and unstable patients and for very urgent cesarean section.

For general anesthesia, prepare, drape and be ready with a knife to start as soon as the endotracheal tube (ET) tube is in. It is believed to be 2 minutes from the intubation to delivery so as to have reduced anesthetic drug effects on the baby. In the past when thiopentone was the anesthetic agent used, it was advisable for extraction of the baby either within 45 seconds or after 4 minutes, as it is a barbiturate with ultra-short action. It crosses the blood–brain barrier and placenta. The reason is redistribution of drug in muscle and fat. So we either act before its action starts (45 seconds) or action is finished (4 minutes); otherwise we may (not necessarily) get a slightly depressed baby.

The advantages of spinal anesthesia over general are that it is quick to perform, reliable dense block, and cheap with little airway risk (NB: having an airway-competent practitioner present is essential).

Generally, it is considered very safe as the mother is awake, so mother–baby bonding can occur rapidly. Neuraxial opioid may be given for postoperative analgesia.

The disadvantages of spinal anesthesia are that duration of block < 2 hours, hypotension, and vasopressors may be needed. Fetal acidosis is associated with high ephedrine use. There is risk of post-dural-puncture headache.

General anesthesia is considered the fastest and the most reliable technique for induction with mother asleep and airway secured once intubated. It can also be used to manage unstable patients. Complex equipment are required and an expert anesthetist is needed for the procedure. Risks of failed intubation/aspiration, uterine atony/increased blood loss, postoperative pain relief, and postoperative nausea and vomiting may be problematic. Drug transfer to baby, neonatal depression, and delayed mother–baby bonding are to be considered.

If intraoperative hemorrhage exceeds 1 L, give additional oxytocics (e.g., oxytocin infusion, misoprostol). When uncontrolled with pharmacologic therapy, consider uterine compression sutures (Hayman), followed if necessary by uterine artery ligation. Internal iliac artery ligation can be tried. Arterial embolization requires specialized facilities and expertise. Adequate and appropriate blood transfusion protocols should be followed to prevent postoperative complications such as shock lung. Thromboprophylaxis is to be considered in all operated cases.

The incidence of placenta accreta has increased in parallel with the increase in the frequency of cesarean section, indicating a direct causal effect. Placenta accreta complicates about 5% of pregnancies with placenta previa and one prior cesarean section. The strongest risk factor for placenta previa and therefore placenta accreta is a prior cesarean section. Ultrasound is the primary tool for the screening and diagnosis of placenta accreta.[1]

■ COMPLICATIONS

The immediate complications are just like any other major abdominal operations. There are certain delayed complications, mainly intestinal obstruction, adhesion formation, and ventral hernia. Intestinal obstruction and the adhesions are more common after classical cesarean section. They usually occur in the second or third week. Small intestines are dragged down into the pelvis by the involuting uterus. This usually occurs in the second or third week. This can occur years later also. Ventral hernia is seen in about 4% of cases coming for follow-up. It is more common in multiparous. Sometimes, we may see cases where the gap is very wide in which case the gravid uterus may herniate through it.

The gynecological complications that can occur are (1) menstrual irregularities, (2) pelvic pain, (3) dysmenorrhea, (4) fistulae, (5) infertility, (6) urinary infection, (7) scar endometriosis, and (8) adenomyosis. Of these, dysmenorrhea is the most important complication.

No two cases are same. Expecting the most unexpected in each and every case with proper preparedness can help the surgeon to tackle the situation successfully.

■ STRATEGIES TO DECREASE LOWER SEGMENT CESAREAN SECTION RATE

Strategies to reduce primary cesarean sections have to be framed after considering the indications for which emergency LSCS are done. Indications in order of frequency are labor dystocia, abnormal or indeterminate (formerly, nonreassuring) fetal heart rate tracing, fetal malpresentation, multiple gestation, and suspected fetal macrosomia.[11]

The strategies suggested by the American College of Obstetricians and Gynecologists (ACOG) are given in the following text.[12]

A prolonged latent phase (e.g., greater than 20 hours in nulliparous women and greater than 14 hours in multiparous women) should not be an indication for cesarean delivery.

Slow but progressive labor in the first stage of labor should not be an indication for cesarean delivery. Cervical dilation of 6 cm should be considered the threshold for the active phase of most women in labor.

A specific absolute maximum length of time spent in the second stage of labor beyond which all women should undergo operative delivery has not been identified.

Operative vaginal delivery in the second stage of labor by experienced and well-trained physicians should be considered a safe, acceptable alternative to cesarean delivery. Training in and ongoing maintenance of practical skills related to operative vaginal delivery should be encouraged.

Amnioinfusion for repetitive variable fetal heart rate decelerations may safely reduce the rate of cesarean delivery.

Scalp stimulation can be used as a means of assessing the fetal acid–base status when abnormal (or indeterminate, formerly nonreassuring) fetal heart patterns (e.g., minimal variability) are present and is a safe alternative to cesarean delivery.

Before 41 0/7 weeks of gestation, induction of labor generally should be performed based on maternal and fetal medical indications.

Fetal presentation should be assessed and documented beginning at 36 0/7 weeks of gestation to allow for external cephalic version to be offered.

Suspected fetal macrosomia: Cesarean delivery to avoid potential birth trauma should be limited to estimated fetal weights of at least 5,000 g in women without diabetes and at least 4,500 g in women with diabetes. The prevalence of birth weight of 5,000 g or more is rare, and patients should be counseled that estimates of fetal weight, particularly late in gestation, are imprecise. Women with excessive maternal weight gain should be counseled about the IOM (Institute of Medicine) maternal weight guidelines in an attempt to avoid excessive weight gain.

Twin gestations: Perinatal outcomes for twin gestations in which the first twin is in cephalic presentation are not improved by cesarean delivery. Thus, women with either cephalic/cephalic-presenting twins or cephalic/noncephalic-presenting twins should be counseled to attempt vaginal delivery.

Other individuals, organizations, and governing bodies should work to ensure that research is conducted to provide a better knowledge base to guide decisions regarding cesarean delivery and to encourage policy changes and protocols that safely lower the rate of primary cesarean delivery.

■ VBAC VERSUS ERCS

The WHO states that no region in the world is justified in having a cesarean rate greater than 10–15%. Despite this advice, in the past 20 years, cesarean section rates have risen to nearly 25% in some countries and still rising. The incidence of cesarean section varies between 8 and 25% at different centers in India.

Vaginal Birth after Cesarean Section (VBAC) versus Elective Repeat Cesarean Section (ERCS) has been one of the most discussed and debated topics over the last several years. ERCS alone contributed to >30% of this rising trend. A potential approach to reverse this rising trend is an attempt to reduce the incidence of ERCS, with increasing VBAC. Neither ERCS nor VBAC is risk free. In properly selected patients, VBAC can be achieved safely and successfully provided adequate facilities are available for monitoring and emergency cesarean section.

Edwin Craigin in 1916 stated, "No matter how carefully the uterine incision is sutured, we can never be certain that the cicatrized uterine wall will stand a subsequent pregnancy and labor without rupture. This means that the usual rule is once a cesarean, always a caesarean." This was true only in that era when classical cesarean sections were done and mostly for nonrecurrent indications.

Schell first reported VBAC in 1923.

VBAC is successful in 60–75% cases selected for trial.

The following terms are recommended and adapted from the National Institutes of Health Consensus Statement (2010):[13]

Trial of labor (TOL): A planned attempt to birth vaginally in a woman who has had a previous cesarean section. This is also sometimes called a "Trial of Vaginal Birth after Cesarean" (TOVBAC) or "Trial of Labor after Cesarean" (TOLAC) (ACOG 2010).

Criteria for Selection for VBAC

- Clinically adequate pelvis
- Period of gestation: 36–41 weeks
- Expected birth weight of baby: 2.5–3.5 kg
- Prior lower segment cesarean section (LSCS; transverse incision)
- Vertex presentation
- Patient's consent, i.e., willingness to take trial after proper understanding of risks, benefits, and success rate of VBAC
- Facility to carry out immediate LSCS must be present (including facility to tackle emergency such as ruptured uterus)
- No associated medical or obstetric complication

Contraindications to VBAC

- Previous classical or inverted "T" uterine scar
- Previous hysterotomy or myomectomy entering the uterine cavity
- Previous uterine rupture
- The presence of a contraindication to labor, such as placenta previa, malpresentation, cephalopelvic disproportion (CPD), or contracted pelvis.
- Presence of any obstetric factor which makes this pregnancy precious, i.e., elderly patient, long-standing secondary infertility, previous perinatal death, severe preeclampsia, uncontrolled diabetes mellitus (DM), and obesity are also contraindications to VBAC.

Healing of Uterine Scar

The uterus heals by formation of smooth muscle and without any fibrous tissue when suturing of the uterine incision is done well with perfect cooptation of incised tissue. Incision heals up by complete muscular regeneration in 80–90% of the cases.

At the end of 3 weeks, it has 30% of its final strength, and at 3 months and beyond, it has approximately 80% of its final strength.

Large amount of tissue included in each suture, inadequate hemostasis, edges of unequal thickness, ragged margins, eversion of the endometrium or inclusion of decidua in scar, and increased levels of corticosteroids are all responsible for a weak scar.

Systemic factors: Age, nutrition, general condition of patient, anemia, diabetes, obesity, ambulation, involution, and lochia drainage will affect scar healing.

Many local factors play a role in scar healing such as location of placenta over previous incision like devitalized uterine muscle, greatly stretched LUS, poorly formed thick LUS, number of previous sections, and adequate blood supply (continuous interlocking technique causes weak scar by tissue ischemia). Thick suture material causes more tissue reaction.

Since the introduction of synthetic suture, one could also reasonably argue that chromic catgut is obsolete due to its marked tissue reactivity, inconsistent tensile strength absorption, and knotting trouble. Chromic catgut has tensile strength for 7–10 days while polyglactin and polyglycolic acid have tensile strength for 30 days.

Polyglycolic acid suture material causes less tissue trauma and induces less intense inflammatory response than catgut. Other important properties such as tensile strength, knot security, thickness or caliber, rate of absorption, and coating are better with delayed absorbable sutures.

Studies by Tucker (1993)[14] and Chapman (1997)[15] showed no relationship between one- and two-layer closure and risk of subsequent uterine rupture.

Durnwald and Mercer (2003)[16] showed that single layer closure has no increased risk of rupture, uterine dehiscence.

Flamm et al. (1997)[17] after a prospective study on patients with previous LSCS proposed a scoring system. The score is based on the age of the patient, prior successful vaginal delivery, history of CPD, and cervical dilatation and effacement. The highest score is 10. The 0–2 range had a 49% VBAC success rate, while the 8–10 group had a 95% VBAC rate.

Scar dehiscence means disruption of part of the scar and not the entire length; the fetal membranes remain intact. Usually the visceral peritoneum is also intact, bleeding is minimal, and small hematoma on the scar line may be present.

Scar rupture is disruption of the entire thickness of scar. complete rupture is when it occurs in its whole length. This is associated with varying amounts of internal and external hemorrhage.

The most reliable first sign of uterine rupture is a nonreassuring fetal heart tracing. Cardiotocography heralds uterine rupture in 50–70% of cases. The changes include bradycardia, tachycardia, reduced baseline variability, and severe late decelerations.

Signs:
- Scar tenderness
- Tachycardia
- Cessation of contractions (even decrease in uterine activity)
- Abdominal pain
- Vaginal bleeding
- Hematuria
- Superficial palpation of fetal parts
- Loss of the presenting part on vaginal examination
- Hypotension

When any of the features suggesting scar dehiscence develops, immediate LSCS is carried out. In case of frank rupture, hypotension and tachycardia are always present, the fetus is usually dead, and uterine contractions have stopped. Immediate resuscitation of the mother is done and preparations for urgent laparotomy are made.

In spite of the risks of uterine rupture, VBAC remains an option for many patients with a success rate of 60–75%. Increasing recourse of VBAC, after careful selection of cases, can potentially reduce the prevailing high cesarean incidence.[18]

Women with a uterine scar should be counseled as to the risks and benefits involved with both TOL and ERCS. They should be given all pertinent information free of bias, in order to make an appropriately informed decision.

▪ REFERENCES

1. Jauniaux E, Grobman WA (Eds). Textbook of Caesarean Section. Oxford: Oxford University Press; 2016. 224 pp.
2. Sewell JE. Cesarean section—a brief history. A brochure to accompany an exhibition on the history of cesarean section at the National Library of Medicine. April 30 to August 31, 1993.
3. Gray H. Gray's Anatomy: With Original Illustrations by Henry Carter. London: Arcturus Publishing; 2009.
4. Torloni MR, Betran AP, Souza JP, Widmer M, Allen T, Gulmezoglu M, et al. Classifications for cesarean section: A systematic review. PLoS One. 2011;6(1):e14566.
5. Williams B. The routine use of the original Pfannenstiel incision. BJOG. 1960;67(5):853-6.
6. Lippert TH. Abdominovaginal delivery in case of impacted head in cesarean section operation. Am J Obstet Gynecol. 1985;151(5):703.
7. Saha PK, Gulati R, Goel P, Tandon R, Huria A. Second stage caesarean section: evaluation of Patwardhan technique. J Clin Diagn Res. 2014;8(1):93.
8. Vinayachandran S, Vedhapriya S. Comparison of two different techniques of uterine closure in caesarean section: Continuous single layer technique versus Babu and Magon technique. IJRCOG. 2017;7(6):2197-2201.
9. CORONIS Trial Collaborative Group. The CORONIS Trial. International study of caesarean section surgical techniques: a randomised fractional, factorial, trial. BMC Pregnancy Childbirth. 2007;7:24.
10. The CAESAR study collaborative group. Caesarean section surgical techniques: a randomised factorial trial (CAESAR). BJOG. 2010;117:1366-76.
11. Barber EL, Lundsberg LS, Belanger K, Pettker CM, Funai EF, Illuzzi JL. Indications contributing to the increasing cesarean delivery rate. Obstet Gynecol. 2011;118(1):29-38.
12. American College of Obstetricians and Gynecologists (College); Society for Maternal-Fetal Medicine; Aaron B Caughey, Alison G Cahill, Jeanne-Marie Guise, Dwight J Rouse. Safe prevention of the primary cesarean delivery. Am J Obstet Gynecol. 2014;210(3):179-93.
13. National Institutes of Health Consensus Development Conference Statement: Vaginal Birth After Cesarean: New Insights, March 8–10, 2010; 27(3). [online] Available from https://consensus.nih.gov/2010/images/vbac/vbac_statement.pdf [Last accessed October, 2020]
14. Tucker JM, Hauth JC, Hodgkins Owen 1. Winkler CL Trial of labor after one or two-layer closure of a low transverse uterine incision. Am J Obstetric Gynecol 1993;168:545-6.
15. Chapman S, Owen J, Hauth J. One versus two-layer closure of low transverse cesarean : the next pregnancy . Obstet and Gynecol. 1997;89:16-8.
16. Durnwald C, Mercer B, Uterine rupture, perioperative and perinatal morbidity after single-layer and double-layer closure at cesarean delivery. American Journal of Obstetrics and Gynecology. 2003;4(189):925-9.
17. Flamm BL,Geiger AM. Vaginal birth after cesarean delivery: an admission scoring system. Obstet Gynecol. 1997;90:907-10.
18. Royal College of Obstetricians and Gynaecologists . (2007). Birth after previous caesarean birth. Green-top Guideline No. 45. [online] Available from https ://www .rcog .org .uk/globalassets/ documents/guidelines/gtg _45 .pdf [Last accessed October, 2020]

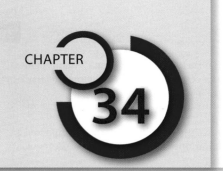

Rupture of the Uterus

Ashok Kumar Behera

■ INTRODUCTION

Rupture of the uterus is an acute obstetric emergency with grave consequences for both the mother and the fetus. There is no standard definition of the condition. However, the condition can be described, as the meaning suggests, as laceration or tear of the uterine wall not due to any surgical incision. Rupture has also been described as primary if it develops in a previously intact or unscarred uterus and secondary when occurs in a previously scarred uterus.[1]

■ INCIDENCE

It is unfortunate that in spite of the obstetric advancements during the last 50 years, uterine rupture cases are still seen. According to a World Health Organization (WHO) multicentric study of 83 reports, the prevalence of uterine rupture reported for population-based studies was lower with a median of 0.053% (range 0.016–0.30%) than facility-based studies with a median of 0.31 (range 0.12–2.9%). The prevalence tended to be lower for developed countries than the less- or least-developed countries as defined by United Nations.[2] In sub-Saharan African countries, the incidence is much higher at 1.3%.[3]

There has been a changing trend in the incidence of uterine rupture. Before 1960, there were more cases of rupture in an unscarred uterus in multiparous women. With ever-increasing rates of cesarean section, the incidence of scar rupture has increased,[4] the overall incidence being between 0.1 and 1%.[5]

In India, it has been reported that the overall incidence of uterine rupture was 0.35%, of which 1.69% were women with a previous cesarean section and 0.152% without it.[6]

■ CLASSIFICATION

There is no standard classification of uterine rupture. The condition is classified clinically according to timing as:
- Rupture during pregnancy
- Rupture during labor

Both the above types may be further classified into spontaneous or traumatic depending on etiology.

According to the extent of involvement of the uterine wall, rupture is classified into complete, when all the layers are involved, and incomplete with the peritoneal layer being intact. As already discussed earlier, rupture can be primary if it occurs in an unscarred uterus and secondary if it occurs in a scarred uterus due to previous operations on the uterus, particularly a prior cesarean section.[1]

■ RISK FACTORS AND ETIOLOGY

The following risk factors and etiological factors are responsible for uterine rupture.

During Pregnancy

Spontaneous rupture:
- In a scarred or weak uterine wall
  - Previous cesarean section
    - Lower segment cesarean section (LSCS)
    - Classical cesarean section (nowadays rare)
  - Previous myomectomy
  - Previous hysterotomy (done very rarely)
  - Previous uterine perforation during dilation and curettage (D&C), dilation and evacuation (D&E), suction evacuation, or hysteroscopy
  - Induction of labor in a scarred uterus
  - Hypoplasia of the uterine wall
  - Mullerian anomalies of the uterus
  - Previous metroplasty operation, even hysteroscopic
  - Sacculation of the uterine wall due to an incarcerated retroverted gravid uterus
  - Ehlers–Danlos syndrome (a very rare condition)
- In a normal unscarred uterus, traumatic rupture due to:
  - Road traffic accidents
  - Fall
  - Direct blow on the abdomen

During Labor

Spontaneous rupture:
- Scarred uterus
  - Previous cesarean section during trial of labor (TOLAC)

- Previous myomectomy
- Previous hysterotomy
  - Previous perforation due to D&C, D&E, suction evacuation, or hysteroscopy
- Normal or unscarred uterus
  - Obstructed labor mostly in multipara due to:
    - Occipitoposterior position, particularly deep transverse arrest
    - Malpresentations, i.e., shoulder presentation, mentoposterior position, and unrecognized brow presentation
    - Cephalopelvic disproportion
    - Tumors in pelvis
  - Grand multiparity
  - Pendulous abdomen
  - *Rigid cervix:* Either developmental or following previous operations.
  - Injudicious use of an oxytocic agent
  - Precipitate labor

Traumatic rupture, usually due to instrumental and assisted vaginal deliveries:

- Version
  - External cephalic version (rare)
  - Internal podalic version
- Forceps and vacuum extraction
- Destructive operations

Post delivery, very rarely seen are:

- Manual removal of placenta
- Intrauterine manipulations (intrauterine balloon)
- Morbidly adherent placenta

The above is a long list of risk factors and etiological factors. In clinical practice, it is commonly seen that in the antenatal period or during labor a previous cesarean section scar is one of the most common causes of uterine rupture. Rupture during labor is more common than during the antenatal period, particularly during TOLAC or acceleration of labor. The risk of uterine rupture based on a classical or T- or J-shaped incision of a prior cesarean delivery is 2–6%, 2% for low vertical incision 2%, and 0.5–1% for low transverse incision.[7]

The other common risk factor is obstructed labor in multipara due to malpresentations, as malpresentations are more associated with high parity. Less common risk factors are iatrogenic such as oxytocic use and obstetric operations for vaginal delivery.

MECHANISM OF UTERINE RUPTURE

The most common mechanism is overdistension of the lower uterine segment. In cases where there is obstructed labor due to cephalopelvic disproportion or malpresentation, the nulliparous and multiparous uterus behave differently.

The nulliparous develops uterine inertia for which the nulliparous uterus has been described as being "virtually immune to rupture."[8] But the multiparous uterus contracts vigorously in order to overcome the obstruction. As a result, the upper segment gradually retracts and the lower segment stretches. There develops a clear-cut demarcation between the upper and the lower segments with formation of the pathological retraction ring, a groove that can be felt near the level of the umbilicus. Gradually, by the powerful contractions and retraction of the upper segment, the fetus is pushed into the lower segment. The fetus gets accommodated in the lower segment by stretching it further which results in rupture of the already thinned-out lower segment.

In cases of a prior cesarean section, the scar is the weakest part of the lower segment. Delayed progress of labor either due to undetectable borderline obstruction or due to an unyielding cervix causes the lower segment to get stretched and thinned out with contraction and retraction of the upper segment leading to maximum stretching of the scar followed by rupture.

Intrauterine manipulations and obstetric operations to achieve vaginal delivery with lack of skill and care cause rupture of a thinned-out lower segment.

MORBID ANATOMY

Uterine ruptures are more commonly complete. Incomplete ruptures are less common. But incomplete ruptures are very commonly associated with prior cesarean section scars. The peritoneum remains intact in incomplete ruptures. Even when the lateral wall of the uterus has undergone rupture leading to formation of a hematoma and extrusion of fetal parts in between the layers of broad ligament, the rupture is described as incomplete.

Rupture invariably starts in the lower segment except for some cases of traumatic rupture. Subsequently, the tear may remain confined to the lower segment or usually extends laterally and then upward into the upper segment. The rupture can extend downward to involve the cervix and vagina in which case the urinary bladder may be involved. While extending laterally, the rupture can injure one or both of the uterine arteries causing massive hemorrhage and shock.

Following complete rupture, usually the fetus and the placenta are extruded into the abdominal cavity. Occasionally, a part of the fetus may be extruded through the ruptured wall and the uterus is retracted over the extruded fetal part.

One characteristic type of incomplete rupture in cases of a prior cesarean section is known as scar dehiscence. In scar dehiscence, the rent is confined to the limits of scar due to which it is usually not associated with any bleeding. But scar rupture extends beyond the limits of the scar and is associated with bleeding.

CLINICAL FEATURES AND DIAGNOSIS

The clinical presentation of the case depends on the rapidity of rupture and amount of hemorrhage. Diagnosis is usually established by recognition of the uterine laceration by palpation.

Symptoms

During pregnancy, usually there is a sudden onset of acute abdominal pain followed by fainting. This may be preceded by trauma, fall, or road traffic accidents. But all the cases are not typical. There may be slight pain and discomfort when the injury is trivial and rupture is incomplete. In such cases, the diagnosis is very easily missed. In cases of intrapartum rupture, however, usually there is a history of prolonged labor. The patients typically complain of cessation of intermittent pains of labor but replaced by continuous acute abdominal pain. When rupture is early in labor, particularly in cases of a prior cesarean section, the patients usually have very strong contractions and suddenly complain of an agonizing sensation of bursting at the height of labor pain followed by relief with cessation of contractions and then continuous pain and discomfort.

On examination:
- The patient usually bears a distressed look.
- There are features of shock which may be severe in some cases depending on the amount of hemorrhage.
- On abdominal examination when the rupture is complete and the fetus and placenta have been extruded into the peritoneal cavity, we will be able to find the following signs:
  - Acute tenderness all over the abdomen
  - Distended abdomen
  - Presence of free fluid depending on the amount of intra-abdominal collection
  - Loss of contour of the uterus
  - Fetal parts felt superficially with ease
  - The retracted uterus may be felt in the lower abdomen.
  - Fetal heart sounds obviously will be absent.

When the rupture is incomplete with the fetus and placenta still in the uterine cavity, the following clinical findings will be elicited:
- There will be maternal tachycardia.
- Abdominal examination will show absence of intermittent contraction of labor with tenderness all over the uterus with severe tenderness over the site of rupture, so much that the patient resists the examining hand. The fetal parts are not palpable and the fetal heart may be absent or will show bradycardia with irregularity.
- *On vaginal examination:*
  - There will be bleeding in both complete and incomplete ruptures.
  - The cervix will be at different stages of dilatation without any progress.
  - The cervix will appear to be closing after being dilated seen earlier.
  - The presenting part will be static at one station in incomplete rupture but will recede higher up in complete rupture.

The diagnosis of uterine rupture is almost always clinical. Imaging investigations are usually not required; however, they may be done.

TREATMENT

Definitive treatment is always laparotomy followed by hysterectomy or repair of the laceration in the uterine wall. However, the patients are usually in shock and not fit for immediate surgery. All such cases must be resuscitated immediately. These cases need to be managed in a high-dependency care unit (HDCU) on an emergency basis. Immediate attention needs to be given to airway, breathing, and circulation (ABC). The patient should be infused with intravenous fluids, preferably Ringer's lactate solution and transfusion with cross matched packed RBC. Any obstruction to the airway is cleared and oxygen inhalation is given by mask. Broad-spectrum antibiotics are given intravenously.

Laparotomy must be always done by subumbilical longitudinal median incision. The fetus, placenta, and collected blood are removed from the abdominal cavity. A quick decision on whether the patient needs hysterectomy or repair can be made based on age, parity, and morbid anatomy of rupture.

Usually, repair is possible in cases of incomplete rupture and majority of scar ruptures and some of the complete ruptures. It is reported that repair is possible in 26–55% of cases.[9,10] However, sometimes even the morbid anatomy of scar ruptures can be so extensive that they are beyond repair.

When repair is decided, all efforts should be made for hemostasis and optimal anatomical restoration.

If repair is not possible, total hysterectomy with conservation of the ovaries is the ideal treatment. But if the general condition of the patient is not favorable and normal anatomy is distorted, subtotal hysterectomy is usually done to avoid injury to the nearby organs and structures, particularly the ureters. In some cases, the rupture extends downward to involve the cervix and the upper vagina. Total hysterectomy is ideal in such cases. If subtotal hysterectomy is done, the rent should be identified and repaired. The angle of the rent in the vagina is to be secured properly for hemostasis.

OUTCOME

Maternal mortality ranges from 1 to 13% and perinatal death varies between 74 and 92% from the developed countries to less-developed countries.[2] A stillbirth rate of 98% has been reported from Ethiopia.[11]

These cases commonly develop postoperative complications such as pyrexia, sepsis leading to wound dehiscence, and paralytic ileus. Long-term complications of urinary fistula are always a possibility.

The cases who undergo repair are likely to develop scar rupture in the next pregnancy and labor. The overall incidence is reported to be 6%; if the rupture involves the upper segment, the risk is increased to 32%.[12]

The age-old proverb of "prevention is better than cure" also holds true for uterine rupture. Preventive measures should not only be taken for prevention of rupture but also taken for prevention of maternal mortality and morbidity by early diagnosis and treatment. Good antenatal care for all pregnant women combined with institutional deliveries will prevent uterine rupture. Care needs to be taken to diagnose cases of malpresentations and cephalopelvic disproportion in late pregnancy for their delivery in specialized centers. Postcesarean pregnancy cases must be admitted at least 2 weeks before the estimated date of delivery (EDD). In these cases, TOL and induction of labor must be done under close and strict supervision. Death due to uterine rupture is absolutely preventable and must be prevented.

KEY POINTS

- Rupture uterus may occur during pregnancy or labor, in an unscarred or previously scarred uterus. However, rupture occurring during labor is commonest, specially in a previously scarred uterus.
- Rupture may be complete (common) or incomplete (commony associated with previous CS)
- Rupture commonly occurs in lower segment (except some cases of traumatic rupture) and then extends either laterally, upwards or downwards involving cervix, vagina and even bladder.
- *Scar dehiscence:* Theoretically, dehiscence means amniotic sac should be intact, incomplete rupture means visceral peritoneum should be intact. Complete rupture: means all layers have given way.
- The clinical presentation of the case depends on the rapidity of rupture and amount of hemorrhage.
- *Evaluation:* H/O trauma, fall or RTA, prolonged labor. Symptoms: sudden onset of acute abdominal pain, cessation of uterine contractions, bleeding P/V. Signs: Acute tenderness all over the abdomen, distended abdomen, free fluid, loss of uterine contour, superficially palpable fetal parts, retracted uterus may be felt separately in the lower abdomen, FHS is generally absent. On P/V examination, frank bleeding along with static station of presenting part or it may be pushed up with ease,
- Definitive treatment is always laparotomy followed by hysterectomy or repair of the laceration in the uterine wall (depending upon extent of rupture and parity). If repair is not possible, total hysterectomy with ovary conservation is the ideal treatment. But if the general condition of the patient is not favorable and normal anatomy is distorted, subtotal hysterectomy is usually done.
- *Prevention:* Timely diagnosis of malpresentations, CPD. Previous C.S. pregnancy cases must be admitted two weeks prior to EDD.

REFERENCES

1. Yheomans ER, Hoffman BL, Gilstrap III LC, Cunningham FG. Cunningham and Gilstrap's Operative Obstetrics, 3rd edition. New York: McGraw-Hill Education; 2017.
2. Justus Hofmeyr G, Say L, Metin Gülmezoglu A. WHO systematic review of maternal mortality: the prevalence of uterine rupture. BJOG;2005:112:1221-8.
3. Guise JN, McDonagh MS, Osterweil P, Nygren P, Chan BKS, Helfand M. Systemic review of the incidence and consequences of uterine rupture in women with previous caesarean section. BMJ. 2004; 329(7456):19-25.
4. Al-Zirqi I, Stray-Pederson B, Forsen L, Daltveit AK, Vangen S. Uterine rupture: trends over 40 years. BJOG. 2016;123(5):780-7.
5. Hofmeyr GJ. Obstructed labour: Using better technologies to reduce mortality. Int J Gynecol Obstet. 2004;85:S62-S72.
6. Singh A, Shrivastava C. Uterine rupture: still a harsh reality. J Obstet Gynaecol India. 2015;65(3):158-61.
7. Landon MB, Hauth JC, Leveno KJ, Spong CY, Leindecker S, Varner MV, et al. Maternal and perinatal outcomes associated with a trial of labour after prior caesarean delivery. N Engl J Med. 2004;351(25):2581.
8. O'Driscoll K, Meagher D, Robson M. Active Management Labour: The Dublin Experience. 4th edition. London: Mosby; 2004.
9. Sharma S, Sharma A, Mathur A, Swarnkar M, Khangarot DS. Uterine rupture: 5 years study in a tertiary care hospital of Western Rajasthan, India. Int J Current Res Rev. 2012;4(15):36-41.
10. Astatikie G, Limenitu MA, Kebede M. Maternal and fetal outcomes of uterine rupture and factors associated with maternal death secondary to uterine rupture. BMC Pregnancy Childbirth. 2017;17:117.
11. Gessessen A, Melese MM. Rupture uterus—eight years retrospective analysis of causes and management outcome in Adigrat Hospital, Tigray Region, Ethiopia. Ethiop J Health Dev. 2002;16(3):241-5.
12. Richie EH. Pregnancy after rupture of pregnant uterus. A report of 36 pregnancies and a study of cases reported since 1932. J Obstet Gynecol Br Commonw. 1971;78:642-8.

Contracted Pelvis and Cephalopelvic Disproportion

Ambarisha Bhandiwad

■ CONTRACTED PELVIS

Obstetric definition: A contracted pelvis is defined as one in which any of the essential diameters is so reduced as to affect the normal mechanism of labor.

Anatomical definition: A contracted pelvis is one in which one or more of its diameters is reduced below the normal by 1 or more centimeters.

The factors influencing the size and shape of the pelvis are:
- *Developmental factor*: Hereditary or congenital
- Racial factor
- *Nutritional factor*: Malnutrition results in small pelvis
- *Sexual factor*: As excessive androgen may produce android pelvis
- *Metabolic factor*: As rickets and osteomalacia
- Trauma, diseases, or tumors of the bony pelvis, legs, or spines

Etiology of Contracted Pelvis

Causes in the Pelvis
- Developmental (congenital)
  - Small gynecoid pelvis (generally contracted pelvis)
  - Small android pelvis
  - Small anthropoid pelvis
  - Small platypelloid pelvis (simple flat pelvis)
  - *Naegele's pelvis*: Absence of one sacral ala
  - *Robert's pelvis*: Absence of both sacral alae
  - *High assimilation pelvis*: The sacrum is composed of six vertebrae.
  - *Low assimilation pelvis*: The sacrum is composed of four vertebrae.
  - *Split pelvis*: Split symphysis pubis
- Metabolic
  - Rickets
  - Osteomalacia (triradiate pelvic brim)
- *Traumatic*: As fractures
- *Neoplastic*: As osteoma

Causes in the Spine
- Lumbar kyphosis
- Lumbar scoliosis
- *Spondylolisthesis*: The 5th lumbar vertebra with the above vertebral column is pushed forward while the promontory is pushed backward and the tip of the sacrum is pushed forward leading to outlet contraction.

Causes in the Lower Limbs
- Dislocation of one or both femurs
- Atrophy of one or both lower limbs

NB oblique or asymmetric pelvis: One oblique diameter is obviously shorter than the other. This can be found in:
- Naegele's pelvis
- Scoliotic pelvis
- Diseases, fractures, or tumors affecting one side

Fetopelvic disproportion may be defined as a clinical mismatch between the size or shape of the presenting part of the fetus and the size or the shape of the maternal pelvis. When the presenting part is head, the same is termed as cephalopelvic disproportion (CPD). The prediction that CPD will adversely influence labor as well as the assessment of its extent is more than matters of mathematical measurement and demands a skill and experience which no textbook can provide. The dynamics of labor are more important than the mechanics and the efficacy of the uterine contractions, and the capacity of the fetal head to mold; and the stamina and the temperamental resilience of the patient contribute more to the outcome of labor in the minor and more common types of disproportion than the pelvic measurements themselves. An appreciation of the mechanism of labor in disproportion is, therefore, essential. CPD may be due to a large baby, contracted pelvis, or a combination of both. In CPD, which is a common cause of dystocia, one or more diameters in one or more of the planes of the pelvis may be shorter than normal, or the diameters of the fetal head may be larger. The contraction maybe at the brim of the pelvis, cavity, or at the outlet, or at all three. The contraction may be symmetrical or asymmetrical, thus causing varieties of deformities. The contractions may affect either the anteroposterior diameter, or the transverse diameter, or both. A contraction in one diameter may be compensated for by an increase in the other diameters. Hence, in assessing the possibility of vaginal delivery, the obstetrician would do well to take into consideration the capacity of the pelvis as a whole at all levels.

DEGREES OF DISPROPORTION

- *Minor disproportion*: The anterior surface of the head is in line with the posterior surface of the symphysis. During labor, the head is engaged due to molding and vaginal delivery can be achieved.
- *Moderate disproportion (first-degree disproportion)*: The anterior surface of the head is in line with the anterior surface of the symphysis. Vaginal delivery may or may not occur.
- *Marked disproportion (second-degree disproportion)*: The head overrides the anterior surface of the symphysis. Vaginal delivery cannot occur.

Successful vaginal delivery will depend to a large extent on good uterine contractions and attitude of good flexion on the part of the fetus. The two, often interlinked as poor flexion, cause poor pains and poor pains aggravate deflexion.

The size of the fetal head can be accurately determined by estimation of biparietal diameter on ultrasound. The molding during labor can reduce the biparietal dimensions by 6–7 mm. However, such gross degrees of fetal head compression are not compatible with the child's safety, and therefore, molding should not cause a reduction of >4 mm.

Disproportion at the brim is often partly countered by the mechanism of asynclitism, whereby the lateral rocking of the head presents a slightly diminished diameter, namely, the subparieto-superparietal diameter of 9 cm as compared to the biparietal diameter of 9.5 cm. There are two types of asynclitism. The more common is the anterior variety, also known as Naegele's obliquity, whereby the anterior parietal bone presents predominantly so that the sagittal suture lies nearer the sacrum. This is a favorable mechanism. The other type is the posterior asynclitism, also known as Litzman's obliquity, in which the posterior parietal bone presents, thereby placing the sagittal suture closer to the pubic symphysis. This is an unfavorable position and affects the chances of spontaneous delivery adversely if it persists.

Disproportion at the outlet is a definite entity. One most important feature is the width of the subpubic arch and the acuteness of the subpubic angle. A narrow arch and angle cause a great wastage of the anteroposterior dimensions of the outlet because the head can only emerge more posteriorly, by negotiating the posterior segment of the outlet, with greater detriment to the maternal pelvic floor. Outlet difficulties are far more often responsible for extreme molding and elongation of the fetal head than the brim dystocia.

When to suspect disproportion?

Major degrees of contracted pelvis should be suspected before the patient reaches term. The main problem is confined to the lesser degrees and borderline cases. A fetal head deeply engaged within the pelvis during the last 4 weeks of pregnancy practically rules out disproportion, for there is no finer pelvimeter than the fetal head. When satisfactory engagement of the head does not occur at term, disproportion is one of the numerous diagnostic possibilities.

CLASSIFICATION OF THE PELVIS

On the basis of X-ray studies, Caldwell and Moloy have classified the types of female pelvis. The pelvic type becomes much more important when contraction in any of the diameters is present. Four parent types of pelvic shapes could be recognized: Gynecoid, android, platypelloid, and anthropoid **(Fig. 1)**. The approximate frequency of the various types are gynecoid (50%), android (18%), anthropoid (26%), and platypelloid (5%). None of these types is pathological unless any of the diameters are substantially reduced below average.

Gynecoid Pelvis

The brim of the pelvis is well rounded and there is a good, full curvature of the fore pelvis. The transverse diameter of the inlet is either slightly greater than or about the same as the anteroposterior diameter. The maximum transverse diameter does not lie far behind the midpoint of the true conjugate with the result that the area of the hind pelvis is only somewhat less than the fore pelvis. The posterior sagittal diameter at the inlet is slightly less than the anterior

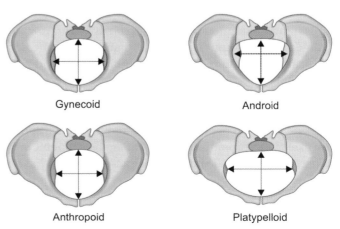

Fig. 1: Classification of pelvic shapes: Gynecoid, android, anthropoid, and platypelloid.

sagittal. The sides of the posterior segment are well rounded and wide. The cavity of the pelvis is almost the segment of a sphere and there is no convergence of the side walls. The side walls are straight and parallel. The ischial spines are not prominent and the sacrosciatic notches are wide and relatively evenly curved. The subpubic arch is normal in shape and the subpubic angle is not <85°, while the descending pubic rami are short and slender. The sacrum is well curved and is neither inclined anteriorly nor posteriorly and the sacral angle exceeds 90°.

Android Pelvis

Android pelvis is more like a triangle with the base toward the sacrum. The fore pelvis is beaked rather like the bows of a ship, and the maximum transverse diameter of the brim intersects the true conjugate very close to the sacrum so that the area of the hind pelvis is only fraction of that of the fore pelvis. Because of the breaking of the fore pelvis, the fetal head is unable to make use of much of the fore pelvis area and has to pass some distance posterior to the symphysis pubis. The posterior sagittal diameter is much less than the anterior sagittal at the inlet limiting the use of the posterior space. The sides of the posterior segment are not rounded and the anterior pelvis is narrow and triangular. In the midpelvis, the side walls tend to converge downward and the ischial spines are often prominent. The sacrosciatic notches are narrow and deep in a vertical direction and highly arched. The length of the symphysis pubis is greater than usual, the subpubic arch tends to be narrow, the subpubic angle is definitely acute, and the descending pubic rami are long and thick. The sacrum is set forward in the pelvis and is usually straight with little or no curvature. The angle of the brim inclination is steep and the sacral angle is <90°.

Anthropoid Pelvis

In anthropoid pelvis, the brim has an anteroposterior diameter which exceeds the transverse giving it an oval appearance. The anterior segment is somewhat narrow and pointed. The maximum transverse diameter may intersect the true conjugate fairly near its midpoint providing a reasonable ratio between the areas of fore pelvis and the hind pelvis, but the normal engagement of the head in the occipitotransverse position is discouraged. In the midpelvis, the side walls are often convergent and the ischial spines are likely to be prominent. At the outlet, the subpubic arch is narrowed but well-shaped. The sacrum usually has six segments and is straight and the sacrosciatic notch is large.

Platypelloid Pelvis

Platypelloid pelvis is the flat type of pelvis. The transverse diameter is very much larger than the anteroposterior

diameter and the sacral promontory tends to encroach upon the area of the hind pelvis. The cavity tends to be more roomy than usual, the side walls of the pelvis diverge downward, the sacral angle is >90°, and the sacrum may be somewhat flattened in the upper portions with a rather sharp curve forward near its tip. The sacrosciatic notches are wide and shallow in the vertical direction and the ischial spines are not prominent. The symphysis pubis is not deep, the subpubic arch is wide, and the subpubic angle is in excess of 90°.

Intermediate or Mixed Type of Pelvis

In this type of pelvis, a posterior segment of one of the four parent types may be associated with the fore pelvis of another. In the mixed types, the posterior segment determines the type of the pelvis.

Clinical Significance

In gynecoid pelvis, the fetal head engages in transverse or oblique diameter, internal rotation occurs anteriorly, and normal delivery occurs.

In anthropoid pelvis, because the posterior segment is roomy, the head engages in the anteroposterior diameter as direct occiput posterior and delivery occurs face to pubis.

In android pelvis, the head engages in transverse diameter and deep transverse arrest is common and difficult instrument deliveries are likely.

In platypelloid pelvis, the head engages in transverse diameter with marked asynclitism. There is a delay at the inlet and in many cases, engagement occurs by exaggerated asynclitism so that super subparietal diameter (8.5 cm) instead of the biparietal diameter (9.4 cm) passes through the pelvic brim. If the head is able to negotiate the inlet by means of asynclitism, there is usually no further problem. However, the internal rotation will occur only when the head is low down in the pelvis.

Assimilation Pelvis

There are two types of assimilation pelvis—the high and the low. In high assimilation pelvis, the last lumbar vertebra is incorporated in the body of the sacrum, thus not only increasing the length of the sacrum but also placing the sacral promontory at a higher level than normal. This has the effect of increasing the angle of the pelvic inclination and reducing the sacral angle well below 90°. It may be a potent cause of dystocia. In low assimilation pelvis, only four pieces comprise the body of the sacrum and there are no obstetrical disadvantages.

Naegele's Pelvis and Robert's Pelvis

In Naegele's pelvis, one sacral ala is not properly developed or absent resulting in profound asymmetry. In Robert's pelvis, the condition is bilateral. However, both these types of pelvis are very rare.

DIAGNOSIS OF CEPHALOPELVIC DISPROPORTION IS THROUGH HISTORY AND EXAMINATION

History

In a parous woman, the history of previous deliveries gives important information. Safe vaginal delivery of a normal-sized, live, undamaged baby at term usually denotes a pelvis of normal capacity. On the other hand, difficult vaginal delivery ending in stillbirth or neonatal death, in the absence of other etiological factors, would be strongly suggestive of contracted pelvis or CPD. An inquiry into the history (e.g., rickets) should be carried out if there is a history of delayed walking and dentition and trauma or diseases of the pelvis, spines, or lower limbs.

Dystocia dystrophia syndrome: A syndrome which was described in the early part of the 20th century is classically associated with disproportion and difficult labor. Typically, the patient is obese with a stocky built, broad shoulders, and short thighs. The bony structure of the pelvis tends to be toward the android type predisposing to deep transverse arrest of the head in the cavity and difficulties at the outlet.

General Examination

A short-stature woman has a tendency to have smaller pelvis and in many cases babies too are smaller. Even so, it is wise to be on guard against pelvic dystocia in women who have less than average height. Pendulous abdomen, deformities of the spine—especially those involving the lower lumbar spinal region, shortening of the lower limb, filling of pelvis, and waddling gait are factors which make the pelvis a suspect and hence must be looked for physical examination.

Abdominal Examination

An unengaged or a floating head in a primigravida at term should always arise a suspicion of a contracted pelvis or CPD. As deflexed attitude of the head prior to the commencement of labor is perhaps a more common cause, pelvis contraction should be ruled out before coming to such a diagnosis. It is also to be remembered that deflexion may simulate or exaggerate disproportion.

Causes of a high head at term: The most common cause is the occipitoposterior position which is an important factor contributing to dystocia and unsuccessful vaginal delivery. A high angle of the inclination of the pelvic brim discourages engagement. It occasionally operates singly but is more commonly associated with compensatory lordosis of the spine and pendulous abdomen. Sometimes, a high head is found which cannot be pushed into the pelvis because

that is already occupied by the presenting part of another twin. Hydramnios is not uncommonly a cause of high head. There may be an adventitious obstacle in engagement of the head in the form of placenta previa or the presence of pelvic tumors, such as fibroid or an ovarian cyst within the pelvis.

Assessment of CPD can be done by abdominal palpation or by bimanual examination.

The various methods used for the assessment of CPD are as follows:

- Assessment of disproportion at brim
- Clinical assessment of the pelvis
- Imaging pelvimetry
- Estimation of fetal weight
- Progress of labor

Assessment of Disproportion at Brim

Pressing the head into the brim, an attempt is made to push the head into the brim, and many methods are employed to execute this maneuver, but because of the resistance of the abdominal muscles and the oblique tilt of the plane of the brim (normally 60° from the horizontal) many of these methods are often unsatisfactory.

Donald's Method

Donald's method consists of the patient lying on a couch with the head supported by a pillow. The knees are not fully raised and fairly widely separated. Standing on the right of the patient and using the third, fourth, and fifth fingers of both hands, the head is gripped at the sinciput and occiput. One of the index fingers, usually the left, now reaches over and identifies the position of the top of the symphysis pubis. The thumb then presses backward against the parietal eminence (**Fig. 2**).

A complete grip of the head is thus obtained and its relationship to the symphysis pubis can be fully appreciated. Now, and not before, an assistant applies his hands to the breech baby and presses the baby toward the pelvis. At the same time, the thumbs which are applied to the parietal

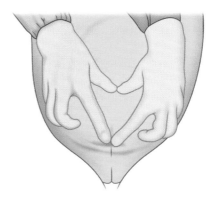

Fig. 2: Donald's method of testing for engagement.

eminence press downward and backward, while the fingers on sinciput and occiput can observe what is happening. The index finger of the left hand is kept as before at the upper margin of the pubic symphysis. If the head is mechanically capable of engagement, it can be now steered into the brim with the thumbs and the whole movement can be fully appreciated.

Equivocal terms such as "engaging" should never be used. Either a head is engaged or it is free, and if it is free it can either be made to engage or it cannot. Only one definition of engagement is acceptable, namely the biparietal diameter has passed the pelvic inlet or brim.

If the head cannot thus be pressed into the pelvis a vaginal examination should be performed, after the 36th week. This should be made with a proper aseptic or antiseptic ritual.

Abdominal Method or Purandare's Method

The woman is asked to lie down in dorsal position with thighs slightly flexed and the fetal head is grasped by the left hand. The index and the middle finger of the right hand are placed on the pubic symphysis and degrees of overlapping are noted and reported as no disproportion of head can be pushed into the pelvis; if slight overlapping is present moderate disproportion is suspected and when the parietal bones overhang the pubic symphysis severe disproportion should be anticipated.

Bimanual Examination

Munro Kerr–Muller Method

The patient is placed in the lithotomy position after explaining the procedure. The bladder and bowel should be empty.

The resistance of the pelvic floor is noted and then the presenting part is identified and the state of the cervix is observed. The fingers are now gently, a bit firmly pressed inward in an attempt to reach the sacral promontory and if reached the diagonal conjugate is measured. If the rest of the pelvis is adequate, the disproportion at the brim is judged by Munro Kerr's method **(Figs. 3A and B)**.

With the help of an assistant pressing upon the fundus of the uterus, an attempt is made to push the head into the pelvis.

The thumb of the examining hand in the vagina palpates the head over the symphysis. By this method, the relative sizes of the fetal head and the maternal pelvis are gauzed. If the head can be pushed down to the level of the ischial spines, brim disproportion can be excluded. If it cannot, the thumb denotes the degree of overlap. In the first-degree overlap, the parietal bone lies flush with the anterior surface of the symphysis pubis. This amounts to about 0.6 cm of overlap, and, given good contractions and a favorable position, delivery is possible. If the head is felt by the thumb to overhang the symphysis pubis, second-degree overlap is diagnosed in which case the outlook for vaginal delivery is very poor.

Remember that it is very difficult to push the head down in the presence of an unfavorable cervix. Therefore, this is only helpful in active labor. Also, only disproportion at the brim can be detected and this method is not useful to detect midpelvic or outlet contraction.

However in clinical practice, it must be remembered that the fetal head is the best pelvimeter. Hence, the relative size of the fetal head to the pelvis is more important than the absolute size of the pelvis.

Hiller–Muller test: This is done when the patient is in labor and performed at the peak of uterine contractions. By pressing the uterine fundus, the presenting part is pushed into the pelvis with one hand and the vaginal hand assesses the pelvis as well as downward mobility of the head. If the

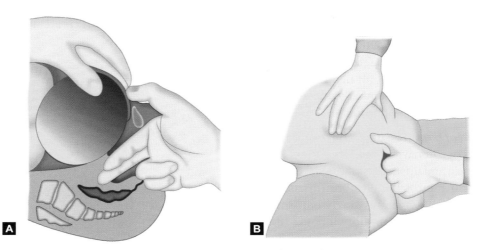

Figs. 3A and B: Munro Kerr–Muller method of testing for disproportion at brim.

presenting part does not move, a probability of CPD should be kept in mind.

Vaginal Examination

Clinical pelvimetry is one of the most valuable methods of assessing the pelvic capacity. During the vaginal examination to assess the pelvic capacity, the following must be looked for:

- Subpubic arch
- *Ischial spines*: There should be no marked projection of ischial spines in the cavity. The ischial bispinal measurement can be roughly gauzed.
- The sacral concavity from the promontory to the sacral tip should be well developed so that at the midpelvic and higher levels, the bone can be reached only with great difficulty.
- The flattening of the sacrum is an unfavorable sign, which may produce "transverse arrest."
- The length of the sacrotuberous ligament (the sacrosciatic notch). Normally, two fingers can easily be placed over this ligament. It serves as a useful index of the adequacy of the pelvis at the lower levels. Less space indicates narrowing of sacrosciatic foramen and diminished capacity of lower pelvis.
- *Pelvic side walls*: These should be palpated. Normally, they are parallel and sometimes diverging. Converging side walls are an ominous sign.
- *Diagonal conjugate*: To obtain this measurement, the middle and the forefinger of the right hand are passed into the vagina until the middle finger impinges on the promontory. The forefinger of the other hand then marks off the lower margin of the subpubic ligament. Both hands are then withdrawn and the distance between the tip of the middle finger and the point marked by the forefinger is measured with the rod or calipers **(Fig. 4)**.

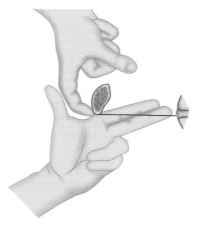

Fig. 4: Method of measurment the diagonal conjugate.

The true conjugate is estimated by deducing 1.5–2 cm from this measurement.

The diagonal conjugate usually measures about 12.5 cm.

It is evident that a vaginal examination gives essential information in assessing the pelvic capacity at all levels.

Contracted inlet: The inlet is said to be contracted, when the shortest anteroposterior diameter is <10 cm or the largest transverse diameter is <12 cm. As the anteroposterior diameter is usu-ally measured by assessing the diagonal conjugate, the inlet contraction is usually said to occur when the diagonal conjugate is <11.5 cm. When there is inlet contraction, the head remains high and this is a common cause of mobile head at term in a nullipara.

Contracted midpelvis: It is suspected if the interspinous diameter is <10 cm, ischial spines are prominent, side walls are convergent, sacrosciatic notch is narrow, and there is loss of the normal sacral curvature. Midpelvis contraction is more common than inlet contraction and may be associated with malrotation of fetal head or deep transverse arrest.

Contracted pelvic outlet: The outlet is said to be contracted when the interischial tuberous diameter is 8 cm or less and there is a consequent narrowing of the subpubic arch. It is clinically suspected when the intertuberous diameter does not admit four knuckles. It is usually associated with contraction of midpelvis.

Degrees of Contracted Pelvis **(Table 1)**

- *Minor degree*: The true conjugate is 9–10 cm. It corresponds to minor disproportion.
- *Moderate degree*: The true conjugate is 8–9 cm. It corresponds to moderate disproportion.
- *Severe degree*: The true conjugate is 6–8 cm. It corresponds to marked disproportion.

TABLE 1: Findings indicating adequate pelvis.	
Parameters	*Findings*
Fore pelvis (pelvic brim)	Round
Diagonal conjugate	≥ 11.5 cm
Symphysis	Average thickness, parallel to sacrum
Sacrum	Hollow, average inclination
Side walls	Straight
Ischial spines	Blunt
Interspinous diameter	≥10.0 cm
Sacrosciatic notch	2.5–3 finger-breadths
Subpubic angle	2 finger-breadths
Bituberous diameter	4 knuckles (>8.0 cm)
Coccyx	Mobile
Anteroposterior diameter of outlet	≥11.0 cm

■ *Extreme degree*: The true conjugate is <6 cm. Vaginal delivery is impossible even after craniotomy as the bimastoid diameter (7.5 cm) is not crushed.

Radiopelvimetry: It can give a precise assessment of the pelvic measurements, but in practice it is almost never done because pelvic capacity is only one of the factors that determine a successful outcome.

If employed, a single erect lateral film is taken. X-ray pelvimetry can be of help in getting an idea of the shape and size of the pelvis. In cephalic presentation with suspected CPD, in breech presentation also, X-ray pelvimetry gives good information regarding pelvic configurations, fetal size, and deflexion or otherwise of the fetal head.

Computed tomography (CT) scanning: CT scan is more accurate than X-ray pelvimetry in assessing the size of maternal pelvis.

Magnetic resonance imaging (MRI): It is associated with lack of ionizing radiation. The fetus can be completely imaged and soft-tissue dystocia can also be diagnosed.

Ultrasound: It is now possible by the ultrasound technique to measure accurately the biparietal diameter.

There are certain unpredictable factors during labor. These are molding of the fetal skull, increase in capacity of the lower pelvis, and uterine action.

The effect of these can be realized only after labor is well established and hence information gained by radiography should only be used to supplement the observations obtained on clinical examination, especially in suspected disproportion in primigravida or in a multigravida with a bad obstetric history and in case of breech presentation.

Prognosis

Early diagnosis and proper management considerably influence the maternal and fetal prognosis. If proper care is not available, the results can be disastrous for both mother and child. As a result of obstructed labor, the mother may die from rupture of uterus and the fetus from asphyxia. With moderate degrees of pelvic contractions, vaginal delivery after prolonged obstructed labor may result in a stillbirth or a badly traumatized baby, which dies in the neonatal period. Trauma to the fetal scalp may result in cephalohematoma. Extreme molding of the fetal head may result in intracranial hemorrhage and neonatal asphyxia.

Due to prolonged pressure by the presenting part—usually the vertex on the vagina and the surrounding structures, the bladder, and rectum—pressure necrosis may occur in the puerperium resulting in vesicovaginal or rectovaginal fistulas. Of these, the former is more common.

Strong expulsive efforts on the part of the mother to effect delivery may result in forcing the fetal head through the pelvis, as a result of which rupture or subluxation of the symphysis pubis may take place. The sacroiliac joints may also be involved in the subluxation. Fracture or fracture dislocation of the coccyx and sacrococcygeal joint is also likely to occur.

Prolonged pressure on the sciatic nerve and nerve roots results in neurological complications confined to the lower limbs; foot drop is not uncommon.

Morbidity is more in the puerperium due to infection.

■ MANAGEMENT OF LABOR

The nulliparous reacts to mechanical problems such as contracted pelvis by uterine inertia or inadequate action and only rarely undergoes spontaneous rupture. In contrast, the multiparous uterus contracts more violently and may lead to rupture. Hence, the two should not be considered in the same manner. In a multipara with a suspected disproportion, earlier recourse to cesarean section would be better and oxytocin, if given, should be with extreme caution.

There are two options in general for managing CPD:
1. Elective cesarean section
2. Trial of labor

Elective Cesarean Section

In cases where the pelvis is markedly contracted or a second-degree CPD is involved, elective cesarean section at term would be the treatment of choice.

First-degree CPD with any other maternal or fetal complications (including all high-risk pregnancies, previous cesarean section, and malpresentation) should also be considered for elective cesarean.

Trial of Labor

The basis of allowing trial of labor is the hope that with good effective uterine contractions, there is a "give way" of the pelvis and the fetal head molds to overcome minor degrees of disproportion. These factors which aid in successful vaginal delivery are impossible to predict before labor and hence the rationale of allowing a trial of labor in such women.

A trial is said to be successful if it results in the birth of a healthy baby vaginally (spontaneously or assisted) with the mother in good condition.

Delivery by cesarean section or delivery of a dead or a deeply asphyxiated or deeply compromised baby is considered as a failed trial.

Selection of Patients

For a trial of labor, the presentation must be vertex. Any other presentation is contraindicated for a trial.

The most favorable pelvis is the one that is contracted only at one level in one diameter, i.e., the flat or platypelloid pelvis.

Conduct of Trial of Labor

The patient must be psychologically prepared. Her general strength must be maintained and supported.

When the labor begins, careful note must be made of the uterine nature and frequency of the uterine contractions, the amount of fluids taken, and the urinary output.

Maternal pulse and fetal heart must be frequently observed. Analgesics should be administered as and when necessary or required. The progress of labor and descent of the head should be observed by abdominal palpation by assessing the part of the fetal head palpable in fifths.

Cardiotocography (CTG) monitoring is ideal and if not available, intermittent auscultation is employed.

The good prognostic signs are good uterine action, early engagement of the head, well thinned out and effaced cervix closely applied to the vertex, and a flat pelvis without any cavity contraction and vertex anterior presentation.

When these are present, trial of labor is almost always successful to the extent that vaginal delivery can be affected with safety to the mother and the child.

On the contrary, the signs of bad prognosis are weak or incoordinate uterine action and slow descent of the head. Prolonged latent phase is >8 hours in primigravida and 6 hours in multigravida. When signs such as premature rupture of membranes, uneffected partially dilated cervix hanging loose like a cuff, occipitoposterior position of the head and android, or a generally contracted pelvis are present, trial of labor seldom results in vaginal delivery of an undamaged, live child, and hence cesarean section may have to be considered.

Augmentation of Labor

Once the patient is in active labor, artificial rupture of membranes (ARM) can be done to hasten progress. In a nullipara with ineffective uterine contractions and slow progress, oxytocin can be used for augmenting labor. In a multigravida, it should be used with caution. Reassessment should be done by a senior obstetrician before augmentation.

When to terminate the trial by emergency cesarean section?

The exact duration of a trial is difficult to define.

Abdominal palpation helps to assess the descent of the head.

- Fetal or maternal distress occurring at any time during a trial of labor is an indication for immediate termination of labor.
- If the progress of labor is unsatisfactory and in spite of good uterine action the descent of the head is slow and cervical dilatation is poor, labor should be terminated by lower segment cesarean section (LSCS). Progress is best monitored by a partogram.

In conducting a trial of labor, the obstetrician must remember that his/her primary responsibility is to the woman and the unborn fetus and so must be willing to intervene when indicated.

The vaginal delivery of a deeply asphyxiated baby is not to be considered a successful trial and such situations are to be deplored.

There is no place for midcavity deliveries in modern obstetrics and if the head is still high, cesarean section is indicated. When instrumental delivery is attempted in the second stage, the obstetrician should not feel committed to completing delivery vaginally and in case of doubt he should recourse to abdominal delivery. It is this balance of judgment that is the hallmark of a good obstetrician.

KEY POINTS
- Contracted pelvis is diagnosed when there is reduction in any one of the essential diameters of pelvis by 1 centimeter or more.
- Contracted pelvis is usually associated with CPD
- Trial of labor may be conducted in a tertiary care setup with borderline CPD in young primigravida with strict monitoring with use of partogram.

■ SUGGESTED READING

1. ACOG Practice Bulletin Number 49, December 2003: Dystocia and Augmentation of Labor. Obstet Gynecol. 2003; 102:1445-54.
2. Benjamin SJ, Daniel AB, Kamath A, Ramkumar V. Anthropometric measurements as predictor of cephalopelvic disproportion. Acta obstet Gynecol Scand. 2012;91:122-7.
3. Bruno D, Roger VC, Thierry L. The value of maternal height as risk factor of dystocia: A meta-analysis. Trop Med Int Health. 1996;1:510-21.
4. Dujardin B, Van Custem R, Lambrechts T. The value of maternal height as a risk factor of dystocia: a meta-analysis. Trop Med Int Health. 1996;1:510-20.

5. Frame S, Moore J, Peters A, Hall D. Maternal height and shoe size as predictors of pelvic disproportion: an assessment. Br J Obstet Gynaecol. 1985;92:1239-45.

6. Helen AB. Anthhropometric measures as a predictor of cephalopelvic disproportion. Trop Doct. 1997;27:135-8.

7. Liselele HB, Boulvain M, Tshibangu CK, Meuris S. Maternal height and external pelvimetry to predict cephalopelvic disproportion in nulliparous African women: a cohort study. Br J Obstet Gynaecol. 2000;107:947-52.

8. Moller B, Lindmark G. Short stature: an obstetric risk factor? A comparison of two villages in Tanzania. Acta Obstet Gynecol Scand. 1997;76:394-7.

9. Munrokerr JM. Pelvic disproportion. BMJ, 1939;857-62.

10. Rossiter CE, Chong H. Relations between maternal height, fetal birth weight and cephalopelvic disproportion suggest that young Nigerian Primigravidae grow during pregnancy. Br J Obstet Gynaecol. 1985;5:40-8.

11. Rozenholc A, Ako SN, Leke RJ, Boulvain M. The diagnostic accuracy of external pelvimetry and maternal height to predict dystocia in nulliparous women: a study in Cameroon. BJOG. 2007;114:630-5.

12. Shagun B, Kiran G, Neera A. Evaluation of sacral rhomboid dimensions to predict contracted pelvis: A Pilot Study of Indian primigravidae. J Obstet Gynecol Ind. 2011;61(5):523-7.

13. Van Roosmalen J, Brand R. Maternal height and the outcome of labor in rural Tanzania. Int J Gynecol Obstet. 1992;37:169-77.

14. World Health Organisation. Maternal anthropometry and pregnancy outcomes. A WHO collaborative study. WHO Bull. 1995;73:1-69.

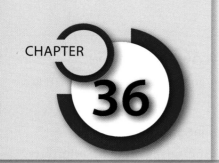

Nonimmune Hydrops Fetalis

Shipra Kunwar

INTRODUCTION

Fetal hydrops is a condition characterized by an increase in the total body water content, whereby the excess fluid collects by ultrafiltration in body cavities (pleural, pericardial, and peritoneal effusions) and/or in subcutaneous tissue.

Placental edema and polyhydramnios are frequently associated (30–70%).

Incidence: Fetal hydrops occurs in 1 in 2,000 births.

Etiology: Fetal hydrops occurs as a nonspecific finding in a wide variety of fetal and maternal disorders.

Classically, fetal hydrops is divided into:
- *Immune (10% cases)*: Occurs due to maternal hemolytic antibodies
- *Nonimmune (90% cases)*: Occurs due to all other etiologies

In this chapter, nonimmune hydrops fetalis (NIHF) has been discussed.

CAUSES OF NONIMMUNE HYDROPS FETALIS

Table 1 enumerates various causes of NIHF.

TABLE 1: Causes of nonimmune hydrops fetalis.

Cause	Cases (%)
Cardiovascular	17–35
Chromosomal	7–16
Hematologic	4–12
Infectious	5–7
Thoracic	6
Twin-to-twin transfusion	3–10
Urinary tract abnormalities	2–3
Gastrointestinal	0.5–4
Lymphatic dysplasias	5–6
Tumors	2-3
Skeletal dysplasias	3–4
Syndromes	3–4
Inborn error of metabolism	1–2
Idiopathic	15–30

MECHANISM

Table 2 summarizes the mechanism involved in various medical conditions to produce NIHF.

PATHOPHYSIOLOGY

In various conditions mentioned above, there is a breakdown of equilibrium between intracapillary and extracapillary pressures, with consequent fluid ultrafiltration in interstitial space.

In NIHF, the etiology being so diverse, precise pathogenesis depends on the underlying cause and remains unclear in many cases.

Various mechanisms proposed are cardiac failures, low output or high output (e.g., structural heart defects, anemia); inadequate diastolic ventricular filling (e.g., arrhythmias);

TABLE 2: Mechanism of nonimmune hydrops fetalis.

Anemia	Alpha thalassemia, G6PD deficiency, fetal infection (especially Parvovirus B19)
Infection	Cytomegalovirus, Parvovirus B19, toxoplasmosis, syphilis, rubella, coxsackievirus
Chromosomal	Turner syndrome, trisomy 21, 13, 18, triploidy
Heart failure	Cardiac defects, dysrhythmias, myocarditis, cardiomyopathy, recipient in TTTS, fetal thyrotoxicosis (maternal Graves' disease)
Arteriovenous shunts	Fetal tumor, vein of Galen aneurysm, placental chorioangioma, acardiac twin
Metabolic disorder	Mucopolysaccharidosis, Gaucher's diseases, Hurler's syndrome, gangliosidosis, sialidosis
Neuromuscular	Fetal akinesia deformation sequence
Brain abnormality	Encephalocele, intracranial hemorrhage, porencephaly with absent corpus callosum
Mediastinal compression	Skeletal dysplasias, diaphragmatic hernia, cystic adenomatoid malformation, pulmonary sequestration, laryngeal obstruction
Hypoproteinemia	Renal defects, gastrointestinal defects
Genetic syndrome	Arthrogryposis, Noonan syndrome, multiple pterygium syndrome, Pena–Shokeir syndrome, tuberous sclerosis
Idiopathic	

(G6PD: Glucose-6-phosphate dehydrogenase; TTTS: twin-to-twin transfusion syndrome)

obstruction of venous or arterial flow (e.g., thoracic masses); hepatic venous congestion leading to decreased hepatic function and hypoalbuminemia (e.g., infections, gastrointestinal abnormalities); lymphatic dysplasias or obstruction (e.g., cystic hygroma, aneuploidies); or reduced osmotic pressures (e.g., congenital nephrosis).

◼ ULTRASOUND DIAGNOSTIC CRITERIA (BOX 1)

Doppler (peak systolic velocity). Elevated value of peak systolic velocity of MCA has been associated with fetal anemia even in cases of NIHF.

◼ MANAGEMENT

Nonimmune hydrops fetalis poses a considerable diagnostic dilemma.

BOX 1: Diagnostic criteria on USG (Figs. 1A to C).

Diagnosis of hydrops:
- Scalp edema—scalp thickness > 5 mm
- Fluid in two or more cavities
- *Other features could include*:
  - Placental thickening > 4 cm in first trimester and 6 mm in third trimester
  - Polyhydramnios

◼ INVESTIGATIONS (FLOWCHART 1)

The investigation tests required to diagnose NIHF are shown in **Flowchart 1**.

Maternal Blood Investigations

- Elaborate history including that of ethnicity, consanguinity (hematological/metabolic disorders), past medical and obstetric history, any history of fetal, neonatal or infantile loss, congenital malformation, and developmental delay (pedigree analysis should be done)
- Complete blood cell count and indices (hematological disorders)
- Indirect Coombs test (ICT) (to rule out Rh isoimmunization)
- Hemoglobin electrophoresis (alpha thalassemia)
- SS-a, SS-B antibodies (fetal rhythm defects)
- Blood chemistry [for maternal glucose-6-phosphate dehydrogenase (G6PD), pyruvate kinase carrier status—to rule out fetal red blood cell enzyme deficiency]
- Kleihauer–Betke test (fetal maternal transfusion)
- Viral titers (fetal infection—coxsackievirus, parvovirus B19, TORCH)

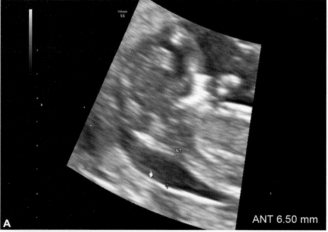
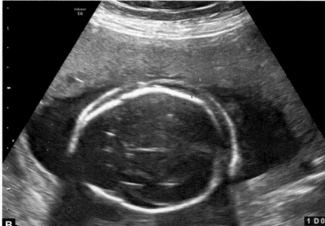
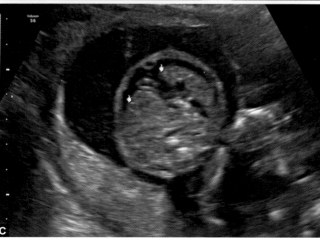

Figs. 1A to C: Ultrasound pictures in hydrops fetalis: (A) Cystic hygroma; (B) Scalp edema; (C) Fetal ascitis.

Flowchart 1: Investigations required to diagnose nonimmune hydrops fetalis.

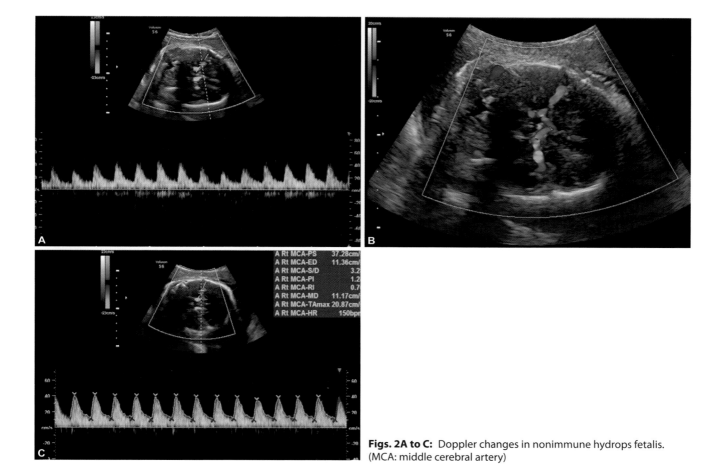

Step 1	Step 2	Step 3
• Detailed ultrasound • Fetal Doppler (MCA, venous, arterial) • Fetal echo	Amniotic fluid testing FISH	• Fetus survives • Physical examination • USG • TORCH test
Maternal blood	Fetal blood sampling	• Fetal death • Placental pathology • Autopsy • DNA analysis

(FISH: fluorescence in situ hybridization; MCA: middle cerebral artery; TORCH: toxoplasmosis, rubella cytomegalovirus, herpes simplex, and HIV)

A Rt MCA-PS	37.28cm/
A Rt MCA-ED	11.36cm/
A Rt MCA-S/D	3.2
A Rt MCA-PI	1.2
A Rt MCA-RI	0.7
A Rt MCA-MD	11.17cm/
A Rt MCA-TAmax	20.87cm/
A Rt MCA-HR	150bpr

Figs. 2A to C: Doppler changes in nonimmune hydrops fetalis. (MCA: middle cerebral artery)

- VDRL (Venereal Disease Research Laboratory; syphilis)
- USG including fetal echocardiography (to assess NIHF and its progression and to exclude congenital heart defects and other malformations, and multiple gestation). Doppler study—MCA peak systolic velocity for fetal anemia.

Amniocentesis

- Fetal karyotype, microarray (chromosomal/certain genetic abnormalities)

- Amniotic fluid polymerase chain reaction (cytomegalovirus, toxoplasmosis, rubella, Parvovirus B19)
- Alfa fetoprotein (fetal tumors such as sacrococcygeal teratoma)
- Specific metabolic tests (metabolic disorders)

Fetal Blood Aspiration

- Karyotype and metabolic tests (chromosomal/metabolic abnormalities)
- Hemoglobin chain analysis (thalassemias)

- Fetal plasma analysis for specific immunoglobulin M (IgM; intrauterine infection)
- Fetal plasma albumin (hypoalbuminemia)
- Complete blood count (fetal anemia)

Postdelivery

In case of fetal demise/termination—autopsy, X-ray, placental histopathology, karyotype, DNA analysis.

Fetal Therapies

Only about 20–30% of NIHF cases are amenable to treatment which include:
- Fetal anemia by intrauterine blood transfusion
- Fetal thyrotoxicosis—transplacental administration of antithyroid agents
- Fetal tachyarrhythmias by transplacental/intraumbilical therapy with antiarrhythmic drugs
- Pleural effusions/pulmonary cysts by insertion of thoracoamniotic shunts
- Teratomas and chorioangiomas by ultrasound-guided laser coagulation of feeding vessels
- Recipient fetus in twin-to-twin transfusion syndrome by fetoscopic laser coagulation of communicating placental vessels
  Follow-up scan every 2–3 weeks is required to monitor progression of hydrops.

■ COMPLICATIONS

Maternal mirror syndrome (MMS) is a rare complication of fetal hydrops appearing as a triple edema (fetal, placental, and maternal). In this syndrome which was first described in 1892 by the Scottish obstetrician John William Ballantyne, the mother "mirrors" the hydropic fetus. MS has been associated with rhesus isoimmunization (29%), twin-to-twin transfusion syndrome, viral infection, fetal malformations, and fetal or placental tumors. The mother's clinical presentation includes peripheral edema, uterine distension, and rapid weight gain. These may lead to a misdiagnosis of preeclampsia. Hypertension is not the usual presentation, but blood pressure can be elevated and proteinuria can appear, resembling the clinical features of preeclampsia. Laboratory findings may include proteinuria, low platelet count, and elevation of creatinine, hepatic enzymes and uric acid levels.

Fetal prognosis in MS is usually worse than in pre-eclampsia, resulting in many cases in intrauterine fetal demise and mortality as high as 50–60%.

The treatment of choice for MS is the resolution of the fetal hydrops. Delivery is required when it is not possible to perform fetal therapy or when it is not successful. Vaginal delivery may be preferred, but complications such as maternal pulmonary edema or deterioration of the fetal condition can lead to an emergent cesarean section.

■ PROGNOSIS

Prognosis depends on etiology and gestation age at diagnosis.

In general, the earlier the hydrops occurs, the poorer is the prognosis. In particular, pleural effusions and polyhydramnios prior to 20 weeks of gestation are poor prognostic signs because of increased risk of pulmonary hypoplasia and preterm labor/premature rupture of membranes respectively. Mostly, NIHF has a poor prognosis with 23–48% survival rate.

■ DELIVERY

- Timing and method of delivery depend on the cause of hydrops.
- Delivery of a hydropic baby can be conducted in a tertiary care center with an experienced resuscitation team as respiratory distress is anticipated. The need for endotracheal intubation, emergency vascular access, thoracocentesis, paracentesis, and other emergent measures might arise.

■ DIFFERENTIAL DIAGNOSIS

Nonimmune hydrops fetalis should be differentiated from isolated effusions (e.g., pericardial effusion in case of congenital heart disease; ascites in case of urinary/gastrointestinal abnormalities).

■ RISK OF RECURRENCE

- *Fetal defects/infections*: No increased risk of recurrence
- *Trisomies*: 1%
- *Metabolic disorders*: 25%

CONCLUSION

All patients with fetal hydrops should be referred to a tertiary care center for evaluation. Evaluation begins with antibody screen (ICT) to differentiate immune from nonimmune. A comprehensive obstetric ultrasound including evaluation of fetus(es), placenta, fetal echocardiography, and MCA Doppler is warranted. Fetal karyotype and chromosomal microarray analysis should be offered in all cases regardless of whether a structural defect is found in the fetus or not. Autopsy should be advised for all cases of fetal/neonatal deaths, more so if no diagnosis is reached prenatally. Prognosis depends on etiology, gestation age at detection, and response to therapy (in treatable cases). Prognosis in most cases is not good.

KEY POINTS

- All patients with fetal hydrops should be referred to a tertiary care center for evaluation.

- Evaluation begins with antibody screen (ICT) to differentiate immune from nonimmune.
- A comprehensive obstetric ultrasound including evaluation of fetus(es), placenta, fetal echocardiography, and MCA Doppler is warranted.
- Fetal karyotype and chromosomal microarray analysis should be offered in all cases regardless of whether a structural defect is found in the fetus or not.
- Autopsy should be advised for all cases of fetal/neonatal deaths, more so if no diagnosis is reached prenatally.
- Prognosis depends on etiology, gestation age at detection, and response to therapy (in treatable cases). Prognosis in most cases is not good.

■ SUGGESTED READING

1. Abrams ME, Meredith KS, Kinnard P, Clark RH. Hydrops fetalis: a retrospective review of cases reported to a large national database and identification of risk factors associated with death. Pediatrics. 2007;120:84-9.

2. Desilets V, De Bie I, Audibert F. No. 363-Investigation and management of nonimmune fetal hydrops. JOGC. 2018;40(8):1077-90.

3. Hernandez-Andrade E, Scheier M, Dezerega V, Carmo A, Nicolaides KH. Fetal middle cerebral artery peak systolic velocity in the investigation of nonimmune hydrops. Ultrasound Obstet Gynaecol. 2004;23(5):442-5.

4. Holzgreve W, Holzgreve B, Curry JR. Nonimmune hydrops fetalis diagnosis and management. Semin Perinatol. 1985;9:52.

5. Laneri GG, Classen DL, Scher MS. Brain lesions of fetal onset in encephalopathic infants with nonimmune hydrops fetalis. Pediatr Neurol. 1994;11:18-22.

6. Machin GA. Hydrops revisited: literature review of 1,414 cases published in the 1980s. Am J Med Genet. 1989;34:366-90.

7. Norton ME, Chauhan SP, Dashe JS. Society of maternal-fetal medicine (SMFM) clinical guideline #7: Nonimmune hydrops fetalis. Am J Obstet Gynecol. 2015;212(2):127-39.

8. Santo S, Mansour S, Thilaganathan B, Homfray T, Papageorghiou A, Calvert S, et al. Prenatal diagnosis of non-immune hydrops fetalis: what do we tell the parents? Prenat Diagn. 2011;31:186-95.

9. Staretz-Chacham O, Lang TC, LaMarca ME, Krasnewich D, Sidransky E. Lysosomal storage disorders in the newborn. Pediatrics. 2009;123:1191-207.

Amniotic Fluid Embolism

Deepa Lokwani Masand

INTRODUCTION

Amniotic fluid embolism (AFE) is a rare but potentially catastrophic obstetric condition. It may present with a mild degree of organ dysfunction as well as sudden and profound maternal cardiovascular collapse, coagulopathy, and death in response to inflow of amniotic components into the maternal circulation. The process is similar to anaphylaxis than the mechanical, so the alternative terms used are "anaphylactoid syndrome of pregnancy" or "sudden obstetric collapse syndrome."

Amniotic fluid embolism accounts for 5–15% of cases worldwide and remains one of the leading causes of maternal death. The case-related maternal mortality is estimated to range between 0.5 and 1.7 deaths per 100,000 deliveries in the developed world and 1.9 and 5.9 deaths per 100,000 deliveries in the developing world.

For the first time, Ricardo Juvenal Meyer in 1926 discovered fetal tissue in the pulmonary vessels of dead mothers. AFE was first reported by Steiner and Lushbaugh (1941) who studied a case series of circulatory collapse, respiratory failure, and severe hypoxia during childbirth and linked them to embolism of amniotic fluid into pulmonary circulation.

ETIOPATHOGENESIS

Majority cases of AFE occur during labor, delivery (vaginal/cesarean), or up to 48 hours postpartum. Rarely, it may present during abortion, abdominal trauma, amniocentesis, or amnioinfusion.

Any break of the barrier between amniotic fluid and maternal blood permits the entry of amniotic fluid components into the maternal circulation and triggers the reaction.

Risk Factors

The triggering events for AFE are artificial rupture of membranes, cesarean section, pre-eclampsia, abruption placentae, hypertonic uterine contractions, placenta previa, dilation and evacuation, amniocentesis, and uterine trauma that allow the exposure of the amniotic fluid components to the maternal circulation **(Box 1)**.

BOX 1: Risk factors of amniotic fluid embolism.

- Older age
- Multiparity
- Physiologic intense uterine contractions
- Medical induction of labor
- Instrumental vaginal delivery
- Prolonged gestation
- Cesarean section
- Uterine rupture
- Polyhydramnios
- High cervical tears
- Premature placental separation
- Intrauterine fetal death
- Large fetal size
- Meconium staining of the amniotic fluid
- Placental abruption
- Eclampsia
- Fetal distress
- Trauma to abdomen
- Surgical intervention
- Saline amnioinfusion
- Male fetus meconium

The other identifiable risk factors are elderly mothers, multiparty, multiple pregnancy, male baby, and fetal demise.

The pathophysiology of AFE is not yet well understood, as fetal material is not present in the maternal circulation of all patients of AFE while not all women with amniotic fluid components in circulation have features of AFE **(Flowchart 1)**.

There are two proposed theories:

1. The first historic idea was entry of amniotic fluid into maternal circulation due to abnormal labor, surgical trauma, or abnormal placentation causing mechanical obstruction of pulmonary vessels.
2. More popular is anaphylactoid reaction theory— amniotic fluid has vasoactive and procoagulant substance leading to endothelial activation and massive inflammatory reaction or complement activation.

Significantly higher levels of beta tryptase (serine protease) at the pulmonary level support "mast cell degranulation" as the pathophysiological mechanism in anaphylactoid theory whereas abnormally low levels of C3 and C4 suggest complement activation through classical or alternative pathways.

The course of events is observed in three phases:

- *Phase 1:* Cardiopulmonary involvement
  - The biochemical mediators result in pulmonary artery vasospasm with sequel of pulmonary hypertension and increase in right ventricular pressure.

Flowchart 1: Components of amniotic fluid and their role in pathophysiology of AFE. Surfactant enhances production of leukotrienes C4 and D4. Endothelin and Prostaglandins E2 and F2-α cause coronary vasoconstriction and negative inotropic effect. Leukotrienes induce hypertension followed by hypotension, pronounced negative inotropic effects and bronchoconstriction. IL-1 and TNF-α induce production of endothelin. Thromboxane A2 causes increases in coronary and pulmonary vascular resistance. Collagen and thromboplastin induce platelet activation.

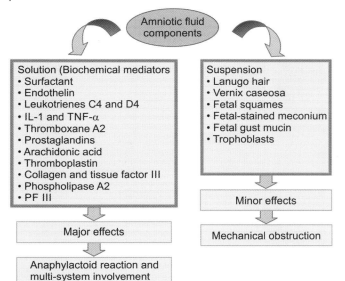

(IL-1: interleukin 1; TNF-α: tumor necrosis factor α)
Source: Gei AF, et al. Anesthesiology. Clin N Am. 2003;21:165-82.

- The hypoxia that occurs results in myocardial capillary damage and left ventricular failure.
- This phase lasts for 30 minutes and surviving patients enter into phase 2.
- *Phase 2:* Hemodynamic phase—The procoagulants cause fatal consumptive coagulopathy characterized by massive bleeding in concordance with uterine atony and disseminated intravascular coagulation (DIC). This may further lead to left ventricular failure and pulmonary edema.
- *Phase 3:* Acute renal failure and neurological symptoms (seizures, coma)

Uszynki has documented symptoms in two forms:
1. Typical/classical presenting with all three phases in sequelae
2. Atypical having first symptom as life-threatening hemorrhage due to DIC

CLINICAL FEATURES (FIG. 1)

Amniotic fluid embolism is known to occur during labor or immediately after vaginal or cesarean delivery or during second-trimester abortions.

Maternal

The patient has prodromal symptoms such as sudden chills, shivering, sweating, and cough progressing to sudden onset of dyspnea and hypotension followed by cardiovascular collapse and respiratory arrest. Hypotension is the most common sign and symptom with diastolic blood pressure which is not measurable.

Disseminated intravascular coagulation is present in about 83% and manifested by petechiae, excess bleeding from surgical sites, hematuria, gastrointestinal bleeding, and excess vaginal bleeding. The onset varies as early as 10–30 minutes and delayed upto 4 hours.

Further, encephalopathy due to hypoxia includes symptoms varying from altered mental state to seizures (tonic–clonic type seen in 10–50% cases).

Fetal

Fetal bradycardia occurs due to hypoxia with a decrease in heart rate of <110 bpm. Terminal bradycardia is indicated in cases with decrease in fetal heart rate < 60 bpm over 3–5 minutes. Among the surviving neonates, persistent neurological deficit is known to occur in about 24–50% neonates.

Diagnosis

Amniotic fluid embolism is diagnosis of exclusion without universal pathological or serological markers. Hence, diagnosis is with traditional clinical features having a triad of respiratory distress, cardiovascular collapse, and coagulopathy in women with ruptured membranes during labor. However, the triad of symptomology is neither sensitive nor specific and considered on ruling out other diagnoses. Recently, Clark had proposed diagnostic criteria to prevent overreporting but the Society for Maternal Fetal Medicine (SMFM) extends its support for current clinical diagnosis.

The diagnosis of AFE is based upon clinical features [less invasive surfactant administration (LISA)], and there is still no pathognomonic marker present for AFE.

In 2016, the uniform diagnostic criteria for AFE reporting were considered to facilitate prompt and early intervention:
- Sudden-onset cardiorespiratory arrest (hypotension of systolic BP < 90 mm Hg, dyspnea, cyanosis, SpO_2 < 90%)
- Overt disseminated intravascular coagulopathy (rule out consumptive coagulopathy)
- Clinical onset during labor or within 30 minutes of placenta delivery
- Absence of raised temperature during labor (>38°C) to exclude sepsis

There are nonspecific and specific diagnostic tests that aid in diagnosis.

Nonspecific Tests

- Complete blood count and peripheral blood smear which shows schistocytes (suggestive of DIC)

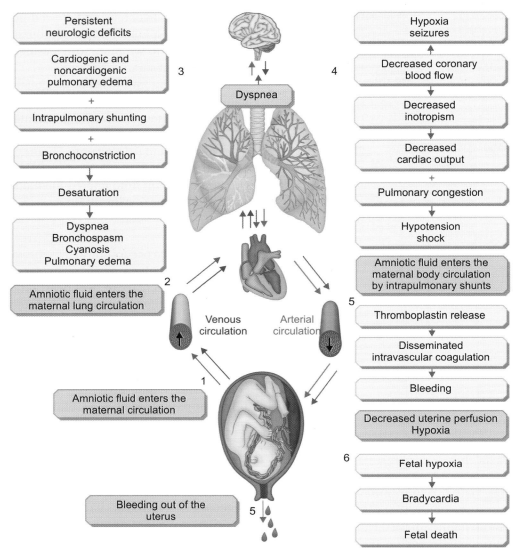

Fig. 1: Pathophysiology of the amniotic fluid embolism.
Source: Gei G, Hankins GDV. Amniotic fluid embolism: an update. Contemp Ob/Gyn. 2000;45:53-66.

- Coagulation profile
- Arterial blood gas analysis (decreased pH, decreased PO_2, increased PCO_2, base excess increased)
- Chest X-ray (nonspecific changes such as bilateral homogeneous or heterogeneous opacities distinguishable from acute pulmonary edema)
- ECG (tachycardia, ST segment, and T-wave changes and findings suggestive of right ventricle stain)
- Ultrasonography

Diagnostic Tests

- On cytological analysis of central venous blood and bronchoalveolar fluid, there is presence of squamous cells, neutrophils, fetal debris such as mucin, and hair that support the diagnosis of AFE.
- Sialyl-Tn antigen test shows monoclonal antibodies TKH-2, MA54, B72.3, and CC49 reacting with meconium

and amniotic fluid-derived mucin. This was first described by Kobayashi and colleagues. The lowest concentration of the antigen can be detected by TKH-2. Sialyl (mucin-type glycoprotein) originates in fetal and adult intestinal and respiratory tracts. It constitutes majority of meconium (10% by weight) and is also present in clear amniotic fluid. If the serum level is >50 U/mL, then sensitivity is between 78 and 100% and specificity is between 97 and 99%.

- Zinc coproporphyrin is a characteristic component of meconium that is elevated in the plasma of suspected AFE.
- Serum tryptase (serine protease) is done in case of AFE suspected due to anaphylaxis.

The tests for detecting AFE like zinc coproporphyrin, sialyl-Tn antigen, tryptase or C3 and C4 complement, and insulin-like growth factor binding protein-1 appears to

TABLE 1: Diagnosis of amniotic fluid embolism.

Test	Possible findings
Non-specific tests • Full blood count • Coagulation • Arterial blood gas • Chest X-ray • ECG • V/Q scans • Echocardiogram	 • Low hemoglobin • Low platelets, increased PT and APTT low fibrinogen • Hypoxemia, raised $PaCO_2$ • Normal, cardiomegaly, pulmonary edema • Right heart strain, rhythm abnormalities • V/Q mismatch • Right or left ventricular dysfunction, low ejection fraction
More specific tests • Pulmonary blood sample • Sialyl Tn antigen • Zinc coproporphyrin • Serum tryptase levels	 • Presence of squamous cells coated with neutrophils and presence of fetal debris • Raised • Raised • Normal or raised

(PT: prothrombin time; APTT: activated partial thromboplastin time; V/Q: ventilation/perfusion)
Source: Dedhia JD, Mushambi MC. Amniotic fluid embolism. Cont Educ Anaesth Crit Care Pain. 2007;7(5):152-6.

be the promising diagnostic markers for AFE but are not established in routine clinical diagnosis **(Table 1)**.

Other specific tests such as transesophageal echocardiography (TEE) and rotational thromboelastometry have a limited role in diagnosis and are generally used for optimization of monitoring and treatment. Bedside TEE shows acute pulmonary vasoconstriction, right ventricular dilation, and a collapsed left ventricle with left-side intraventricular septum deviation.

Hence, diagnosis of AFE is by exclusion and needs consideration in cases of sudden maternal cardiovascular collapse and/or unexplained etiology leading to maternal death in childbirth.

DIFFERENTIAL DIAGNOSIS

Conditions mimicking AFE should be excluded while managing the cases that include obstetric, nonobstetric, and anesthetic etiologies.

Obstetric

- *Eclampsia*: Hypertension, proteinuria, and convulsions are pathognomonic of eclampsia but shock is seen in AFE.
- Hemorrhagic shock in obstetric patients (ruptured uterus, uterine inversion, abruption placenta, and placenta previa)
- Septic shock

Nonobstetric

- *Thrombotic pulmonary embolism*: It occurs in the postpartum period and has associated chest pain with definite evidence of venous thrombosis.
- *Air embolism*: Auscultation reveals water-wheel murmur over pericardium and associated chest pain is present in both.

- Cholesterol embolism
- *Acute left heart failure*: Patient presents with a previous history of cardiac illness and associated murmur. Echocardiography will confirm the diagnosis.
- Myocardial infarction
- *Cerebrovascular accidents (CVAs)*: Hypoxemia, pulmonary edema, and cyanosis will be absent.

Anesthetic

- Drug reaction to anesthetic drugs
- Aspiration of gastric contents
- High spinal anesthesia
- Inadvertent intravascular injection of local anesthetics

MANAGEMENT (FLOWCHART 2)

Amniotic fluid embolism traditionally has been viewed as a condition with poor outcomes and high maternal and fetal mortality.

Early recognition, multidisciplinary approach, and effective supportive treatment along with early involvement of senior experienced staff, including obstetrician, anesthetist, hematologist, and intensivist, are essential for optimizing the outcome. The woman requires intensive care unit (ICU) admission and the following measures are taken.

The treatment comprises supportive and obstetric management that are done simultaneously.

Supportive Management

- Airway and oxygenation
  - Protection of airway via endotracheal intubation
  - Use of PEEP (positive end-expiratory pressure) decreases the risk of aspiration
  - Nonarterial extracorporeal membrane oxygenation is therapeutic treatment for patients with refractory

Flowchart 2: Management of amniotic fluid embolism.

Suspected AFE
(Sudden cardiovascular collapse, respiratory distress, coagulopathy)

Emergent Management
- Intubation (High PEEP, low TV strategy)
- Follow ACLS protocol
- Establish 2 large bore IVs
- Monitor BP, SpO$_2$, EKG for acute changes
- Emergent C-section within 3–5 minutes (fetus ≥23 weeks)
- Initiate mass transfusion protocol, if large hemorrhage occurs

Stat Labs and Echocardiogram
- ABG, CBC with differential
- CMP
- Fibrinogen, fibrin degradation products, D-dimer, anti-thrombin III
- INR, PTT
- Blood type and cross
- Rotational thromboelastometry, if avaiable

Activate Care Team
Contact: Obstetrician, Neonatologist, Critical Care Physician, Anesthesia, and Hemotologist,
Call in additional Nursing staff

Obstetrics Management
Uterotonic–stepwise management for uterine atony

Uterine massage
Methylergonovine
Carboprost
Vaginal misoprostol
Hysterectomy

Pulmonary
- Hyperventilation if acidotic on ABG
- Sildenafil, Inhaled NO, inhaled Prostacycline for ARDS prevention
- Consider ECMO if no coagulopathic issues

Monitoring:
- Repeat echocardiogram
- Monitor Hb, plt, fibrinogen, coage, ionized calcium q2h

Cardiology/Hemodynamic

Coagulation

Hemodynamic Support:
- Crystalloid fluids
- Add NE, Vasopressin
- Add Dobutamine

Hemorrhagic Support:
- Continue to transfuse pRBCs, as needed

If elevated INR, PTT, or PT → Administer FFP

Hyperfibrinolysis ([fibrinogen] <2) → Cryoglobulin and fibrinogen with transexamic acid

Thrombocytopenia (Ph <20,000) → Platelets

(ABG: arterial blood gas; ACLS: advanced cardiac life support; AFE: amniotic fluid embolism; ARDS: acute respiratory distress syndrome; CBC: complete blood count; CMP: comprehensive metabolic panel; ECMO: extracorporeal membrane oxygenation; EKG: electrocardiogram; FFP: fresh frozen plasma; INR: international normalized ratio; NO: nitric oxide; PEEP: positive end-expiratory pressure; PT: prothrombin time; PTT: partial thromboplastin time)
Source: Elsey RJ, Moats-Biechler MK, Faust MW, Cooley JA, Ahari S, Summerfield DT. Amniotic fluid embolism: A case study and literature review. Southwest J Pulm Crit Care. 2019;18(4):94-105

acute respiratory distress syndrome. However, its usage is controversial and routinely not recommended in the management of AFE.

– Hyperoxia worsens ischemia-perfusion injury. The inspired oxygen fraction is gradually weaned to maintain a pulse oximetry value of 94–98%.

TABLE 2: Recommended doses for agents commonly used in cases of acute right ventricular failure.

Agent	Dose
Sildenafil	20 mg tid PO or through nasogastric/orogastric tube
Dobutamine	2.5–5.0 µg/kg/min. Higher doses may compromise right ventricular filling time caused by tachycardia
Milrinone	0.25–0.75 µg/kg/min. Most common side effect is systemic hypotension
Inhaled nitric oxide	5–40 ppm. Follow methemoglobin levels every 6 h, and avoid abrupt discontinuation
Inhaled prostacyclin	10–50 ng/kg/min
Intravenous prostacyclin	Start at 1–2 ng/kg/min through a central line and titrate to desired effect. Side effects include systemic hypotension, nausea, vomiting, headache, jaw pain, and diarrhea
Norepinephrine	0.05–3.3 µg/kg/min

(PO: per os; tid: twice a day)

Source: Society for Maternal-Fetal Medicine (SMFM), Pacheco LD, Saade G, Hankins GDV, Steven S. SMFM Clinical Guidelines No. 9: Amniotic fluid embolism: Diagnosis and management. Am J Obst Gynecol. 2016;215(2):PB16-B24.

- Circulation
  - Check for pulse to assess the volume and insert two large-bore intravenous cannulas. Rapid administration for crystalloid fluid administration
  - *Utilization of vasopressors (norepinephrine, vasopressin)*: Maintains perfusion and optimizes cardiac preload
  - *Inotropes (dobutamine, milrinone)*: Increase left ventricular contractility, right ventricular output is improved, and lead to pulmonary vasodilation
  - *For right-sided heart failure*: Sildenafil, inhaled or injectable prostacyclin, inhaled nitrous oxide (dosage as shown in **Table 2**).

The dosage of vasopressors, antiarrhythmic agents, and defibrillators is the same as utilized in nonpregnant individuals.

- The mean arterial blood pressure recommended is 65 mm Hg.
- Therapeutic hypothermia (32–34°C for 12–24 hours) in post cardiac arrest is avoided in patients with AFE due to increased risk of hemorrhage which leads to predisposition for DIC. However, in patients not with DIC, targeted temperature management to 36°C and hyperthermia should be prevented.

Correction of coagulopathy: Disseminated intravascular coagulation is manifested in majority of cases with AFE with variable onset either immediately following cardiopulmonary collapse or in later phases.

The recommended measures are as follows:
- Early corrective management of coagulopathy should be aggressive in nature.
- Treatment of hyperfibrinolysis by tranexamic acid and fibrinogen concentrate (fibrinogen level < 20 mg/dL)
- Hemostatic resuscitation with packed red cells, fresh frozen plasma, and platelets at a ratio of 1:1:1 administration

BOX 2: Components of high-quality cardiopulmonary resuscitation in pregnancy.

Components
- Rapid chest compressions (100 × minute)
- Perform hard compressions, achieving a depth of at least 2 inches
- Assure adequate chest recoil between compressions
- Minimize interruptions of chest compressions
- Avoid prolonged pulse checks (no more than 5–10 seconds)
- Resume chest compressions immediately after defibrillating
- Switch provider of compressions every 2 minutes to avoid fatigue
- Lateral displacement of uterus during resuscitation

Source: Society for Maternal-Fetal Medicine (SMFM), Pacheco LD, Saade G, Hankins GDV, Steven S. SMFM Clinical guidelines No. 9: Amniotic fluid embolism: Diagnosis and management. Am J Obst Gynecol. 2016;215(2):PB16-B24.

- Transfusion of platelets is done at 1–3 U/10 kg/day if platelet count < 20,000/µL and in cases of bleeding with platelet count < 50,000/µL.
- Cryoprecipitate replacement for consumptive nature of DIC (fibrinogen level < 100 mg/dL). Each unit of cryoprecipitate raises fibrinogen by 10 mg/dL
- Overtransfusion to be avoided
- Factor VIIa procoagulant increases thrombin formation and its use is considered if hemostasis is not attained even after replacement of massive coagulation factors and is considered effective if other clotting factors are replaced.
- Gastrointestinal support
  - Pregnancy is a high calorific state and hence starvation leads to ketosis. Hence, prolonged starvation is to be avoided and extra allowance is preferably given by the enteral route.
- Newer therapeutic modalities are nitric oxide, steroids, continuous hemofiltration, C1 esterase inhibitor concentrate, cardiopulmonary bypass, and plasma exchange transfusion. Also, serum glucose is maintained between 140 and 180 mg/dL with the use of insulin infusion if needed.

Flowchart 3: Summary of suspected amniotic fluid embolism.

Sources: Adapted from Society for Maternal-Fetal Medicine (SMFM), Pacheco LD, Saade G, Hankins GDV, Steven S. SMFM Clinical guidelines No. 9: Amniotic fluid embolism: Diagnosis and management. Am J Obst Gynecol. 2016;215(2):PB16-B24.
Adapted from: Clark SL. Amniotic fluid embolism. Clin Obstet Gynecol. 2010;53;322-8.
Adapted from: Clark Amniotic fluid embolism. Obstet & Gynecol 2008;123(2):337-48.

Obstetric Management

- Patient is placed in left lateral position to improve the venous return to heart and prevent air migration to the pulmonary artery
- Continuous fetal monitoring is to be done.
- Steroids should be considered for fetal lung maturity—betamethasone (12 mg, 2 doses 24 hours apart).
- Delivery of the fetus should be expedited.

- Recommendations include initiation of cesarean section in simultaneous to performance of cardiopulmonary resuscitation.
- In laboring patients with a favorable obstetric condition, operative vaginal delivery (vacuum-assisted or forceps) is performed. If vaginal delivery is contraindicated or obstetric condition is unfavorable, then emergency cesarean section is indicated.

- Uterine atony management is by aggressive use of uterotonics during postpartum (oxytocin, ergot derivatives, prostaglandins).
- Refractory cases require uterine packing, uterine artery ligation, B-lynch sutures, or in severe cases hysterectomy.
- Breast-feeding is encouraged even when on ventilatory support. Early maternal bonding facilitates rapid weaning from mechanical support.

■ CARDIOPULMONARY RESUSCITATION IN PREGNANCY (BOX 2)

In patients with cardiopulmonary arrest, the resuscitation is immediately initiated and immediate cesarean section is performed in 3–5 minutes if the fetus is of ≥23 weeks of gestation. Due to improvisation of venous return to the heart by emptying uterus and reduced inferior vena cava pressure, there is a decrease in the risk of infant having long-term neurologic injury secondary to hypoxia.

During cardioversion or use of defibrination, electric arching may occur if fetal monitors are placed. Hence, such fetal monitors should be removed while cardiopulmonary resuscitation is in progress.

■ PROGNOSIS

There is significant improvement in survival rates after AFE due to early recognition and prompt resuscitative measures. About 56% patients die in the initial phase (0–24 hours) of clinical manifestations. The prognosis is very poor and majority do not survive. Among survivals, persistent neurological impairment is seen in about 6–61% women.

The infant survival rate is 70% and its neurological state depends upon the time elapsed between maternal arrest and delivery.

The risk of recurrence in subsequent pregnancy is still unknown.

(**SUMMARY**)

Amniotic fluid embolism has been summarized in **Flowchart 3** that facilitates the strategized manner management.

■ SUGGESTED READING

1. Amniotic fluid embolism. (2017). [online] Available from https://derangedphysiology.com/main/required-reading/pregnancy-obstetrics-and-gynaecology/Chapter%203.1.3/amniotic-fluid-embolism [Last accessed October, 2020]
2. Benson MD. A hypothesis regarding complement activation and amniotic fluid embolism. Med Hypotheses. 2007;68:1019-25.
3. Clark SL. Amniotic fluid embolism. Clin Obstet Gynecol. 2010;53:322-8.
4. Dedhia JD, Mushambi MC. Amniotic fluid embolism. Cont Educ Anaesth Crit Care Pain. 2007;7(5):152-6.
5. Elsey RJ, Moats-Biechler MK, Faust MW, Cooley JA, Ahari S, Summerfield DT. Amniotic fluid embolism: A case study and literature review. Southwest J Pulm Crit Care. 2019;18(4):94-105.
6. Elsey RJ, Moats-Biechler MK, Faust MW, Cooley JA, Ahari S, Summerfield DT. Amniotic fluid embolism: A case study and literature review. Southwest J Pulm Crit Care. 2019;18(4):94-105. doi: https://doi.org/10.13175/swjpcc105-18 PDF
7. FOGSI. (2010). Medical disorders in pregnancy. [online] Available from www.fogsi.org/wp-content/uploads/fogsi-focus/medical_disorders_pregnancy.pdf [Last accessed October, 2020]
8. Hauora Tairawhiti. (2019). Amniotic fluid embolism. [online] Available from https://www.hauoratairawhiti.org.nz/assets/Uploads/Amniotic-Fluid-Embolism.pdf [Last accessed October, 2020]
9. Kaur K, Bhardwaj M, Kumar P, Singhal S, Singh T, Hooda S. Amniotic fluid embolism. J Anaesthesiol Clin Pharmacol. 2016;32:153-9.
10. NHS. (2017). Management of amniotic fluid embolism. [online] Available from http://www.meht.nhs.uk/EasysiteWeb/getresource.axd?AssetID=17593&type=full&servicetype=Attachment [Last accessed October, 2020]
11. Pandya ST, Mangalampally K. Critical care in obstetrics. Indian J Anaesth. 2018;62:724-33.
12. Piva I, Scutiero G, Greco P. Amniotic fluid embolism: An update of the evidence. Med Toxicol Clin Forens Med. 2016;2:2.
13. Rezai S, Hughes AC, Larsen TB, Fuller PN, Henderson CE. Atypical amniotic fluid embolism managed with a novel therapeutic regimen. Case Rep Obstet Gynecol. 2017;8458375.
14. Royal College of Obstetricians & Gynaecologists. Maternal collapse in pregnancy and the puerperium (Green–top Guideline No. 56). [online] Available from https://www.rcog.org.uk/globalassets/documents/guidelines/gtg_56.pdf [Last accessed October, 2020]
15. Society for Maternal-Fetal Medicine (SMFM), Pacheco LD, Saade G, Hankins GDV, Steven S. SMFM Clinical guidelines No. 9: Amniotic fluid embolism: Diagnosis and management. Am J Obst Gynecol. 2016;215(2):PB16-B24.
16. Tamura N, Farhana M, Oda T, Itoh H, Kanayama N. Amniotic fluid embolism: Pathophysiology from the perspective of pathology. J Obstet Gynaecol Res. 2017;43(4):627-32.
17. Tuffnell D, Knight M, Plaat F. Amniotic fluid embolism – an update. Anaesthesia. 2011;66:3-6.
18. Tuffnell DJ.United Kingdom amniotic fluid embolism register. BJOG. 2005;112:1625-9.
19. Uszyñski M. Amniotic fluid embolism: Literature review and an integrated concept of pathomechanism. Open J Obstet Gynecol. 2011;1:178-83.
20. Viswanathan M, Venkateswaran VK, Daniel S. Amniotic fluid embolism: a comprehensive review. Int J Reprod Contracept Obstet Gynecol. 2014;3(2):304-9.

Immunization in Pregnancy

Chandrakant Madkar, Madhukar Shinde

■ INTRODUCTION

Definition: The immune status of a person is defined when he/she possesses specific protective antibodies of cellular immunity as a result of previous infection or immunization or is so conditioned by such previous experiences as to respond adequately for preventing infection or clinical illness following exposure to a specific infectious agent.[1]

The above immune status is acquired through the immunity system in the body. According to the British Society for Immunology, the immune system is defined as a complex system of structures and processes that has evolved to protect us from diseases. The systematic and scientific study of this immune system is called immunology. Immunology covers a wide spectrum of disorders due to the dysfunction of the immune system, for example, HIV, allergies, autoimmunity, organ transplants, cancer,[2] and vaccination. Immunization/vaccination is one of the important components of this system. In medical history, this word came into focus after germ theory of the disease[3] by Louis Pasteur when the science of immunology began to explain how bacteria cause disease and how following infection the human body can acquire the ability to resist future infection from the same organism. The words "immunization" and "vaccination" are used synonymously or have similar meaning in day-to-day language, but there is a technical difference as given in the following text.

Immunization is an immune status of the body acquired by vaccinating agents, with a stimulation of the immune system. Immunization was called vaccination, because it was derived from a virus affecting cows (in Latin, *vacca* means Cow) in experiments done by Edward Jenner, who is known as the founder of vaccination.[4] Edward Jenner in 1796 inoculated a 13-year-old boy with vaccinia virus (cowpox) and demonstrated immunity to smallpox.

Though few other scientists in the world were also trying for it, he was the first person who published a classic text in the annals of medicine under the head *Inquiry into the Causes and Effects of Variolae Vaccine*.[5] His assertion that the cowpox protects the human from the infection of smallpox led to the foundation of modern vaccinology.

Following this, the smallpox vaccine was developed in 1798.

Systematic implementation of mass-scale smallpox immunization in the 18th and 19th centuries culminated eradication of smallpox in 1979, and smallpox got the honor of being the first disease that was eradicated. Following this, many other diseases were also eradicated one by one.

There is no doubt that development of vaccination is one of the greatest accomplishments in the history of medicine, which has the credit of saving countless millions of lives and continues to save millions more each year. The American Centre for Disease Control and Prevention (CDC) has described immunization as one of the 10 greatest public health achievements in the 20th century.

As per the Indian statistics, the disease burden due to vaccine-preventable disease (VPD) was very high before 1978, i.e., before the start of the expanded program of immunization in 1978. The figure of 6 lakh cases of VPD in 1978 has come down to only 71,000 causing drastic reduction by 90%.[6]

■ VACCINE[7]

Active immunity can be obtained through immunizing agents in different ways as follows:

- Live attenuated organisms, e.g., measles, BCG (Bacillus Calmette-Guérin), and others. These are contraindicated during pregnancy.
- Inactivated killed vaccines, e.g., influenza and hepatitis A, which are safe in pregnancy
- *Toxoids*: They cause detoxification and neutralization of toxins produced after vaccination, e.g., diphtheria and tetanus. They are safe during pregnancy.
- Subunit conjugate vaccines such as hepatitis B, pneumococcal, and meningococcal vaccines.
- *Recombinant vaccines*: These are produced through recombinant DNA technology, e.g., human papillomavirus (HPV).

Passive immunity can be obtained by:

- Human normal immunoglobulins, e.g., rabies and mumps

- Human-specific immunoglobulins, e.g., varicella and hepatitis B
- Nonhuman antisera, e.g., diphtheria, tetanus, and rabies

IMMUNIZATION RECOMMENDATIONS

All the drugs including vaccines are categorized by the Food and Drug Administration (FDA) into different risk categories such as A, B, C, D, and X on the basis of the risk of reproductive and developmental adverse effects. A is safest and X is contraindicated. In fact, it is very difficult and challenging to formulate a policy for guiding vaccination of women during pregnancy and breast feeding because the evidence base to guide decisions is extremely limited. Fortunately, the world's most reputed and standard institutes FOGSI (Federation of Obstetric and Gynaecological Societies of India) and CDC have done this valuable work and prepared guidelines for us. The CDC published Advisory Committee on Immunization Practices (ACIP) guidelines in 2011 and recently updated them in March 2014 whereas the guideline development group of FOGSI uploaded their recommendations in September 2014. They are based on the facts that (1) risk to developing a fetus from vaccination is theoretical, (2) inactivated viral and bacterial vaccines and toxoids are safe, (3) live attenuated vaccines are contraindicated during pregnancy, and (4) benefits of vaccinating pregnant women usually outweigh the risk of disease and infection to mother and fetus.

FOGSI Recommendations—Vaccination in Women[8]

FOGSI recommends that pregnancy should be planned according to vaccination status and all vaccination should be completed as per the recommendation in childhood or adolescent period (and if missed under any condition, 3 months prior to conception). The list includes MMR, HepB, HPV, HepA, and tetanus-diphtheria-influenza.

FOGSI insists on administration of Rubella vaccine to all adolescent girls to prevent the incidence of congenital rubella syndrome (CRS) which occurs through vertical transmission if the woman gets infected during the first 3 months of pregnancy. In a study from Vellore, CRS was reported in 9.8% of all children with suspected congenital infection.[9]

The HPV vaccine should be given as early as 9 years.

VACCINATION DURING PREGNANCY

All unvaccinated women should be counseled, and a history of occurrence of VPDs, previous vaccination, and allergic reactions to vaccination must be recorded. Rubella, HepB, and varicella vaccines should be given during the postmenstrual period and should be deferred 3 months before conception. HepB vaccination with ongoing pregnancy is safe. If pregnancy occurs after the first dose of HPV, the remaining doses should be given after delivery.

FOGSI strongly recommends immunization against tetanus, diphtheria, pertussis, and influenza during pregnancy.

Two doses of tetanus toxoid 28 days apart are to be given to all pregnant mothers commencing from the second trimester. If the subsequent pregnancy occurs after 5 years, only one booster is required; this is because India is a developing country and tetanus is an endemic disease here. In 2012, the World Health Organization (WHO) reported 2,404 cases of tetanus in India.

Tetanus, Diphtheria, and Acellular Pertussis (Tdap) vaccination can be considered instead of the second dose of tetanus toxoid. The regular pertussis vaccination is contraindicated if Tdap is not available, and Td-Vac (diphtheria and tetanus) can be given in such cases.

Context: Since 1998, the cases of diphtheria reported to WHO from India have increased from 1,378 to 2,525 in 2012 with a steady rise. The Indian Association of Pediatrician insists on Tdap during the third trimester in every pregnancy, preferably 27–36 weeks of gestation.[10] The influenza vaccine is recommended to mothers from 26 weeks onward and in case of pandemic it can be given earlier.

Context: Influenza A, B are important with an annual global attack rate of 5–10% in adults and 20–30% in children and are caused by H1N1, H3N2, and influenza B virus. The inactivated vaccine is recommended instead of live attenuated vaccine. This offers protection to mothers who are supposed to be at high risk for acute respiratory distress syndrome and to newborns who cannot be vaccinated for the first 6 months. In 2009 H1N1 pandemic, higher rates of influenza-related complications were recorded.

Studies have also shown 63% reduction in influenza illness amongst infants up to 6 months whose mothers were vaccinated.

Postnatal vaccination: FOGSI recommends postnatal rubella, varicella, HepB, influenza, tetanus, and HPV to all nonimmunized mothers. The clinician should be well informed about correct doses, storage, recommendations, contraindications, and adverse reactions of all vaccines.

ACOG GUIDELINES

The American College of Obstetricians and Gynecologists (ACOG) has nicely summarized different vaccines under three groups as given in **Table 1**.[11]

TABLE 1: ACOG guidelines for vaccination.

Vaccines which are indicated and given	Vaccines which may be given due to high risk	Vaccines which are contraindicated
• Influenza • Tetanus • Diphtheria • Whooping cough (pertussis) (Tdap, Td)	• Hepatitis A (HepA) • Hepatitis B (HepB) • Hib (*Haemophilus influenzae* type b) • Meningococcal ACWY (MenACWY, MCV4) • Meningococcal B (MenB) • Pneumococcal (Pneumovax, PPSV; Prevnar, PCV)	• Human papillomavirus (HPV) • Measles, mumps, rubella (MMR) • Varicella (Chickenpox)

(ACOG: American College of Obstetricians and Gynecologists; PCV: pneumococcal conjugate vaccine; PPSV: pneumococcal polysaccharide vaccine)

TABLE 2: CDC guidelines for vaccination.

Recommended	May be used if otherwise indicated	Base decision on risk versus benefit	Not recommended	Inadequate data for specific recommendation
Hepatitis B, Influenza (Inactivated), Tdap	Meningococcal (ACWY), Polio, Td, Anthrax, Rabies, Yellow fever	Hepatitis A, Meningococcal (B)	Human papillomavirus (HPV), Influenza (LAIV), MMR, PCV13, Varicella, Zoster, BCG, Smallpox	PPSV23, Japanese encephalitis, typhoid

◼ CDC GUIDELINES[12]

The general recommendations on immunization are given by the ACIP.

All the diseases and their vaccines are discussed in detail under respective text for recommendations in pregnancy and listed under different categories as shown in **Table 2**.

Breastfeeding and Vaccination

According to the ACIP guidelines, inactivated and live virus vaccines can be given safely, although live virus can replicate in a vaccine recipient. Majority of viruses are not demonstrated in human milk except Varicella and Rubella vaccine. If infection occurs, it is well tolerated since the virus is attenuated. Breastfeeding is contraindication for smallpox vaccination and yellow fever vaccine should be avoided by postponing travel to an endemic area.

◼ GOVERNMENT OF INDIA PROGRAMS

▪ *Mission Indradhanush* is a health mission of the government of India. It was launched by the union Health Minister J P Nadda on December 25, 2014. It is aimed toward covering 90% full immunization by 2020. Though basically it was focused on children, protection to pregnant women in future was also taken into consideration. Initially, it included 7 vaccines, but after addition of few more vaccines, the package now has 12 vaccines.[13]

▪ The *Measles and Rubella (MR) campaign* is an ambitious public health initiative of the government of India to eliminate measles and rubella by 2020 and control CRS. In this project, children ageing from 9 months to 15 years are covered.[14,15]

◼ ROLE OF WHO IN IMMUNIZATION PROGRAM

Recently, the WHO celebrated World Immunization Week under the theme *Vaccines Work* for all, in the last week of April 2020 (April 24–30, 2020).[16]

It aims to promote the use of vaccines to protect people of all ages against diseases. Immunization saves millions of lives every year and is widely recognized as one of the world's most successful and cost-effective health interventions.

WHO's theme for World Immunization Week in 2019 was Protected Together: Vaccines Work!, and the campaign will celebrate Vaccine Heroes from around the world, from parents and community members to health workers and innovators, who help ensure that we are all protected through the power of vaccines.

2019 Campaign Objectives

Goal: The main goal of the campaign is to raise awareness about the critical importance of full immunization throughout life.

As a part of this campaign, the WHO and partners aim to:
▪ Demonstrate the value of vaccines for the health of children, communities, and world
▪ Highlight the need to build on immunization progress while addressing gaps including through increased investments
▪ Show how routine immunization is the foundation for strong, resilient health systems and universal health coverage

According to WHO, immunization is also a fundamental strategy in achieving other health priorities, from controlling viral hepatitis to curbing antimicrobial resistance and providing a platform for adolescent health and improving antenatal and newborn care.

At the end, it concludes that expanding access to immunization is vital for achieving sustainable development goals, poverty reduction, and universal health coverage.

2020 Campaign Objectives

The main goal of campaign is to urge greater engagement around immunization globally and the importance of vaccination in improving the health and wellbeing of everyone and everywhere throughout life.

As a partner of 2020 campaign WHO and partners aim to :

- Demonstrate the value of vaccines for health of children communities and the world.
- Show how the routine immunization is the foundation for strong, resilient health systems and universal health coverage.
- Highlight the need to build on immunization progress while addressing the gaps, including thorough investment in vaccines and immunization

KEY POINTS

- Obstetrician–gynecologists and other obstetric care providers should routinely access the vaccination status, recommend and, when possible, administer needed vaccines to their pregnant patients.
- There is no evidence of adverse pregnancy outcomes from the vaccination of pregnant women with inactivated virus, bacterial vaccine, or toxoid. Therefore, pregnancy should not preclude women from immunization with these vaccines, if medically indicated
- Live vaccines may pose a theoretical risk to the fetus. However, there is a substantial literature describing the safety of live attenuated vaccines, including monovalent rubella vaccines, combined measles-mumps-rubella vaccines, yellow fever and oral poliovirus vaccines. No significant adverse effects on the fetus have been reported following administration of these live attenuated vaccines. Thus, the contraindication of MMR containing vaccines can be considered a purely precautionary measure. Inadvertent vaccination of pregnant women with MMR-containing vaccines is not considered an indication for termination of the pregnancy.
- The benefits of vaccinating pregnant women generally outweigh the potential risks, if they are at high risk of being exposed to a particular infection and the disease would pose a risk for the woman or her unborn child, and if the vaccine is unlikely to cause harm
- Recently, vaccination with dTap (Boostrix) combined with inactivated poliovirus vaccine (IPV) has been recommended for pregnant women (between 28 and 36 weeks) protect their newborn infants against pertussis.
- Other vaccines may be recommended during pregnancy depending on the patient's age, prior immunizations, comorbidities, or disease risk factors.
- Postnatal vaccination should include rubella, varicella, HepB, influenza, tetanus, and HPV to all non-immunized mothers

■ REFERENCES

1. Benson AS. Control of Communicable Diseases in Man, 13th edition. New York: American P H Association; 1981.
2. O'Byrne KJ, Dalgleish AG. Chromic immune activation and inflammation as a cause of malignancy. Br J Cancer. 2001;85(4):473-83.
3. The history of germ theory. Br Med J. 1888;1(14-15):312.
4. Lombard MF, Pastoret PP, Moulin AM. A brief history of vaccines and vaccination. Revue scientifique et technique (International Office of Epizootics). 2007;26(1):29-48.
5. Stern AM, Markel H. The history of vaccines and immunization, familiar patterns, new challenges. Health Affairs. 2005;(24)3 [online] Available from https://doi.org/10.1377/hlthaff.24.3.611 [Last accessed October, 2020].
6. Sundar Lal, Adarsh, Pankaj (eds). Textbook of Community Medicine: Preventive and Social Medicine, 4th edition. New Delhi: GBS Publishers & Distributors; 2016. p. 557.
7. Park K. Principals of epidemiology and epidemiologic methods. In: Park's Textbook of Preventive and Social Medicine, 17th edition. Jabalpur: Banarasidas Bhanot Publishers; 2002. pp. 91-3.
8. Online available at http://www.fogsiorg/wp-content/uploads/2015/11/vaccination_women.pdf
9. Abraham M, Abraham P, Jana AK, Kuruvilla KA, Cherian T, Moses PD, et al. Serology in congenital infections: Experience in selected symptomatic infants. Indian Pediatri. 1999;36:697-700.
10. Indian Academy of Pediatrics, Advisory Committee on Vaccines and Immunization Practices (ACVIP); Vashishtha VP, Kalra A, Bose A, Choudhury P, Yewale VN, et al. Indian Academy of Pediatrics (IAP) recommended immunization schedule for children aged 0 through 18 years, India, 2013 and updates on immunization. Indian Pediatr. 2013;50(12):1095-81.
11. American College of Obstetricians and Gynecologists. (2018). ACOG Guidelines for Vaccination for Pregnant Women, Women Heath Care Physician. Maternal Immunization. No. 741. [online] Available from https://www.acog.org/clinical/clinical-guidance/committee-opinion/articles/2018/06/maternal-immunization [Last accessed October, 2020]
12. Centers for Disease Control and Prevention. (2017). CDC General recommendations on immunization by Advisory Committee on Immunization Practices (ACIP). [online] Available from https://www.cdc.gov/mmwr/preview/mmwrhtml/rr6002a1.htm [Last accessed October, 2020]
13. Government of India. (2014). Mission Indradhanush. Online Available from https://www.nhp.gov.in/mission-indradhanush1_pg
14. Ministry of Health and Family Welfare. (2017). Introduction of Measles-Rubella Vaccine Guidelines (campaign and routine immunization). [online] Available from https://main.mohfw.gov.in/sites/default/files/195431585071489665073.pdf [Last accessed October, 2020]
15. Shreedevi A. MR vaccination campaign, a trust deficit. J. Post-Graduate Med. 2018;64(4):202-3.
16. available online at http://www.who.int/campaigns/world-immunization-week/2020.

CHAPTER 39

Obstetric Analgesia and Anesthesia in High-risk Pregnancies

Mridul M Panditrao, Minnu M Panditrao

■ INTRODUCTION

Pregnancy is a state of altered physiology. Generally it is well accepted that, as a part of physiological activity, the entire process will start at a specific point in time, run its stipulated course, and will culminate in its finite outcome, namely birth of the fetus and the afterbirths. The desired outcome is obviously the birth of an alive, full-term, and a normal newborn by the natural process of vaginal delivery followed by the complete expulsion of placenta and membranes. However, in nature, this seemingly simple physiological process does not necessarily always run the normal course. The process of conception, growth, maturity, and expulsion of the fetus may get deviated from normal and will be labeled as a "high-risk or complicated pregnancy." A high-risk pregnancy is defined as "the pregnancy which, due to altered physiological or pathological conditions of the mother or fetus or both, preexisting or acquired during the course of pregnancy, is associated with a compromised outcome, in terms of the well-being of the mother or growth/delivery of the fetus/placenta or all of them."[1]

These patients will require some kind of intervention, logically analgesia and/or anesthesia in most cases. It would be very pertinent to give due considerations to the specific conditions and their needs and make necessary changes in anesthetic and related management.

As already mentioned, pregnancy does lead to changes in the entire maternal body. The discussion of this entire spectrum is beyond the scope of this chapter. So, the focus shall be mainly "high-risk pregnancy," the specific problems encountered in such a case, and the necessary and suitable modalities of analgesia and anesthesia.

■ CLASSIFICATION OF PATIENTS TO BE INCLUDED AS "HIGH-RISK PREGNANCY"

Broadly, patients of high-risk pregnancy can be classified into six main categories as follows:
1. Peripartum/obstetric hemorrhage spectrum disorders
2. Hypertensive disorders associated with pregnancy
3. Metabolic diseases coexisting/preexisting with pregnancy

4. Systemic diseases coexisting/preexisting with pregnancy
5. Miscellaneous disorders affecting/associated with pregnancy
6. Fetal conditions/factors complicating pregnancy

Accordingly, they are further subclassified as follows:
1. Peripartum/obstetric hemorrhage spectrum disorders
   1.1 Antepartum hemorrhage (APH)
      1.1.1 *Abnormal placement of placenta:* Placenta previa
      1.1.2 Abruptio placentae
         1.1.2.1 Visible hemorrhage
         1.1.2.2 Concealed hemorrhage and Couvelaire uterus
   1.2 Postpartum hemorrhage (PPH)
      1.2.1 Uterine atony
      1.2.2 Placenta accreta
      1.2.3 Retained placenta and other products of conception
      1.2.4 Inversion of uterus
2. Hypertensive disorders associated with pregnancy (older description)[2]
   Pregnancy-induced hypertension (PIH)
   2.1 Preeclamptic toxemia (PET)
   2.2 Eclampsia
   2.3 HELLP (Hemolysis, Elevated Liver enzymes, Low Platelet count) syndrome
   The newer categorization as per the guidelines by the American College of Obstetricians and Gynecologists (ACOG), which has been endorsed by the National High Blood Pressure Education Program of the National Heart, Lung, and Blood Institute (NHLBI),[3,4] is as follows:
   2.1 Gestational hypertension
   2.2 Chronic hypertension
   2.3 Chronic hypertension with superimposed preeclampsia
   2.4 Preeclampsia/eclampsia
   2.5 HELLP syndrome
3. Metabolic diseases coexisting/ preexisting with pregnancy
   3.1 *Diabetes mellitus*: Gestational diabetes and preexisting
   3.2 Obesity

4. Systemic diseases coexisting/preexisting with pregnancy
   4.1 Cardiac diseases
      4.1.1 Congenital heart diseases
      4.1.2 Acquired heart diseases
   4.2 Pulmonary diseases
   4.3 Renal diseases
   4.4 Endocrine diseases
5. Miscellaneous disorders affecting/associated with pregnancy
   5.1 Elderly mothers or advanced maternal age
   5.2 Peripartum infections/sepsis
   5.3 Premature rupture of membranes and/or cord prolapse
6. Fetal conditions/factors complicating pregnancy
   6.1 Prematurity/postmaturity
   6.2 Intrauterine growth retardation
   6.3 Multiple gestations
   6.4 Problems of liquor production
      6.4.1 Polyhydramnios
      6.4.2 Oligohydramnios
   6.5 Fetal malpositions
   Let us try to deal with each of these individually.

Peripartum/Obstetric Hemorrhage Spectrum Disorders

These disorders of disparate etiologies present as a bleeding *per vaginum*, in the perinatal period, namely during pregnancy and childbirth, or in the postpartum period. So, they are collectively called major obstetric hemorrhage or hemorrhagic disorders of obstetrics.[5] In peripartum hemorrhage spectrum disorders, the main causes may be:

- Abnormal placement of placenta
- Abnormality of the tone of the myometrium
- Coexistence or emergence of coagulopathy
- Trauma

These factors may complicate pregnancy individually or collectively. These disorders will present in the form of excessive bleeding *per vaginum* in the peripartum period.

Antepartum Hemorrhage

Antepartum hemorrhage is one of the leading causes of perinatal mortality.

Both of the main causes, placenta previa or abruptio placentae, are fairly common in occurrence.

Placenta previa: The incidence of placenta previa worldwide varies between 2.7 and 12.2 per 1,000 pregnancies depending on the region.[6] There seems to be an obvious correlation between the higher incidence of placenta previa and the history of a previous lower segment cesarean section (LSCS) and increasing parity. Clinically, it can be suspected when a pregnant patient presents in the third trimester with painless bright red vaginal bleeding with no history of trauma. The management from an obstetrician's point of view mainly gives stress on the conservative approach, especially in milder cases, till the maturity of the fetus is achieved with supportive measures such as absolute bed rest, transfusion of cross-matched blood, and strict monitoring of coagulation profile. In severe cases, especially with severe APH, termination of pregnancy is done by performing the LSCS.

Anesthetic management: Patients presenting for a cesarean section with minimal bleeding or earlier after onset with hemodynamic stability or a well-planned, electively posted patient may be managed with subarachnoid/spinal analgesia. In larger centers, where obstetric analgesia is prevalent, an epidural catheter may already be in place and the analgesia may be converted into anesthesia, by increasing the concentration of the local anesthetic being used. The only indication for general anesthesia (GA) may be a patient presenting with a severe hemorrhage and associated hemodynamic instability.

Abruptio placentae: Abruption occurs in 0.4–1% of pregnancies.[7] The patient presenting with abruptio placentae is a real emergency. These patients may have associated precipitating factors such as PET, hypertension, history of smoking, substance abuse, and multiple gestation. A very high degree of mortality is associated with abruption, because of acute, catastrophic blood loss, in addition to the complications such as acute renal failure (ARF); "Couvelaire uterus," a condition in which, there is intramyometrial bleeding or blood dissects out the myometrial fibers/wall; and coagulopathy culminating into disseminated intravascular coagulation (DIC). By the time the patient is brought to the labor room/obstetric unit, the fetus may have been seriously compromised. In all such cases, emergency LSCS would be indicated, with the exception that fetal death may have happened. If the maternal hemodynamic stability is not compromised, then normal vaginal delivery may be tried.

Postpartum Hemorrhage

By definition, postpartum hemorrhage is:[8]

"Loss of blood > 500 mL, post normal vaginal delivery or >1,000 m: post caesarean section." There may be multiple associated and/or predisposing factors, which can cause the PPH, such as PET, hypertension, infection, induction of labor, multiple pregnancies, multiple gestations, and polyhydramnios. The main causes or reasons of PPH are given in the following text.

Uterine atony: It is by far the most prominent cause of PPH. It can be defined as "the failure or inability of the myometrium to contract after complete expulsion or removal of all the products of conception." From the obstetrician's point of view, two drugs are used, either oxytocin in the infusion form or synthetic ergot derivatives such as methylergometrine or methyl ergonovine.

Placenta accreta spectrum:[9] In olden days, what was called "morbidly adherent placenta" is now renamed as "placenta accreta spectrum" disorders. In this condition, there is an abnormal and invasive adherence of the placental tissue with the uterine wall. As per the depth of its adherence, it has been classified into three different types: accreta vera, where the adherence is only up to the surface of the myometrium; increta, where the entire thickness of the myometrium is invaded; and percreta, where the adherence has crossed the myometrium, and even the serosal covering, and into the surrounding tissues. Irrespective of the type, the only therapeutic intervention indicated is hysterectomy. By taking into consideration all the precautions, and carrying out resuscitation, the anesthetic management is similar to the other conditions of obstetric hemorrhage.

Retained placenta and other products of conception: These are one of the more common problems faced in the peripartum period, where anesthetic intervention is often needed. This is when, after the delivery of the fetus, both the entire placenta and the membranes or may be the fragments of placenta and parts of the membranes may remain behind. In the case of an entire placenta, manual removal of placenta is to be undertaken. Logically, the relaxation of uterine body and cervical opening are essential aspects. As a result, a myometrial relaxant such as glyceryl trinitrate in the boluses of 50–100 µg intravenously may be needed. Invariably, GA with endotracheal intubation, muscle relaxant, and addition of an inhalational agent is the modality of anesthesia to be employed, especially if the patient is about to go into or is already in hemorrhagic hypovolemic shock. In the bygone days, halothane was the inhalational agent of choice, specifically for manual removal of placenta, because of its myometrial relaxant properties. In general, in normal obstetric patients requiring GA, it was rather relatively contraindicated, because of this property and possibility of PPH.

However, if only fragments/minor products of conception are retained and are to be surgically removed, the complete relaxation of the uterus may not be needed, as the intervention to be carried out is curettage. The choices of the anesthetic technique remain any of the following three: (1) the spinal/subarachnoid block may be given or of already labor analgesia with the epidural catheter in situ, (2) convert the analgesia to anesthesia by increasing the concentration of the local anesthetic, or (3) short GA using a supraglottic airway device (SAD) such as the laryngeal mask airways (LMA) or I-Gel may be employed.

Injuries (lacerations) to the birth canal: In the course of vaginal delivery, during the passage of the fetus, due to application of obstetric forceps and precipitate labor, injuries might get inflicted upon cervical os, vagina, and perineum, thus contributing to a significant amount of PPH. The anesthetic considerations would be on the similar lines to those employed for curettage and removal of fragments.

Inversion of the uterus: This is one of the rarer complications, which can present as one of the "real, life-threatening obstetric emergencies." Acute management of shock, resuscitation, as discussed below, under GA with endotracheal intubation and controlled ventilation is the choice.

Management of ensuing hemorrhagic, hypovolemic shock: For the convenience of understanding and remembering, the American College of Surgeons in the Advanced Trauma Life Support (ATLS) has given various classes of hemorrhage as shown in **Table 1**.[10]

There have been serious attempts to rationalize and logisticate this classification in relation to the clinical features. The well accepted of these are given in **Table 2**.[11]

As the basic pathophysiology involved in any major obstetric hemorrhage or peripartum/obstetric hemorrhage spectrum disorder is almost similar to the hypovolemia/hemorrhage secondary to trauma, the same guidelines can also be applied to these patients and they can be classified, monitored, and managed accordingly.

Principles of management of hemorrhagic shock: It is directed toward optimizing perfusion of the vital organs and thereby optimizing oxygen delivery. Rapid diagnosis and treatment of the underlying hemorrhage are a must with concurrent management of shock.

Supportive therapy:
- Oxygen administration
- Monitoring
- Establishment of intravenous access (two large-bore cannulas in peripheral lines, central venous access)

Intravascular volume and oxygen-carrying capacity should be optimized.

In addition to crystalloids, some colloid solutions, hypertonic solutions, and oxygen-carrying solutions [hemoglobin (Hb)-based and perfluorocarbon emulsions] may be administered.
- Blood products in severe hemorrhagic shock
- Replacement of lost components using red blood cells (RBCs), fresh frozen plasma (FFP), and platelets
- Recent combat experience has suggested that aggressive use of FFPs may reduce coagulopathies and improve outcomes.
- Determination of the site and etiology of hemorrhage are must.

TABLE 1: ATLS classification of hemorrhagic shock.

Class	Percentage blood volume loss	Clinical signs and symptoms	Necessary intervention
Class I hemorrhage	Up to 15% of blood volume	Typically no change in vital signs	Fluid resuscitation is not usually necessary
Class II hemorrhage	15–30% of total blood volume	Tachycardia, decreased pulse pressure, peripheral vasoconstriction, pale and cool skin, altered behavior	Volume resuscitation and no blood transfusion
Class III hemorrhage	30–40% of circulating blood volume	Hypotension, tachycardia, shock with decreased capillary refill, mental state worsens	Crystalloids and blood
Class IV hemorrhage	>40% of circulating blood volume	The limit of the body's compensation is reached	Aggressive resuscitation is required to prevent death

(ATLS: Advanced Trauma Life Support)

TABLE 2: Clinical presentation according to the class of hemorrhagic shock: For a 70-kg man.

	Class I	Class II	Class III	Class IV
Blood loss (mL)	Up to 750	750–1,500	1,500–2,000	>2,000
Blood loss (% blood volume)	Up to 15	15–30	30–40	>40
Pulse rate (bpm)	<100	100–120	120–140	>140
Systolic blood pressure (mm Hg)	Normal	Normal	Decreased	Decreased
Pulse pressure	Normal or increased	Decreased	Decreased	Decreased
Respiratory rate	14–20	20–30	30–40	>40
Urine output (mL/h)	0.30	20–30	5–15	Negligible
CNS/ mental status	Slightly anxious	Mildly anxious	Anxious confused	Confused, lethargic
Initial fluid replacement	Crystalloid	Crystalloid	Crystalloid and blood	Crystalloid and blood

(CNS: central nervous system)

- Control of hemorrhage may be achieved in the emergency department.
- Control may require a multidisciplinary approach and special interventions.

Recently, there has been rekindled interest in the management of hemorrhagic hypovolemic shock. A Pan-European, multidisciplinary Task Force for Advanced Bleeding Care in Trauma was founded in 2004. This included representatives of six relevant European professional societies. The group used a structured, evidence-based consensus approach to address scientific queries that served as the basis for each recommendation and supporting rationale. The existing recommendations were reconsidered and revised based on new scientific evidence and observed shifts in clinical practice; new recommendations were formulated to reflect the current clinical concerns and areas in which new research data have been generated. This guideline represents the fourth edition of a document first published in 2007 and updated in 2010 and 2013.[12]

The same guidelines can be equated and appropriately implemented in the management of the bleeding parturient, both antepartum and postpartum.
- Avoidance of hypoxemia
- Oxygen supplementation by mask is useful, but if required early intubation and controlled ventilation

may be an ideal thing to do, to avoid maternal as well as, and if possible, fetal complications. Normoventilation is the norm.

Initial survey: The anesthesiologist clinically assesses the extent of hemorrhage using a combination of patient physiology, clinical presentation, and the patient's response to initial resuscitation.

High degree of suspicion of coagulopathy:
- A low initial Hb can be considered an indicator for severe bleeding associated with coagulopathy.
- Use of repeated Hb measurements as a laboratory marker for bleeding, as an initial Hb value in the normal range, may mask bleeding.
- Serum lactate and/or base deficit measurements as sensitive tests to estimate and monitor the extent of bleeding and shock
- Routine practice to include the early and repeated monitoring of coagulation profile,
  - Prothrombin time (PT), PTI, international normalized ratio (INR), activated partial thromboplastin time (APTT), platelet counts and fibrinogen and/or a viscoelastic method (thromboelastogram)
- A target systolic blood pressure (SBP) of 80–90 mm Hg until major bleeding has been stopped.

Volume therapy:

- In the presence of life-threatening hypotension, administration of vasopressors in addition to fluids to maintain target arterial pressure
- Infusion of an inotropic agent in the presence of myocardial dysfunction
- Fluid therapy using isotonic crystalloid solutions be initiated
- *"3:1 rule"*: 3-cc crystalloid for every 1 cc of blood loss
- Excessive use of 0.9 % NaCl solution be avoided
- The use of colloids be restricted due to the adverse effects on hemostasis
- A target Hb of 7–9 g/dL
- Early application of measures to reduce heat loss and warm the hypothermic patient in order to achieve and maintain normothermia.

Damage control management: Urgent emergency surgery in a patient presenting with deep hemorrhagic shock, signs of ongoing bleeding, and coagulopathy.

Pharmacological control over bleeding:

- Monitoring and measures to support coagulation be initiated immediately upon hospital admission
- In the initial management of patients with expected massive hemorrhage, one of the two following strategies, to maintain PT and APTT < 1.5 times the normal control:
  - FFP in a plasma–RBC ratio of at least 1:2 as needed
  - Fibrinogen concentrate and RBC according to Hb level
- Tranexamic acid (TXA) be administered as early as possible (within 3 hours) at a loading dose of 1 g infused over 10 minutes, followed by an IV infusion of 1 g over 8 hours
- Resuscitation measures be continued using a goal-directed strategy guided by standard laboratory coagulation values and/or viscoelastic tests.

Component therapy:

- Plasma transfusion be avoided in patients without substantial bleeding
- Fibrinogen concentrate or cryoprecipitate, if significant bleeding along with:
  - Viscoelastic signs of a functional fibrinogen deficit
  - Plasma fibrinogen level of <1.5–2.0 g/L
- Initial fibrinogen supplementation of 3–4 g
  - This is equivalent to 15–20 single donor units of cryoprecipitate or
  - Repeat doses must be guided by viscoelastic monitoring and laboratory assessment of fibrinogen levels.
- Platelets be administered to maintain a platelet count above 50×10^9/L

- Maintenance of a platelet count above 100×10^9/L in patients with ongoing bleeding and/or traumatic brain injury (TBI)
- If administered, an initial dose of four to eight single-platelet units.

Other modalities to control the bleeding:

- Ionized calcium levels be monitored and maintained within the normal range during massive transfusion
- *Administration of platelets in patients with*:
  - Substantial bleeding
  - Continued microvascular bleeding
- Desmopressin is not to be used routinely.
- Desmopressin (0.3 µg/kg) be administered only in patients treated with platelet-inhibiting drugs or with von Willebrand disease (Grade 2C).

Miscellaneous

- If bleeding is life-threatening, treatment with TXA 15 mg/kg (or 1 g) intravenously and high-dose (25–50 U/kg) prothrombin complex concentrate (PCC)/activated PCC (aPCC) until specific antidotes are available
- *Off-label use of activated recombinant factor VII (rFVIIa) to be considered*

Role of rFVIIa:

A very lucid review[13] describes in detail the role of rFVIIa in various bleeding disorders as well as acute episodes during surgical and traumatic conditions.

The recommendations are as follows:

- Replace lost/consumed hemostatic factors with FFP, cryoprecipitate, platelets, and RBCs.
- Full blood count, PT, APTT, and fibrinogen level monitoring
- The use of rFVIIa should be considered:
  - If bleeding continues when more than one blood volume has been transfused (approximately 10 units of red cells in an adult)
  - When no identifiable surgical source of bleeding has been found
  - If it is felt that rFVIIa may be of benefit
- It should normally only be requested by a consultant anesthetist.
- It should normally be used only following discussion with a consultant hematologist.
- One 4.8-mg vial should be given (50–100 µg/kg for a 50–100-kg patient). If bleeding does not diminish in 30–60 minutes, then a further 4.8-mg vial can be given.
- If bleeding continues after the second dose, there is little evidence to support the use of a third dose, and surgical exploration should be considered.

Hypertensive Disorders Associated with Pregnancy

Among the high-risk pregnancies, hypertensive disorders of pregnancy are one of the most common disorders, especially in developing countries such as India, with the incidence ranging between 3 and 10%, and one of the most common causes of maternal morbidity and mortality ranging from 10 to 15% worldwide.[14] Even according to the World Health Organization (WHO), hypertensive disorders of pregnancy account for up to 13–16% of mortality associated with pregnancy.[15] The associated predisposing factors are elderly primigravida, diabetics, obesity, or women with other chronic metabolic/systemic diseases.

According to the ACOG classification, there are four categories of hypertensive disorders associated with pregnancy:[3,4]

1. Gestational hypertension
2. Chronic hypertension
3. Chronic hypertension with superimposed preeclampsia
4. Preeclampsia/eclampsia

Gestational Hypertension

Gestational hypertension is defined as a rise in blood pressure above 140 mm Hg systolic and 90 mm Hg diastolic, which occurs after 20 weeks of gestation in a previously normotensive woman, but there is no proteinuria or other severe features of preeclampsia.

Chronic Hypertension

In this condition, there is a preexisting hypertension, before the onset of pregnancy or appears before 20 weeks of pregnancy. This condition can progress to chronic hypertension with superimposed preeclampsia.

Chronic Hypertension with Superimposed Preeclampsia

In this condition, there is elevated blood pressure associated with proteinuria and/or other features of PET.

Preeclampsia/Eclampsia

There is elevated blood pressure with proteinuria of >300 mg in 24 hours or any of the severe features of preeclampsia such as severe hypertension with SBP of >160 mm Hg and diastolic of >110 mm Hg, epigastric or right upper quadrant abdominal pain, vomiting, thrombocytopenia of platelet count of <1 lakh/mL, impairment of liver function, renal insufficiency indicated by serum creatinine > 1.1 mg/dL, pulmonary edema, and visual or cerebral disturbances. The cerebral disturbances may present as headache, giddiness, confusion, cortical blindness, and hyperreflexia.

In eclampsia, there is occurrence of seizures. It is one of the most severe forms of the obstetric emergencies observed in late pregnancy near to term/delivery. In 50% of cases, there may be associated signs and symptoms of severe preeclampsia; however, in rest of the cases, the classical triad of hypertension, proteinuria, and edema may be very mild or even absent. In almost two thirds of cases, the onset of seizure/coma precedes before delivery, while in the rest of the patients it may occur in the postpartum period. In most of the postpartum cases, the signs and symptoms develop in the first 24 hours but they can occur even up to 3 weeks after delivery. The risk of maternal and perinatal morbidity and mortality is higher when signs and symptoms of eclampsia appear before 32 weeks' gestation.

A typical eclamptic fit starts in the form of facial muscle twitching followed by a tonic/clonic seizure, associated with a brief period of apnea. This progresses into a postictal phase of variable duration, where the patient is spontaneously breathing but is comatose. The number of seizures may be variable ranging from 1–2 to up to 100 in untreated cases. The exact etiology of seizures is not very clear, but various factors which are implicated may be cerebral vasospasm, ischemia, hemorrhage, or edema and hypertensive encephalopathy. Unless other causes are proven, a fit during late pregnancy should be labeled as eclamptic fit. The differential diagnoses of eclampsia are cerebrovascular accident, meningitis, encephalitis, epilepsy, or cerebral tumor.

Common maternal complications are placental abruption, DIC, HELLP syndrome, neurological deficits, tongue-bite, retinal detachment, pulmonary aspiration of blood/gastric contents, pulmonary edema, ARF, and cardiac arrest.

Management of preeclampsia/eclampsia: The latest ACOG guidelines recommend the initiation of antihypertensive treatment only when the SBP rises above 160 mm Hg and/or DBP rises above 110 mm Hg.

Management of an eclamptic fit: The first priority is to have an unobstructed airway and adequate oxygenation. An oropharyngeal or nasopharyngeal airway should be inserted, and administration of oxygen via a face mask must be started at the earliest. This is followed by ventilatory support if the patient is not breathing adequately. The tongue-bite should be prevented by inserting a bite block or an oropharyngeal airway and aspiration is to be prevented by positioning the patient in lateral and head-low positions and suctioning of the oral cavity. Injection Midazolam in incremental doses of 1–2 mg (maximum up to 20 mg) may be given to control the seizures. If this is not effective, then Injection Thiopentone 5–10 mg/kg, along with a muscle relaxant (succinylcholine or atracurium), may be required to control the seizures. This situation logically must be followed up with laryngoscopy/endotracheal intubation and controlled ventilation. So, all the equipment/

instruments required for endotracheal intubation and ventilation should be kept ready before giving thiopentone and muscle relaxant.

Monitoring of ECG, SpO_2, noninvasive blood pressure (NIBP), and $EtCO_2$ should be started at the earliest. Displacement of uterus to the left with help of a bolster under the right hip should be maintained throughout the resuscitation and till the delivery of the baby.

Injection Magnesium sulfate is to be given as soon as possible to prevent further seizures. A loading dose of 4–6 g given in intravenous infusion over 30 minutes is followed by a maintenance dose of 1–2 g/h. Continuous monitoring of the urine output, deep tendon reflexes, and respiratory rate should be carried out to prevent magnesium toxicity.

Unless there is a specific contraindication, the fetus must be delivered as early as possible because that is the definitive treatment of preeclampsia/eclampsia. The labor is induced and allowed to progress. The indications for LSCS are fetal distress, abruptio placentae, unfavorable cervical dilation, uncontrolled seizures, or persistent postictal agitation.

Choice of anesthesia for LSCS: Unconscious, delirious patients or patients having frank seizures should not be given spinal/subarachnoid or regional anesthesia. Here, GA is indicated for LSCS or any other operative intervention. However, if the patient is conscious, well oriented, behaving normally, and is seizure free for >24 hours, with the normal coagulation profile, then regional anesthesia/analgesia can be used for the labor and delivery. At the end of the surgery under GA, if the patient has stable vitals and becomes conscious after switching off of inhalational anesthetic, she can be given the reversal and extubated. However if the patient was unconscious at the beginning, and has had seizures and very high blood pressures in the perioperative period, she should be left intubated in the postoperative period and transferred to an intensive care unit (ICU) for elective ventilatory support, monitoring, and control of blood pressure and seizures. She should be weaned off slowly after neurological assessment and improvement of consciousness and other parameters. Magnesium should be tapered off only after blood pressure becomes normal and remains stable and the central nervous hyperexcitability has disappeared.

An uncommon complication of pulmonary edema may complicate the postpartum period in preeclamptic/eclamptic patients. The etiological factors in the development of this condition are high intravascular hydrostatic pressure, low plasma oncotic pressure, and increased pulmonary capillary permeability. In addition, these patients receive hypotonic intravenous infusion, namely 5% dextrose with Pitocin for the induction and enhancement of the labor. So, there will be overhydration/overload if the patient has low urinary output and peripheral vasoconstriction. In such patients, supplemental oxygen should be immediately started. The fluid administration should be restricted and guided with the central venous pressure (CVP) monitoring. The loop diuretics such as Frusemide or Torsemide may have to be given as a loading dose followed by maintenance doses, serially. If the diuretics have not been effective and the patient is unable to maintain adequate oxygen saturation and the respiratory distress is increasing, urgent endotracheal intubation and intermittent positive-pressure ventilation may have to be started to push back the fluid into the intravascular compartment and improve gaseous exchange. In resistant cases, hemodialysis may be required to remove excessive fluid volume and prevent/treat congestive heart failure. The supportive treatment in the form of appropriate antibiotics, colloid infusion such as Injection Albumin 20%, or FFPs may be needed.

HELLP Syndrome

HELLP syndrome consists of a triad of *H*emolysis, *E*levated *L*iver *E*nzymes and *L*ow *P*latelets, thus the reason behind the acronym HELLP. It is a severe form of preeclampsia, with very high maternal and perinatal mortality. The exact etiology is not understood, but in this condition there is microvascular endothelial damage, leading to intravascular activation of platelets. The main features are microangiopathic hemolysis and anemia with an abnormal peripheral blood smear and elevated levels of serum bilirubin (≥1.2 mg/dL). There are increased levels of aspartate aminotransferase (≥70 U/L) and lactate dehydrogenase (≥600 U/L), and platelet count is also decreased. Therefore, according to the platelet count it has been classified into three categories:

- *Class I*: When the platelet count is <50,000/mm³
- *Class II*: When the platelet count is between 50,000 and 1 lakh/mm³
- *Class III*: When the platelet count is >1 lakh/mm³

For making the diagnosis of the classical HELLP syndrome, all the three criteria must be present. If only one or two of the three are present, it is called a partial HELLP syndrome. Most cases occur before the term, with only about 20% cases occurring after the term and delivery. The full HELLP syndrome carries a high incidence of morbidity and mortality. The complications include cerebrovascular accidents, DIC, abruptio placentae, ARF, pleural effusion, septicemia, and wound infections. Postpartum cases are more prone to pulmonary edema and renal failure.

Management: Delivery of the fetus and placenta are the only definitive treatment. But if delivery is not possible, then steroid therapy in the form of Inj. Dexamethasone 10 mg twice a day is carried out till there is clinical improvement in the form of adequate control of blood pressure (≤150/100 mm Hg), urine output (≥30 mL/h for 2 consecutive hours, without the use of diuretics or fluid bolus), platelet count >50,000/mm³, and declining lactate dehydrogenase (LDH) levels. The management should also include bed rest, antithrombotic agents, and fresh blood and platelet concentrates. If the platelet counts rise above 100,000/mm³ and INR comes within normal limits (1–1.3), then one can opt for the regional techniques of anesthesia. In the rest of the patients, GA would be the method of choice.

Metabolic Diseases Coexisting/Preexisting with Pregnancy

The coexistence as well as the preexistence of certain metabolic conditions and diseases along with the pregnancy may add to an unfavorable outcome. These are mainly diabetes mellitus and obesity.

Diabetes Mellitus

While discussing diabetes in relation to pregnancy, one has to consider both the possibilities, occurrence of gestational diabetes and occurrence of pregnancy in a woman with preexisting diabetes, type I as well as type II.

Gestational diabetes: This is defined as the occurrence of impaired glucose metabolism with the onset of pregnancy. The fetal developmental problems such as macrosomia, intrauterine fetal death, and large babies complicating the course of labor are some of the associated problems. As such, there is enough evidence that the females presenting with gestational diabetes have a higher risk of developing maturity onset diabetes or type II diabetes later on in their life.

Preexisting diabetes type I as well as type II: The pregnancy in already diagnosed/confirmed diabetic mothers, with either of the types, is not only also associated with the high risk of abnormal fetal outcomes but in addition there is a high propensity for end-organ damage in the mothers. Especially in type I, juvenile onset diabetic (JOD) mothers, even without having significantly higher blood sugar levels, there is an increased tendency to developing diabetic ketoacidosis (DKA). This can also add to increase in fetal demise.

In comparison to nonpregnant counterparts, the euglycemic control in pregnant patients needs to be much more stringent with lower target fasting blood levels with the maximum permissible up to 120 mg/dL. Again, in comparison to nonpregnant diabetics, the blood sugar level of >100 mg/dL is an indication for initiating the insulin therapy.

Anesthetic management: Generally, many of these patients may require assisted delivery or even LSCS. The continuation of analgesia and converting it into an anesthesia of the pre-emptively placed epidural catheter would be an ideal modality. But in our country, this may not be the possible solution, because of lack of acceptance of epidural by routine patients. In such a situation, if it is an elective well-planned procedure, spinal/subarachnoid anesthesia is and will be the method of choice. Preoperative preparation includes serial blood glucose estimation, preferably by the laboratory method, and maintaining the blood glucose levels to <120 mg/dL. The bedside handheld devices using paper or plastic sticks, also called point-of-care tests (POCTs), are fraught with inherent fallacies[16] so they are not recommended for the monitoring of the glucose levels in these patients. In an unforeseen situation, necessitating emergency surgery, it is still possible to use spinal anesthesia but if there are extenuating circumstances, in the best interests of both the mother and the fetus, GA may have to be employed.

Obesity

As in the western world, even in India, the incidence of obesity is increasing. As a result, obesity in pregnancy, or pregnancy in obese women, is a major area of concern, especially in bigger cities/metros. In these patients, there is an association of other comorbid conditions such as chronic hypertension, diabetes mellitus, and PET. Logically, the fetal consequences found in patients with diabetes mellitus such as a large-sized fetus, fetal congenital anomalies, and prolonged/abnormal labor are to be anticipated. In the immediate antepartum period, the problems for which one must be prepared for are as follows:

- The common occurrence of abnormalities of labor culminating into possible elective or emergency LSCS, and thus the anticipatory preanesthetic checkup and preparation are necessary.
- Because of anatomical changes related to obesity, anticipate "difficult airway management" and make suitable alternative plans and preparation.
- If labor analgesia is requested by the patient or is to be opted for, then because of the obesity, anticipate the "technical difficulties" in achieving neuraxial blocks such as insertion of an epidural needle, identifying space, and epidural catheter placement. In the case of requirement for achieving spinal analgesia, regular length spinal needles may not be enough to reach the prerequisite depth. As a result, extra-long spinal needles are needed.

The obese patients, in the immediate postoperative period, may have higher predisposition for complications, i.e., delayed awakening, airway obstruction, increased blood loss, sepsis, and subsequent maternal morbidity/mortality.

Systemic Diseases Coexisting/Preexisting with Pregnancy

With the advances taking place in the treatment modalities of various systemic diseases and the increased survival of these patients, more and more of them tend to go ahead and fulfill their desire of becoming pregnant. The pre- as well as the coexistence of one or multiple systemic diseases with pregnancy complicates the already tumultuous progress of each of these conditions.

Cardiac Diseases

This spectrum includes two disparate classes:
1. Patients with congenital heart disease, either operated or nonoperated
2. Patients with acquired heart disease

Pregnancy in preexisting congenital cardiac disease patients: As already mentioned, due to tremendous advances in the cardiac surgeries, and because of associated advances in cardiac anesthesia, especially in pediatric patients, the total corrections of many of the previously thought to be uncorrectable congenital anomalous conditions have been happening in the childhood itself. In addition, with advances in the postoperative monitoring/care, the survival has also increased. The classic examples of such conditions are the left-to-right shunt/acyanotic congenital heart diseases group, atrial septal defect (ASD), ventricular septal defect (VSD), and patent ductus arteriosus (PDA).

In cyanotic heart diseases/right-to-left shunt group, mainly the tetralogy of Fallot, with primary defects such as right outflow obstruction like pulmonary valve/canal stenosis, a large VSD, overriding of the aorta and the right ventricular hypertrophy, corrective surgeries in the form of opening of the pulmonary tract and closure of VSD are being carried out, generally, in infancy itself. As more and more of these females are growing up and attaining adulthood, they are now defying the old belief or dictum that patients with such lesions may not survive the pregnancy. With careful and vigilant monitoring and planning, they can be given proper peripartum care. Epidural analgesia is recommended in these patients, because of its advantages in obviating the labor pains and ensuing consequences.

The patients who have not been operated upon for their primary pathology or the condition has a milder form of the disease, but have survived up to adulthood and present for the LSCS, can pose challenges. The author can still recollect successfully managing a patient with trilogy of Fallot, with pulmonary stenosis, right ventricular hypertrophy and ASD for two consecutive LSCSs under balanced GA.

Acquired heart diseases: Although the incidence of rheumatic heart disease and its most common consequence, mitral stenosis, in the western world has become almost nonexistent, in our country, it is still a major problem. Mitral stenosis with its low fixed cardiac output state is a serious problem, especially during pregnancy, with its hyperdynamicity of circulation and increased blood volume, and often leads to the increased tendency for precipitation of left ventricular failure (LVF). But with advances in the cardiac surgical techniques, patients with prosthetic valve replacements have a better life expectancy. When such patients are encountered for pregnancy and related management, the most important factor to be taken into consideration is that majority of these patients would be on some form of anticoagulant therapy making neuraxial blocks a relative contraindication.

Pulmonary Diseases

Patients with childhood-onset bronchial asthma, bronchiectasis, or even interstitial lung disease (ILD) may rarely be encountered with pregnancy and its management. The important considerations in these cases are the compromised pulmonary function in the form of impaired gaseous exchange, decreased ability of removing the respiratory secretions, increased bronchomotor tone leading to tendency for developing bronchospasm, and propensity of landing into acute respiratory failure, which must be actively anticipated and the anesthetic management is to be suitably adjusted. For these patients, the most suitable form of anesthesia logically would be the regional/neuraxial block, unless there is a contraindication for it. As far as possible, GA is to be avoided, for obvious reasons.

Miscellaneous Disorders Affecting/Associated with Pregnancy

Elderly Gravida

As is prevalent in the western countries, even in India, with a more career-oriented approach and liberalization, the age of marriage in females and subsequent pregnancy is gradually increasing. In addition, advent of newer technologies such as in-vitro fertilization (IVF), in the older or elderly females, has started posing the challenges of management of elderly pregnant mothers. Many of these patients may have preexisting or coexisting systemic and metabolic conditions, which can complicate the course of pregnancy. Some of these conditions include diabetes, both gestational and preexisting diabetes mellitus, chronic hypertension and associated coronary artery disease, thyroid dysfunctions, rheumatoid arthritis, obesity, etc. In addition, in these patients there is an increased incidence of PET, intrauterine growth retardation, oligohydramnios, abruptio placentae, and increased requirement of surgical intervention (LSCS). So, planned LSCS would be the method of choice for the delivery. Taking into consideration the multiple factors, a detailed preanesthetic checkup is required with suitable adjustment in the anesthetic plan, accordingly.

Fetal Conditions/Factors Complicating Pregnancy

These conditions, although do complicate the pregnancy and are categorized under "high-risk pregnancy," do not per se make any significant impact on the analgesic and anesthetic management. The standard management of an obstetric patient in terms of labor analgesia with epidural and anesthetic management in the case of LSCS, either elective or emergency with either GA or regional depending upon the general condition of the patient, remains the same. However, there have been reports of acute morbidity as well as near mortality such as "sudden cardiac arrest" in the multiple-pregnancy patients, coming for emergency LSCS and receiving myometrial stimulants such as carboprost tromethamine.[17] So, caution needs to be exercised while administering such agents.

SUMMARY

"High-risk pregnancy" is a very challenging situation, not only to the obstetrician but also to the "anesthesiologist." The gravity of situation depends upon multiple factors: whether an emergency or elective procedure, primigravida or multigravida, single fetus or multiple pregnancies, pre-/coexisting and associated obstetric as well as other systemic disorders, to mention a few. With more advances in the understanding of pathophysiology, diagnostic tools, monitoring devices, and methods of intervention, the outcomes have and are becoming more positive. But the fundamental principles of multispecialty or team approach, with mutual trust/respect, understanding, and cooperation, go a long way in gaining favorable outcomes for both the mother and the fetus, out of these dire, difficult circumstances.

KEY POINTS

- Regional anesthesia, with its high safety profile, is the most common method of providing anesthesia to a parturient. While GA is largely avoided in pregnant patients, it is the preferred mode of anesthesia in certain situations.
- It is essential to take into account the physiological changes of pregnancy and administer a safe GA that minimises risks, such as failed intubation, aspiration and awareness.

■ REFERENCES

1. The Free Dictionary. High-risk pregnancy care. [online] Available from https://medical-dictionary.thefreedictionary.com/high-risk+pregnancy [Last accessed October, 2020].
2. Mammaro A, Carrara S, Cavaliere A, Ermito S, Dinatale A, Pappalardo EM, et al. Hypertensive disorders of pregnancy. J Prenat Med. 2009;3(1):1-5.
3. American College of Obstetricians and Gynecologists. (2013). Hypertension in pregnancy. [online] Available from http://www.spog.org.pe/web/phocadownloadpap/HypertensioninPregnancy.pdf. [Last accessed October, 2020].
4. Roccella EJ. Report of the National High Blood Pressure Education Program Working Group on high blood pressure in pregnancy. Am J Obstet Gynecol. 2000;183(1):S1-22.
5. Trikha A, Singh PM. Management of major obstetric haemorrhage. Indian J Anaesth. 2018;62(9):698-703.
6. Cresswell A, Ronsmans C, Calvert C, Filippi V. Prevalence of placenta praevia by world region: a systematic review and meta-analysis. Trop Med Int Health. 2013;18(6):712-24.
7. Sengodan SS, Palanivelu A, Pandian A. A study on perinatal outcomes in antenatal mothers with abnormal pulmonary function tests. Int J Reprod Contracept Obstet Gynecol. 2017;6(10):4389-92.
8. Royal College of Obstetricians and Gynaecologists. (2016). Postpartum Haemorrhage, Prevention and Management (Green-top Guideline No. 52). [online] Available from https://www.rcog.org.uk/en/guidelines-research-services/guidelines/gtg52/ [Last accessed October, 2020].
9. American College of Obstetricians and Gynecologists. (2018). Placenta accreta spectrum. [online] Available from https://www.acog.org/Clinical-Guidance-and-Publications/Obstetric-Care-Consensus-Series/Placenta-Accreta-Spectrum [Last accessed October, 2020].
10. Committee on Trauma, American College of Surgeons. Advanced Trauma Life support for Doctors-Student Course Manual, 8th edition. Chicago: American College of Surgeons; 2008.
11. Mutschler A, Nieber U, Brockamp T, Wafaisade A, Wyen H, Peiniger S, et al. A critical appraisal of the ATLS classification of hypovolemic shock: does it really reflect clinical reality. Resuscitation. 2013;84:309-13.
12. Rossaint R, Bouillon B, Cerny V, Coats TJ, Duranteau J, Fernández-Mondéjar E, et al. Crit Care. 2016;20:100.
13. Panditrao M, Panditrao M, Shamsah M. Massive bleeding in trauma and surgery: Role of rFVIIa. Kuwait Med J. 2011;43(3):176-88.
14. Mehta B, Kumar V, Chawla S, Sachdeva S, Mahopatra D. Hypertension in pregnancy: A community-based study. Indian J Community Med. 2015;40(4):273-8.
15. World Health Organization. (2003). Global burden of hypertensive disorders of pregnancy in the year 2000. [online] Available from https://www.who.int/healthinfo/statistics/bod_hypertensivedisordersofpregnancy.pdf [Last accessed October, 2020].
16. Panditrao MM, Panditrao MM. Strict glycemic control: The demise of another good strategy? Anaesthesia. 2015;2(2):69-73.
17. Panditrao MM, Singh C, Panditrao M. An unanticipated cardiac arrest and unusual post-resuscitation psycho-behavioral phenomena/near death experiences in a patient with pregnancy induced hypertension and twin pregnancy undergoing elective lower segment caesarian section: a case report. Indian J Anaesth. 2010;54:467-9.

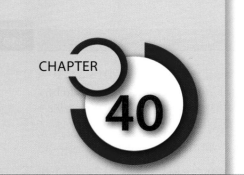
Cord Around Neck

Priyanka A Dahiya

■ INTRODUCTION

The nuchal cord was first defined as one that is "wrapped 360 degrees around the fetal neck" by J Selwyn Crawford MD from the British Research Council in 1962.[1] Although the implications of nuchal cords are controversial, several studies have noted an association between nuchal cords and adverse perinatal outcome. Its prevalence is reported to be 6–30%, and the incidence of nuchal cord increases with advancing gestation.[2] The occurrence of nuchal cords from 24 weeks on was demonstrated by Clapp et al.[3] The nuchal cords are often referred to as "tight" or "loose" depending on whether the loop of cord can be easily manually released over the fetal head or not. Male fetuses and polyhydramnios have a greater propensity of cord around neck (CRN).[4]

The incidence of the number of loops found in nuchal cord is as follows:

- One loop: 20%
- Two loops: 2.5–3.5%
- Three loops: 0.5%
- Four loops: <0.5%
  Almost 50% of CRN resolve spontaneously.

■ CLASSIFICATION

Two types of nuchal cord have been described by Giacomello et al. depending upon the manner in which they encircle the fetal neck (**Figs. 1A and B**).[5] They are:

1. *"Type A"*: The nuchal cord is wrapped around the neck but is free sliding, meaning that the cord encircles the neck in an unlocked pattern.

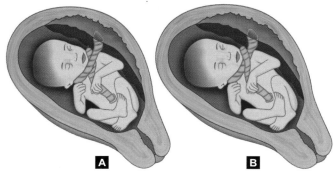

Figs. 1A and B: Types of nuchal cords. (A) Type A: Encircling the neck in an unlocked pattern; (B) Type B: Encircling the neck in a locked manner.

2. *"Type B"*: This pattern is described as a hitch which cannot be undone and ends up as a true knot, i.e., the cord encircles the neck in a locked pattern.

■ ETIOPATHOGENESIS

The umbilical cord formation starts as early as 5 weeks after conception and cord twisting can be seen as early as the 6th week. Normally as the cord grows longer, it coils around itself. The cords are helical in nature, with as many as 380 helices. Then it continues to grow longer until 28 weeks of pregnancy, reaching an average length of 22–24 inches. The length of the umbilical cord varies from no cord (achordia) to 300 cm, with the diameter ranging from 1 to 3 cm. On an average, the umbilical cord is 55 cm long, with a diameter of 1–2 cm and 11 helices, but diameters up to 3 cm and helices of as many as 380 per cord have been described.

A cord >70 cm in length is defined as a *long cord* and a cord <30 cm in length is taken as a *short cord*. The presence of short cords seems to double and triple the predictive values of low Apgar scores, low IQ values, neurologic abnormalities, and stillbirths whereas long cords have association with poor fetal outcome, higher fetal entanglements, and true knots and they are prone to torsion.[6,7] The in-utero movement of fetus controls the cord twisting, in addition to controlling umbilical cord length. The left twisting of cord outnumbers the right by a ratio of 7:1 (85% are left twisted while 15% are right twisted). While the exact causes for left twists are unknown, one of the possible mechanisms seems to be that the right umbilical artery is usually larger than the left, which creates differential flow patterns resulting in a left twist of the umbilical cord. Another proposed theory is subsequent re-entry of physiologically herniated gut which usually is anticlockwise. Excessive twisting can lead to intrauterine fetal death by compressing the fetal vessels beyond the capacity of Wharton's jelly.

It is proposed that the biometrics patterns of uterine, fetal, and umbilical cord lengths coupled with placental and amniotic fluid volumes could possibly be playing a role in the formation of nuchal cords. Most of the nuchal cords (>80%) are wrapped right to left around the fetal neck.

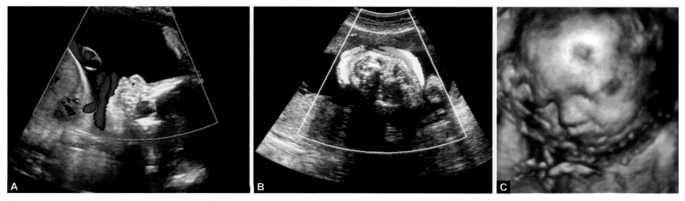

Figs. 2A to C: (A and B) Early recognition of a single loop relies on the demonstration of a section of cord between head and shoulder in a sagittal section, and the demonstration of a complete loop in an axial section of neck. This is often difficult due to shadowing and a compound image is often required. (C) 4D demonstration of a cord around neck.

Almost 5–18% of all fetal asphyxia cases are attributed to nuchal cord accidents. The nuchal cords were increased with true knots; the frequency of knots and encirclement is 0.5%. An encirclement of 14.2% was found with cords ranging from 27 to 122 cm in length. Many studies have proved that although the nuchal cord is not associated with 1-year neurologic status or stillbirths, growth restriction was often associated. A nuchal cord at the onset of labor is very unlikely to correct itself whereas in the absence of nuchal cord during prelabor, it is unlikely to occur during labor. Tightly wrapped nuchal cords seem to have some similar physical features to those seen in strangulations such as duskiness of face, facial petechiae, and conjunctival hemorrhage.

Morarji Pessay[8] recommends developing the grading system of tight nuchal cords as follows:

- *Grade 1*: Conjunctival hemorrhage and petechiae
- *Grade 2*: Duskiness of face, facial suffusion, and pallor
- *Grade 3*: Respiratory distress, stupor, and hypotonia requiring resuscitation.

tCAN Syndrome

The "*tCAN (tight Cord Around the Neck Syndrome) syndrome*" refers to a cluster of cardiorespiratory and neurological signs and symptoms associated with tight cord-round-the-neck of the fetus.[9] The umbilical cord compression occurring due to *tCAN* first obstructs the blood flow in the umbilical vein while the fetal blood continues to be pumped out through the thick umbilical arteries finally resulting in hypovolemia and hypotension, hence acidosis, anemia, and respiratory distress.

Such newborns may have facial/conjunctival petechiae, facial puffiness, skin abrasion around neck, petechiae of the neck and upper part of the chest, and suffusion of face as well as head.

Babies born with nuchal cords are more often deprived of placental blood transfusion, because of very early cord

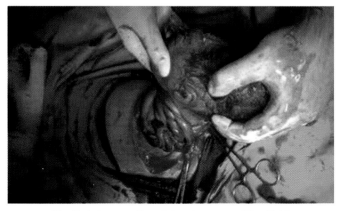

Fig. 3: Intraoperative picture in a case of five tight loops of cord around neck.

cutting, and they are significantly more anemic than controls because of reduced venous return from placenta secondary to compression of the umbilical vein. Cerebral palsy is a probable consequence of this hypovolemic shock. Increased pulmonary perfusion because of tCAN results in pulmonary hemorrhages and fetomaternal hemorrhages. "Compression asphyxia" term which is an established terminology in forensic medicine has been proposed for description of such cases because of the similarities in their pathophysiological mechanisms and clinical findings. This can help differentiating birth asphyxia from infant with the effects of a tight nuchal cord.

■ MANAGEMENT

Antenatal diagnosis of CRN can easily be done by ultrasonography. A study was published in 2004, which was carried out to establish the sensitivity of ultrasound in the diagnosis of a nuchal cord. Each of 289 women, induced the same day, underwent a transabdominal ultrasonography with an Aloka 1700 ultrasound machine (3.5-MHz abdominal probe, using gray-scale and color Doppler) imaging immediately prior to induction of labor.

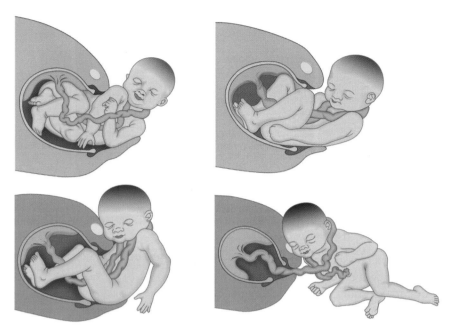

Fig. 4: Somersault maneuver for nuchal cords.

In this study, ultrasound was only 35% accurate at finding a single loop **(Figs. 2A to C)** and 60% accurate at detecting a nuchal cord wrapped multiple times around the fetal neck **(Fig. 3)**.[10] On gray-scale machines, a "divot" sign which appears as a circular indentation of the fetal nuchal skin can diagnose nuchal cord. Nuchal cord is best detected using color Doppler with a sensitivity of around 90% with advancing gestational age.[11]

Clinically, at term fetal bradycardia and late returning to baseline while trying to push floating head in pelvis can give a hint of tCRN.[12] During labor, variable fetal heart decelerations with uterine contractions indicate tCRN.

A close monitoring is required in cases where a prolonged persistent nuchal cord with poor fetal growth is observed and delivery as appropriate. The goal in management is directed toward preventing the compression of the umbilical cord whenever possible. The decision of vaginal delivery or a cesarean section should be individualized.

Several case reports and an integrated literature by Mercer et al. suggest an increase in an infant's risk of birth asphyxia and even neonatal death, if the cord is cut before birth, more so in cases of severe shoulder dystocia.[13] Immediate cord clamping results in 25% reduction in a neonate's blood volume and about 50% reduction in red cell volume.[14] Techniques to preserve an intact nuchal cord depend on how tightly the cord is wrapped around the baby's neck. The cord can be easily slipped over the baby's head during delivery, if the cord is loose followed by delivering rest of the body and placing over the maternal abdomen. If the cord is too tight to go over the baby's head, it may be possible to slip it over the infant's shoulders and deliver the body through the cord. Unwrapping the cord from around the baby may be done after birth. Finally, if the cord is too tight to even slip back over the shoulders, "*Somersault maneuver*" may be carried out if one does not want to severe the cord **(Fig. 4)**.[15] Schorn and Blanco first described the Somersault maneuver. It involves slow delivery of baby and bringing the fetal head as it is borne toward the maternal thigh in flexion. The baby is kept tucked near the perineum so that the body rolls out and the feet are away from mother, with the head still up toward the introitus. If shoulder dystocia is suspected, keeping the cord intact, *Somersault maneuver* is recommended. While performing this maneuver, since the baby's head is kept very close to the perineum as the body delivers, very little traction is exerted on the cord. A delayed cord clamping is needed to equalize the blood volume after birth and stabilize the baby to early neonatal life.

If not feasible, clamping and cutting the umbilical cord can be done to facilitate vaginal delivery. But one may perform milking of the cord to restore the newborn's blood volume especially after shoulder dystocia if immediate cutting of the cord is required.

CONCLUSION

tCAN are a potential cause for perinatal distress and an important risk factor for long-term neurodevelopmental consequences. Nuchal cords can be diagnosed antenatally by use of ultrasound with color Doppler, middle cerebral

- False-positive and false-negative results can occur as with any other test. Therefore, another practical learning point to remember is that CVS or amniocentesis is strongly recommended for diagnostic purposes in cases of all pregnant women who have abnormal cell-free fetal DNA results.

Management of Screening Results

Combined First-trimester Screening Test (Flowchart 1)

Screen-negative or low-risk result: A screen-negative report does not exclude the possibility of aneuploidy; however, it just implies that the fetus is at low risk of Down syndrome as predefined by the specific laboratory cutoff (<1 in 250). It is seen in 80–85% of all women who undergo screening. Further testing after a low-risk aneuploidy screen is not recommended and only routine prenatal care is offered.

Screen-positive or high-risk result: A screen-positive report implies an increased risk of Down syndrome as predefined by the specific laboratory cutoff (>1 in 250), and it is seen in about 3–5% of all women who undergo prenatal screening. Invasive prenatal testing for definitive fetal chromosomal analysis by CVS or amniocentesis is the most widely used approach following a high-risk result; however, NIPT as a secondary screen can also be a reasonable alternate approach in certain circumstances. It should be noted that repeat testing or multiple biochemical screening tests are not recommended in these cases as repeat testing might lead to a very small increase in detection rates, but it often leads to confusion and is not cost effective.[15]

Intermediate-risk result: This group includes pregnant women with risk between 1:251 and 1:1,000 and is seen in about 10–15% of the pregnant women screened. After counseling, such women are offered NIPT as a preferred approach or can be offered quadruple test for integration of final result. In cases where NIPT is also positive, invasive testing is advised.

Screening Tests in Second Trimester (Flowchart 2)

In cases where no biochemical screening test is done, a-priori risk is taken as her age risk unless modified by a genetic sonogram.

Screen-positive Cell-free DNA-based Test

Invasive testing is offered for definitive diagnosis to all pregnant women who undergo NIPT as their initial screening test and are tested positive by test.

Ultrasound in Prenatal Screening: Role of Genetic Sonogram

There are various soft markers, which can be noted on ultrasound and can act as markers for aneuploidy, especially trisomy 21. These include increased nuchal fold thickness, echogenic bowel, ventriculomegaly, echogenic heart focus, choroid plexus cyst, and short long bones. The risk of aneuploidy is calculated based on the a-priori risk of the patient and it is increased by the presence of a specific likelihood ratio or decreased if no markers are present.[8] However, screening in the second trimester using soft markers should not be used alone. Also, it is important to note that the presence of two or more soft markers on ultrasound does warrant an invasive testing. Genetic sonogram should be used with caution if proper first- or second-trimester biochemical screening test or NIPT has already been done **(Flowcharts 3 and 4)**.[8]

When to Offer a Diagnostic Test?[9]

An invasive prenatal diagnostic test should be offered in the following conditions:

- A positive screening test

Flowchart 1: Antenatal screening in the first trimester.

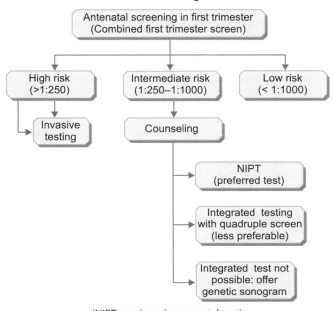

(NIPT: noninvasive prenatal test)

Flowchart 2: Antenatal screening in the second trimester.

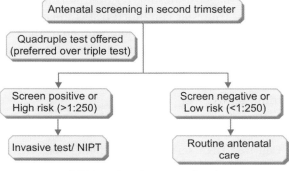

(NIPT: noninvasive prenatal test)

Flowchart 3: Management for soft markers on ultrasound in cases where no biochemical screening has been done.

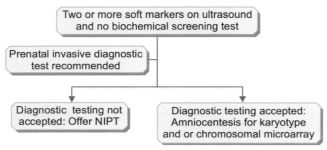

(NIPT: noninvasive prenatal test)

Flowchart 4: Management of soft markers on ultrasound in cases where biochemical screening has been done.

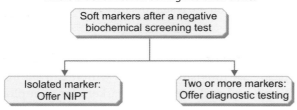

(NIPT: noninvasive prenatal test)

- A previous pregnancy complicated by fetal trisomy
- At least one major or two minor fetal structural anomalies in the current pregnancy
- Chromosomal translocation, inversion, or aneuploidy in the pregnant woman or her partner.

The choice of a prenatal diagnostic test to be performed depends on the period of gestation. CVS is performed in the first trimester and amniocentesis is performed in the second trimester for analysis of karyotype. The rapid aneuploidy test report [quantitative fluorescence-polymerase chain reaction (QF-PCR)] can be available as early as 2 days; however, it takes 10–14 days for full karyotype results from cultured cells.

KEY POINTS

- Prenatal screening for Down syndrome should be offered to all pregnant women.
- All pregnant women should have the option of invasive diagnostic testing, regardless of maternal age.
- The first-trimester combined test is the best serum screening option for pregnant women as the risk of Down syndrome can be estimated early in pregnancy.
- The quadruple test is the best serum screening test for women who present for prenatal care in the second trimester.
- Maternal plasma cell-free DNA testing, also called NIPT, is a screening test and not a diagnostic test. Cell-free DNA screening has higher sensitivity for

detection of Down syndrome and a lower FPR, which in turn leads to more cases detected with reduction in invasive procedures.
- NIPT can be offered for secondary screening after a positive biochemical marker screening test.

■ REFERENCES

1. American College of Obstetricians and Gynecologists' Committee on Practice Bulletins—Obstetrics; Committee on Genetics; Society for Maternal–Fetal Medicine. Practice Bulletin No. 162: Prenatal Diagnostic Testing for Genetic Disorders. Obstet Gynecol. 2016;127(5):e108-22.
2. Palomaki GE, Lee JE, Canick JA, McDowell GA, Donnenfeld AE; ACMG Laboratory Quality Assurance Committee. Technical standards and guidelines: prenatal screening for Down syndrome that includes first-trimester biochemistry and/or ultrasound measurements. Genet Med. 2009;11(9):669-81.
3. Kuppermann M, Pena S, Bishop JT, et al. Effect of enhanced information, values clarification, and removal of financial barriers on use of prenatal genetic testing: a randomized clinical trial. JAMA. 2014;312:1210.
4. American College of Obstetricians and Gynecologists. ACOG Practice Bulletin No. 88, December 2007. Invasive prenatal testing for aneuploidy. Obstet Gynecol. 2007;110:1459.
5. ACOG Committee on Practice Bulletins. ACOG Practice Bulletin No. 77: screening for fetal chromosomal abnormalities. Obstet Gynecol. 2007;109:217.
6. Palomaki GE, Knight GJ, Ashwood ER, et al. Screening for down syndrome in the United States: results of surveys in 2011 and 2012. Arch Pathol Lab Med. 2013;137:921.
7. Alldred SK, Takwoingi Y, Guo B, et al. First and second trimester serum tests with and without first trimester ultrasound tests for Down's syndrome screening. Cochrane Database Syst Rev 2017;3:CD012599
8. Audibert F, De Bie I, Johnson JA, Okun N, Wilson RD, Armour C, et al. No. 348-Joint SOGC-CCMG Guideline: Update on Prenatal Screening for Fetal Aneuploidy, Fetal Anomalies, and Adverse Pregnancy Outcomes. J Obstet Gynaecol Can. 2017;39(9):805-81.
9. Committee on Practice Bulletins—Obstetrics, Committee on Genetics, and the Society for Maternal-Fetal Medicine. Practice Bulletin No. 163: Screening for Fetal Aneuploidy. Obstet Gynecol. 2016;127(5):e123-37.
10. Odibo AO, Stamilio DM, Nelson DB, et al. A cost-effectiveness analysis of prenatal screening strategies for Down syndrome. Obstet Gynecol. 2005;106:562.
11. Society for Maternal-Fetal Medicine (SMFM) Publications Committee. Electronic address: pubs@smfm.org. #36: Prenatal aneuploidy screening using cell-free DNA. Am J Obstet Gynecol. 2015;212(6):711-6.
12. Committee Opinion No. 640: Cell-Free DNA Screening For Fetal Aneuploidy. Obstet Gynecol. 2015;126(3):e31-7
13. Bianchi DW, Parker RL, Wentworth J, et al. DNA sequencing versus standard prenatal aneuploidy screening. N Engl J Med. 2014;370:799.
14. Gregg AR, Gross SJ, Best RG, Monaghan KG, Bajaj K, Skotko BG, Thompson BH, Watson MS. ACMG statement on noninvasive prenatal screening for fetal aneuploidy. Genet Med. 2013;15(5):395-8.
15. Hackshaw AK, Wald NJ. Repeat testing in antenatal screening for Down syndrome using dimeric inhibin-A in combination with other maternal serum markers. Prenat Diagn. 2001;21:58.

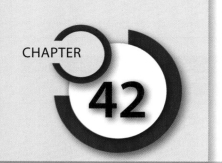
Amniotic Fluid Abnormalities

Sujatha Patnaik

■ INTRODUCTION

Amniotic fluid surrounds the developing embryo throughout the pregnancy. It acts as a cushion, protecting the fetus from trauma while allowing mobility for promoting structural growth and development.[1] The pathological conditions associated with excess of amniotic fluid and diminished amniotic fluid volume are polyhydramnios and oligohydramnios, respectively. An understanding of the normal amniotic fluid dynamics and measurement techniques of amniotic fluid is essential before discussing the amniotic fluid abnormalities.

■ AMNIOTIC FLUID DYNAMICS

There are three major determinants influencing amniotic fluid volume: transfer of solutes within and across the membranes, fetal regulation through swallowing, and urine production and transplacental fluid movement.[2]

During the first half of pregnancy, amniotic fluid mainly consists of water through transfer from mother across amnion (transmembranous) fetal vessels on the placental surface (intramembranous) and fetal skin (transcutaneous).[3]

Later, in the second trimester, when fetal skin keratinization occurs beyond 22–25 weeks four pathways play a major role in amniotic fluid volume regulation: fetal urine production, lung liquid secretion, fetal swallowing, and intramembranous absorption.[4]

As the hypotonic fetal urine enters the amniotic fluid from 11 weeks of gestation, it creates a potential osmotic force for outward flow of water across transmembranous pathways.[4,5] Changes in aquaporins with advancing gestation have a role in controlling transmembranous water flow and amniotic fluid volume.[6]

Fetal lung secretions enter the amniotic fluid on an average rate of 165 mL/day near term because under physiologic conditions, half of the fetal lung fluid is swallowed by the fetus.[7]

Swallowing is the major pathway of amniotic fluid removal. Studies of near-term pregnancies suggest that a normal human fetus swallows an average of 210–760 mL/day.[8]

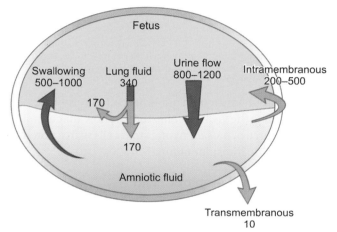

Fig. 1: Pathway for daily fluid production and resorption in a term fetus.

Figure 1 shows the pathway for daily fluid production and resorption in a term fetus.[1,5]

Normal Amniotic Fluid Volume and Composition

Amniotic fluid volume increases steadily in early gestation and remains stable between 22 and 38 weeks averaging 0–800 mL; thereafter, amniotic fluid declines by 8% per week with a mean volume of approximately 500 mL at 40–42 weeks gestation.[9-11]

Figure 2 shows the normograms for amniotic fluid volume which were developed by Queenan et al. (dye-determined method),[9] Brace and Wolf (direct measurement and dye dilution),[10] and Magann et al. (dye dilution, direct measurement, and sonographic measurement).[11]

However, the reference range of amniotic fluid index (AFI) used in clinical practice should be based on data from local population.[12]

Amniotic Fluid Composition

Amniotic fluid composition reflects the composition of its source: fetal urine and fetal lung liquid. It has a pH of 7.0–7.5 with an osmolality of 260 mmol/kg which is slightly lower than blood (280 mmol/kg).[13]

Initially, the amniotic fluid mainly contains water and electrolytes but after 12–14 weeks it also contains protein,

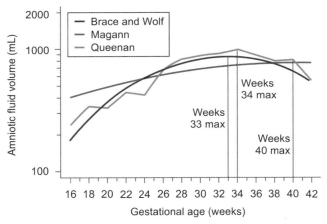

Fig. 2: Normograms for amniotic fluid volume developed by Queenan et al., Brace and Wolf, and Magann et al.

TABLE 1: Various amniotic fluid estimates and their interpretation.

Ultrasound estimate	Oligohydramnios	Normal values	Polyhydramnios
AFI	<5 cm	5–25 cm	>25 cm
SDP	<2 cm	2–8 cm	>8 cm
Two-diameter pocket	<4 cm²	4–50 cm²	>50 cm²
Subjective assessment	Reduced	Normal	Excess

(AFI: amniotic fluid index; SDP: single deepest pocket)

carbohydrates, lipids, phospholipids, and urea which help in growth of the fetus.[14] Recent studies show that amniotic fluid is a source of mesenchymal stem cells with a potential for therapeutic transplantation.[15]

Measurement of Amniotic Fluid

Amniotic fluid volume should be assessed at every prenatal ultrasound as disorders in amniotic fluid are associated with an adverse perinatal outcome.[16]

The most accurate method to assess amniotic fluid volume is by direct measurement[17] at hysterotomy or cesarean delivery and indirect dye dilution technique.[18] These methods are invasive and only used for research purposes and have helped us to develop normograms[19] for understanding normal amniotic fluid volume. Rapid magnetic resonance projection hydrography has been used for assessment of amniotic fluid volume; however, this is an impractical approach for everyday setting.[20]

Sonographic Assessment

Sonographic techniques to estimate amniotic fluid volume include subjective (qualitative) estimation and semiquantitative methods: measurement of two-diameter pocket (2 × 2), maximum vertical or single deepest pocket (SDP), and AFI.[1] Semiquantitative assessment of amniotic fluid is preferable because it is reproducible, easy to teach, and can be followed over a time (ACOG 2016).[21]

Using either technique, the fluid pocket must be at least 1 cm in width, to be considered adequate, and fetal parts and cord loops are not included in measurement.[22] Color Doppler is generally used to identify cord loops in the pocket.

Single Deepest Pocket

Chamberlain et al. originally described this method where vertical dimensions of the largest pocket of amniotic fluid

are taken.[23] The measurement is done at a right angle to the uterine surface.

Amniotic Fluid Index

Phelan and Rutherford[24] proposed this technique where amniotic fluid volume is calculated by adding the SDP from each quadrant. Here, the uterus is divided into four quadrants using linea nigra and umbilicus as surface markings.

Moore and Cayle[25] established the mean and outer boundaries (5th and 95th percentiles, respectively) for the AFI from 16 to 42 weeks of gestation in a study of 791 normal pregnancies.

Two-diameter Amniotic Fluid Pocket

The two-diameter amniotic fluid pocket is the product of the vertical depth multiplied by the horizontal diameter of the largest pocket.[26] A normal two-dimensional measurement is 15.1–50 cm². However, this technique is a component of biophysical profile (BPP) and is not clinically useful to predict pregnancy outcome.[27]

Subjective Assessment

It is the subjective visual interpretation of amniotic fluid volume during ultrasound. The amniotic fluid volume is reported as reduced, normal, or excess.[28] These impressions appear to be reliable and reproducible among experienced observers.

Table 1 shows the various amniotic fluid estimates and their interpretation.

Comparison of Sonographic Assessment Methods

According to the Canadian task force[29] guidelines on preventive health care:

- Accurate quantification of amniotic fluid volume using the current sonographic technique is challenging. *(II-2)*
- No technique is universally considered superior at predicting perinatal outcome.[30] *(II-1)*
- It is proposed that SDP should always be used for the initial assessment during routine scanning because AFI

over diagnoses amniotic fluid abnormalities leading to unnecessary interventions. *(1-A)*

- For assessment of amniotic fluid volume before 20 weeks and in twin gestation, the SDP technique should be used.

POLYHYDRAMNIOS

Definition and Incidence

Polyhydramnios has been classically *defined* as an accumulation of amniotic fluid within the uterus, usually >2,000 mL.[26] Its incidence varies from 0.2 to 3.9%.[1,31] With the advent of ultrasonography, polyhydramnios is best defined as an SDP > 8 cm,[32] AFI > 24 cm[27,33] [grade 2C, Society for Maternal-Fetal Medicine (SMFM) 2018] above the 95th percentile for gestational age17 or a subjective assessment28 of excessive liquor within the uterus.

Figure 3 shows the ultrasound image of polyhydramnios.

The *degree* of polyhydramnios is often stratified as mild, moderate, or severe based on an AFI of 25–29.9, 30–34.9, or >35 cm or an SDP of 8–11, 12–15, or >16 cm, respectively.[34] Mild polyhydramnios is more common, frequently benign, and accounts for 65–70% of cases; moderate polyhydramnios for 20%; and severe polyhydramnios for <15%. Mild hydramnios is often idiopathic and has a benign course whereas severe polyhydramnios has an underlying etiology and adverse pregnancy outcome.[35,36]

Etiology

The etiology of polyhydramnios is often multifactorial and in >50% of cases, the cause remains unexplained.[1,37]

- *Maternal diabetes*: This accounts for approximately 25% cases of polyhydramnios in singleton pregnancies. Maternal hyperglycemia results in fetal hyperglycemia with subsequent osmotic diuresis and increased

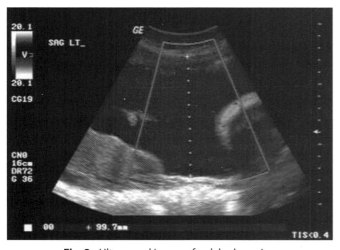

Fig. 3: Ultrasound image of polyhydramnios.

amniotic fluid volume. Bar-Hava et al.[38] showed that amniotic fluid volume reflects the glycemic status in gestational diabetes mellitus. However, rescreening for glucose intolerance in pregnancies with polyhydramnios is not beneficial if the second-trimester glucose tolerance test (GTT) was normal.[39]

- *Fetal anomalies*: In singleton pregnancies, fetal anomalies account for 35% of cases of polyhydramnios. The basic pathophysiology behind these anomalies[30,40,41] and fluid increase is impaired fetal swallowing (gastrointestinal obstruction, neuromuscular) or excess urine production [cardiac, ureteropelvic junction (UPJ) obstruction].

Dashe et al.[42] noted that the risk of aneuploidy is 10% in a sonographically abnormal fetus and 1% in a normal fetus. The risk of anomalies increases with the severity of hydramnios.[42]

- *Multifetal gestation*: Hydramnios was identified in 18% of twin pregnancies by Hernandez et al.[43] Fetal surveillance should be considered in monochorionic twins with polyhydramnios because of risk of twin-to-twin transfusion syndrome (TTTS) and stillbirths.

- *Idiopathic hydramnios*: It is more often seen in a male fetus[44] than in a female fetus. Approximately 60–70% of cases of polyhydramnios are idiopathic.[45,46] The mean gestational age at diagnosis is between 32 and 35 weeks. The rate of spontaneous resolution is 37%, especially if diagnosed early in pregnancy.[47] However, there is an increased risk of macrosomia, preterm delivery, and fetal aneuploidy[48] in the persistent group.[47]

- *Others*: Other causes of polyhydramnios are mainly fetal conditions associated with a high output cardiac state.[37] In general, any condition known to cause nonimmune hydrops fetalis (NIHF) may result in polyhydramnios, e.g., fetal alloimmunization, congenital infections with parvovirus, cytomegalovirus (CMV), or syphilis.[46] Rare causes include maternal smoking,[49] maternal use of lithium,[50] and vascular placental chorioangioma.

Table 2[37] shows the causes of polyhydramnios in a singleton pregnancy.

Clinical Significance

Polyhydramnios has both maternal and fetal sequalae. *Maternal symptoms* usually consist of abdominal discomfort and slight dyspnea in mild cases. There can be marked respiratory distress, orthopnea, and edema of lower limbs in severe cases. The increased amniotic fluid volume causes *overstretching of myometrium* and hence complications such as preterm labor, uterine dystocia, preterm premature rupture of the membranes (PPROM), and postpartum hemorrhage.[51] *Rapid decompression* of distended uterus during membrane rupture can predispose to abruption

TABLE 2: Causes of polyhydramnios in a singleton pregnancy.

Maternal	Fetal	Others
Uncontrolled diabetes mellitus	Structural or congenital malformations	Placental tumors (chorioangioma)
Rhesus and other blood group isoimmunization	Multifetal gestation	Idiopathic
Drug exposure to lithium	Chromosomal and genetic abnormalities	
Maternal smoking	Congenital infections (toxoplasma, CMV, rubella, parvovirus)	
	Macrosomia	
	Fetal tumors (teratomas, nephromas)	

(CMV: cytomegalovirus)

Flowchart 1: Polyhydramnios detected on ultrasound.

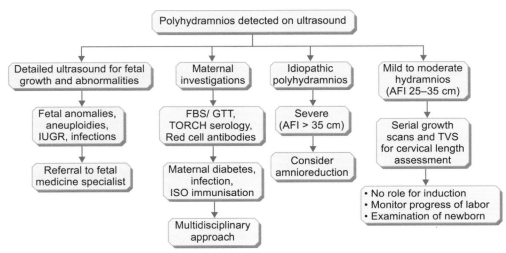

(AFI: amniotic fluid index; FBS: fasting blood sugar; GTT: glucose tolerance test; IUGR: intrauterine growth restriction; TVS: transvaginal scan; TORCH: toxoplasmosis, other agents, rubella, cytomegalovirus, and herpes simplex)

and cord prolapse.[37] *Fetal complications* include congenital malformations,[40] aneuploidies,[42] and fetal malpresentations during labor.

Pregnancy Outcome

Pregnancies with idiopathic hydramnios have been associated with infant birth weight >4,000 g in approximately 25% of cases, more often in moderate and severe hydramnios.[47,52] Mild isolated polyhydramnios was independently associated with increased incidence of induction of labor and *cesarean delivery*[53] due to prolonged first stage of labor, abnormal fetal heart rate (FHR) tracing, and shoulder dystocia.[54]

In nonanomalous pregnancies affected by polyhydramnios, the risk of *intrauterine fetal demise (IUFD)* is greater at every gestational age compared with unaffected pregnancies with a 7–10-fold risk at term gestation.[55]

Genetic syndromes, neurological disorders, and *developmental delay* in children were more common in pregnancies affected by polyhydramnios.[56]

Evaluation and Investigations (Flowchart 1)

Clinically, polyhydramnios is suspected when there is rapid growth in symphysial fundal height (SFH), tense uterus, and difficulty in palpating fetal parts.[57]

Initial evaluation should include a targeted *ultrasound* for detection of structural fetal *anomalies*. Assessment of *fetal growth* is important because idiopathic hydramnios is associated with large-for-dates baby[47] and there is increased risk of aneuploidy in a growth-restricted fetus.[58] While doing ultrasound, we should also search for markers of aneuploidy and *signs of congenital infections* such as NIHF, placentomegaly, and organomegaly in a structurally normal fetus with polyhydramnios.

Maternal screening for diabetes, alloimmunization, and prenatal testing for syphilis is done. If there are signs of NIHF or additional sonographic features suggesting congenital infections, then TORCH (Toxoplasmosis, Other agents, Rubella, Cytomegalovirus, and Herpes simplex) serology is advisable and evaluation of fetal anemia is done.[33]

Evaluation of detailed cardiac anatomy of fetus along with *fetal echo* is helpful to detect cardiac abnormalities in the fetus.[46]

Fetal karyotyping should be considered for severe polyhydramnios with a growth-restricted fetus[58] and structurally abnormal fetus[42] in ultrasound and in persistent polyhydramnios.

Antepartum Management

Treatment of polyhydramnios depends on the underlying etiology. In cases of poorly controlled maternal diabetes, a multidisciplinary approach with involvement of dietician and endocrinologist is essential.

Referral to a *maternal fetal medicine specialist [Royal Australian and New Zealand College of Obstetricians and Gynaecologists (RANZCOG)][60]* should be considered when fetal karyotyping is necessary. The risk of preterm delivery should be assessed with serial cervical length measurements,[37] and administration of antenatal steroids for lung maturity is advisable in high-risk patients.

The most recent guidelines from the American College of Obstetricians and Gynecologists (ACOG) on *antepartum fetal surveillance* does not include polyhydramnios as an indication for testing (ACOG 2014,[60] SOGC[61]). Even though antepartum fetal surveillance does not decrease perinatal mortality, it is often done to detect fetal growth abnormalities.

Amnioreduction should be considered as a treatment option for severe maternal discomfort and dyspnea in cases with severe polyhydramnios (grade 1B, SMFM 2018).[33] It is usually done using a three-way stopcock with a 50-mL syringe or using a vacuum-assisted drainage system under ultrasound guidance.[62]

The volume of fluid removed in each sitting is limited to <2,000–2,500 mL; however, serial amniocentesis is often required as the amniotic fluid tends to reaccumulate quickly.[63]

The complications of amnioreduction are preterm labor, PPROM, abruption, and risk of intraamniotic infection in 1–3% cases. It is a safe palliative procedure in severe hydramnios with median prolongation of pregnancy by 3.7 weeks from the first amnioreduction until delivery.[62]

Maternal administration of prostaglandin synthetase inhibitors such as *indomethacin* can decrease amniotic fluid, primarily by reducing fetal urine output and by enhancing the resorption of lung fluid. Indomethacin is usually given at a dose of 25 mg orally four times a day.[64] The primary concern with the use of indomethacin is premature closure of ductus arteriosus, especially after 32 weeks of gestation.[65] Other fetal complications are intraventricular hemorrhage, necrotizing enterocolitis, and impaired renal function. In view of these potential adverse effects, indomethacin is not recommended for the sole purpose of decreasing amniotic fluid in cases of polyhydramnios (grade 1B, SMFM).[33]

Timing of Delivery

There is no evidence which suggests that induction of labor improves the pregnancy outcome in polyhydramnios alone;[66] however, labor can be induced for other coexisting obstetric and maternal indications. Due to the increased risk of stillbirth in polyhydramnios, if induction is planned it should be done at >39 weeks gestation.[57] Labor should be allowed to occur spontaneously at term and the mode of delivery is determined by the obstetric indication (grade 1c, SMFM).[33]

Intrapartum Management

It is important to confirm fetal lie, presentation, and position during labor. An external version for nonvertex position can be considered if there are no contraindications to this procedure.[37] The progress of labor and fetal heart rate should be carefully monitored as rates of dysfunctional labor are high with polyhydramnios.

Safe obstetric practices such as controlled amniotomy in theater are advisable. We should be prepared for complications such as cord prolapse, abruption, shoulder dystocia, postpartum atony, and embolism.[67]

Newborn Management

Thorough neonatal examination with checking of patency of the upper gastrointestinal tract is recommended as esophageal atresia and trachea esophageal fistula can be missed in ultrasound.

As the likelihood of genetic syndromes and major abnormalities being detected in the idiopathic polyhydramnios group is 9% in the neonatal period and up to 28% in infancy, these children need close follow-up.[45]

Since the NICU admission rates are also high, pediatric support should be available at delivery. Women with severe polyhydramnios should deliver in a tertiary care center level (grade 1C, SMFM).[33]

▪ OLIGOAMNIOS

Definition and Incidence

Oligoamnios is defined as a decrease in the amniotic fluid relative to the gestational age. Its incidence varies from 1 to

4%.[68] It is best defined as AFI < 500 mL, AFI < 5 cm,[42] SDP < 2 cm,[26] below the 5th percentile for gestational age[25] or a sonographic assessment of crowding of fetal parts, two-diameter pocket method <1 × 1 cm^2 or <15 cm^2.[32]

The ACOG recommends that SDP should be used for diagnosis of oligoamnios as it reduces the number of unnecessary interventions without any effect on the adverse perinatal outcome (Level 1-A, ACOG 2016).[21]

Borderline oligoamnios has been defined as an AFI of 5–8 cm[69] and when no measurable pocket is identified, it is known as anhydramnios.

Etiology and Risks

Oligoamnios may be either acute or chronic. Acute-onset oligoamnios is due to rupture of membranes whereas chronic oligoamnios is due to either structural abnormality of fetus, placental insufficiency, or chronic hypoxia.

Table 3 shows the list of common etiologies of oligoamnios.[57]

First-trimester Oligoamnios

It is usually rare with an uncertain etiology. The diagnosis is based on a smaller mean sac diameter (MSD) than expected at gestation.[70]

Second-trimester Oligoamnios

In a fetus with severe oligoamnios between 13 and 24 weeks' gestation, 51% have fetal abnormalities (4% have aneuploidy), 34% have PPROM, 7% abruption, and 5% growth restriction.[71-73]

Third-trimester Oligoamnios

The etiology of oligoamnios varies between second and third trimesters not in the actual type of anomaly but in the prevalence of each anomaly.[72]

- *PROM*: The incidence of premature rupture of membranes is 2–4% in preterm pregnancies.

PROM at <20 weeks is associated with poor prognosis. About 40% miscarry due to infection and in the remaining 60%, >50% of neonates die due to pulmonary hypoplasia.[74]

- *IUGR*: Approximately 6% of growth-restricted fetuses have associated oligoamnios.[75] Low amniotic fluid volume is due to chronic hypoxia and brain-sparing effect resulting in decreased fetal urine output.
- *Fetal anomaly*: Congenital anomalies occur in 4.5–37% of fetuses with oligoamnios with a higher incidence in the second-trimester fetus.[74] The risk of fetal aneuploidy is 14% in an anomalous fetus with oligoamnios.[76]

The malformations commonly associated with oligoamnios are urinary, musculoskeletal, digestive, and cardiac.[76] Urinary tract abnormalities such as bilateral renal agenesis and multicystic or polycystic kidney and urethral obstruction decrease fetal urine output and reduce amniotic fluid volume.

- *Postdate pregnancy*: Oligoamnios is more common in post-term pregnancies due to placental aging and decreased fluid production.[77]
- *Idiopathic oligoamnios*: This occurs in 1–5% of pregnancies at term. Zhang et al. concluded that isolated oligoamnios at term is not associated with either adverse perinatal outcome or impaired fetal growth.[78] However, antepartum fetal surveillance with Doppler velocimetry[79] is indicated in this group to avoid early induction of labor.
- *Maternal medication*: Oligoamnios has been associated with exposure to drugs which block the renin—angiotensin system and cause renal hypoperfusion in the fetus and subsequently low amniotic fluid volume. Examples include angiotensin-converting-enzyme (ACE) inhibitors, NSAIDs (nonsteroidal anti-inflammatory drugs), and angiotensin receptor blockers.[80] Maternal administration of indomethacin also decreases amniotic fluid volume by reducing fetal urine output.[62]

TABLE 3: Common etiologies of oligoamnios.

Fetal	Maternal	Placental	Iatrogenic	Others
Fetal urinary tract abnormalities	Hypertensive disorders of pregnancy	TTTS	Drugs (ACE inhibitors, NSAIDs)	Rupture of membrane
Fetal growth restriction	Post-date pregnancy	Abruptio placenta	Fetal diagnostic procedure—amniocentesis	Idiopathic
	Diabetes			
	SLE			
	APLA syndrome			

(ACE: angiotensin-converting-enzyme inhibitor; APLA: antiphospholipid antibody; NSAIDs: nonsteroidal anti-inflammatory drugs; SLE: systemic lupus erythematosus; TTTS: twin-to-twin transfusion syndrome)

- *Iatrogenic*: Invasive fetal procedures such as genetic amniocentesis, diagnostic, and operative fetoscopy can cause decrease in amniotic fluid volume. Borgida et al. noted that after amniocentesis, amniotic fluid volume usually returns to normal in 2 weeks.[81]
- *Maternal disorders*: Maternal conditions causing uteroplacental insufficiency (chronic hypertension, preeclampsia, diabetes) or vascular disorders (APLA, systemic lupus erythematosus) cause chronic hypoxia which impairs fetal growth and reduces fetal urine output.[82]
- *Twins*: Oligoamnios has been associated with donor twin, in TTTS. TTTS complicates 8–10% of twin pregnancies with monochorionic diamniotic (MCDA) placentation. Even laser-treated TTTS is associated with a perinatal mortality rate of 30–50% and permanent neurological handicap of 5–20% in donor twin.[83]

Clinical Significance

Regardless of etiology, fetuses in pregnancies complicated by oligoamnios are at an increased risk of adverse outcomes. Severe and persistent mid-trimester oligoamnios causes contractures,[84] *Potter syndrome*,[85] and *lung hypoplasia*.[86]

Decreased amniotic fluid is associated with a higher incidence of *small-for-gestational-age infants*, variable and late decelerations during labor, *cesarean section* for *nonreassuring FHR*, low APGAR scores, *stillbirths*, IUFD,[69] and high perinatal mortality rate.[87]

Pregnancy Outcome

Pregnancies with *borderline AFI* have a good prognosis; however, the perinatal mortality rate noted in one study was 3.7%.[23]

Oligoamnios in the *second trimester* usually has a poor pregnancy outcome with high perinatal mortality rates.[88] In the *third trimester*, oligoamnios increases induction and cesarean delivery rates.[68,69] Idiopathic isolated oligoamnios at term has a more favorable prognosis.[89]

The most significant risk to the newborn is iatrogenic prematurity resulting from sudden rush to delivery.[90]

Evaluation and Investigations

Clinically, oligoamnios is suspected when fetal parts are easily palpable, height of uterus is less than the period of gestation, difficulty in ballottement of fetal head, and absence of amniotic fluid at the time of amniotomy.[31]

Initial evaluation consists of thorough review of maternal history and clinical conditions, to search for medical problems that are related to oligoamnios. Maternal screening for diabetes, hypertension, and vascular disorders should be done.

Rupture of membranes should be excluded. Most facilities combine ultrasound evaluation with other modalities for diagnosis of PPROM such as evaluation of vaginal fluid with nitrazine, fern test, or monoclonal antibody to detect placental alpha macroglobulin-1 (PAMG-1) (AmniSure test).[91]

A thorough *sonographic evaluation* should be done. Ultrasound helps in diagnosis of amniotic fluid volume, fetal anatomic survey focusing on the genitourinary tract, abruptio placenta, abnormalities of twinning, and assessment of fetal growth. Transabdominal amnioinfusion can be considered to improve the diagnostic accuracy of ultrasound in second-trimester severe oligoamnios.[92]

Antepartum Management

First-trimester oligoamnios is managed with serial ultrasound.[70]

The most common causes of *mid-trimester* oligoamnios are *PPROM* and *fetal anomalies*. *Karyotyping* should be done in anomalous and growth-restricted fetus and the option of termination of pregnancy should be discussed.

PPROM can be spontaneous or iatrogenic. The chance of spontaneous sealing is 6–11% after spontaneous rupture as opposed to 40% after iatrogenic rupture.[93] The traditional *expectant* obstetric management includes administration of broad-spectrum antibiotics and steroids for lung maturity. The use of tocolysis is controversial. During expectant management, the signs of chorioamnionitis, labor, and fetal compromise must be screened.[94]

Antepartum *amnioinfusion* of isotonic 0.9% saline solution or Ringer's lactate is a treatment option in the second trimester and it increases the chance of perinatal survival.[95] The technical equipment is similar to genetic amniocentesis and the volume of fluid infused depends on gestational age with an aim to re-establish the normal amniotic fluid volume (>8 cm).[92,93]

Another accepted novel technique is the use of *amniopatch* in iatrogenic PPROM where a platelet or cryoprecipitate plug is used to seal the membrane defect (ranging from 0.72 to 3.8 mm).[96] However, the role of these techniques is still experimental.

The presence of oligoamnios is an indication for *antepartum fetal surveillance* (ACOG 2014).[59] Serial ultrasound for assessment of fetal growth, Doppler velocimetry, and BPP and weekly assessment of amniotic fluid volume should be done in the third trimester **(Flowchart 2)**. Antenatal steroids are given for lung maturity.

In *isolated oligoamnios, maternal hydration* either oral (2 L in 24 hours) or intravenous solution (1,500–2,500 mL/day) has been shown to increase amniotic fluid by fetal

Flowchart 2: Oligoamnios detected in ultrasound.

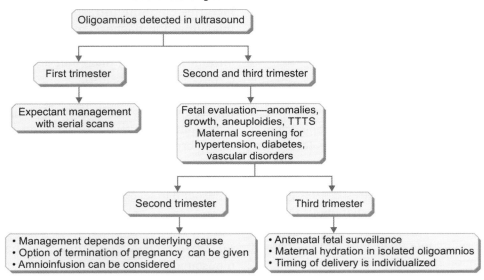

(TTTS: twin-to-twin transfusion syndrome)

diuresis and improving placental perfusion.[97] Gizzo et al. showed that maternal oral hydration, with hypotonic solutions,[98] is effective to improve amniotic fluid volume and this improvement is time dependent (RCOG Evidence Level 1a).

In some studies, L-arginine[99] (3-g sachets daily for 2–4 weeks) and intravenous aminoacid[100] solution have been shown to improve amniotic fluid volume in idiopathic oligoamnios. Nitric oxide released from L-arginine is a potent vasodilator which improves uteroplacental perfusion.

Timing of Delivery

The timing of delivery depends on the underlying cause, gestational age, and results of antenatal testing. Based on an expert opinion, in uncomplicated isolated and persistent oligoamnios [deepest vertical pocket (DVP) < 2 cm], delivery at 36–37 weeks of gestation is recommended (ACOG 2014).[59] In pregnancies at <36 weeks of gestation with *intact membranes* and oligoamnios, the decision regarding expectant management or delivery should be individualized depending on maternal and fetal conditions.[101] In cases associated with *postmaturity*, review the pregnancy dating and deliver the fetus (ACOG 2014).[69,102] In cases of *membrane rupture* at *term* and oligoamnios, the recommendation is to induce labor at 24 hours in the absence of other risk factors since majority of women are likely to go into labor before this time (NICE 2014).[103]

Intrapartum Management

Once labor is established, the fetal heart rate should be continuously monitored as chances of cord compression

and variable decelerations are high during labor. Amnioinfusion[104] can be used during labor as it provides a cushion effect and relieves umbilical cord compression. It has also been used to reduce the risk of meconium aspiration syndrome[105] though evidence of benefit is mixed.

The progress of labor should be carefully monitored as chances of arrest of labor are also high in oligoamnios.[106]

Newborn Management

A careful examination and follow-up of neonate should be done because the risk of chromosomal anomalies is 13%.[76] Term infants with oligoamnios detected near birth have a higher prevalence of renal malformations (mild hydronephrosis).[87]

KEY POINTS

- The pathological conditions associated with excess of amniotic fluid and decreased volume are polyhydramnios and oligohydramnios respectively.
- The extremes of volume—too much or too little may be associated with an unfavorable prognosis.
- The three major determinants of amniotic fluid volume are transfer of solutes across fetal membranes, fetal regulation through swallowing and fetal urine production.
- SDP should always be used for initial assessment during scanning because AFI over diagnoses amniotic fluid abnormalities leading to unnecessary intervention.
- Obstetric management is based on the gestational age at diagnosis and underlying cause of abnormal amniotic fluid volume.

- Important management issue in both the groups is to detect any fetal congenital malformations. Referral to a fetal medicine unit should ideally be done when associated with major structural anomaly or genetic syndrome.

▨ REFERENCES

1. Dubill EA, Magann EF. Amniotic fluid as a vital sign for fetal wellbeing. AJUM. 16(2); 62-70.
2. Chandrasekharan N, Bhide A. Fetal dysmorphology. In: Arias F, Bhide A, Arulkumaran S, Damani K, Daftary S (Eds). Arias' Practical Guide to High-risk Pregnancy & Delivery, 4th edition. India: Elsevier; 2014.
3. Gulbius B, Jauniaux E, Cotton F, Stordeur P. Protein and enzyme patterns in the fluid cavities of the first trimester gestational sac: relevance to the absorptive role of secondary yolk sac. Mol Hum Reprod. 1998;4:857-62.
4. Brace RA, Cheung CY. Regulation of amniotic fluid volume: evolving concepts. Adv Exp Biol. 2014;814:49-68.
5. Gibert WM, Brace RA. The missing link in amniotic fluid volume regulation : intramembranous absorption. Obstet Gynecol. 1989;74(5):748-54.
6. Beall MH, Wang S, Yang B, Chaudhri N, Amidi F, Ross MG. Placental and membrane aquaporin water channels: correlation with amniotic fluid volume and composition. Placenta. 2007;28(5-6):421-8.
7. Brace RA, Wlodek ME, Cock ML, Harding R. Swallowing of lung liquid and amniotic fluid by the ovine fetus under normoxic and hypoxic conditions. Am J Obstet Gynecol. 1994;171:764-70.
8. Pritchard JA. Fetal swallowing and amniotic fluid volume. Obstet Gynecol. 1966;28:606-10.
9. Queenan JT. Thompson W, Whitfield CR, Shah CI. Amniotic fluid volumes in normal pregnancies. Am J Obstet Gynecol. 1972;114:34.
10. Brace RA, Wolf E. Normal amniotic fluid volume changes throughout pregnancy. Am J Obstet Gynecol. 1989;161:382.
11. Magann EF, Bass JD, Chauhan SP, Young RA, Whitworth NS, Morrison JC. Amniotic fluid volume in normal singleton pregnancies. Obstet Gynecol. 1997;90(4):524.
12. Adebayo FO, Onafowokan O, Babalola A, Adewole N, Nggada B. Comparison of amniotic fluid index at different gestational age in normal pregnancy. J Women's Health Care 2017;6:4.
13. Beall MH, Van Din Wijngaard JPHM, Ross MG. Amniotic fluid water dynamics. Placenta. 2007;28(8-9):816-23.
14. Wikipedia. (2019). Amniotic fluid. [online] Available from https://en.wikipedia.org/wiki/Amniotic_fluid. [Last accessed October, 2020].
15. in't Anker PS, Scherjon SA, Kleijburg-van der keur C, Noort WA, Frans HJ Class, Willemze R. Blood. 2003;102(4):1548-9.
16. Reddy UM, Abuhamad AZ, Levin D, Fetal Imaging Workshop Invited Participants. Fetal imaging: executive summary of a joint Eunice Kennedy Shriver National Institute of Child Health and Human Developmental Society of Maternal – Fetal Medicine, American Institute of Ultrasound in Medicine, American College of Obstetricians and Gynecologists, American College of Radiology, Society for Pediatric Radiology, and Society of Radiologists in Ultrasound Fetal Imaging Workshop. Obstet Gynecol. 2014;123(5):1070.
17. Horsager R, Nathan L, Leveno K. Correlation of measured amniotic fluid volume and sonographic prediction of oligohydramnios. Obstet Gynecol. 1994;83:955-8.
18. Charles D, Jacoby HE. Preliminary data on the use of sodium aminohippurate to determine amniotic fluid volumes. Am J Obstet Gynecol. 1966;95:266-9.
19. Dildy GA, Lira N, Moise KJ, Riddle GD, Detes RL. Amniotic fluid assessment: comparison of ultrasonographic estimates versus direct measurements with a dye dilution technique in human pregnancy. Am J Obstet Gynecol. 1992;167:986-94.
20. Hilliard NJ, Hawkes R, Patterson AJ, Graves MJ, Priest AN, Hunter S, et al. Amniotic fluid volume: Rapid MR-based assessment at 28-32 weeks gestation. Eur Radiol. 2016;26(10):3752-9.
21. Committee on Practice Bulletins—Obstetrics and the American Institute of Ultrasound in Medicine. Practice Bulletin No. 175: Ultrasound in Pregnancy. 2016;128(6):241-56.
22. Gandhi MR. A prospective study of critical methods of amniotic volume assessment. Int J Reprod Contracept Obstet Gynaecol. 2017;6(7):3021-5.
23. Chamberlain PF, Manning FA, Morrison I, Harman CR, Lange IR. Ultrasound evaluation of amniotic fluid. The relationship of marginal and decreased amniotic fluid volumes to perinatal outcome. Am J Obstet Gynecol. 1984;150:245.
24. Phelan JP, Smith CV, Broussard P, Small M. Amniotic fluid volume assessment with the four quadrant technique at 36-42 weeks gestation. J Reprod Med. 1987;32:540-2.
25. Moore TR, Cayle JE. The amniotic fluid index in normal human pregnancy. Am J Obstet Gynecol. 1990;162(5):1168.
26. Magann EF, Morton ML, Nolan TE, Martin JN Jr, Whitworth NS, Morrison JC. Comparative efficacy of two sonographic measurements for the detection of aberrations in the amniotic fluid volume on pregnancy outcome. Obstet Gynecol. 1994;83:959-62.
27. Chauhan SP, Magann EF, Morrison JC, Whitworth NS, Hendrix NW, Devoe LD. Ultrasonographic assessment of amniotic fluid does not reflect actual amniotic volume. Am J Obstet Gynecol. 1997;177:291-6.
28. Goldstein RB, Filly RA. Sonographic estimation of amniotic fluid volume: subjective assessment versus pocket measurements. J Ultrasound Med. 1988;7(7):363-9.
29. Lim KI, Butt K, Naud K, Smithies M. Amniotic fluid: Technical update on physiology and measurement. J Obstet. Gynecol Can. 2017;39(1):52-8.
30. Coombe-Patterson J. Amniotic fluid assessment: amniotic fluid index versus maximum vertical pocket. J Diagn Med Sonogr. 2017;33(4):280-3.
31. Fischer R. Glob libr. women's med. (ISSN: 1756-2228) 2008; DOI 10.3843/GLOWM.1028.
32. Magann EF, Nevils BG, Chauhan SP, Whitworth NS, Klausen JH, Morrison JC. Low amniotic fluid volume is poorly identified in singleton and twin pregnancies using the 2x2 cm pocket technique of the biophysical profile. South Med J. 1999;92:802-5.
33. Dashe JS, Pressman EK, Hibbard JU. SMFM Consult Series #46: Evaluation and management of polyhydramnios. Am J Obstet Gynecol. 2018;219(4):B2-B8.
34. Rasuli B, Refaey M. Polyhydramnios. Radiology Reference Article. [online] Available from https://www.radiopaedia.org/articles/polyhydramnios [Last accessed November, 2020].
35. Pri Paz S, Khalek N, Fuchs KM, Simpson LL. Maximal amniotic fluid index as a prognostic factor in pregnancies complicated by polyhydramnios. Ultrasound Obstet Gynecol. 2012;39(6):648.
36. Lazebink N, Hill LM, Guzick D, Martin JG, Mary A. Severity of polyhydramnios does not affect the prevalence of large for gestational newborn infants. J Ultrasound Med. 1996;15(5):835-88.

37. Karkhanis P, Patni S. Polyhydramnios in singleton pregnancies: perinatal outcomes and management. Obstetrician Gynaecologist. 2014;16:207-13.

38. Bar-Hava I, Scarpelli SA, Barnhard Y, Divon MY. Amniotic fluid reflects recent glycemic status in gestational diabetes mellitus. Am J Obstet Gynecol. 1994;171(4):952-5.

39. Wolf MF, Peleg D, Stahl-Rosenzweig T, Kurzweil Y, Yogev Y. Isolated polyhydramnios in the third trimester: is a gestational diabetes evaluation of value? Gynecol Endocrinol. 2017;33(119):84.

40. Kouamé N, N'goan-Domoua AM, Nikiéma Z, Konan AN, N'guessan KE, Sétchéou A, et al. Polyhydramnios: a warning sign in the prenatal ultrasound diagnosis of foetal malformation? Diagn Interv Imaging. 2013;94(4):433-7.

41. Nabhan AF, Abdelmoula YA. Amniotic fluid index versus single deepest vertical pocket: a meta-analysis of randomized controlled trials. Int J Gynaecol Obstet. 2009;104:184-8.

42. Dashe JS, McIntire DD, Ramus RM, Santos-Ramos R, Twickler DM. Hydramnios: anomaly prevalence and sonographic detection. Obstet Gynecol. 2002;100(1):134-9.

43. Hernandez JS, Twickler TM, McIntire DD, Dashe JS. Hydramnios in twin gestation. Obstet Gynecol. 2012;120(4):759-65.

44. Stanescu AD, Banica R, Olaru G, Ghinda E, Birdir C. Idiopathic polyhydramnios and fetal gender. Arch Gynecol Obstet. 2015;291(5):987-91.

45. Abele H, Starz S, Hoopmann M, Yazdi B, Rall K, Lagan KO. Idiopathic polyhydramnios and postnatal abnormalities. Fetal Diagn Ther. 2012;32(4):251.

46. Kollmann M, Voetsch J, Koidl C, Schest E, Haeusler M, Lang U, et al. Etiology and perinatal outcome of polyhydramnios. Ultraschell Med. 2014;35(4):350-6.

47. Odibo IN, Newville TM, Ounpraseuth ST, Dixon M, Lutgendorf MA, Foglia LM, et al. Idiopathic polyhydramnios: persistence across gestation and impact on pregnancy outcomes. Eur J Obstet Gynecol Reprod Biol. 2016;199:175-8.

48. Glantz JC, Abramoicz JS, Sherer DM. Significance of idiopathic mid trimester polyhydramnios. Obstet Gynecol. 1990;76:517-9.

49. Myhra W, Davis M, Hickok D. Maternal smoking and the risk of polyhydramnios. Am J Public Health. 1992;82(2):176-9.

50. Ang MS, Thorp JA, Parisi VM. Maternal lithium therapy and polyhydramnios. Obstet Gynecol. 1990;76:517-9.

51. Ross MG, Beloosesky R, Queenan JT. Polyhydramnios and oligohydramnios. In: Queenan JT, Sponge CY, Lockwood CJ (Eds). Management of High – Risk Pregnancy: An Evidence Based Approach, 5th edition. Massachusetts: Blackwell Publishing; 2007. pp. 316-23.

52. Luo QQ, Zou L, Gao H, Zheng YF, Zhao Y, Zhang WY. Idiopathic polyhydramnios at term and pregnancy outcomes: a multicentric observational study. J Matern Fetal Neonatal Med. 2017;30(14):1755.

53. Khan S, Donelly J. Outcome of pregnancy in women diagnosed with idiopathic polyhydramnios. Aust NZ J Obstet Gynaecol. 2017;57(1):57.

54. Aviram A, Salzur L, Hiersch L, Ashwal E, Golan G, Pardo J, et al. Association of isolated poyhydramnios at or beyond 34 weeks of gestation and pregnancy outcome. Obstet Gynecol. 2015;125(4):825-32.

55. Pilloid RA, Page JM, Burwick RM, Kaimal AJ, Cheng YW, Caughey AB. The risk of fetal death in nonanomalous pregnancies affected by polyhydramnios. Am J Obstet Gynecol. 2015;213(3):410.e1-e6.

56. Yefet E, Spiegel ED. Outcomes from polyhydramnios with normal ultrasound. Paediatrics. 2016;137(2):e 20151948.

57. MacOnes GA. Disorders of amniotic fluid. In: James D, Steer P (Eds). Late Prenatal – Fetal Problems. Cambridge: Cambridge University Press; 2017. pp. 269-80 (Chapter 11).

58. Biggio JR Jr, Wenstrom KD, Dubbard MB, Cliber SP. Hydramnios prediction of adverse perinatal outcome. Obstet Gynecol. 1999;94:773.

59. Practice bulletin no. 145: antepartum fetal surveillance. Obstet Gynecol. 2014; 124(1):182-92.

60. RANZCOG. (2018). Maternal suitability for models of care, and indication for referral within and between models of care (C-Obs 30). [online] Available from https://ranzcog.edu.au/RANZCOG_SITE/media/RANZCOG-MEDIA/Women%27s%20Health/Statement%20and%20guidelines/Clinical-Obstetrics/Maternal-suitability-for-models-of-care-(C-Obs-30)-March-18.pdf?ext=.pdf [Last accessed November, 2020]

61. Liston R, Sawchuck D, Young D. Fetal health surveillance: antepartum and intrapartum consensus guidelines. J Obstet Gynaecol Can. 2007;29:S3-S6.

62. Halfhill JE, Smith CV, Thomas RL, Talavera F. (2019). Amnioreduction technique. [online] Available from https://emedicine.medscape.com>article [Last accessed October, 2020].

63. Dickinson JE, Tijioe YY, Jude E, Kirk D, Franke M, Nathan E. Amnioreduction in the management of polyhydramnios complicating singleton pregnancies. Am J Obstet Gynecol. 2014;211(4):434.e1-e7.

64. Kramer WB, Van den Veyver IB, Krishon B. Treatment of polyhydramnios with indomethacin. Clin Perinatol. 1994;21:615-30.

65. Loudon JA, Groom KM, Bennet PR. Prostaglandin inhibitors in preterm labor. Best Pract Res Clin Obstet Gynecol. 2003;17:731-44.

66. Boulvain M, Marcoux S, Bureau M, Fortier M, Fraser W. Risks of induction of labour in uncomplicated term pregnancies. Paediatr Perinat Epidemiol. 2001;15:131-8.

67. Hamza A, Herr D, Solomayer EF. Polyhydramnios: Causes, diagnosis and therapy. Geburtshilfe Fraunenheiiskid. 2013;73(12):1241-6.

68. Casey BM, McIntire DD, Bloom SL, Santos R, Twickler DM, Ramus RM, et al. Pregnancy outcome after antepartum diagnosis of oligohydramnios at or beyond 34 weeks gestation. Am J Obstet Gynecol. 2000;182:909-12.

69. Petrozella LN, Dashe JS, McIntire DD, Leveno KJ. Clinical significance of borderline amniotic fluid index and oligohydramnios in preterm pregnancy. Obstet Gynecol. 2011;117(2 Pt 1):338-42.

70. Bromley B, Harlow BL, Laboda LA, Benacerraf BR. Small sac size in the first trimester: a predictor of poor fetal outcome. Radiology. 1991;178:375-7.

71. Richard Beukema et al. Complications of pregnancy. Family Medicine Obstetrics 3rd edition. 2008.

72. Shipp TD, Bromley B, Pauker S, Frigoletto FD, Benaceraff BR. Outcome of singleton pregnancies with severe oligoamnios in the second and third trimesters. Ultrasound Obstet Gynaecol. 1996;7:108-13.

73. Moore TR, Longo J, Leoppld GR, Casola G, Gosink BB. The reliability and predictive value of an amniotic fluid scoring system in severe second-trimester oligohydramnios. Obstet Gynecol. 1989;73:739-42.

74. The Fetal Medicine Foundation. Fetal abnormalities » Amniotic fluid. [online] Available from https://fetalmedicine.org/education/fetal-abnormalities/amniotic-fluid/polyhydramnios [Last accessed November, 2020]

75. Chauhan SP, Taylor M, Shields D. IUGR and oligoamnios among high risk patients. Am J Perinatol. 2007;24(4):215-21.

76. Stoll C, Alembik Y, Roth MP, Dott B. Study of 224 cases of oligohydramnios and congenital malformations in a series of 225,669 consecutive births. Community Genet. 1998;1:71-7.

77. ACOG Practice Bulletin Number 146: Management of late-term and post term pregnancies. Obstet Gynecol. 2014;124:390-6.

78. Zhang J, Troendle J, Meikle S, Klebanoff MA, Rayburn WF. Isolated oligohydramnios is not associated with adverse perinatal outcome. BJOG. 2004;111:220-5.

79. Caroll BC, Bruner JP. Umbilical artery Doppler velocimetry in pregnancies complicated by oligohydramnios. J Reprod Med. 2000;45:562-6.

80. Bullo M, Tschumi S, Bucher BS. Pregnancy outcome following exposure to angiotensin – converting enzyme inhibitors or angiotensin receptor antagonists: a systematic review. Hypertension. 2012;60:444..

81. Borgida AF, Mills AA, Feldman DM, Rodis JF, Egan JF. Outcome of pregnancies complicated by ruptured membranes after genetic amniocentesis. Am J Obstet Gynecol. 2000;183(4):937-9.

82. Cunningham FG, Leveno KJ, Bloom SL, Dashe JS, Hoffman BL, Casey BM, et al. Amnionic fluid. Williams Obstetrics. New York: Mc Graw Hill Education; 2018. pp. 225-32 (Chapter 11).

83. Simpson LL. Society for Maternal Fetal Medicine: Twin–twin transfusion syndrome. Am J Obstet Gynecol. 2013;208(1):3-18.

84. Oyelese Y. Placenta, umbilical cord and amniotic fluid: the not-less-important accessories. Clin Obstet Gynecol. 2012;55:307-23.

85. Nimrod C, Varela-Gittings F, Machen G, Campbell D, Wesenberg R. The effect of very prolonged membrane rupture on fetal development. Am J Obstet Gynecol. 1984;148:540.

86. Lawrence F, Rosenfeld CR. Fetal pulmonary development and abnormalities of amniotic fluid volume. Semin Perinatol. 1986;10:142.

87. Leibovitch L, Kuint J, Rosenfeld E, Schushan-Eisen I, Weissmann-Brenner A, Maayan-Metzger A. Short term outcome among term singleton infants with intrapartum oligohydramnios. Acta Paediatr. 2012;101:727-30.

88. Ashley H, Elizabeth L. Outcomes in oligohydramnios: The role of etiology in predicting pulmonary morbidity or mortality (28R). Obstet Gynecol. 2017;129(5):190.

89. Ashwal E, Hiersch L, Melamed N, Aviram A, Wiznitzer A, Yogev Y. The association between isolated oligohydramnios at term and pregnancy outcome. Arch Gynecol Obstet. 2014;290:875-81.

90. Melamed N, Pardo J, Milstein R, Chen R, Hod M, Yogev Y. Perinatal outcome in pregnancies complicated by isolated oligohydramnios diagnosed before 37 weeks of gestation. Am J Obstet Gynecol. 2011;205(3):241.e1-6.

91. Cousins LM, Smok DP, Lovetti SM, Poeltler DM. AmniSure placental alpha microglobulin-1 rapid immunoassay versus standard diagnostic methods for detection of rupture of membranes. Am J Perinatol. 2005;22(6):317-20.

92. Fisk NM, Ronderos-Dummit D, Soliani A, Nicolini U, Vaughan J, Rodeck CH. Diagnostic and therapeutic transabdominal amnioinfusion in oligohydramnios. Obstet Gynecol. 1991;78: 270-8.

93. Devlieger R, Millar LK, Deprest JA. Fetal membrane healing after spontaneous and iatrogenic membrane rupture: A review of current evidence. Am J Obstet Gynecol. 2006;195(6):1512-20.

94. Kozinszky Z, Sikovanyecz J, Pasztor N. Severe midtrimester oligohydramnios treatment strategies. Curr Opin Obstet Gynecol. 2014;26:67-76.

95. Gramellini D, Fieni S, Kaijura C, Faiola S, Vadora E. Transabdominal antepartum amnio- infusion. Int J Gynecol Obstet. 2003;83:171-8.

96. Quintero RA. Treatment of previable premature membranes. Clin Perinatol. 2003;30:573-89.

97. Hofmeyer GJ, Gulmezoglu AM. Maternal hydration for increasing amniotic fluid volume in oligohydramnios and normal amniotic fluid volume. Cochrane Database Syst Rev. 2002:CD ind000134.

98. Gizzo S, Noventa M, Vitagliano A, Dall'Asta A, D'Antona D, Aldrich CJ, et al. An update on maternal hydration strategies for amniotic fluid improvement in isolated oligoamnios and normohydramnios. Evidence from a systematic review of literature and meta-analysis. PLoS One. 2015;10(12):e0144334.

99. Qureshi FU, Yusuf AW. Intravenous amino acids in third trimester isolated oligohydramnios. Ann King Edw Med Univ. 2011;17(2):140.

100. Soni A, Garg S, Patel L. Role of L-arginine in oligohydramnios. J Obstet Gynaecol India. 2016;66(1):279-83.

101. Chauhan NS, Namdeo P, Modi JN. Evidence based management of oligohydramnios. J Gynecol. 2018;3(3):000160.

102. Carter BS, RL Boyd. (2017). Polyhydramnios and oligohydramnios. [online] Available from https://reference.medscape.com/article/975821-overview [Last accessed November, 2020].

103. National Institute for Health and Clinical Excellence. (2014). Intrapartum care for healthy women and babies. Clinical guideline [CG190]. London: NICE. [online] Available from https://www.nice.org.uk/guidance/cg190 [Last accessed November, 2020]

104. Amnio infusion ICD-9-CM. Coordination and Maintenance committee. volume 3, December 4, 1997.

105. Hofmeyer GJ, Xu H. Amnio infusion for meconium stained liquor in labour. Cochrane Database System Rev. 2014;1:CD000014.

106. ACOG Committee on Practice Bulletins – Obstetrics. ACOG Practice Bulletin No. 107: Induction of labor. Obstet Gynecol. 2009;114:386-97.

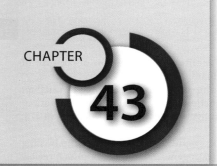

Obesity and Pregnancy

Srinivas Krishna Jois

■ INTRODUCTION

Obesity, once a problem of affluence, is now assuming epidemic proportions, especially in developing countries. The irony in some developing countries is that a group of population is struggling with malnutrition whereas at the other end of the spectrum, we see obesity and its associated noncommunicable disease morbidity.

The proportion of global adult women who are overweight increased to 38.0% in 2013 over a period of 33 years (from 29.8%). Across the globe, it has been estimated that in 2014 there were 38.9 million overweight and 14.6 million obese pregnant women. 21.7% of the women in India were overweight or obese and 4.3 million of the pregnant women are obese, largest (11.1%) in the world.[1]

■ HISTORY[2]

In the famous work "Little Women" by Louisa May Alcott (1832–1888), Margaret is described as a very pretty girl as she was plump and fair and her suitor is shown to be very happy with her, "He pressed the plump hand gratefully". Charles Dickens in his characterization of Joe calls him "A wonderfully fat boy".

If we try to search for the history of obesity, we frequently encounter the problem of starvation than obesity. However, some of the sculptures and depiction of some Greek gods and goddesses such as Venus bring this concept of obesity as an entity of antiquity.

The Indian surgeon *Sushrutha* related obesity to diabetes and heart diseases way back in the 6th century BC. The Greeks were the first to recognize obesity as a medical disorder by about the 4th century BC.

Hippocrates, the great Greek physician, had recognized the fact that sudden deaths could happen more frequently in the fat people than lean ones. Littre, a physician, in 1839 had noted that obesity could be responsible for oligomenorrhea and infertility in women.

There are many countries across the globe which still consider female and male obesity as a sign of beauty, prosperity, and fertility. Some of the African countries have a practice of rearing girls in special places called "fattening huts" for a couple of years and once they are certified by

elders to be well grown, they will be let out of the place. The 20th-century actress Lillian Russell, weighing around 200 pounds, was considered as a sex symbol.

■ DEFINITION AND CLASSIFICATION

The Centers for Disease Control and Prevention (CDC) defines obesity as weight which is above the normal healthy limit prescribed for a given height. This is assessed by *Quetelet's index* or body mass index (BMI).

Based on BMI, obesity is classified by the World Health Organization (WHO) as follows:[3]

- *BMI < 18.5 kg/m²*: Underweight
- *BMI 18.5–24.9 kg/m²*: Normal
- *BMI 25.0–29.9 kg/m²*: Overweight
- *BMI 30.0 kg/m² or higher*: Obese

> Adolphe Quetelet, born in 1796, a Belgian mathematician, devised the BMI calculation method, which is followed even today.
>
> BMI = Weight in kg/height in meter square

Obesity is subdivided into the following categories:

- *Class 1*: BMI of 30–34.9 kg/m²
- *Class 2*: BMI of 35–39.9 kg/m²
- *Class 3*: BMI of 40 kg/m² or higher

The WHO has also suggested a different classification for Asians[3] that incorporates the waist measurements too to calculate the risk of comorbidities **(Table 1)**.

The term "super-obesity" appears in many of the studies and the classification followed is class I obesity (BMI = 30–34.9 kg/m²), class II obesity (BMI = 35–39.9 kg/m²), class III obesity (BMI = 40–49.9 kg/m²), or super-obesity (BMI ≥ 50 kg/m²). In the past 2 decades, it has been observed that the proportion of super obese population has increased by five times.[4]

■ EPIDEMIOLOGY OF OBESITY IN WOMEN AND IN PREGNANCY[5]

- Since 1975, the obese population has increased by about three times.
- In 2016, out of the 1.9 billion overweight population (>18 years), over 650 million were obese.

TABLE 1: Suggested classification for obesity by WHO for Asians including waist circumference.

Category	BMI (kg/m²)	Risk of comorbidities	
		Waist circumference (Women)*	
		<80 cm	>80 cm
Underweight	<18.5	Low	Average
Normal range	18.5–22.9	Average	Increased
Overweight	23 and above		
At risk	23–24.9	Increased	Moderate
Obese I	25–29.9	Moderate	Severe
Obese II	30 and above	Severe	Very severe

*For men, it is 90 cm.[3]
(BMI: body mass index: WHO: World Health Organization)

TABLE 2: Possibility of adverse events happening during pregnancy with obesity.

Events	Incidence
GDM	2–3 times
Hypertensive disorders	3 times[4]
Depression	1.4 (Odds ratio)[7]
Congenital anomalies	1.3 (Odds ratio)[7]
Cesarean section rate	2.26 (Odds ratio)[7]
Macrosomia	2.42 (Odds ratio)[7]
VTE	1.7–2.3 (Odds ratio)[8]

(GDM: gestational diabetes mellitus; VTE: venous thromboembolism)

- Under-5 child obesity was to the tune of 46 million in 2016.
- Amongst the 5–19-year age group, over 340 million were overweight or obese in 2016.

Women living in urban areas (23.5%), those belonging to a higher socioeconomic state (30.5%), and literates (23.8%) are more likely to be obese as per the National Family Health Survey 3 (NFHS-3) survey.[6]

Also, childhood obesity which is fast increasing in India could contribute for obesity later in life and a woman entering pregnancy with obesity.

Pregnancy and Obesity

The global problem of obesity has made the obstetrician to consider obesity as a risk factor in pregnancy and thus look for adverse outcomes, other morbidities, and challenges associated with managing a pregnant woman with obesity. The Royal College of Obstetricians and Gynaecologists too has come out with a separate guideline for managing pregnancy with obesity. Ample literature is coming up on obesity in pregnancy.

The problems and challenges associated could be as follows (summary given in **Table 2**):

- Adverse pregnancy outcomes such as abortions, stillbirth, preterm labor, postpartum hemorrhage (PPH), cesarean delivery, need for induction of labor, failure of induction, or trial of labor
- Associated morbidity such as hypertension, diabetes, ischemic heart disease (IHD), venous thromboembolism problems
- Fetal issues such as macrosomia, shoulder dystocia, anomalous babies, instrumental deliveries, perinatal morbidity and mortality
- Anesthesia challenges about epidural or subarachnoid block placement, operation theater arrangements, shifting of the woman
- Wound healing, lactation problems, contraception issues, prolonged hospitalization, etc.

Thus, pregnancy with obesity is to be considered as a high-risk pregnancy.

The complications associated with obesity in pregnancy are given in **Table 2**.

Amongst the obese population, the risk of developing gestational diabetes mellitus (GDM) is two times more in overweight women, four times more in class 1 and 2 obesity, and eight times more in class 3 obesity, as per the reports of a meta-analysis.[9]

It has been also found that as the obesity class goes up, the risk of pre-eclampsia also increases, the highest incidence of about 13% being found in super-obese women. A study by Mbah et al.,[4] also observes the fact that more the weight gain during pregnancy in obese women, more the possibility of pre-eclampsia. When a comparison has been made between early and late-onset pre-eclampsia, the incidence of early onset pre-eclampsia is not much affected by the class of obesity, shown in **Figure 1**. The study quotes a three-times increase in the risk of pre-eclampsia amongst obese mothers.[4]

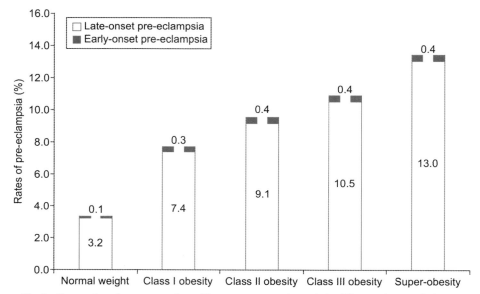

Fig. 1: Comparison between early and late-onset pre-eclamspia in different classes of obesity.
Source: Reproduced with permission from Mbah A, Kornosky J, Kristensen S, August E, Alio A, Marty P, et al. Super-obesity and risk for early and late pre⊠eclampsia. BJOG. 2010;117:997-1004.

FACTORS

- Childhood obesity
- Retention of weight after delivery
- Endocrine problems such as hypothyroidism
- Sedentary lifestyle, urban dwelling, higher strata of socioeconomic state
- Polycystic ovary syndrome (PCOS)
- Genetic predisposition

DIAGNOSIS

Diagnosis of obesity is purely based on clinical examination. As discussed earlier, the BMI is taken into account to classify a subject as either overweight or obese of various classes. For Asian population, the recommendation by the WHO may be considered **(Table 1)**.

While applying this to the pregnant women, the prepregnancy weight or the weight recorded during the first antenatal visit (booking visit in the first trimester) may be taken. It is ideal to document the BMI of every pregnant woman which can help to formulate the weight gain recommendations for them during pregnancy.

The waist circumference could be a good parameter for the classification. Truncal obesity noticed during prepregnancy or in the first trimester could also be considered to categorize a woman as obese.

Prepregnancy Considerations

If the woman meets the obstetrician during the pre-pregnancy period and if she is found to be overweight or obese and planning pregnancy, consider the following in prepregnancy counseling:[8]

- Optimizing the weight before planning pregnancy
- The consequences of obesity with pregnancy to be discussed
- Lifestyle modifications to be suggested
- Folic acid 5 mg to be started at least a month before attempting pregnancy.

> Weight optimization before pregnancy is known to reduce the chances of hypertensive disorders, stillbirth, and macrosomia and also increases the success of vaginal birth after cesarean.[7]

CARE DURING PREGNANCY

Whenever an obese pregnant woman walks into the consultation chamber for the antenatal care, the following are the practical issues faced during the examination:

- Blood pressure measurement may be difficult or fallacious.
- Pedal edema interpretation could be problematic.
- Weighing machines may not withstand the weight.
- Spine may not be palpable to know if there is any deformity.
- Auscultation for abnormalities in respiratory and cardiovascular systems may not be very informative.
- Obstetric examination may be difficult—size of the uterus, obstetric grips, liquor quantity, presenting part may not be accurately interpreted.
- Measurements such as abdominal girth and symphysio-fundal height may not be very accurate.

The above problems may have to be tackled with:

- BP apparatus with a special size cuff usage
- Special weighing machines

In pregnancies with absent or reversed end-diastolic (ARED) flow, the capillary loops in placental tertiary villi are reduced, longer, and with fewer branches than in normal pregnancies. Therefore, there is a strong association between ARED velocity and hypoxia/acidosis.

- *Fetal vessels*: The Doppler modifications in the fetal circulation associated with fetal hypoxia include increased resistance in both the UA and the fetal peripheral vessels, in association with decreased resistance in the fetal cerebral vessels. Study of MCA gives important information for detection of fetal distress. In some growth-restricted fetuses, the cerebral vessels are dilated. Usually, these are fetuses with reduced UA flow velocity. This proves that fetuses with mild hypoxia will have dilated cerebral vessels as a compensatory response: "brain-sparing" effect. Brain-sparing effect is a phenomenon where fetuses that are hypoxic preferentially perfuse brain, heart, and adrenals at the expense of viscera, gut, kidneys, and integument. A high MCA peak systolic velocity (PSV) predicts fetal distress and perinatal mortality better than a low MCA-PI.
- *Cerebroplacental ratio (CPR)*: CPR is the ratio of MCA-PI to UA-PI. CPR is emerging as an important predictor of adverse perinatal outcome. Fetuses with an abnormal CPR have a higher incidence of fetal distress during labor requiring emergency cesarean delivery, a lower cord pH, and an increased admission rate to neonatal intensive care unit (NICU) when compared with fetuses with a normal CPR.
- *Ductus venosus*:[7] Increasing venous Doppler indices are the hallmark of increasing circulatory deterioration as they indicate a decreased ability of heart to accommodate venous return. In response to hypoxia, the DV becomes more dilated and there is reduced flow during ventricular diastole, resulting in increased DV-PI, followed by increasing retrograde flow during atrial systole, seen as absent or reversed a-wave.

During Labor Surveillance

Identification of Fetal Distress

Maternal blood flow to the placenta may be severely reduced by uterine contractions, so the potential for fetal hypoxia increases during labor. Intrapartum Doppler velocimetry is used as an adjunct to conventional intrapartum fetal monitoring.

Monitoring of Fetal Heart Rate

The pattern of fetal heartbeat during labor is a good indicator of fetal well-being. A normal heart rate suggests that the fetus is receiving adequate oxygen from the mother's blood. Abnormal variations in the FHR can indicate decreased oxygen in the blood and tissues that can damage the fetus. FHR can be monitored either intermittently by auscultation or continuously by CTG.[10-12]

Monitoring of Fetal Oxygenation

- *Pulse oximetry*: Fetal pulse oximetry is used as a means of improving the specificity of CTG in intrapartum fetal surveillance. It is a less traumatic and invasive method of assessing fetal oxygenation than fetal scalp sampling. It uses a probe that stays inside the vagina during labor and is possible only if the membranes have been ruptured as the probe has to be placed in contact with the fetal skin. A value of 30% is considered pathological and is associated with acidosis and a poor fetal outcome.
- *Fetal scalp blood sampling*: A sample of blood is taken from the fetal scalp during labor to test for the acidity of the blood. In case of severe hypoxia, the blood becomes highly acidic. It is an invasive procedure and requires a cervical dilatation of at least 2–3 cm.
- *Fetal electrocardiography (ECG)*: The fetal ECG is a reflection of fetal myocardial metabolism and acid-base balance. It can be used as a supplement to continuous electronic FHR recording during labor. Fetal acidemia is associated with fetal ECG ST-segment elevation and increased T-wave amplitude.

▓ TREATMENT

The primary treatment (active management) for fetal distress is intrauterine resuscitation.

The aim of intrauterine fetal resuscitation is to increase oxygen delivery to the placenta and umbilical blood flow in an attempt to reverse fetal hypoxia and acidosis.

Means of Intrauterine Resuscitation[9-12]

- *Changing the mother's position (i.e., left lateral position)*: To correct any supine hypotension (a low blood pressure which some pregnant women can develop in late pregnancy when they lie flat on the back).
- *Ensuring the mother is well hydrated*: To improve blood flow to the placenta.
- *Ensuring the mother has adequate oxygenation*: Oxygen lessens fetal distress by increasing the available oxygen from the mother.
- Amnioinfusion (the insertion of fluid into the amniotic cavity to alleviate compression of the umbilical cord)
- *Tocolysis (a therapy used to delay preterm labor by temporarily stopping uterine contractions)*: To relax the uterus and improve blood flow to the placenta.

Nevertheless, there are cases in which an emergency cesarean section is necessary. Due to overdiagnosis of fetal distress and misinterpretation of FHR, it is recommended to confirm a fetal distress diagnosis with a fetal blood acid—base study.[14]

KEY POINTS

- Fetal distress is defined as depletion of oxygen and accumulation of carbon dioxide, leading to a state of hypoxia and acidosis during intrauterine life.
- Several factors—maternal, placental, umbilical and drug-induced lead to fetal distress.
- Fetal distress can be acute or chronic.
- Decreased fetal movement, abnormal fetal heart rate, abnormal amniotic fluid level and abnormal results of biophysical profile (BPP) are signs of fetal distress.
- Fetal distress can be identified in antepartum as well as intrapartum testing.
- Changing the mother's position to left lateral, adequate hydration and oxygenation, amnioinfusion and tocolysis are various means of intrauterine resuscitation for fetal distress.

■ REFERENCES

1. Alfirevic Z, Stampalija T, Gyte GM. Fetal and umbilical Doppler ultrasound in high-risk pregnancies. Cochrane Database Syst Rev. 2013;11:CD007529.
2. Alfirevic Z, Devane D, Gyte GM. Continuous CTG as a form of electronic fetal monitoring for fetal assessment during labour. Cochrane Database Syst Rev. 2013;31(5):CD006066.
3. Alfirevic Z, Stampalija T, Medley N. Fetal and umbilical Doppler ultrasound in normal pregnancy. Cochrane Database Syst Rev. 2015;4:CD001450.
4. Allen RM, Bowling FG, Oats JJ. Determining the fetal scalp lactate level that indicates the need for intervention in labour. Aust N Z J Obstet Gynaecol. 2004;44:549-52.
5. American College of Obstetricians and Gynecologists. Practice Bulletin No. 116. Management of intrapartum fetal heart rate tracings. Obstet Gynecol. 2010;116:1232-40.
6. Amer-Wahlin I, Hellsten C, Noren H, Hagberg H, Herbst A, Kjellmer I. Cardiotocography only versus cardiotocography plus ST analysis of fetal ECG for intrapartum fetal monitoring: a Swedish randomised controlled trial. Lancet. 2001;358: 534-8.
7. Baschat AA. Ductus venosus Doppler for fetal surveillance in high-risk pregnancies. Clin Obstet Gynecol. 2010;53:858-68.
8. Berkley E, Chauhan SP, Abuhamad A. Doppler assessment of fetus with IUGR. Am J Obstet Gynecol. 2012;206:300-8.
9. Chandraharan E. Fetal scalp blood sampling during labour: is it a useful diagnostic test or a historical test that has no longer a place in modern clinical obstetrics? BJOG. 2014;121:1056-62.
10. Committee on Obstetric Practice, American College of Obstetricians and Gynecologists. ACOG Committee Opinion. Number 326, December 2005. Inappropriate use of the terms fetal distress and birth asphyxia. Obstet Gynecol. 2005;106(6):1469-70.
11. Hofmeyr GJ, Novikova N. Management of reported decreased fetal movements for improving pregnancy outcomes. Cochrane Database Syst Rev. 2012;4:CD009148.
12. Fetal Heart Monitoring: What's Normal, What's Not? (2018). [online]Available from: http://www.healthline.com/health/pregnancy/abnormal-fetal-heart-tracings[Last accessed October, 2020]
13. American Pregnancy Association. (2016). Fetal distress: Diagnosis, conditions & treatment. [online] Available from: http://americanpregnancy.org/laborand-birth/fetal-distress/ [Last accessed October, 2020]
14. Fetal Distress- American Pregnancy Association http://americanpregnancy.org/healthy-pregnancy/labor-and-birth/fetal-distress-9221.

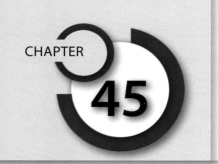

Corticosteroids for Fetal Lung Maturity

Janki Pandya, Munjal Pandya

INTRODUCTION

Preterm births are on the rise, making it difficult for the newborn to survive because of premature lungs. Preterm prelabor rupture of membranes, multiple pregnancies, advancing maternal age, and artificial reproductive techniques are known risk factors for preterm labor. Globally, preterm labor has been accepted as the most common cause for perinatal and neonatal mortality and morbidity.[1] Increased risk of septicemia and difficult breathing and feeding have been contributing factors for increased morbidity and mortality in preterm neonates.[2,3]

Prevention of preterm birth by correcting the preventable cause is of utmost importance, but in cases of inevitable preterm births, special care must be given to improving neonatal outcomes by utilizing the available resources in the form of corticosteroids for fetal lung maturity, magnesium sulfate, and antibiotics.[4]

Liggins and Howie conducted the first randomized trial in 1972, which concluded that antenatal corticosteroids did reduce respiratory distress syndrome (RDS) and neonatal mortality.[5]

CORTICOSTEROIDS FOR FETAL LUNG MATURITY

Fetal lungs are last to mature. Surfactant is proven to get released in amniotic fluid before delivery, and analyzing it in the form of lecithin—sphingomyelin (L/S) ratio helps in measuring fetal lung maturity. Before 32–33 weeks of gestation, the L/S ratio is around 1, but as pregnancy advances, the lecithin concentration increases significantly, making a ratio of 2.0 at term. The surfactant plays an important role in preventing collapse of pulmonary alveoli, by maintaining intra-alveolar tension. The presence of phosphatidylglycerol (a constituent of surfactant) also confirms fetal lung maturity, which becomes detectable several weeks after increase in lecithin.

MECHANISM

Antenatal steroids work by thinning alveolar walls, thus increasing lung volume available for gas exchange, followed by stimulation of surfactant production in alveolar spaces, improvement of lung compliance, clearance of fluid from lung, and maturation of parenchymal structure.

At the molecular level, glucocorticosteroids increase enzymes and proteins, including surfactant, via gene transcription. Antenatal glucocorticosteroids are found to have maturational effect on brain, kidney, gut, circulation, hypothalamus, and thyroid, which are essential support for postnatal adaptation.

OTHER FETAL EFFECTS

After administration of antenatal corticosteroids, transient reduction in fetal breathing and body movement has been noted, which may alter biophysical profile finding. The effect lasts for 48–72 hours after the second dose.

MATERNAL EFFECTS

A transient rise in maternal platelets and white blood cell count has been noted, which lasts for 72 hours.

TIMING OF ADMINISTRATION

Antenatal corticosteroids are recommended between 24 and 34 weeks of gestation to women who are at risk of preterm birth. The administration of corticosteroids therapy needs the following conditions to be fulfilled:[6]

- Accurate measurement of gestational age
- When preterm birth is inevitable
- No maternal infection
- Adequate resources for proper management of preterm neonate

Caution needs to be taken while administering steroid therapy to women with systemic infections such as tuberculosis or sepsis.[7]

Correct diagnosis of preterm labor is essential for avoiding overtreatment of patients. It was concluded that at least 40–50% of women who were thought to have imminent preterm labor, and were administered steroids for fetal lung maturity, did not deliver even after 7 days of steroid administration. So, international clinical guidelines were published by the European Association of Perinatal Medicine, making biochemical markers (fetal fibronectin) and ultrasonography necessary along with clinical uterine contractions and cervical changes to conclude a case as preterm labor.[8,9]

According to the Royal College of Obstetricians and Gynaecologists (RCOG), antenatal corticosteroids should be administered to all women at risk of preterm birth before 34 weeks of gestation as well as women whose elective cesarean section is planned before 39 completed weeks.[7]

PREMATURE RUPTURE OF MEMBRANES

Women presenting with premature rupture of membranes (PROM) between 24 and 32 weeks of gestation are candidates for antenatal steroid administration but in absence of clinical findings of chorioamnionitis.

The American College of Obstetricians and Gynecologists (ACOG) recommends a single course of corticosteroids for pregnant women between 24 and 34 weeks of gestation, who are at risk of preterm delivery within the next 7 days, including those having multifetal gestation and ruptured membranes.[10]

Delaying delivery in PROM may prove detrimental to fetus as well as to mother, so repeat or rescue dose in preterm PROM is controversial, and any guideline for or against cannot be made due to insufficient evidences.[11]

GESTATIONAL DIABETES MELLITUS

Women with gestational diabetes have increased chances of fetus with lung immaturity as compared to nondiabetic women. Such a fetus is more likely to lag behind in lung maturity, and use of antenatal steroids with close glycemic control has been found to reduce RDS. Maternal hyperglycemia is a responsible factor, for adversely affecting fetal lung maturity, making additional insulin necessary for women receiving antenatal steroid.[7]

Caution needs to be taken with antenatal steroid administration, along with close glycemic monitoring during 3 days after steroid administration. The effect was found to begin approximately 12 hours after the dose and would last for the next 5–6 days.[12]

LATE PRETERM BIRTH

Antenatal steroids can also be given after 34 weeks of gestation, when there is evidence of fetal lung immaturity. A significant reduction was noted in need for respiratory support, along with significant reduction in transient tachypnea of newborn, bronchopulmonary dysplasia, and need for postnatal surfactant, when antenatal steroids were administered between 34 and 36 6/7 weeks of gestation. There was no increase in chorioamnionitis, endometritis, or neonatal sepsis in such cases.[10] In one

of the studies, neonatal hypoglycemia was noted in the group who received betamethasone, but the findings were clinically nonsignificant. The American Academy of Pediatrics recommends neonatal blood sugar monitoring as late preterm birth is a known independent risk factor for neonatal hypoglycemia.[13]

The ACOG recommends administration of glucocorticosteroids to pregnant women between 34 and 36 6/7 weeks of gestation, who are at risk of preterm delivery within the next 7 days and have not received any previous dose.[10]

Tocolysis should not be administered to delay the delivery of corticosteroids' administration nor such late preterm delivery be delayed for steroid administration.[14]

MULTIFETAL GESTATION

Multiple pregnancy attenuates the effects of antenatal steroids, but administration of antenatal corticosteroids in multifetal gestation between 24 and 34 weeks of gestation is associated with significant reduction in neonatal morbidity and mortality.[15] Thus, antenatal administration is recommended for women with gestational age between 24 and 34 weeks, who are at risk of preterm delivery within 7 days, irrespective of the fetal number.[16,17]

ELECTIVE CESAREAN SECTION

Cesarean section itself is considered a risk factor for respiratory morbidity. The risk declines with advancing gestational age. Neonates born at 37–37 6/7 weeks of gestation are at 1.7 times more risk of developing respiratory complications than neonates born at 38–38 6/7 weeks of gestation. Neonates at 38–38 6/7 weeks of gestation are at 2.4 times more risk of developing respiratory morbidity than those born at 39–39 6/7 weeks of gestation. Respiratory morbidity during cesarean section is mainly due to fluid retention in lungs and lack of catecholamines surge, as against vaginal delivery, where vaginal squeeze and activation of pulmonary epithelial sodium channels are thought to facilitate alveolar fluid drainage.

Glucocorticoids are thought to increase the number and function of sodium channels, along with increasing responsiveness toward catecholamines and thyroid hormones, specifically in relation to their usage in cesarean delivery. Elective cesarean section is usually done at around 39 completed weeks of gestation, assuming that the fetus achieves maximum lung maturity at 39 completed weeks. Antenatal corticosteroids are recommended to women undergoing elective cesarean section before 39 completed weeks of gestation, to reduce respiratory morbidity in neonates.[7]

HYPERTENSIVE DISORDERS OF PREGNANCY

Antenatal corticosteroids are found to reduce RDS, neonatal death, and intraventricular hemorrhage (IVH).[18] In the absence of a previous course, and with the possibility of buying time till delivery, antenatal corticosteroids are recommended for women with hypertensive disorders of pregnancy (HDP), irrespective of a plan for expectant/conservative management. No aggravation of maternal blood pressure has been found with antenatal steroid usage.

When the patient is on a tocolytic agent, administration of betamethasone may increase the chances of pulmonary edema; thus, caution needs to be exercised while dealing with patients with HDP/preeclampsia/eclampsia.

FETAL GROWTH RESTRICTION

Intrauterine fetal growth restriction (IUGR) is associated with redistribution of blood flow, directing more blood to vital organs, at the cost of splanchnic circulation. Antenatal steroids may alter vascular tone, resulting in detrimental effect on fetal brain. Antenatal betamethasone in sheep model was found to demonstrate significant carotid blood reperfusion, leading to increased chances of cell death in fetal brain, along with detrimental effects on placenta and fetoplacental perfusion, increasing the chances of neurological damage to fetus. IUGR fetuses have been found to have accelerated lung maturity as compared to their non-IUGR counterparts.

But, with proper selection of cases with fetal lung immaturity, the RCOG recommends administration of a single course of antenatal steroid between 24 and 36 weeks of gestation.[7]

PATIENT LIVING WITH HIV/AIDS

In the absence of any indication for scheduled cesarean section, vaginal delivery can be timed as per routine obstetric indication. The ACOG recommends scheduled cesarean section to be done at 38 weeks, to avoid the patient from going into labor or any possibility of rupture of membranes, thus reducing perinatal transmission of human immunodeficiency virus (HIV). Along with the decision of antiretroviral therapy (ARV), according to viral load, antenatal corticosteroids are recommended in preterm HIV-positive cases, as there has been no data indicating necessity of any change for women living with HIV/acquired immunodeficiency syndrome (AIDS).

PREGNANCY WITH HEPATITIS B INFECTION

Chronic hepatitis B infection has been found to be significantly associated with increased risk of preterm birth (21% increased chances), as compared to noninfected pregnant women. An optimal maternal and fetal outcome can be achieved in such pregnancies by monitoring and controlling maternal viral load as well as by interventions to prevent preterm labor and measures for fetal lung maturity. Hepatitis B DNA virus can get reactivated during pregnancy as well as in postpartum phase due to reduced maternal immunity. In approximately 4–6% of cases, "HBV flare" is also a possibility. Starting of antiviral therapy is usually indicated in the third trimester when hepatitis B virus (HBV) DNA levels are >2,00,000 IU/mL to reduce perinatal transmission as well as to reduce the viral load, thus reducing chances of preterm labor. Antenatal corticosteroids are recommended for optimal fetal lung maturity, in women with hepatitis B infection, with preterm labor, after making sure that there is absence of HBV flare and after confirmation of viral load control.

DOSE

Dexamethasone 6 mg 12 hours apart for four doses or betamethasone 12 mg 24 hours apart for two doses are the current recommendations. The administration of steroids should depend on the timing of expected preterm birth, making it optimally effective when the birth occurs within 7 days of their administration.

After proper diagnosis of imminent preterm labor, even a single incomplete dose of antenatal corticosteroids has been found to be effective, when delivery occurs at least 1 hour after the injection.[18,19]

Steroid therapy even within 24 hours was associated with significant reduction in neonatal morbidity and mortality, resulting in recommendation of the first dose, even if delivery is supposed to happen before the timing of the second dose.[20,21]

DURATION OF BENEFIT

The effect of antenatal steroids is thought to start as early as after 1 hour of the first dose. The study of duration between the dose and the time taken for fetal effects is a difficult process, as the interval between treatment and delivery varied in previous trials. The optimal effect in the form of fetal lung maturity usually starts 24 hours after the last dose. These transient yet beneficial effects last for at least 7 days after the course and are found to sustain till at least 14 days.

TIMING OF EFFECTS

- The RDS risk was found to be lower in neonates born within 48 hours and between 1 and 7 days after a single course, but not those born within 24 hours and after 7 days of the administration of the last dose.

- Neonatal deaths have been reduced in neonates born within 24 hours and within 48 hours after administration of the last dose, but not in neonates born between 1 and 7 days and after 7 days of the last dose.
- IVH was found to be reduced in a group of neonates born within 48 hours of the last dose, but not in any other groups (within 48 hours, 1–7 days, and after 7 days).
- No difference has been found in neonates delivered within 1–7 days and those delivered within 8–14 days after the last dose.

■ REPEAT COURSES

There have been trials demonstrating no benefit of antenatal steroids when delivery occurred after 7 days of steroid administration.[5,18,22]

Thus, the need to repeat the course was felt. Few trials on animals and humans with multiple doses of steroids concluded with detrimental outcomes, in the form of impaired myelination, impaired brain growth, and neurodevelopmental issues.[23-27]

Repeat doses not only were found to reduce the incidence and severity of neonatal respiratory problems but were also associated with reduction in some measurements of weight and head circumference at the time of birth.[28] Neonatal birth weight reduction along with an increase in the number of small-for-gestation infants was noted with four courses of antenatal steroids.[29] With serial courses, there are increased chances of maternal infections and suppression of the hypothalamic-pituitary-adrenal axis.[30,31]

The Maternal-Fetal Medicine Units (MFMU) study suggested that four or more courses of steroids may be associated with cerebral palsy,[32] but no strong association could be established.

As per the ACOG, a repeat course of antenatal corticosteroids is considered for women having <34 weeks of gestation, who are at risk of preterm delivery within 7 days, and whose previous course was given at least 14 days back.[33] The rescue course can be given earliest only after 7 days of the first course, as benefits are maximum within 2–7 days from the initial dose.[34]

Regular repeat or serial courses (more than two) are not recommended currently.[20]

■ BETAMETHASONE VERSUS DEXAMETHASONE

Though both dexamethasone and betamethasone have been equally effective in promoting fetal lung maturity, there has been no conclusive evidence over one being superior to the other.[35] Other corticosteroids are not suitable for fetal lung maturity, due to decreased placental transfer and lack of any demonstrable benefits.

Both cross placenta and have equal biological activity. Betamethasone has a longer half-life while dexamethasone has been found to be cheaper and widely available in comparison to betamethasone.

One study concluded that a significant reduction was noted in neonatal mortality, with betamethasone as compared to dexamethasone.[36] One more observational study concluded that betamethasone was associated with a less adverse neurological outcome after 18–22 months of exposure.[37] Betamethasone was also found to reduce the risk of periventricular leukomalacia in premature infants in a couple of studies, as compared to dexamethasone.[38,39]

Another study compared oral versus intramuscular dexamethasone, and it was concluded that neonatal sepsis was significantly higher in patients who received oral dexamethasone.[35] Oral dexamethasone was found to produce increased risk of adverse effects in comparison to the intramuscular route.

Various studies compared antenatal corticosteroids versus placebo or no treatment, which concluded that there was no increase in maternal morbidity nor in mortality in the group receiving steroids as compared to the placebo or no-treatment group.[6] Fetal and neonatal deaths were significantly reduced in the steroids group as compared to the other group. Significant reductions were noted in the steroid group when it came to neonatal morbidity, including RDS, cerebrovascular hemorrhage, and necrotizing enterocolitis.

An analysis of gestational age at therapy concluded that chorioamnionitis was significantly reduced in the steroid group between 30 and 33 weeks of gestation; the rest of the gestational age categories did not have any difference. Significant reduction was noted in neonatal morbidity and mortality when the gestational age at therapy was between 26 and 34 weeks. Neonatal mortality was not reduced when infants were born after 34 weeks of gestation. Similarly, there was no significant reduction in RDS, when infants were born after 34 weeks of gestation, between steroid and placebo groups.

A large Cochrane review which included 21 randomized trials, conducted in 2006, also concluded that antenatal corticosteroids did not increase maternal risks including mortality, chorioamnionitis, and sepsis. Antenatal corticosteroids significantly reduced neonatal mortality, RDS, IVH, necrotizing enterocolitis, respiratory support, intensive care admissions, and systemic infections.[18]

■ OTHER ROUTES FOR ANTENATAL CORTICOSTEROID ADMINISTRATION

Few other routes have also been studied for antenatal steroids administration. Fetal intravascular steroid injections by cordocentesis were found to be ineffective.[40]

Betamethasone was injected intra-amniotically, but it was found to increase fetal morbidity and mortality, due to its prolonged presence.[41]

Intramuscular injection to fetus was found to be as effective in maturing lung as maternal injection, but fetal neuroprotection effect was reduced as compared to conventional maternal administration.[42,43]

■ POTENTIAL COMPLICATIONS

A single course of antenatal steroids in women with <34 weeks of gestation showed no deleterious effect on the mother as well as the fetus.[44]

KEY POINTS

- Confirmed diagnosis of preterm labor by clinical as well as biochemical and sonography findings is essential before opting for antenatal steroid.
- Glucocorticosteroids are to be administered to women between 24 and 34 weeks of gestation, having imminent preterm delivery in 7 days.
- Delaying delivery for antenatal steroids in PROM is not advisable, and the first dose of corticosteroids should be given, even if the possibility of the second dose is not there.
- Proper glycemic control is required in gestational diabetes when antenatal steroids are administered.
- Antenatal steroids between 34 and 38 6/7 weeks of gestation are not harmful and are found to be effective in cases of fetal lung immaturity.
- Multiple fetus in utero may dilute the effectiveness of steroids, but they were found to be benefited with a single course of corticosteroids.
- Women undergoing elective cesarean section before 39 completed weeks need to be administered antenatal corticosteroids.
- Systemic infections need to be ruled out before antenatal steroid administration.
- Rescue dose can be administered, only after 14 days from the first course of antenatal corticosteroids, and no more than two courses are recommended.

■ REFERENCES

1. Kinney MV, Lawn JE, Howson CP, Belizan J. 15 million preterm births annually: what has changed this year? Reprod Health. 2012;9:28.
2. Escobar GJ, McCormick MC, Zupancic JAF, Coleman-Phox K, Armstrong MA, Greene JD, et al. Unstudied infants: outcomes of moderately premature infants in the neonatal intensive care unit. Arch Dis Child Fetal Neonatal Ed. 2006;91(4):F238-44.
3. Wang ML, Dorer DJ, Fleming MP, Catlin EA. Clinical outcomes of near-term infants. Pediatrics. 2004;114(2):372-6.
4. Iams JD, Romero R, Culhane JF, Goldenberg RL. Primary, secondary and tertiary interventions to reduce the morbidity and mortality of preterm birth. Lancet. 2008;3711(9607):164-75.
5. Liggins G, Howie R. A controlled trial of antepartum gluco-corticosteroid treatment for prevention of the respiratory distress syndrome in premature infants. Pediatrics. 1972;50:515-25.
6. World Health Organization. (2015). WHO recommendation on antenatal corticosteroid therapy for women at risk of preterm birth from 24 weeks to 34 weeks of gestation. [online] Available from https://extranet.who.int/rhl/topics/preconception-pregnancy-childbirth-and-postpartum-care/pregnancy-complications/preterm-birth/who-recommendation-antenatal-corticosteroid-therapy-women-risk-preterm-birth-24-weeks-34-weeks [Last accessed October, 2020]
7. Royal College of Obstetricians and Gynaecologists. (2010). Antenatal Corticosteroids to Reduce Neonatal Morbidity (Green-top Guideline No. 7). [online] Available from https://www.rcog.org.uk/en/guidelines-research-services/guidelines/gtg7/ [Last accessed October, 2020]
8. Di Renzo GC, Al Saleh E, Mattei A, Koutras I, Clerici G. Use of tocolysis: what is the benefit of gaining 48 hours for the fetus? BJOG. 2006;113:72-7.
9. Di Renzo GC, Roura LC, European Association of Perinatal Medicine-Study Group on "Preterm Birth". Guideline for the management of spontaneous preterm labour. J Perinat Med. 2006;34:359-66.
10. American College of Obstetricians and Gynecologists. Committee Opinion No. 713: Antenatal corticosteroid therapy for fetal maturation. Obstet Gynecol. 2017;130(2):e102-9.
11. Gyamfi-Bannerman C, Son M. Preterm premature rupture of membranes and the rate of neonatal sepsis after two courses of antenatal corticosteroids. Obstet Gynecol. 2014;124:999-1003.
12. Mathiessen ER, Christensen AB, Hellmuth E, Hornnes P, Stage E, Damm P. Insulin dose during glucocorticoid treatment for fetal lung maturation in diabetic pregnancy: test of an algorithm. Acta Obstet Gynecol Scand. 2002;81:835.
13. Adamkin DH. Postnatal glucose homeostasis in late preterm and term infants. Committee on fetus and newborn. Pediatrics. 2011;127:575-9.
14. Society for Maternal-Fetal Medicine (SMFM) Publications Committee. Implementation of the use of antenatal corticosteroids in the late preterm birth period in women at risk for preterm delivery. Am J Obstet Gynecol. 2016;215(2):PB13-5.
15. Quist-Therson EC, Myhr TL, Ohlsson A. Antenatal steroids to prevent respiratory distress syndrome: multiple gestation as an effect modifier. Acta Obstet Gynecol Sacnd. 1999;78:388-92.
16. American College of Obstetricians and Gynecologists. Practice Bulletin No. 169: Multifetal gestations: twin, triplet, and higher-order multifetal pregnancies. Obstet Gynecol. 2016;128:e131-46.
17. NIH. Effect of corticosteroids for fetal maturation on perinatal outcomes. NIH Consens Statement. 1994;12:1-24.
18. Roberts D, Dalziel S. Antenatal corticosteroids for accelerating fetal lung maturation for women at risk of preterm birth. Cochrane Database Syst Rev. 2006;(3):CD004454.
19. Elimian A, Figuera R, Spitzer AR, Ogburn PL, Wiencek V, Quirk JG. Antenatal corticosteroids: are incomplete courses beneficial? Obstet Gynecol. 2003;102:352.
20. American College of Obstetricians and Gynaecologists. Practice Bulletin No. 171: Management of preterm labour. Obstet Gynecol. 2016;128:e155-64.
21. NIH. Antenatal corticosteroids revisited: repeat courses. NIH Consens Statement. 2000;17:1-18.
22. McLaughlin KJ, Crowther CA, Walker N, Harding JE. Effects of a single course of corticosteroids given more than 7 days before birth: a systemic review. Aust N Z J Obstet Gynaecol. 2003;43:101.
23. Aghajafari F, Murphy K, Metthews S, Ohlsson A, Amankwah K, Hannah M. Repeated doses of antenatal corticosteroids in animals: a systemic review. Am J Obstet Gynecol. 2002;186:843-9.

24. Dunlop SA, Archer MA, Quinlivan JA, Beazley LD, Newnham JP. Repeated prenatal corticosteroids delay myelination in the ovine central nervous system. J Matern Fetal Med. 1997;6:309-13.

25. French NP, Hagan R, Evans SF, Mullan A, Newnham JP. Repeated antenatal corticosteroids: effects on cerebral palsy and childhood behavior. Am J Obstet Gynecol. 2004;190:588-95.

26. Huang WL, Harper CG, Evans SF, Newnham JP, Dunlop SA. Repeated prenatal corticosteroid administration delays astrocyte and capillary tight junction maturation in fetal sheep. Int J Devel Neuroscience. 2001;19:487-93.

27. Seidner SR, Ikegami M, Yamada T, Rider ED, Castro R, Jobe AH. Decreased surfactant dose-response after delayed administration to preterm rabbits. Am J Resp Crit Care Med. 1995;152:1256-61.

28. Miracle X, Di Renzo GC, Stark A, Fanaroff A, Carbonell-Estrany X, Saling E. Guideline for the use of antenatal corticosteroids for fetal maturation. J Perinat Med. 2008;36:191-6.

29. Wapner RJ, Sorokin Y, Thom EA, Johnson F, Dudley DJ, Spomng CY, et al. Single versus weekly courses of antenatal corticosteroids: evaluation of safety and efficacy. National Institute of Child Health and Human Development Maternal Fetal Medicine Units Network. Am J Obstet Gynecol. 2006;195:633-42.

30. Abbasi S, Hirsch D, Davis J, Stouffer N, Debbs R, Gerdes JS. Effect of single versus multiple courses of antenatal corticosteroids on maternal and neonatal outcome. Am J Obstet Gynecol. 2000;182:1243-9.

31. McKenna Ds, Wittber GM, Nagaraja HN, Samuels P. The effects of repeat doses of antenatal corticosteroids on maternal adrenal function. Am J Obstet Gynecol. 2000;183:669-73.

32. Wapner RJ, Sorokin Y, Mele L, Johnson F, Dudley DJ, Spong CY, et al. Long term outcomes after repeat doses of antenatal corticosteroids. National Institute of Child Health and Human Development Maternal Fetal Medicine Units Network. N Engl J Med. 2007;357:1190-8.

33. Garite TJ, Kurtzman J, Maurel K, Clark R, Obstetrix Collaborative Research Network. Impact of a 'rescue course' of antenatal corticosteroids: a multicentric randomized placebo-controlled trial. Am J Obstet Gynecol. 2009;200:248:e1-9.

34. Crowther CA, McKinlay CJ, Middleton P, Harding JE. Repeat doses of prenatal corticosteroids for women at risk of preterm birth for improving neonatal health outcomes. Cochrane Database Syst Rev. 2015;7:CD003935.

35. World Health Organization. (2015). WHO recommendation on use of either dexamethasone or betamethasone as the antenatal corticosteroids of choice. [online] Available from https://extranet. who.int/rhl/topics/preconception-pregnancy-childbirth-and-postpartum-care/pregnancy-complications/preterm-birth/who-recommendation-use-either-dexamethasone-or-betamethasone-antenatal-corticosteroid-choice [Last accessed October, 2020]

36. Lee BH, Stoll BJ, McDonald SA, Higgins RD, National Institute of Child Health and Human Development Neonatal Research Network. Adverse neonatal outcomes associated with antenatal dexamethasone versus antenatal betamethasone. Pediatrics. 2006;117:1503-10.

37. Lee BH, Stoll BJ, McDonald SSA, Higgins RD, National Institute of Child Health and Human Development Neonatal Research Network. Neurodevelopmental outcomes of extremely low birth weight infants exposed prenatally to dexamethasone versus betamethasone. Pediatrics. 2008;121:289-96.

38. Baud O, Foix-L'Helias L, Kaminski M, Audibert F, Jarreau PH, Papiernik E, et al. Antenatal glucocorticosteroid treatment and cystic periventricular leukomalacia in very premature infants. N Engl J Med. 1999;341:1190-6.

39. Spinillo A, Viazzo F, Colleoni R, Chiara A, Cerbo RM, Fazzi E. Two-year infant neurodevelopmental outcome after single or multiple antenatal courses of corticosteroids to prevent complications of prematurity. Am J Obstet Gynecol. 2004;191:217-24.

40. Jobe AH, Polk D, Ikegami M, Newnham J, Sly P, Kohen R, et al. Lung responses to ultrasound-guided fetal treatments with corticosteroids in preterm lambs. J Appl Physiol. 1993;75:2099-105.

41. Moss TJM, Mulrooney NP, Nitsos I, Ikegami M, Jobe AH, Newnham JP. Intra-amniotic corticosteroids for preterm lung maturation in sheep. Am J Obstet Gynecol. 2003;189:1389-95.

42. Jobe A, Newnham J, Willet K, Sly P, Ikegami M. Fetal versus maternal and gestational age effects of repetitive antenatal glucocorticosteroids. Pediatrics. 1998;102:1116-25.

43. Newnham JP, Evans SF, Godfrey M, Huang W, Ikegami M, Jobe A. Maternal, but not fetal, administration of corticosteroids restricts fetal growth. J Matern Fetal Med. 1999;8:81-7.

44. Sotiriadis A, Tsiami A, Papatheodorou S, Baschat AA, Sarafidis K, Makrydimas G. Neurodevelopmental outcome after a single course of antenatal steroids in children born preterm: A systemic review and met-analysis. Obstet Gynecol. 2015;125:1385-96.

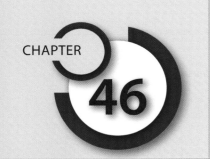

CHAPTER

46

Progesterone in Pregnancy

Nilesh Balkawde

"Where flowers bloom, so does hope"
—Lady Bird Johnson

INTRODUCTION

Progesterone is an enigmatic but a feel-good hormone. It has given us hope to treat many disorders in obstetrics and gynecology. Many studies have validated its use in pregnancy in different scenarios.

On September 23, 1929, Willard Allen, PhD, published the first paper on extracting progesterone from the corpus luteum.[1] Historically, it was obtained from natural sources such as Mexican yam and was used in contraceptive preparations in the mid-20th century. As more and more research was done, newer functions of progesterone were studied. It came to be used in various forms, different molecules, and varying combinations and applications in treating different conditions. It can be used to treat many conditions of estrogen excess such as abnormal uterine bleeding (AUB), fibroids, adenomyosis, endometriosis, endometrial hyperplasia, and endometrial cancer.

The role of progesterone in maintaining uterine quiescence and preventing preterm labor is extensively studied, so is its use as corpus luteal support and in prevention of first-trimester bleeding. Extensive studies have already been done already, and many are underway to decide the molecule best suitable for use in pregnancy. In this chapter, we will study the uses of progesterone in pregnancy and various guidelines for its use.

In 2011, the US Food and Drug Administration (FDA) approved the use of progesterone supplementation [17-hydroxyprogesterone caproate (17OHP)] during pregnancy to reduce the risk of recurrent preterm birth in women with a history of at least one prior spontaneous preterm delivery.

FUNCTIONS OF PROGESTERONE IN OBSTETRICS

- Progesterone decreases the maternal immune response to allow for the acceptance and implantation of the pregnancy.
- It decreases contractility of the uterine smooth muscle and maintains pregnancy till term. A drop in progesterone levels is possibly one step that facilitates the onset of labor.
- It inhibits lactation during pregnancy. The fall in progesterone levels following delivery is one of the triggers for milk production.

Its *role in pregnancy* includes its use in:
- Luteal phase defect (LPD)
- Recurrent pregnancy loss (RPL)
- Preterm labor
- Multiple pregnancy
- Assisted reproduction technique (ART)

PROGESTERONE AND PREGNANCY: PHYSIOLOGY

Progesterone is very necessary for the occurrence and pregnancy maintenance. It helps the endometrium for the process of implantation. The preovulatory increase in the secretion of 17β-estradiol (E2) promotes the proliferation and differentiation of uterine epithelial cells. Then the production of progesterone takes place causing the proliferation and differentiation of stromal cells. Progesterone acts on the endometrium via specific receptors. It causes conversion of Th1 to Th2 as response produces progesterone-induced blocking factor (PIBF) and performs reduction of natural killer (NK) cells activity.

At the molecular level, the following is the mode of action (**Box 1**):
- Progesterone exerts its primary action through the intracellular progesterone receptor although a distinct, membrane-bound progesterone receptor has also been postulated.
- The mechanism includes (1) steroid hormone diffusion across the cell membrane, (2) steroid hormone binding to receptor protein, (3) interaction of a hormone-receptor complex with nuclear deoxyribonucleic acid (DNA), (4) synthesis of messenger ribonucleic acid (mRNA), (5) transport of the mRNA to the ribosomes, and finally (6) protein synthesis in the cytoplasm that results in specific cellular activity.

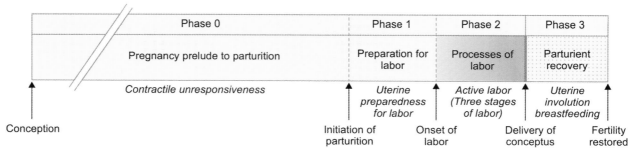

Fig. 1: Mode of action of progesterone.

BOX 1: Mechanism of action of progesterone to prevent preterm birth.

- Stimulate transcription of ZEB1 and ZEB2. They inhibit connexin 43 (gap junction protein that helps synchronize contractile activity) and oxytocin receptor gene.
- Decrease prostaglandin synthesis—infection-mediated cytokine production by fetal membranes
- Decreases PR-A/PR-B ratio which makes the uterus quiescent
- Membrane-bound progesterone in myometrium
- Interfere with cortisol-mediated regulation of placental gene expression
- Nongenomic pathways
- Prevent cervical stromal degradation
- Alter barrier to ascending inflammation in cervix
- Reduce myometrial contractility
- Attenuate response to inflammation in deciduas
- Alter estrogen synthesis in fetal membranes/placenta
- Alter fetal endocrine-mediated effects

- In addition, progesterone is a highly potent antagonist of the mineralocorticoid receptor (MR). It reduces the sodium-retaining activity of aldosterone.

Initiation of Parturition

Progesterone is thought to enhance uterine quiescence by inhibiting uterine contractions (**Box 1**).[2] It has been shown that the progesterone receptor antagonizes nuclear factor-K-beta-activation of cyclooxygenase-2 (COX-2)–induced contractility in the uterus.[3] Progesterone causes Th2 shift.[4] PIBF decreases decidual NK cell activity. Progesterone stimulates transcription of ZEB1 and ZEB2 (zinc finger E box binding homeobox proteins) which inhibit connexin 43 and oxytocin receptor gene.[5] It decreases PR-A/PR-B (progesterone receptor) ratio which makes the uterus quiescent. It reduces levels of inducible nitric oxide synthase (iNOS) and COX-2, which are associated with cervical ripening.[6] It possibly also works by modulating gene expression in the cervix.[7] Basal and interleukin-1 (IL-1) induced IL-8 production in uterine cervical fibroblasts is downregulated by progesterone at the transcriptional level.[8] 17-Hydroxyprogesterone caproate (17-OHP-C) suppresses the maternal immune response (IL-6 decreased).[9]

Progesterone in Implantation and First Trimester

Corpus luteum is the only source of progesterone during the luteal phase of the normal/routine menstrual cycle, and in pregnancy the corpus luteum and trophoblast are the sources of progesterone.[10]

Cyclic secretion of estrogens and progesterone causes physiological and morphological changes of the endometrium and creates the implantation window [5–10 days after the luteinizing hormone (LH) surge]. Progesterone in turn inhibits release of both follicle-stimulating hormone (FSH) and LH from pituitary.

If progesterone production is lower than normal, then there will not be a suitable endometrial environment for embryo implantation and maintenance of early pregnancy. Progesterone deficiency leads to increased levels of proinflammatory IL-8, COX-2, and monocyte chemoattractant protein-1 which destabilize the endometrium.[11] Thus, progesterone has important immune-modulatory functions, i.e., decreasing proinflammatory and increasing anti-inflammatory cytokines in early pregnancy to maintain it (**Box 2**).

■ PROGESTERONE IN RECURRENT PREGNANCY LOSS

Recurrent pregnancy loss is defined as the occurrence of three or more consecutive spontaneous clinically detectable pregnancy losses prior to the 20th week of gestation.

The American Society for Reproductive Medicine (ASRM) now considers two or more consecutive losses as RPL.[12]

Immunology of Recurrent Pregnancy Loss

- *Number and activity of CD56+ NK cells*: Increase in RPL[13]
- Ratio of CD4+/CD8+ in endometrium increases in RPL
- No change in CD3+ T cells in both peripheral blood and fetomaternal interface in patients with RPL

Placenta
Umbilical cord
At placenta, Regulates timing of labor via controlling stress hormone—CRH
At fetal membrane, blocks pro-inflammatory cytokines induced apoptosis, ↓PPROM
Uterus
Fetus
Amniotic sac
In amniotic fluid, limits prostaglandin production
At myometrium and cervix, suppresses inflammatory response and myometrial contractility
Uterine wall
Cervix
Vagina
Anus

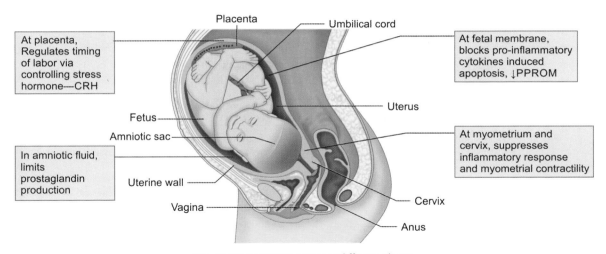

Fig. 2: Progesterone action at different places.
(CRH: corticotropin-releasing hormone; PPROM: preterm premature rupture of the membranes)

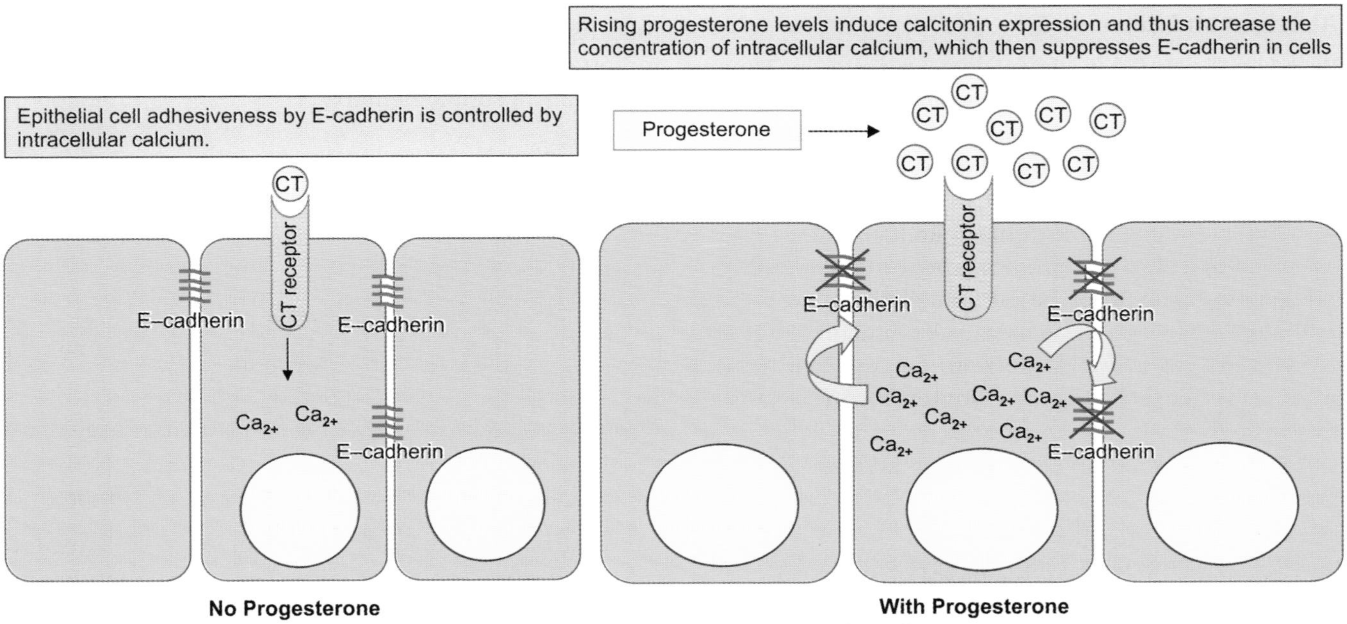

Rising progesterone levels induce calcitonin expression and thus increase the concentration of intracellular calcium, which then suppresses E-cadherin in cells
Epithelial cell adhesiveness by E-cadherin is controlled by intracellular calcium.
Progesterone
CT
CT receptor
E–cadherin
Ca2+
No Progesterone
With Progesterone

Fig. 3: Blastocyst invasion aided by dissolution of E-cadherin.

BOX 2: Positive effects of progesterone in implantation and pregnancy maintenance.

- Preparation of endometrium for implantation (secretory changes)
- Regulation of cellular immunity
- Stimulation of prostaglandin E2 production
- Stimulation of lymphocyte proliferation at fetomaternal interface
- Suppression of cellular cytotoxicity from increased interleukin-2
- Suppression of T-cell and killer-cell activity
- Shift from Th1 to Th2 cells
- Synthesis of progesterone-induced blocking factor
- Suppression of matrix metalloproteinases

Cochrane Data

There is no evidence to support the routine use of progestogen to prevent miscarriage in early to mid-pregnancy.

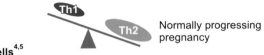

Th1
Th2
Normally progressing pregnancy
Th1 cells[4,5]
Pro-inflammatory cytokines[4]
Cell-mediated immunity[4]
Rheumatoid arthritis (Th1-mediated disease)[5]
• Improves in pregnancy as less Th1 cytokines[5]
Th2 cells[4,5]
Anti-inflammatory cytokines[4]
Humoral immunity[4]
Systemic lupus erythematosus (Th2-mediated disease)[5]
• Worsens in pregnancy as more Th2 cytokines[5]

Fig. 4: Th1–Th2 paradigm in pregnancy.

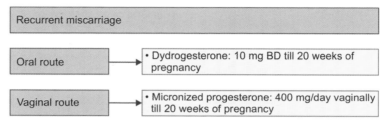

Fig. 5: FOGSI Position Statement 2015. (FOGSI: Federation of Obstetric and Gynaecological Societies of India)
Source: FOGSI. (2015). FOGSI GCPR. [online] Available from https://www.fogsi.org/fogsi-gcpr/ [Last accessed October, 2020]

However, there seems to be evidence of benefit in women with a history of recurrent miscarriage.

For women with unexplained recurrent miscarriages, supplementation with progestogen therapy probably reduces the rate of miscarriage in subsequent pregnancies.[14]

FOGSI Stand on Use of Progesterone in Threatened Abortion and RPL (Fig. 5)[15]

Based on the available clinical data, progesterone support (vaginal micronized progesterone and dydrogesterone) is beneficial in women presenting with a clinical diagnosis of threatened miscarriage with relative risk reduction in the miscarriage rate of 47% with the use of progesterone.

There is no evidence of harm and some evidence of benefit, although not coming from huge multicentric trials. The decision should be based on a clinician's discretion until strong evidence is available to recommend routine use.

There is no role of progesterone supplementation in normal healthy pregnant women for prevention of miscarriage.

(FOGSI: Federation of Obstetric and Gynaecological Societies of India)

◼ PROGESTERONES USED IN LUTEAL PHASE DEFECT AND PRETERM BIRTH

Progesterone should be started as early as immediately after ovulation for the treatment of LPD.

Progesterone is of two types: (1) Natural and (2) synthetic.
- *Natural progesterone (micronized progesterone):* Micronization and lipid coating cause rapid absorption and dissolution. It has got increased bioavailability.
  - *Route:* Oral, intramuscular, transdermal, vaginal, or rectal suppository
  - *Dose:* 100–400 mg
- *Derivatives of progesterone (dydrogesterone):* Properties closest to native progesterone. Free from androgenic, estrogenic, and anabolic effects. Complete secretory transformation with no glandular stromal asynchrony. No adverse metabolic effect.
  - *Dose:* 10–20 mg/day

- *Synthetic progestins:* Esters of 17α-hydroxyprogesterone (Pregnane steroids), 17α-OH progesterone acetate (acetoxy progesterone), 6α-methyl-17 α-OH progesterone (Medroxyprogesterone), and 17α-OH progesterone caproate (Proluton Depot).

17OHP-treated women had a significantly lower incidence of preterm delivery who were at a particularly high risk (37, 35, 32 weeks) and babies had a lower incidence of intraventricular hemorrhage, necrotizing enterocolitis, and need for supplemental O_2.[16]

Side effects:
- Injection site reaction, urticaria (65%), vaginal discharge (4–9%)
- No teratogenic effects
- No rise in mid-trimester loss
- No risk of gestational diabetes
- Body weight < 2,500 g but no increase in neonatal morbidity/mortality

Progesterone gel 8%: Dose 90 mg every night for vaginal use

◼ MECHANISM OF ACTION OF PROGESTERONE

Compared with natural progesterone, the synthetic progesterone may have luteolytic action on corpus luteum and can produce glandular stromal disparity. Progesterone is lipophilic in nature and diffuses freely into cells where it binds to receptors and produces its activity. Progesterone has a distribution phase half-life of 3–6 minutes followed by an elimination phase half-life of 19–95 minutes. After metabolism, it gets converted to Pregnanediol. It is excreted in feces and urine.

Doses
- *Oral:* 200–400 mg in two doses with an interval of 12 hours. Best to be taken 1 hour before or after meals
- *Vaginal/rectal:* 200–600 mg. It has to be started immediately after the ovulation and continued till 12th week completion. (Vaginal progesterone induces secretary transformation.)[17]
- Injectable route is best as bioavailability and the dose is 50–100 mg daily till the 12th week.

BOX 3: Micronized versus injected progesterone.

- Maximal serum concentrations achieved more rapidly (Simon et al., 1993).
- Does not adversely affect pregnancy outcome (Cornet et al., 1990).
- No decrease in HDL cholesterol levels (PEPI Trial, 1995)
- No effect on mood (Sherwin et al., 1991)
- Fewer side effects Micronized Vs synthetic progestins

TABLE 1: Common and uncommon side effects of dydrogesterone.

Common	Uncommon
Migraines/headache Nausea Menstrual disorders (e.g., metrorrhagia, menorrhagia, oligo/amenorrhea, dysmenorrhea, and irregular menstruation)	Depressed mood Increase in size of progestogen-dependent neoplasms Dizziness Hemolytic anemia Vomiting Hypersensitivity

TABLE 2: Guidelines for use of progesterone in preterm birth.

Source	Criteria	Route, dose	Duration	Evidence level
French guidelines 2016	Undilated os, CL < 25 mm	Vaginal progesterone, 90–200 mg/d	24–34 weeks	A
FIGO 2015	CL < 25 mm screened between 19 and 24 weeks	Vaginal progesterone, 90–200 mg/d	Till 34 weeks	A
StratOG 2015	CL < 25 mm	Vaginal progesterone	Till 37 weeks	
ACOG 2012	Prior preterm birth OR CL < 20 mm before 24 weeks	Vaginal or IM progesterone	16–34 weeks	A
SOGC	Prior preterm birth OR CL < 15 mm at 22–26 weeks	Vaginal or IM progesterone		1-A, 1-B

(ACOG: American College of Obstetricians and Gynecologists; CL: cervical length; FIGO: International Federation of Obstetrics and Gynecology; SOGC: Society of Obstetricians and Gynaecologists of Canada)

Micronized Progesterone (Box 3)

- It is a natural progesterone (decreasing the particle size increases absorption and bioavailability).
- Dose-dependent increase of serum progesterone can be achieved.
- 300 mg/day in divided doses (mostly 100 mg by day and 200 mg at night as sedation is a side effect) is required.
- Maximum absorption is obtained after food than on an empty stomach.
- It is short acting and needs multiple doses.
- It is lipid friendly.
- It favors diuresis.

Dydrogesterone

- First marketed in 1961
- The only retroprogesterone commercially available
- Molecular structure closely related to natural—progesterone
- Orally active at lower doses than micronized progesterone[18]
- No estrogenic, androgenic, or glucocorticoid effects
- T1/2= 4–5 hours

Compared with oral micronized progesterone, dydrogesterone has:

- More rigid structure (positively influences selectivity)
- Better oral bioavailability

- Requires a 10–20-times lower oral dose
- Has good receptor-binding selectivity
- Has metabolites with progestogenic activity

Side Effects

The side effects of dydrogesterone are given in **Table 1**.

Use

Dydrogesterone is used in threatened abortion, recurrent abortion, and luteal phase support in in vitro fertilization (IVF).

■ GUIDELINES FOR USE OF PROGESTERONE IN THREATENED ABORTION (TABLE 2)

NICE Guidelines

Threatened abortion: The evidence for the effectiveness of this treatment has been inconclusive, but data from a meta-analysis of several small studies suggest that progestogens are better than placebo.

2013 Australian and New Zealand Guidelines

For women presenting with a clinical diagnosis of threatened miscarriage, there is now preliminary evidence of a reduction in the rate of spontaneous miscarriage with the use of progestins (Consensus-based recommendation Reference: Wahabi 2011).

Cochrane 2013 (Haas and Ramsey 2013)

- No evidence of reduction of miscarriage by progestogen
- No evidence of reduction by route of administration (oral, vaginal, intramuscular)

Dark is not opposite of light. It is just the absence of light. Similarly, a problem is the absence of an idea. Not absence of a solution.

It's better to light a candle than curse the darkness....

So, as a doctor spreads the light into the lives of millions!

KEY POINTS

- Progesterone plays vital role for occurrence and maintenance of pregnancy.
- Corpus luteum is the only source of progesterone during the luteal phase of the normal menstrual cycle, and whereas during pregnancy the corpus luteum and trophoblast, both are sources of progesterone.
- There is no evidence to support the routine use of progestogen to prevent miscarriage in early to mid-pregnancy.
- Progesterone support is beneficial in women presenting with a clinical diagnosis of threatened miscarriage with relative risk reduction in the miscarriage rate of 47% with the use of progesterone.
- It can be synthetic or natural and used via oral, vaginal, rectal or intramuscular route.
- Compared with oral micronized progesterone, dydrogesterone has better oral bioavailability, has lower oral dose, better receptor selectivity and has metabolites with progestogenic activity
- Progesterone is mostly used in threatened abortion, recurrent abortion (RPL), and luteal phase support in IVF.
- There is no evidence of reduction in miscarriage by route of administration (oral, vaginal, intramuscular).

■ REFERENCES

1. Allen WM. Physiology of the corpus luteum, V: the preparation and some chemical properties of progestin, a hormone of the corpus luteum which produces progestational proliferation. Am J Physiol. 1930;92:174-88.
2. Ruddock NK, Shi SQ, Jain S, Moore G, Hankins GDV, Romero R, et al. Progesterone, but not 17-alpha-hydroxyprogesterone caproate, inhibits human myometrial contractions. Am J Obstet Gynecol. 2008;199(4):e391.
3. Hardy DB, Janowski BA, Corey DR, Mendelson CR. Progesterone receptor plays a major antiinflammatory role in human myometrial cells by antagonism of nuclear factor-κB activation of cyclooxygenase 2 expression. Mol. Endocrinol. 2006;20(11): 2724-33.
4. Choi BC, Polgar K, Xiao L, Hill JA. Progesterone inhibits in-vitro embryotoxic Th1 cytokine production to trophoblast in women with recurrent pregnancy loss. J Hum Reprod Sci. 2012;5(3): 248-51.
5. Peltier MR, Tee SC, Smulian JC. Effect of progesterone on proinflammatory cytokine production by monocytes stimulated with pathogens associated with preterm birth. Am J Reprod Immunol. 2008;60:346-53.
6. Marx SG, Wentz MJ, Mackay LB, Schlembach D, Maul H, Fittkow C, et al. Effects of progesterone on iNOS, COX-2, and collagen expression in the cervix. J Histochem Cytochem 2006;54(6): 623-39.
7. Xu H, Gonzalez JM, Ofori E, Elovitz MA. Preventing cervical ripening: the primary mechanism by which progestational agents prevent preterm birth? Am J Obstet Gynecol. 2008;198(3): e311– 8.
8. Ito A, Imada K, Sato T, Kubo T, Matsushima K, Mori Y. Suppression of interleukin 8 production by progesterone in rabbit uterine cervix. Biochem J. 1994; 301(Pt 1):183-6.
9. Foglia LM, Ippolito DL, Stallings JD, Zelig CM, Napolitano PG. Intramuscular 17α-hydroxyprogesterone caproate administration attenuates immunoresponsiveness of maternal peripheral blood mononuclear cells. Am J Obstet Gynecol. 2010;203(6):561.e1-5.
10. Mesen TB, Young SL. 2015. Progesterone and the luteal phase: a requisite to reproduction. Obstet Gynecol Clin N Am. 2015;42(1):135-51.
11. Hussain M, El-Hakim S, Cahill DJ. Progesterone supplementation in women with otherwise unexplained recurrent miscarriages. 2012;5(3):248-51.
12. American Society for Reproductive Medicine. Evaluation and treatment of recurrent pregnancy loss: a committee opinion. [online] Available from https://www.asrm.org/.../asrm/asrm.../evaluation and treatment of recurrent pregnancy [Last accessed October, 2020]
13. Clifford K, Flanagan AM, Regan L. Endometrial CD56+ natural killer cells in women with recurrent miscarriage: A histomorphometric study. Hum Reprod. 1999;14(11):2727-30.
14. Haas DM, Hathaway TJ, Ramsey PS. Progestogen for preventing miscarriage in women with recurrent miscarriage of unclear etiology. Cochrane Database Syst Rev. 2018;10(10):CD003511.
15. FOGSI. (2015). FOGSI Position Statement on the use of progestogens. [online] Available from https://www.fogsi.org/wp-content/uploads/2017/07/Progesterone-position-paper-Oct-2015.pdf [Last accessed October, 2020]
16. Meis PJ, Klebanoff M, Thom E, Dombrowski MP, Sibai B, Moawad AH, et al. Prevention of recurrent preterm delivery by 17 alpha-hydroxyprogesterone caproate. N Engl J Med. 2003;348(24): 2379-85.
17. Cicinelli E, De Ziegler D, Bulletti C, Matteo MG, Schonauer LM, Galantino P. Direct transport of progesterone from vagina to uterus. Obstet Gynecol. 2000;95(3):403-6.
18. Lee HJ, Park TC, Kim JH, Norwitz E, Lee B. The influence of oral dydrogesterone and vaginal progesterone on threatened abortion: A systematic review and meta-analysis. Biomed Res Int. 2017;2017:3616875.

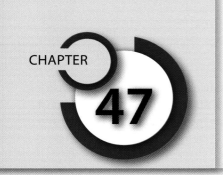

Varicose Veins in Pregnancy

Rajendra P Shitole

■ INTRODUCTION

Lower extremities chronic venous disease (CVD) is a spectrum of diseases ranging from visible varicosities, spider veins, lower leg edema, itching, leg ulcer leading to severe disability. It occurs when the valves in the venous system get damaged as a result of which the vein gets distended leading to a variety of symptoms. The disease involves a superficial venous system of the lower limb. In this chapter, we will be studying about the development of CVD in pregnancy, the course of disease, and the treatment aspect.

■ INCIDENCE

The prevalence of CVD is high during pregnancy, affecting almost 70% of population in various forms.[1]

■ ETIOPATHOLOGY

Multiple theories have been explained for the development and worsening of varicose veins in pregnancy.[1]

Mechanical Compression

The oldest theory is that of mechanical compression. It was assumed that the mechanical compression due to gravid uterus on pelvic veins leads to development of varicosities. But there is very little evidence to support this theory. Varicose veins begin to develop from the first trimester when the uterus is not big enough to cause compression on the varicose vein. Also, the pelvic tumor of the size of a gravid uterus does not cause varicose veins and neither worsens the preexisting varicose veins as compared to gravid uterus. However, there is some correlation between the development of valvular varicosities and mechanical compression of gravid uterus on inferior vena cava (IVC) and iliac veins later in pregnancy.[2,3]

Hormonal Theory

The hormonal theory is the most widely accepted theory.[4,5] There is a significantly increased level of estrogen and progesterone during pregnancy. Progesterone causes increase in hypotonia in the smooth muscles. This leads to increase in the vein distension. On the other hand, estrogen increases the arterial supply to the uterus. This leads to increase in venous return from pelvic organ. This increase in venous return leads to functional obstruction of venous drainage of the lower limb. Both these conditions hamper the venous drainage of lower limb leading to development of varicose veins.

Hereditary Predisposition

According to a study conducted by Bertone C,[6] family history plays a significant role in the development of varicose veins during pregnancy.

Other Risk Factors

Increased Age

Age is one of the important risk factors for the development of varicose veins. The incidence of varicose vein increases with increasing age. According to Basle study III conducted by A. Adhikari et al,[7] there is a 6–10 times higher prevalence of varicose vein in 70-year-old persons than in 30-year-old persons.

Multiple Pregnancies

It has been observed that there is a higher incidence of varicose vein in multiparous women as well as in multifetal gestation.

■ CLINICAL EVALUATION

The most common symptom of varicose veins is edema. Other symptoms are pain, night cramps, numbness, tingling, and heaviness of leg; achy and visible varicosities may also be seen. The patient may have itching around the vein. Pain is severe at the end of the day or after standing for longer duration and is relieved by rest.

Evaluation is done using the clinical status, etiology, anatomy, and pathophysiology (CEAP) classification system. The CEAP scale grades the patients based on the physical observations of disease severity as shown in **Table 1**.[8]

TABLE 1: CEAP classification.

Class	Description
C0	No visible or palpable signs of venous disease
C1	Telangiectasias or reticular veins
C2	Varicose veins, distinguished from reticular veins by a diameter of 3 mm
C3	Edema
C4	Changes in skin and subcutaneous tissue
C4a	Eczema, pigmentation (and additionally corona phlebectasia)
C4b	Lipodermatosclerosis or atrophie blanche
C5	Healed venous ulcer
C6	Active venous ulcer

(CEAP: clinical status, etiology, anatomy, and pathophysiology classification)

■ DIAGNOSIS

Duplex ultrasonography is the most common imaging test for the evaluation of patients with CVD. Gray-scale imaging and Doppler imaging are used for the evaluation of blood flow in veins and for identifying the reflux.

■ TREATMENT

Treatment for varicose veins during pregnancy is divided into nonpharmacological, pharmacological, and surgical.

Nonpharmacological

Compression Stocking

Compression stockings provide graduated compression which is highest at the ankle and gradually loosens further up. These need to be worn during daytime and removed at night.

Rest

Women are advised to take rest in between when standing for longer duration. In addition when resting for longer duration, the left lateral position is advised so that the pressure on IVC is decreased.

Reflexology

Reflexology may be used to relieve the pain in the lower limb.[9]

Water Immersion Technique

Water immersion technique has been traditionally used to relive the lower limb edema. It helps to displace the fluid from the extravascular compartment to the intravascular compartment, thus reliving the leg edema. During this treatment, the individual is subjected to an external water gradient which is slightly higher than venous pressure leading to decrease in leg edema.[10]

Foot Massage

This technique has been used traditionally to decrease leg edema. Massage helps to shift the fluid from the extravascular compartment to the intravascular compartment.[11]

Pharmacological

Phlebotonics

Phlebotonics are the naturally occurring flavonoids, most of them being extracted from plants. Few of these drugs are synthetically prepared with flavonoid-like properties. These drugs act either by improving the venous tone[12] or may decrease capillary hyperpermeability.[13] These are known to decrease the symptoms of night cramps, heaviness of leg, and edema. However, the safety of these drugs during pregnancy is not proved.

Surgery

Surgery mainly consists of ablation of great saphenous and short saphenous veins using thermal energy. It is a minimally invasive surgery done under either local anesthesia or spinal anesthesia. The other traditional form of surgery is venous stripping and ligation.

However, surgery is avoided during pregnancy. For majority of women, the symptoms subside within 3–4 months of delivery.

Data Review on Treatment

All the above treatment options have not been adequately assessed within the context of a randomized controlled trial. No significant differences were found in lower leg edema with compression stockings when they were compared against rest or foot massage with routine care.

There was a significant reduction in symptoms of CVD with reflexology (relaxing and lymphatic) compared with rest alone.[9]

A trial by Irion and Irion,[14] suggesting that water immersion for 20 minutes in a swimming pool compared with sitting upright in a chair with legs elevated for 20 minutes reduced leg volume significantly.

Phlebotonics appear to help women with CVD. However, the safety profile of drug during pregnancy is not yet clear.[15,16] All the above conclusions are drawn from a single study.

Because of paucity of trials, and the absence of relevant and important information from available trials, no reliable conclusions can be made regarding the management of women with varicose veins in pregnancy.

WHO Recommendation for Treatment of Varicose Vein During Pregnancy

Nonpharmacological options, such as compression stockings, leg elevation, and water immersion, can be

TABLE 2: Associated maternal complications after liver transplantation.

Pregnancy-induced hypertension	2–43%
Preeclampsia	2–22%
Gestational diabetes mellitus	0–37.5%
Graft rejection	0–20%

TABLE 3: Fetal complications after liver transplant.

Spontaneous/missed abortions	4.9–19%
Stillbirths	0–2%
Low birth weight (<2,500 g)	4.8–57%
Fetal distress	10.3–40%
Congenital abnormalities	0–16.7%

organ transplant recipients. For this reason, it is highly recommended that women who have undergone lung transplantation avoid getting pregnant in the first 2–3 years after surgery.

Risks of Pregnancy Post-transplant

The most common risks associated with pregnancy after a lung transplant include:
- Premature birth
- Low birth weight
- Declined lung function and rejection
- Preeclampsia
- Hypertension
- Diabetes
- Infection
- Complications associated with some common anti-rejection medications (especially birth defects and premature delivery)

It is important to assess the patient's health and make sure that risk-related factors such as liver function, blood sugar, and graft function are adequately controlled.

■ RENAL TRANSPLANT

In most of the patients who undergo renal transplant, pregnancy is possible. During childbearing age, pregnancy occurs in 12% of women. After the first trimester, >90% pregnancies reach term. In women who are close to the end of their childbearing years and undergo renal transplantation, pregnancy becomes least likely.

The first successful pregnancy reported occurred in a recipient of a kidney transplant from an identical twin sister performed in 1958. Since then, numerous successful pregnancies were reported in renal transplant patients. Conception is rare for women on dialysis.

Complications in Women with Chronic Renal Failure
- Loss of libido
- Anovulatory vaginal bleeding or amenorrhea
- High prolactin levels
- Decreased libido and reduced ability to reach orgasm

■ EFFECT OF PREGNANCY ON GRAFT FUNCTION

Pregnancy causes an increase in the glomerular filtration rate (GFR), which causes increased plasma flow, with no concomitant increase in intraglomerular pressure.

In most of the recipients, pregnancy does not appear to cause excessive or irreversible problems with graft function if the function of the transplant organ is stable prior to pregnancy.

■ IMMUNOSUPPRESSIVE DRUGS IN PREGNANCY

Glucocorticoids

The most commonly used glucocorticoids are the short-acting agents—prednisone, prednisolone, and methyl prednisolone. Radiolabeled prednisone and prednisolone can cross the placenta, but maternal-to-cord-blood ratios are approximately 10:1.

Complications
- Adrenal insufficiency and thymic hypoplasia have been occasionally seen in infants of transplant recipients (if the dose of prednisolone is >15 mg/day).
- Cleft palate or mental retardation has also been described in humans after in utero corticosteroid exposure.
- Premature rupture of membranes (PROM) intransplant recipients. Also, the incidence of hypertension is more in such patients.
- Maternal infection (if doses of Prednisolone >20 mg/day)

Azathioprine

Azathioprine is used during pregnancy in many transplant recipients. Radioactive labeling studies show that 64–93% of azathioprine administered to mothers appears in fetal blood as inactive metabolites and the fetus is relatively protected from the effects of the drug.

Complications
- Low-birth-weight babies
- Prematurity
- Jaundice
- Respiratory distress syndrome and aspiration in kidney transplant recipients
- Myelosuppression in the fetus (usually dose-related)

Cyclosporin

The dose of cyclosporin is 2–4 mg/kg/day.

Complications

- Graft dysfunction after pregnancy
- Low-birth-weight babies
- Maternal diabetes
- Hypertension/preeclampsia
- Renal allograft dysfunction

Tacrolimus

There is limited data concerning the effect of tacrolimus on pregnancy. The dose is significantly reduced to prevent toxicity.

Mycophenolate Mofetil

The risk of birth defects or abortion is increased in pregnant women exposed to mycophenolate mofetil (MMF). Data is limited at the moment; hence, its use is not recommended.

OKT3 and Polyclonal Antibodies

OKT3 is an immunoglobulin G (IgG) that crosses the placenta.

The National Transplantation Pregnancy Registry (NTPR) has reported treating five women with OKT3 during pregnancy, with four surviving infants. The effect of polyclonal antibodies on the developing fetus is not known.

◼ MANAGEMENT GUIDELINES

All women who desire a pregnancy after kidney transplantation should be counseled regarding the possibility and risks of pregnancy. Before transplantation, patients who are not rubella immune should receive the rubella vaccine as live virus vaccines are contraindicated post-transplantation.

Patients are usually advised to wait at least 1-year post living/related donor transplantation and 2 years after cadaveric transplantation. However, waiting 5 years or more is not advisable as this may result in impaired renal function postpartum that fails to recover, because of gradually deteriorating renal function secondary to chronic rejection.

Contraceptive counseling should be done immediately post-transplantation, because in women with well-functioning grafts, ovulatory cycles may begin within 1–2 months post-transplantation.

Low-dose estrogen–progesterone oral contraceptive pills (OCPs) are advised.

Due to risk of infection in immunocompromised patients, use of intrauterine devices is not advised.

BOX 1: Criteria for transplant recipients planning a pregnancy.

- At least 1-year post-transplantation
- Stable renal function with creatinine <2 mg/dL
- No recent episodes of acute rejection
- BP ≤140/90 mm Hg on medications
- Proteinuria <500 mg/day
- Prednisone ≤15 mg/day
- Azathioprine ≤2 mg/kg/day
- Cyclosporin ≤4 mg/kg/day
- Normal allograft ultrasound

◼ CRITERIA FOR TRANSPLANT RECIPIENTS PLANNING A PREGNANCY

The criteria for transplant recipients planning a pregnancy are given in **Box 1**.

◼ MANAGEMENT OF HYPERTENSION

Women who have undergone renal transplantation, and who are pregnant, should be watched closely for mild-to-moderate hypertension and also warned about signs of early preeclampsia. Such patients should ideally be delivered at 37 weeks of gestation.

Antihypertensive Drugs Used in Pregnancy

- *α-Methyldopa*: It is most safe and best in efficacy in post-transplant pregnant women.
- *Beta-blockers*: Cardiovascular beta blockers, such as atenolol and metoprolol, if started in early or midgestation, cause fetal growth retardation. But when started in late pregnancy, they prove to be safe and efficacious.
- Nonselective beta-blockers can cause uterine contractions; hence, they should not be used.
- *Hydralazine*: It is safe and frequently used as an adjunctive therapy along with α-methyldopa and beta blockers.
- *Calcium channel blockers*: Nifedipine, nicardipine, and verapamil can be used in cases of severe hypertension during pregnancy. When used in the first trimester, they do not cause any increase in congenital anomalies. They should be used with caution in women who are at risk of developing preeclampsia.
- *Labetalol*: It is thought to be as effective as methyldopa.
- *Angiotensin-converting enzyme (ACE) inhibitors*: The fetal outcome is good in women who have taken ACE inhibitors in early pregnancy. Exposure to ACE inhibitors during the second and third trimesters may be associated with serious adverse fetal effects such as oligohydramnios, neonatal anuria, renal failure, and death. Hence, continued administration of an ACE inhibitor during pregnancy is contraindicated.

- *Diuretics*: If prescribed before gestation, use of thiazide diuretics has been approved in women with chronic hypertension. However, they are not recommended in preeclamptic women, who often manifest decreased intravascular volumes and poor placental perfusion.

MANAGEMENT OF INFECTION

Bacterial

The most common bacterial infections are urinary tract infections, which occur in up to 40% of pregnant transplant recipients. They are particularly common in patients who develop end-stage renal disease due to pyelonephritis. Urine cultures should be done on a monthly basis. If asymptomatic bacteriuria is found, the patient should be treated for 2 weeks and may be treated with suppressive doses of antibiotics for the rest of the pregnancy.

In case there is any need for invasive procedures such as fetal monitoring with scalp electrodes or intrauterine pressure monitoring, prophylactic antibiotics should be given.

Penicillins are the preferred antibiotic agents. The potential risk of fetal toxicity should be considered while selecting any antibiotics.

Viral

The most frequent cause of viral infection post-transplantation is cytomegalovirus (CMV).

Amniotic fluid culture can be used in diagnosing infection of the fetus.

Herpes simplex virus (HSV) infection prior to 20 weeks of gestation is associated with an increased rate of miscarriage. A positive HSV cervical culture at term is an indication for cesarean section. This minimizes the risk for neonatal herpes. Acyclovir is the drug of choice and can be safely used in pregnancy.

Any infant born to an HBSAg-positive mother should be given hepatitis B immunoglobulin within the first 12 hours of birth and hepatitis B virus (HBV) vaccine at another site within 48 hours followed by a booster injection at 1 and 6 months.

For >90% of infants, this combination of immunoglobulin and vaccine offers protection for vertical transmission and is believed to be <7%, with hepatitis C unless the patient has a coexisting human immunodeficiency virus infection.

LABOR AND DELIVERY

Vaginal delivery is preferred in most transplant recipient women. Indications for a cesarean section should be obstetric reasons only. Fluid overload and infection should be taken care of. At the time of delivery, instrumentation should be minimized. Oxytocin should be used with caution in patients with renal insufficiency, as this may increase the risk of water retention.

In the perinatal period, the dose of steroids should be augmented to cover the stress of labor and to prevent postpartum rejection. During labor and delivery, injection Hydrocortisone, 100 mg 6 hourly, should be given. Patients on immunosuppressive drugs should avoid breastfeeding.

CONCLUSION

Pregnancy usually does not appear to have any adverse effect on the long-term survival of renal allografts. It is advisable to treat end-stage renal disease patients with transplantation and wait until renal function has been stable for 1–2 years before undertaking a planned pregnancy. Planned pregnancies offer favorable outcomes to the mother and the fetus.

SUGGESTED READING

1. Brännström M, Dahm Kähler P, Greite R, Mölne J, Diaz-Garcia C, Tullius SG. Uterus transplantation: A rapidly expanding field. Transplantation. 2018;102:569-77.
2. Costa ML, Surita FG, Passini R, Jr, Cecatti JG, Boin IF. Pregnancy outcome in female liver transplant recipients. Transplant Proc. 2011;43:1337-9.
3. Erman Akar M, Ozkan O, Aydinuraz B, Dirican K, Cincik M, Mendilcioglu I. Clinical pregnancy after uterus transplantation. Fertil Steril. 2013;100(5):1358-63.
4. Jabiry-Zieniewicz Z, Szpotanska-Sikorska M, Pietrzak B, et al. Pregnancy outcomes among female recipients after liver transplantation: Further experience. Transplant Proc. 2011;43:3043-7.
5. Jarvholm S, Johannesson L, Brannstrom M. Psychological aspects in pre-transplantation assessments of patients prior to entering the first uterus transplantation trial. Acta Obstet Gynecol Scand. 2015;94(10):1035-8.
6. Kociszewska-Najman B, Pietrzak B, Cyganek A, et al. Intrauterine hypotrophy and premature births in neonates delivered by female renal and liver transplant recipients. Transplant Proc. 2011;43:3048-51.
7. Ozkan O, Akar ME, Erdogan O, Ozkan O, Hadimioglu N. Uterus transplantation from a deceased donor. Fertil Steril. 2013;100(6):e41.
8. Shaner J, Coscia LA, Constantinescu S, McGrory CH, Doria C, Moritz MJ, Armenti VT, Cowan SW. Pregnancy after lung transplant. Prog Transplant. 2012;22(2):134-40.
9. Tendron A, Gouyon JB, Decramer S. In utero exposure to immunosuppressive drugs: experimental and clinical studies. Pediatr Nephrol. 2002;17(2):121-30.

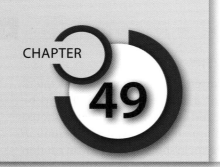

CHAPTER 49

Human Milk Banking— Need of the Time

Shailaja Mane

INTRODUCTION

Neonatal morbidity and mortality are public health challenges all over the globe with 3.1 million babies dying worldwide, each year, in the first month of life. In India, approximately 1.72 million children die annually before reaching their first birthday, which is highest for any country in the world. Out of these, 72% die during the neonatal period. *India contributes to one-fifth of global live births and more than a quarter of neonatal deaths.* The World Health Organization (WHO) ascertains that breastfeeding is the most effective way for preserving child health and survival. Every infant and child have the right to good nutrition as per the Convention on the Rights of the Child. The WHO recommends breast milk as the optimum exclusive source of nutrition for the first 6 months of life and may remain part of the healthy infant diet for the first 2 years of life and beyond. Human milk is species-specific and thus it is superior to all the alternate newborn feeds. Breast milk is solely excellent nutrition for the newborns. When none is available, human milk bank (HMB) can help.

EVIDENCE IN LITERATURE

The first evidence in the support of human milk sharing is from ancient India. "Yashodha" was a wet nurse (human milk donor) to Lord Krishna. Not only in Indian mythology, wet nursing is also depicted in tomb paintings of ancient Egypt. It is also found in the Code of Hammurabi from 2250 BC in which appropriate wet nurses are described. Providing donor milk from another woman is not a new concept; wet nursing was a fairly common practice a few decades ago.

Sushruta, an ancient Indian surgeon, has beautifully described mother's milk in his Samhita, "One just cannot compare even water of seven seas with mother's milk, which is nothing but water ensuring optimum growth, nutrition and healthy life of hundred years."

In the 18th century, wet nursing was widely practiced by mothers of nobility who refused to feed their babies to guard their beauty and figure. In the latter half of the 18th century, a law controlling wet nursing was introduced where the wet nurses were registered and had to be disease free and were not permitted to nurse more than two infants at a time.

Later, the wet nursing practice declined due to fear of infections and diseases such as HIV and syphilis, and the same is the reason why wet nursing is not encouraged today. So, members of the healthcare system introduced the concept of pasteurized donor human milk (PDHM) banks.

WHO and UNICEF (United Nations Children's Fund) has made a joint statement: "Where it is not possible for the biological mother to breast feed, the first alternative, if available, should be the use of human milk from other sources. Human milk banks should be made available in appropriate situations."

For achieving Millennium Development Goals: The goal of Under-five Mortality Rate (U5MR) of 20 or less by 2035 set in the "Committing to Child Survival: A promise renewed" initiative that India co-hosts states that HMB is imperative.

HUMAN MILK BANKING

Human milk banking is a service for collection, screening, processing, storing, and distributing human milk from donors. Human milk is the suitable source of nutrition for the first 6 months and may remain as part of the infant nutrition for the first 2 years of life and beyond.

The world's first official HMB was opened in Vienna at the outset of the 20th century in 1909. Asia's first HMB was established at SION Hospital, Mumbai, India, in November 1989 under the name "*Sneha.*"

After decades of research and evidence, it is proved that breast milk is the safest source for infant feeding with no disadvantage. WHO and UNICEF had supported promotion of breastfeeding across the globe by launching Baby-Friendly-Hospital-Initiative (BFHI).

When a mother's own breast milk is not available for any reason for the sick, hospitalized newborn, pasteurized human donor breast milk should be accessible as the best alternative source of nutrition.

WHO and UNICEF have also studied that donor human breast milk should be the first alternative rather than commercial formulas available in the market when mother's milk is not available. HMBs have done their best so far in these situations. In milk bank, breast milk is collected through voluntary donation from mothers, which is pasteurized by using scientific equipment. This pasteurized milk is then examined to make sure that it is free from any infection source and then stored in containers in hospital-grade authentic deep freezers. Many of the breast milk's nutritional and protective components are not altered or only minimally reduced through the process of pasteurization. Human breast milk provides various optimum proteins, energy, and micro- and macronutrients that enhance immunity in the premature infant and normal neonates. Human milk is also known to decrease many morbidities such as diarrhea, respiratory infections, and necrotizing enterocolitis (NEC) and lower the incidence of mortality in term and preterm newborns. It also reduces the future incidence of chronic diseases such as obesity, hypertension, and diabetes in adulthood. Lactating mothers who breastfeed also benefit as it is known to reduce chances of breast cancer and various other morbidities.

Milk banking is approved as a cost-effective nutritional source for hospitalized neonates because it lessens disease incidence, severity, and length of stay in hospital.

Need of Human Milk Banking

- Proper nutrition for newborns is a concern all across the world; HMB can serve to ease this concern by being a consistent source of nutrition to the needy babies, especially the ones in neonatal intensive care units (NICUs).
- India faces its own unique challenges, having the highest number of low-birth-weight (LBW) babies. The annual incidence of very low birth weight (VLBW) babies in India is about 7 million which account for significant morbidity and mortality in the country. Feeding VLBW babies is a challenge because most of these babies are either admitted to NICUs or have some limitations for feeding.
- PDHM can be prescribed on priority for:
  - Extremely low birth weight (ELBW; <1,000 g), VLBW (<1,500 g), congenital cardiac diseases, insufficient lactation, etc., and for mothers with multiple gestation and those who cannot secrete adequate breast milk for their neonates initially
  - Babies of nonlactating mothers, mothers who adopt neonates, and where induced lactation is not possible
  - Abandoned and sick neonates in the NICU
  - Temporary interruption of breastfeeding due to any cause
  - Infant at health risk from breast milk of the biological mother
  - Babies of mother who died in the immediate postpartum period.

Human milk bank is an organization that screens, collects, stores, processes (to exclude the risk of viral and bacterial transmission), and distributes donated human milk. The recipient is a hospitalized preterm or ill infant. Donor human milk (DHM) is an alternative to infant formula for special needs' infants and not a substitute for the mother's own milk.

Definitions

- *HMB*: It is an organized service for selection of donors, collection, processing, storage, or distribution of human breast milk for the sick newborn or low-weight or premature babies.
- *Donor*: It means a lactating woman who voluntarily contributes milk to a HMB for use by a newborn or an infant or a child other than her own.
- *Human milk collection center*: It means the location at which containers of human breast milk are held temporarily between the donation site and human milk.

The *aims and objectives of human milk banking* are to increase breastfeeding practices to reduce neonatal and infant mortality and morbidity and improve maternal health by providing safe human milk to babies whose mothers are unable to breast feed.

- The conceptual framework of HMB is shown in **Figure 1**.

Training of staff includes expression and collection of milk, cleaning, using pumps, sterilization of containers, storing donated milk, cooling, freezing, thawing, labeling milk, documentation, distribution of milk, transportation of milk, counseling for donation in local language and according to cultural beliefs, etc.

Process of Collecting, Testing, and Storing of Breast Milk

The mothers offering their breast milk for collection and storage need to be informed about the concept of HMB and its benefits to the other babies and herself. She should be informed of its benefits if the milk is expressed regularly from her breast via a breast pump. It is to be carried out by training herself or under supervision of proper trained and qualified persons to do the job. A written, informed consent of donors and parents of recipients should be taken. The milk collection depends on the willingness of mothers who want to donate. The records of the milk collected, tested, and disbursed are maintained to keep the track record of the donors and consumers.

Potential Donors

Mothers of premature, sick, and cleft palate babies; mothers with flat or inverted nipple, and mothers who have recently lost their baby can be potential donors.

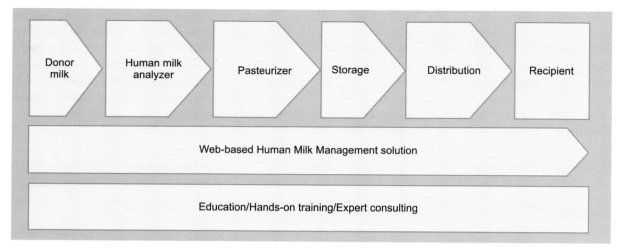

Fig. 1: Conceptual framework of human milk banking.

The breast milk of the lactating mothers is collected hygienically by breast pumps. This is collected after her own baby had his/her share of feed. Then excess milk retained in the breast is expressed hygienically by the breast pumps.

The milk collected is stored, marked, and recorded separately every time the milk is expressed. The milk collected is then pasteurized and tested for its safe consumption. The tests carried on daily collection of breast milk are to find out if there is presence of any infectious growth after the culture test is performed. The donor mother is also informed accordingly. The safe milk is stored in the refrigerators and deep freezers as per need.

The milk after removing from the deep freezer needs to be thawed and brought to room temperature before giving it to the baby for consumption. Only smaller proportion of milk should be removed as per need. Once the milk is thawed and again stored for freezing, it loses its vital contents.

The milk collected can be ready for use only after 24 hours after confirmation of safety. It is ready to use for consumption after culture tests.

Breast milk can be collected and stored:
- At normal room temperature of 15–25°C (66–72°F) for 10 hours
- In a refrigerator up to 8 days with temperature well below 15°C
- In refrigerator deep freezer for 3–4 months
- In a specialized deep freezer (–20°C) for 6–12 months.

Ten tips for pumping and storing breast milk:
1. Always wash hands before expressing or handling breast milk.
2. Store breast milk in jars with tight-fitting lids or in nursery plastic bags. Do not store milk in ordinary plastic bags or formula bags.
3. Discard all milk that has been refrigerated >72 hours.
4. If you freeze milk, keep it at 0° for 3–6 months of storage.
5. Try to freeze milk in single servings—roughly 2–4 ounces, the average amount needed for one feeding.
6. Do not add fresh milk to milk that has been frozen.
7. To thaw frozen milk, let it stand in the refrigerator or place the container in a bowl of warm water.
8. Never use a microwave oven to defrost milk or heat it to feed your baby. Heating can destroy some of the nutrients in the milk and can scald your baby's mouth and tongue.
9. Never refreeze breast milk. Discard what your baby does not finish in a feeding; milk that is thawed in a refrigerator should be used in 24 hours.
10. Do not save milk from a used bottle or refrigerate what your baby did not finish for a later feeding.

Donor screening criteria and training: Donors are screened as per the International Screening Criteria. Healthy mothers without any acute or chronic illness can donate their breast milk voluntarily. They must be screened for hepatitis B, HIV, syphilis, tuberculosis, etc.

Training for new donors includes counseling and promotion, milk donation and its benefits and importance, handwashing and its importance, good personal hygiene, mother support group work, etc.

The electronic and manual breast pumps are shown in **Figures 2 and 3**, respectively.

Method of Milk Banking

- Milk expressed into autoclaved, labeled, steel containers with caps
- Babies fed their own mother's unprocessed milk
- Excess milk and milk from voluntary donors collected in larger containers, refrigerated, and transferred to a milk bank

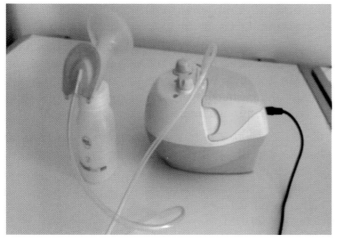

Fig. 2: Electronic breast pump.

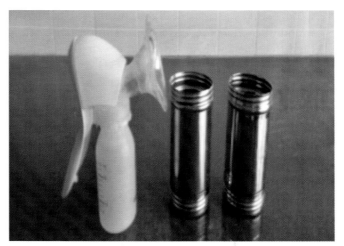

Fig. 3: Manual breast pump.

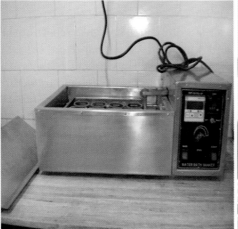

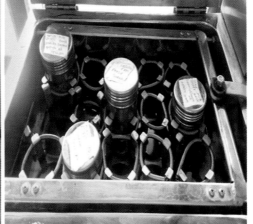

Fig. 4: Water shaker bath pasteurizer.

Holder Pasteurization of Milk

Milk is expressed into autoclaved (steel)/ETO sterile (plastic)/glass containers with corkscrew caps. Milk is stored separately in different containers. A hot air oven can be used for sterilization of steel containers. Expression of milk is done with breast pumps in a painless way. Pasteurization of milk is done in a holder water shaker bath pasteurization. As per the recommendations of Human Milk Banking Association of North America (HMBANA), expressed breast milk is pasteurized at 62.5°C for 30 minutes in a shaker water bath. After pasteurization, milk is rapidly cooled to 4°C or lower. A sample of milk should be sent for culture of pathological bacterial growth. Extra milk is frozen at –20°C. Culture-negative milk can be used for babies. Common organisms cultured in milk are *Staphylococcus aureus, Acinetobacter, Klebsiella, Pseudomonas, Bacillus subtilis, Escherichia coli,* etc. Culture-positive milk should be discarded or re-pasteurized. Milk is used on "first in first out" basis. Milk is thawed by standing container in lukewarm water. After thawing, milk is used within 4–6 hours only.

Water shaker bath pasteurizer is shown in **Figure 4** and advanced equipment used for pasteurization of milk are shown in **Figure 5**.

COMPREHENSIVE LACTATION MANAGEMENT CENTER

- Comprehensive lactation management center (CLMC) is an elaborate setup established for the purpose of collecting, screening, processing, storing, and distributing DHM.
- CLMCs are established at the government medical colleges or district hospitals with high delivery load and availability of newborn treatment units such as NICUs/special newborn care units (SNCUs).

- CLMC serves as an ancillary support to the baby-friendly hospital practices of promoting and supporting breastfeeding and kangaroo mother care (KMC). It is a nonprofit setup.
- CLMC should be located in the vicinity of the neonatal units (NICU/SNCU) and preferably be situated within the Maternal and Child Health (MCH) building in the vicinity of the obstetrics–neonatology complex.

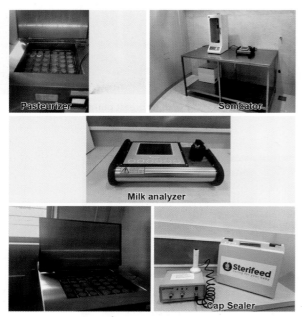

Fig. 5: Advanced equipment used for pasteurization of milk.

Functions of Comprehensive Lactation Management Center

Comprehensive lactation management center promotes and supports breastfeeding for all newborns including preterm, low birth weight, and sick newborns through support of breastfeeding by skilled counseling, lactation management through human milk donation, and KMC.

*The processes in CLMC have six basic steps (**Fig. 6; Flowchart 1**):*

1. Screening of donor mothers
2. Milk expression and collection
3. Processing of DHM
4. Testing of DHM
5. Storage of pasteurized DHM
6. Dispensing of processed Milk

Benefits of Human Milk Banking

Benefits Noted for Mothers

Painless milk extraction gives relief from breast engorgement and pain. Fever, back pain, and breast pain get reduced. HMB can be used by working mothers in hospital. Milk from HMB is useful during problem in feeding baby—preterm, extremely preterm, NICU babies, etc. HMB helps in milk establishment as frequent expression helps maintain lactation and prevents mastitis and breast abscess. Donor mothers feel contented and have great satisfaction by helping other babies when in need.

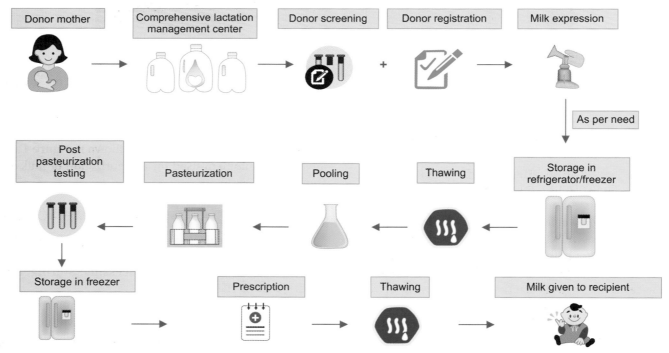

Fig. 6: Summary of process for a comprehensive lactation management center.

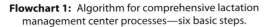

Flowchart 1: Algorithm for comprehensive lactation management center processes—six basic steps.

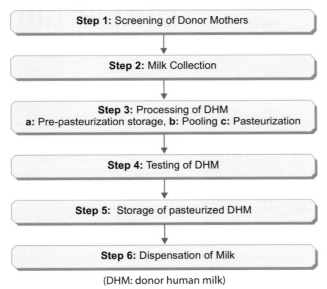

(DHM: donor human milk)

Benefits Noted for Newborns

Human milk bank shows a reduced incidence of neonatal morbidities, such as sepsis and NEC, and increased feed tolerance. It reduces time to full feeds, helps in better weight gain, and reduces the duration of hospital stay and expenses. Neonatal morbidity and mortality is reduced by ensuring continuous supply of safe human milk for sick and preterm babies. It has a positive influence on breastfeeding practices in hospital and community. HMB is the best way of ensuring a safe supply of human milk to all the needy neonates. It ensures optimum health and development of infants at minimum cost. Studies suggest that use of PDHM shows lower risk of NEC (which remains a disease of high morbidity and mortality with adverse long-term effects) as opposed to artificial formula.

Advantages to Community and Nation

Human milk bank reduces the incidence of morbidity and mortality in neonates, infants, and mothers. It saves the energy of mother and caretaker. HMB has a positive influence on breastfeeding practices. It reduces burden on health system, saves extra cost of top milk, fuel, and avoids environmental pollution.

Conclusion and Recommendation

Human milk banking is a boon for newborns. Every large NICU and medical college hospital should establish HMB. Awareness of HMB should be increased in community. Establishment of HMBs will help to improve neonatal care in developing countries.

Mobile milk banking: It collects and distributes breast milk from various collection centers, homes and work places of women, offices, etc. A mobile milk van will be of great help to working mothers.

KEY POINTS

- *Human milk banking is a strong way to promote breast-feeding and should be integrated with breastfeeding promotion*: HMBs are most successful when developed as part of a package to promote breastfeeding by various means.
- HMBs would be a boon to mothers and newborns by helping the society at large.
- HMBs help to reduce the incidence of sepsis, NEC, and jaundice which are the leading neonatal morbidities worldwide.
- Thus, HMB will help in reducing neonatal morbidity and mortality rates. HMB is imperative for the achievement of the *Millennium Development Goals*.
- Not only babies, but also the *donating mothers* get benefits due to reduced incidence of *breast engorgement, breast abscess, mastitis,* and *lactation failure*.
- HMBs thus helps in reducing the economical and disease burden by improving neonatal care in developing countries such as India.
- HMB is a feasible, cost-effective measure as a *boon for newborns*.
- *Human milk banking—NEED OF TIME!!*

SUGGESTED READING

1. Bharadva K, Tiwari S, Mishra S, Mukhopadhya K, Yadav B, Agarwal RK, et al. Human milk banking guidelines. Indian Pediatr. 2014;51(6):469-74.
2. IAP-IYCF Chapter. (2015). Infant and Young Child Feeding and Human Milk Banking Guidelines[online] Available from http://idamumbaichapter.com/wp-content/uploads/2017/07/Infant-and-Young-Child-Feeding-and-Human-Milk-Bank-guideline-2015.pdf [Last accessed November, 2020].
3. Kim JH, Unger S. Human milk banking-. Paediatr Child Health. 2010;15(9):595-8.
4. Registrar General of India. (2013). Sample Registration System (SRS) statistical report 2012. [online] Available from https://censusindia.gov.in/vital_statistics/SRS_Report_2012/1_Contents_2012.pdf [Last accessed November, 2020]
5. Resource Centre. (2012). Nutrition in the First 1,000 Days: State of World's Mothers. [online] Available from https://resourcecentre.savethechildren.net/library/state-worlds-mothers-2012-nutrition-first-1000-days [Last accessed November, 2020]
6. UNICEF. (2005). The baby-friendly hospital initiative. [online] Available from https://www.unicef.org/nutrition/index_24806.html [Last accessed November, 2020]
7. UN Inter-Agency Group for Child Mortality Estimation. Estimates developed by the UN Inter-Agency Group for Child Mortality Estimation (UNICEF, WHO, World Bank, UN DESA Population Division). [online] Available from www.childmortality.org [Last accessed November, 2020]
8. World Health Organization. (2015). Breastfeeding. [online] Available from www.who.int/features/factfiles/breastfeeding/en/ [Last accessed November, 2020]
9. World Health Organization. (2020). Infant and young child feeding. [online] Available from www.who.int/mediacentre/factsheets/fs342/en/ [Last accessed November, 2020]

Oncofertility

Veena Ranjan

INTRODUCTION

Teresa K Woodruff termed the coin "oncofertility" at the Oncofertility Consortium in 2006. "Oncofertility is a subfield that bridges oncology and reproductive research to explore and expand options for the reproductive future of cancer survivors." It is an important aspect of supportive care among young cancer survivors.[1]

Occurrence of cancers in young women has two main concerns: Present fertility and future fertility. The young woman may be currently pregnant or may be aspiring to become pregnant later on in life. These two are different entities and shall be discussed in two separate sections: "Pregnancy in genital malignancies" and "Preserving fertility in women with malignancies."

PREGNANCY IN GENITAL MALIGNANCIES

When a pregnant woman is diagnosed with malignancy, it leads to a contradicting situation of birth of a new life and a life-threatening illness. Fortunately, this is a very rare situation, the incidence being 0.05–0.1%.[2] But when it occurs, it leads to dilemmas in management as there is lack of randomized studies to choose the appropriate therapeutic methods and the care providers have to depend entirely on knowledge derived from case reports, registries, and observational studies. We will be seeing more of these cases as women are increasingly postponing their pregnancies for the sake of their career growth. Most common malignancies seen among pregnant women are gynecological cancers (especially cervical and ovarian cancer), breast cancer, lymphatic system neoplasm, and melanoma.[3,4]

Initially, the diagnosis of malignancy in pregnancy was seen as a clear indication for termination of pregnancy. But today, termination of pregnancy is not the only solution and it is possible for the woman to hope for cure for herself and for the birth of a healthy baby, albeit the treatment is more complex and needs the coordination of a multidisciplinary team for the management consisting of oncologist, obstetrician, and neonatologist. Therapeutic abortion for cancer during the pregnancy can be recommended for locally advanced-stage cervical carcinoma, advanced breast cancer or breast cancer necessitating adjuvant systemic treatment, stage III-IV aggressive non-Hodgkin's lymphoma (NHL) or Hodgkin's disease, and acute leukemia.[5]

Gynecological Cancers Coexisting with Pregnancy

The most common gynecological cancers diagnosed during pregnancy are cervical and ovarian cancers. Endometrial cancer and vulvar and vaginal cancer are very rare in pregnancy.

Cervical Cancer

Cervical cancer is the most common gynecological cancer during pregnancy (1–12 cases per 10,000 pregnancies).[6] Noninvasive lesions diagnosed after complete evaluation do not need any treatment till delivery of the baby, and treatment can be postponed until after birth of the baby. But monitoring in each trimester with colposcopy for progression of the disease is a must.[7,8]

In case of invasive disease, the management mainly depends on the stage of the disease, the status of the lymph nodes, and gestational age at diagnosis.[7] Accurate staging of the disease is very important and can be achieved by clinical examination and MRI to assess cervical growth, uterus, bladder, rectum, parametrium, and lymph nodes. Gadolinium can be used as a contrast medium for MRI use only if it is absolutely essential.[9] Other than assessment of pelvic lymph nodes by imaging, laparoscopic lymphadenectomy is possible between the 13th and the 22nd weeks of pregnancy for histopathological confirmation of lymph node involvement.[10]

For stage 1A cervical cancer without lymph node involvement, waiting for fetal maturity is a valid option with close monitoring and treatment after birth of the baby. Similar treatment is acceptable for stage 1B1 cancers with <2-cm growth and negative lymph nodes. In locally advanced cervical cancer, chemoradiation is the treatment of choice and this necessitates termination of pregnancy. If surgical termination of pregnancy is not possible due to large cervical growth, radiation can be started and this will lead to embryonic/fetal death. If the patient is keen to continue pregnancy, neoadjuvant chemotherapy with intensive monitoring is an option and definitive treatment can be started after birth of the baby. Cisplatin/carboplatin and paclitaxel are the preferred drugs for neoadjuvant chemotherapy. It is extremely important to keep the patient well informed about all treatment options and the need for close monitoring. It is equally important to obtain a written informed consent from the patient for the therapy chosen.[7,8,10,11]

Ovarian Cancer

Most of the ovarian masses during pregnancy are diagnosed on USG done for pregnancy itself and majority of them are benign masses. For further evaluation of the mass to differentiate between the benign and malignant nature of the mass, USG with or without color Doppler and MRI are preferred. Contrast-enhanced computed tomography (CECT) is contraindicated in pregnant patients. Tumor markers such as CA-125 are elevated due to pregnancy itself and are not helpful in differentiating benign from malignant masses.

Among malignant tumors, germ cell tumors are the most common, followed by sex cord stromal tumors, borderline tumors, and finally invasive epithelial cancers.[12] Early stage ovarian cancers can be treated surgically in second and early third trimesters. Surgical staging consisting of peritoneal washings for cytology, adnexectomy of the affected side, random peritoneal biopsies, omentectomy, and removal of suspicious lymph nodes should be performed. Both laparoscopy and laparotomy are acceptable, but it is essential to avoid peritoneal spillage in both the cases. Adjuvant chemotherapy with paclitaxel and carboplatin can be safely given in the second and third trimesters. For germ cell tumors, the bleomycin, etoposide and platinum (BEP) regimen is associated with severe growth restriction and other neonatal complications; as a result, the European Society for Medical Oncology (ESMO) recommends weekly paclitaxel and cisplatin in these patients.[13]

Advanced ovarian malignancy in the first and second trimesters of pregnancy needs complete cytoreduction followed by adjuvant therapy disregarding the pregnancy. If advanced disease is diagnosed in the third trimester, neoadjuvant chemotherapy can be given and cesarean delivery and complete cytoreduction can be done after achieving fetal maturity. It is essential to remember that chemotherapy should not be given 3 weeks prior to delivery as it known to be associated with increased risk of infections in the mother and increased neonatal complications such as pancytopenia due to myelosuppression.

Placental Metastases

Placental metastases in gynecological cancers occurring during pregnancy are very rare (3%) when compared to other malignancies such as malignant melanoma (32%), leukemia and lymphoma (15%), and breast cancer (13%). The placenta should be sent for histopathological examination and if found positive for metastasis, the infant should be evaluated.[14,15]

■ DIAGNOSIS OF CANCER

Unfortunately, diagnosis of cancer in pregnancy is often delayed due to various reasons; many symptoms of malignancy are similar to the symptoms of pregnancy, including nausea/vomiting, breast changes, abdominal pain, anemia, and fatigue. Physical examination may be difficult due to dense breasts and the enlarged gravid uterus. In addition, the clinician may be more hesitant to get the appropriate tests because of concerns that laboratory results may be inaccurate or that radiologic testing is harmful. Owing to its rarity, cancer might not even be considered in the differential diagnosis of many symptoms.

Safety of Diagnostic Work-up

Imaging Procedures

Imaging in pregnancy to diagnose and stage cancer may create conflict between maternal benefit and fetal risk. Radiation exposure of >100 mGy is associated with fetal malformation and childhood cancer. Imaging tests for the purpose of staging among pregnant women should be limited to those associated with the lowest exposure to ionizing radiation. Abdominal plain X-rays, isotope scans, and computerized tomography should be avoided. In contrast, chest X-ray, MRI, and abdominal ultrasound should be used for staging procedures. Positron-emission tomography (PET) imaging in pregnancy is not recommended in pregnancy due to high dose of radiation for the fetus.[16-18]

Laboratory Testing

The utility of tumor markers in pregnancy is debatable as there is significant alteration in the levels of various tumor markers due to pregnancy itself. Many tumor markers such as CA 15-3 used in breast cancer, CA-125 used in epithelial ovarian cancer, and alpha-fetoprotein used in germ cell tumors are physiologically elevated in pregnancy. Physiological changes in pregnancy lead to alteration of commonly used laboratory values such as hemoglobin and hematocrit values which will appear lower, whereas alkaline phosphatase and lactate dehydrogenase are typically higher in pregnancy.[19-21]

■ ADJUVANT TREATMENT

Chemotherapy

During pregnancy, chemotherapy used in gynecological malignancies is relatively safer after the first trimester. Two main concerns with chemotherapy in pregnancy are fetal malformations (12.7–17%) and growth restriction (40%), respectively. It mainly depends on the transplacental transfer of chemotherapeutic drugs which is lower for certain drugs (paclitaxel) and higher for some (carboplatin). In spite of this, carboplatin administered after the first trimester causes little harm to the developing fetus. However, cisplatin is implicated in growth restriction and hearing loss, whereas etoposide is implicated in pancytopenia.[20-22]

Radiotherapy

The main problems with radiotherapy during pregnancy are embryonic/fetal death, gross malformations, growth retardation, sterility, cataracts, and other neuropathology and secondary malignancies. The fetal dose should not exceed 50–100 mGy.[23,24]

■ PRESERVING FERTILITY IN WOMEN WITH MALIGNANCY

Diagnosis of cancer in a young patient can be a devastating situation. Cancers by themselves and the treatments used to cure them have significant negative effects on the fertility of young patients. Major diagnostic and therapeutic advances have improved survival rates of cancer patients markedly over the past years. One of the major sequelae of cytotoxic chemotherapy and/or radiotherapy in young girls and women is premature ovarian failure which depends on the age and follicular reserve of the patient and the type and dose of the drugs used. Eventhough majority of young cancer survivors are interested in parenthood, very few access fertility preservation techniques prior to treatment. While cancer elsewhere in the body affects the reproductive system mainly due to effects of therapies, cancer of reproductive organs is a difficult situation due to the complexity involved. Patients should be made aware of possible effects their treatment could have on sexual function, reproductive function, and their future potential for having children. The woman should also discuss about birth control during treatment and also about the possibility of premature menopause. Several strategies aimed at the preservation of fertility have been developed in these groups of patients: gonadal protection or fertility-sparing approaches using both medical and surgical strategies.

Medical Strategies

Hormone Suppression

Both GnRH agonists (GnRHas) and antagonists (which function with identical end-results) have been used in gonadal protection during cytotoxic chemotherapy. GnRH simulate a prepubertal hormonal milieu and, through this mechanism, and/or possibly others, might minimize the gonadotoxic effect of chemotherapy and increase the chances of spontaneous ovulations.[25] It is essential to remember that treatment with GnRH should begin at least one week before the beginning of chemotherapy as the initial flare-up effect causes undesirable ovarian stimulation. The application should continue in the form of depot injections during the whole duration of chemotherapy, so that the downregulating effect remains for at least 2 weeks after the chemotherapy. Although this therapy is found to have significant protective effect on postchemotherapy ovulation and resumption of menses, subsequent pregnancy rates have been inconsistent.[26] An interesting downside of GnRH was hypothesized by Emons et al.,[27] who noted that a variety of cells including those of the breast, ovary, and endometrium express GnRH receptors and the direct effects of GnRH on human cancer cells are not sufficiently understood. These receptors mediate several effects, such as inhibition of proliferation, induction of cell-cycle arrest, and inhibition of apoptosis, induced by cytotoxic drugs. So they reported that GnRH, a therapy concomitant with cytotoxic chemotherapy, might actually reduce the efficacy of chemotherapy.

Progestins and endometrial cancer: Endometrial cancer in a young nulliparous woman desirous of pregnancy is a difficult situation for the treating gynecologic oncologist. Standard management would involve removal of the uterus and ovaries which will obviously preclude any hope of pregnancy. Fortunately, this is not a common scenario; <10% of endometrial cancers occur in women <40 years of age and very few of them will be desirous of fertility. Fertility-sparing options using conservative treatment are possible only in well-differentiated early endometrial cancer in the absence of any myometrial invasion or adnexal disease seen on imaging. These options include treatment with hormones with different routes of administration based on the hormone sensitivity of these tumors. Hormones include progestogens, antiestrogens, GnRH, and aromatase inhibitors, while the most widely used are progestogens, especially high-dose medroxyprogesterone acetate (600 mg/day orally) and megestrol acetate (160–320 mg/day orally). Endometrial sampling every 3 monthly has to be done to assess the response to treatment. The side effects of such high-dose progestins include thrombus formation, mood alterations, headaches, weight gain, and breast pain and/or tenderness. To circumvent these side effects due to systemic high dose of progestins, the progesterone-releasing intrauterine device (IUD) is used to generate a localized effect within the endometrium. Response to treatment has been high (rates of 73–81%), but not absolute. Recurrence rates are also appreciable (18–40% with follow-up times up to 358 months).[28] Assisted reproductive technologies (ARTs) may be necessary for conception in these women after achieving complete remission.[28] The biggest concern with conservative management of endometrial carcinoma is disease progression while on treatment or after initial response to medical treatment. Women opting for conservative management should be aware that hormonal therapy is not the standard form of management and regular follow-up is essential. A potential adverse oncologic outcome should be considered before deciding for conservative treatment.

Surgical Strategies

Ovarian Transposition and Gonadal Shielding

Irradiation to the ovaries can be quite damaging, and successful ovarian protection in this circumstance has been achieved through ovarian transposition. In this technique, the ovaries are transposed, laparoscopically or in a laparotomy, to a location outside of the field of radiation. This procedure has the advantage not only of sparing fertility, but also of maintaining ovarian function and evading premature menopause. The procedure precludes spontaneous pregnancy, requiring ART.

Cervical Cancer

Although 40% of all cases of invasive cervical cancer in the United States are diagnosed in women younger than 45 years of age, the scenario in India is not the same. In our country, women complete their family quite early and the need for fertility preservation in treatment of cervical cancer is not that frequent. Standard treatment of invasive cancer in early stages includes radical hysterectomy and pelvic radiotherapy, both of which are incompatible with fertility. Cervical conization, simple trachelectomy (cervicectomy), and radical trachelectomy (resection of parametrial tissue with cervix) are being used in women with early stage disease.[29] Radical trachelectomy combined with pelvic lymphadenectomy, open or laparoscopic, has been proposed by Dargent et al. as a conservative treatment for cervical cancer in stage 1A or 1B tumors (<2 cm).[29] It is a must to assess the pelvis for the extent of disease and perform pelvic lymphadenectomy before proceeding with radical trachelectomy. They suggest that the vaginal approach limits the parametrial resection to tissue in the medial half of the broad ligament, restricting radical vaginal trachelectomy to those women with tumors <2 cm and with invasion of <10 mm. Because the abdominal radical trachelectomy procedure appears to be equivalent to the traditional radical procedure, this limitation may not be applicable to abdominal trachelectomies. Successful pregnancies after abdominal radical trachelectomy procedure have been reported. In a study of 236 women reported to have undergone radical vaginal trachelectomy, 63 liveborn babies have been reported.[30] Although there were no recurrences in patients treated with abdominal radical trachelectomy, concerns about long-term adverse events limit the possibility of recommendation of this technique for general use. Adverse effects of the treatment include cervical stenosis, dysmenorrhea, infertility, hematoma, hematosalpinx, or endometriosis. Obstetric adverse events such as second-trimester miscarriages and preterm births have led to propose a more conservative treatment, the simple trachelectomy for very early lesions.

Ovarian Cancer

In the case of ovarian neoplasms, certain factors such as tumor histologic subtype, stage, extent of disease, preexisting ovarian reserve, and willingness of the patient decide the possibility of fertility-sparing surgery. But it is extremely important to remember that we are handling a potentially recurrent disease and the patient should be counseled accordingly regarding the need for strict follow-up.

The most-suited ovarian tumors for fertility-sparing surgery are nonepithelial malignant ovarian tumors, particularly germ-cell tumors. Germ-cell tumors are routinely managed by conservative surgery, unilateral salpingo-ovariotomy, but it has to be emphasized about the need for adequate staging. Cure rates are quite high (90–95%), and despite the usual need for postoperative chemotherapy, resumption of menstruation occurs in at least 80% of patients.[31]

Eventhough epithelial tumors occur at a later age, borderline ovarian tumors, neoplasms of controversial biologic potential and clinical significance, occur at a younger age and deserve a special mention. More than 30% of borderline tumors of the ovary affect women under 40 years of age. They share a risk profile similar to that of malignant ovarian tumors but are associated with a much better prognosis. Surgical staging followed by conservative surgery may be considered among young women who wish to preserve fertility in borderline cases. Although recurrence rates for early borderline tumors have been reported to be similar to or slightly higher than those for traditional surgical management, survival rates are not compromised as recurrences are well treated with repeat and definitive surgical management.[32]

A small proportion of invasive epithelial cancer occurs in women younger than 35 years of age. Conservative treatment can be considered for young women who desire to preserve their fertility and have stage 1A well-differentiated disease. Unilateral salpingo-oophorectomy along with adequate surgical staging is considered an appropriate therapy in these women. The results of unilateral salpingo-

TABLE 1: Fertility conservation in gynecological cancers.[42]

Gynecological cancer	Stage	Recommendation
Cervical cancer	Up to stage IB1 (<2 cm growth)	Radical trachelectomy, simple trachelectomy, cervical conization
Endometrial cancer	Stage IA, grade 1	Hormonal therapy: Progestins
Ovarian cancer	Stage IA, grade 1	Unilateral salpingo-ovariotomy
Others	–	GnRHa during chemotherapy, ovarian transposition, gonadal shielding, mature oocyte cryopreservation, embryo cryopreservation
Prepubertal girls	–	Ovarian cryopreservation and transplantation (experimental)[40]

oophorectomies have been compared with hysterectomies and bilateral salpingo-oophorectomies, and 5-year survival rates are found to be similar in both groups.[33]

Endometrial Cancer

There are few case reports from Europe about hysteroscopic resection of early endometrial cancer followed by progestin therapy as an option for conservative surgical management.[34] The procedure included hysteroscopic resection of the tumor followed by resection of the adjacent endometrium and myometrium. As of now, there are no data to recommend this method as superior to the medical method of progestins' use in conservative management of endometrial cancer. Among women with low-risk endometrial cancer, hysterectomy without removing ovaries is another option to preserve fertility. Evidences from the Korean Gynecology Oncology Group and a recent population-based study have confirmed the safety of this ovarian conservation as a viable option for women with low-risk endometrial cancer. They found that there was no significant difference in recurrence-free survival or overall survival among those who had their ovaries removed along with hysterectomy and those who did not.[35,36]

Other Fertility-preservation Strategies

Advances in medicine and technology have led to increasing survival rates in patients affected by oncological disease, and this is paralleled by advances in reproductive medicine leading to the development and increasing use of various fertility-preservation techniques. For children, adolescents, women without partners, or women wishing to retain their ability for paternity selection at the time of fertilization, oocyte cryopreservation is the only fertility-sparing option. Embryo cryopreservation is a widely used method of fertility preservation and has been available to cancer patients with partners for years. But there are few downsides of controlled ovarian stimulation (COS) which is a part of these methods of fertility preservation; the stimulation protocol takes approximately 2 weeks from the 2nd day of the period, and this may cause delay in initiating cancer treatment, high estradiol levels during stimulation may have a stimulatory effect on tumors with estrogen receptors, and partner's or

donor's sperm is required for embryo cryopreservation which limits reproductive autonomy of the woman. Ovarian tissue cryopreservation and transplantation of ovarian tissue seem to be the most promising way of future fertility. This method does not require ovarian stimulation and can be performed immediately so as to enable starting cytotoxic chemotherapy in aggressive cancers. It also has an added advantage of not requiring sexual maturity and hence may be the only method available in children. It is also an important option for women with hormone-sensitive tumors. As of now, the only established methods for fertility prevention in female cancer patients are in vitro fertilization and embryo cryopreservation and oocyte cryopreservation.[37-41]

KEY POINTS

- Various medical and surgical strategies have been developed to preserve fertility in young women afflicted with cancers, especially gynecological cancers **(Table 1)**.
- GnRH produce a prepubertal hormonal milieu reducing the gonadotoxic effect of chemotherapy. Progestins play an important role in the conservative management of early stage well-differentiated endometrial cancer.
- Radical trachelectomy and more recently even simple trachelectomy have been used with promising results for early stage cervical cancer.
- Conservative surgery with adequate surgical staging can be used in germ cell ovarian tumors, borderline epithelial ovarian tumors, and early invasive cancers.
- It is extremely important to emphasize on the need for strict follow-up.
- Ovarian transposition, gonadal shielding, oocyte cryopreservation, and embryo cryopreservation are being used in women with cancers before embarking on definitive treatment.
- Ovarian tissue cryopreservation and transplantation after cytotoxic chemotherapy are found to be a promising option in future.

■ REFERENCES

1. Teresa K. Woodruff. The Oncofertility Consortium—addressing fertility in young people with cancer. Nat Rev Clin Oncol. 2010;7(8):466-75.

2. Teran-Porcayo MA, Gomez-Del Castillo-Rangel AC, Barrera-Lopez N, Zeichner-Gancz I. Cancer during pregnancy: 10-year experience at a regional cancer reference center in Mexico. Med. Oncol. 2007;24:297-300.

3. Eibye S, Kjaer SK, Mellemkjaer L. Incidence of pregnancy-associated cancer in Denmark, 1977–2006. Obstet Gynecol. 2013;122:608-17.

4. Parazzini F, Franchi M, Tavani A, Negri E, Peccatori FA. Frequency of pregnancy related cancer: A population based linkage study in Lombardy, Italy. Int J Gynecol Cancer. 2017;27:613-9.

5. Pavlidis NA. Coexistence of pregnancy and malignancy. Oncologist. 2002;7:279-87.

6. Skrzypczyk-Ostaszewicz A, Rubach M. Gynaecological cancers coexisting with pregnancy – a literature review. Contemp Oncol (Pozn). 2016;20(3):193-8.

7. Morice P, Uzan C, Gouy S, Verschraegen C, Haie-Meder C. Malignancies in pregnancy 1. Gynaecological cancers in pregnancy. Lancet. 2012;379:558-69.

8. Ilancheran A, Low J, Ng JS. Gynaecological cancer in pregnancy. Best Pract Res Clin Obstet Gynaecol. 2012;26:371-7.

9. Balleyguier C, Fournet C, Ben Hassen W, Zareski E, Morice P, Haie-Meder C, et al. Management of cervical cancer detected during pregnancy: role of magnetic resonance imaging. Clin Imaging. 2012;37:70-6.

10. Amant F, Halaska MJ, Fumagalli M, Steffensen KD, Lok C, Van Calsteren K, et al. Gynecologic cancers in pregnancy: guidelines of a second international consensus meeting. Int J Gynecol Cancer. 2014;24:394-403.

11. Hoellen F, Reibke R, Hornemann K, Thill M, Luedders DW, Kelling K, et al. Cancer in pregnancy. Part I: basic diagnostic and therapeutic principles and treatment of gynaecological malignancies. Arch Gynecol Obstet. 2012;285:195-205.

12. Leiserowitz GS, Xing G, Cress R, Brahmbhatt B, Dalrymple JL, Smith LH. Adnexal masses in pregnancy: How often are they malignant? Gynecol Oncol. 2006;101:315-21.

13. Zagouri F, Dimitrakakis C, Marinopoulos S, Tsigginou A, Dimopoulos MA. Cancer in pregnancy: Disentangling treatment modalities. ESMO Open. 2016;1:e000016.

14. Pavlidis N, Pentheroudakis G. Metastatic involvement of placenta and foetus in pregnant women with cancer. Recent Results Cancer Res. 2008;178:183e94.

15. Miller K, Zawislak A, Gannon C, Millar D, Loughrey MB. Maternal gastric adenocarcinoma with placental metastases: what is the fetal risk? Pediatr Dev Pathol. 2012;15:237e9.

16. McCollough CH, Schueler BA, Atwell TD, Braun NN, Regner DM, Brown DL, et al. Radiation exposure and pregnancy: When should we be concerned? Radiographics. 2007;27:909-17; discussion 917–918.

17. Wang PI, Chong ST, Kielar AZ, Kelly AM, Knoepp UD, Mazza MB, et al. Imaging of pregnant and lactating patients: Part 2, evidence-based review and recommendations. AJR Am J Roentgenol. 2012;198:785-92.

18. Almuhaideb A, Papathanasiou N, Bomanji J. 18F-FDG PET/CT imaging in oncology. Ann Saudi Med. 2011;31:3-13.

19. Han SN, Lotgerink A, Gziri MM, Van Calsteren K, Hanssens M, Amant F. Physiologic variations of serum tumour markers in gynaecological malignancies during pregnancy: A systematic review. BMC Med. 2012;10:86.

20. Sarandakou A, Protonotariou E, Rizos D. Tumor markers in biological fluids associated with pregnancy. Crit Rev Clin Lab Sci. 2007;44:151-78.

21. Moore RG, Miller MC, Eklund EE, Lu KH, Bast RC Jr, Lambert-Messerlian G. Serum levels of the ovarian cancer biomarker HE4 are decreased in pregnancy and increase with age. Am J Obstet Gynecol. 2012;206:349.e1-349.e7.

22. Cordeiro CN, Gemignani ML. Gynecologic malignancies in pregnancy: Balancing fetal risks with oncologic safety. Obstet Gynecol Surv. 2017;72:184-93.

23. Shaw P, Duncan A, Vouyouka A, Ozsvath K. Radiation exposure and pregnancy. J Vasc Surg. 2011;53(Suppl.1):28S-34S.

24. Stovall M, Blackwell CR, Cundiff J, Novack DH, Palta JR, Wagner LK, et al. Fetal dose from radiotherapy with photon beams: Report of AAPM Radiation Therapy Committee Task Group no. 36. Med Phys. 1995;22:63-82.

25. Blumenfeld Z. How to preserve fertility in young women exposed to chemotherapy? The role of GnRH agonist co-treatment in addition to cryopreservation of embryo, oocytes, or ovaries. Oncologist. 2007;12(9):1044-54.

26. Bedaiwy MA, Abou-Setta AM, Desai N, Hurd W, Starks D, El-Nashar SA, et al. Gonadotropin releasing hormone analog co-treatment for preservation of ovarian function during gonadotoxic chemotherapy: a systematic review and meta-analysis. Fertil Steril. 2011;95:906-14.e1–4.

27. Emons G, Grundker C, Gunthert AR, Westphalen S, Kavanagh J, Verschraegen C. GnRH antagonists in the treatment of gynaecological and breast cancers. Endocrine-Related Cancer. 2003;10(2):291-9.

28. Gotlieb WH, Beiner ME, Shalmon B, Korach Y, Segal Y, Zmira N, et al. Outcome of fertility-sparing treatment with progestins in young patients with endometrial cancer. Obstet Gynecol. 2003;102:718-25.

29. Dargent D, Martin X, Sacchetoni A, Mathevet P. Laparoscopic vaginal radical trachelectomy: a treatment to preserve the fertility of cervical carcinoma patients. Cancer. 2000;88(8):1877-82.

30. Roy M, Plante M. Pregnancies after radical vaginal trachelectomy for early-stage cervical cancer. Am J Obstet Gynecol. 1998;179(6 Pt 1):1491-6.

31. Gershenson DM. Fertility-sparing surgery for malignancies in women. J Natl Cancer Inst Monogr. 2005;(34):43-7.

32. Nam JH. Borderline ovarian tumours and fertility. Curr Opin Obstet Gynecol. 2010;22:227-34.

33. Schilder JM, Thompson AM, DePriest PD, Ueland FR, Cibull ML, Kryscio RJ, et al. Outcome of reproductive age women with stage IA or IC invasive epithelial ovarian cancer treated with fertility-sparing therapy. Gynecol Oncol. 2002;87(1):1-7.

34. Mazzon I, Corrado G, Masciullo V, Morricone D, Ferrandina G, Scambia G. Conservative surgical management of stage IA endometrial carcinoma for fertility preservation. Fertil Steril. 2010;93: 1286-9.

35. Lee TS, Lee JY, Kim JW, Oh S, Seong SJ, Lee JM, et al. Outcomes of ovarian preservation in a cohort of premenopausal women with early-stage endometrial cancer: a Korean Gynecologic Oncology Group study. Gynecol Oncol. 2013;131:289-93.

36. Wright JD, Jorge S, Tergas AI, Hou JY, Burke WM, Huang Y, et al. Utilization and outcomes of ovarian conservation in premenopausal women with endometrial cancer. Obstet Gynecol. 2016;127:101-8.

37. Maltaris T, Boehm D, Dittrich R, Seufert R, Koelbl H. Reproduction beyond cancer: a essage of hope for young women. Gynecol Oncol. 2006;103(3):1109-21.

38. Mahajan N. Fertility preservation in female cancer patients: An overview. J Hum Reprod Sci. 2015;8(1):3-13.

39. Oktay K, Harvey BE, Partridge AH, Quinn GP, Reinecke J, Taylor HS, et al. Fertility Preservation in Patients with Cancer: ASCO Clinical Practice Guideline Update. J Clin Oncol. 2018;36:1994-2001.

40. Practice Committee of American Society for Reproductive Medicine. Ovarian tissue cryopreservation: a committee opinion. Fertil Steril. 2014;101(5):1237-43.

41. Suzuki N. Ovarian tissue cryopreservation and transplantation using thawed ovarian cortex for fertility preservation. Onco Fertil J. 2018;1:3-8.

42. Chan JL, Wang ET. Oncofertility for women with gynecologic malignancies. Gynecol Oncol. 2017;144(3):631-6.

Partogram

Kishor Rajurkar

■ DEFINITION

The partogram is defined as a pictorial assessment of the progress of normal labor. With the use of a partogram, the progress in labor can be seen at a glance on one sheet of paper and slow or obstructed labor can be recognized readily and described more easily.[1]

■ EVOLUTION OF A PARTOGRAPH

EA Friedman first described a partogram in 1954 by graphically plotting cervical dilatation against time. The curve obtained was a sigmoid curve.[2] In 1972, Philpot and Castle introduced the alert and action line. Responding to recommendations made during the Safe Motherhood Conference held in Nairobi in 1987, the World Health Organization (WHO) produced a partograph and tested its practical value to decrease maternal and perinatal morbidity and mortality. Since 1987, the WHO has published three different types of partographs. The WHO modified the partogram in 2000; the latent phase was excluded and the active phase commenced at 4-cm cervical dilatation. The WHO further modified the partograph with color coding.[3]

■ COMPONENTS OF A PARTOGRAPH[5]

The WHO partograph records the following points:

- *Patient information*: Name, age, parity, hospital registration number, date and time of admission, time of rupture of membranes, record of actual time **(Fig. 1)**
- *Fetal condition*:
  - Fetal heart rate (FHR)
  - Membrane (presence/absence), color of amniotic fluid

Molding of fetal skull
- Progress of labor
  - Cervical dilatation
  - Descent of head
  - Uterine contractions
- Maternal condition
  - Pulse, BP, temperature
  - Urine output, urine for protein, and acetone
  - Drugs, intravenous fluids, and oxytocin

Fetal Heart Rate

Record the FHR with a dot, half-hourly although it is checked every 15 minutes in the first stage and every 5 minutes in the second stage of labor.

Amniotic Fluid

In the box that correlates with the correct time according to the vertical lines, record half-hourly absence or presence and color of fluid as follows:

I: Membranes are intact.
C: Amniotic fluid is clear.
B: Amniotic fluid is blood stained.
M: Amniotic fluid has meconium staining.

Molding

0: Bones are separated and suture felt easily.
+: Bones are just touching each other.
++: Bones are overlapping.
+++: Bones are overlapping severely.

Progress of Labor

Cervicograph

The cervicograph is the section of the partogram which depicts cervical dilatation and descent of the presenting part in relation to time. Use of the cervicograph enables the progress of labor to be ascertained and delay in the progress readily recognized.

Cervical Dilatation

When a woman is admitted in the active phase, record X for the cervical dilatation on the alert line and at the time the examination is carried out. Vaginal examination is recommended every 4 hours. If the progress of labor is normal, then plotting of cervical dilatation will remain on the left of the alert line.

Descent of Fetal Head

Descent of the head is measured by abdominal palpation and is expressed in terms of fifths above the pelvic

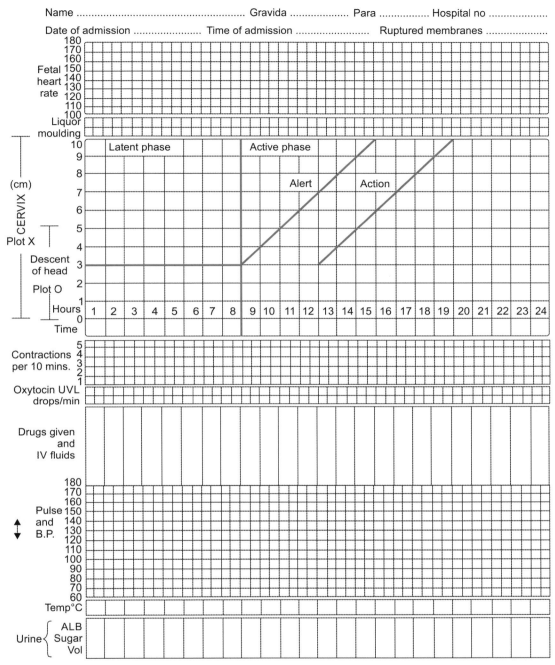

Fig. 1: Information of a patient.[3]

brim. Record O for the level of descent at each vaginal examination.

Alert and Action Lines

The Alert line starts at 4 cm of cervical dilatation and it travels diagonally upward to the point of expected full dilatation (10 cm) at the rate of 1 cm/hr.

The Action line is parallel to the Alert line and 4 hours to the right of the Alert line. These two lines are designed to warn you to take action quickly if the labor is not progressing normally **(Fig. 2)**.

The Action line is for making decisions at the health-facility level.

Uterine Contraction

Contractions are recorded every 30 minutes. Each square represents one contraction, so if two contractions are felt in 10 minutes, you should shade two squares.

On each shaded square, one must also indicate the duration of each contraction by using the symbols shown in **Figure 3**.

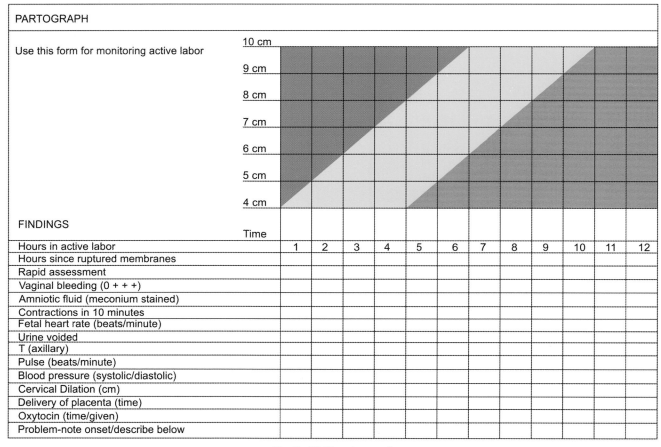

Fig. 2: WHO partogram.[3]

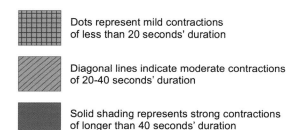

Dots represent mild contractions of less than 20 seconds' duration

Diagonal lines indicate moderate contractions of 20-40 seconds' duration

Solid shading represents strong contractions of longer than 40 seconds' duration

Fig. 3: Symbols to show the duration of each contraction.[5]

Oxytocin, Drugs, and Intravenous Fluids

They are given to the mother.

Blood Pressure, Pulse, Temperature, and Urine Output

Blood pressure is measured every 4 hours. Pulse is recorded every 30 minutes. Temperature is recorded every 2 hours. Urine output is recorded every time urine is passed.

■ CLINICAL UTILITY OF PARTOGRAMS[6]

- The partograph is a valuable tool to help you detect abnormal progress of labor, fetal distress, and signs that the mother is in difficulty.

- Refer the woman to a health center or hospital if the cervical dilatation mark crosses the Alert line on the partograph.

- When you identify +3 molding of the fetal skull with poor progress of labor, this indicates labor obstruction, so refer the mother urgently.

- FHR below 120/min or above 160/min for >10 minutes is an urgent indication to refer the mother, unless the labor is progressing too fast.

- Even with a normal FHR, refer if you see amniotic fluid (liquor) lightly stained with meconium in the latent first stage of labor.

- Moderately stained in the early active first stage of labor, or thick amniotic fluid in all stages of labor, unless the labor is progressing too fast.

■ PAPERLESS PARTOGRAPH[3]

Dr AK Debdas from India has proposed paperless partograph. In paperless partograph, the birth attendant calculates two times an ALERT ETD (estimated time of delivery) and ACTION ETD. If the woman does not deliver at the time of ACTION ETD, the diagnosis for abnormal labor is made.

ePARTOGRAPH[3]

Jhpiego and the John Hopkins Center for Bioengineering Innovation and Design developed a handheld device and software platform on the current partograph recommended by the WHO. The ePartogram improves timeliness of care and supported decision-making and improves quality of care in resource-constrained labor and delivery settings.[7]

MOBILE PARTOGRAPH[3]

Founded in 2002 out of MIT'S lab, Dimagi is a software social enterprise that develops technologies.

ZHANGE GUIDELINES[8]

Recently, a new curve has been developed to assess the progress of labor called the Zhange guidelines. It showed that the pattern of labor progression in contemporary practice differs significantly from the Friedman curve. The diagnostic criteria for protraction and arrest disorders of labor may be too stringent in nulliparous women. However, there is no significant difference in the frequency of intrapartum need of cesarean section between the obstetric units assigned to adhere to the WHO partograph and those assigned to adhere to Zhange's guideline.[9]

> ### KEY POINTS[4]
> - Charting of partograph starts when the woman is in the active phase of labor.
> - Active phase commences at 4-cm cervical dilatation.
> - Alert line differentiates women into two groups, women with cervical dilatation:
>   - ≥1 cm/hr
>   - Slower than 1 cm/hr who are more likely to require an intervention

> - WHO partograph does not differentiate between nulliparous and multiparous women.

REFERENCES

1. Friedman EA. Primigravid labor: a graphicostatistical analysis. Obstet Gynecol. 1955;6:567.
2. National Institute for Health and Care Excellence. (2019). Overview. Intrapartum care for healthy women and babies. Clinical guideline [CG190]. [online] Available from https://www.nice.org.uk/guidance/cg190 [Last accessed November, 2020]
3. Dalal A, Purandare A. The partograph in childbirth: An absolute essentiality or a mere exercise? J Obstet Gynecol India. 2017;68(1):3-14.
4. King Edward Memorial Hospital Obstetrics and Gynaecology. Labour: Partogram. (2019). [online] Available from http://www.wnhs.health.wa.gov.au/~/media/Files/Hospitals/WNHS/For%20health%20professionals/Clinical%20guidelines/OG/WNHS.OG.Labour-Partogram.pdf [Last accessed November, 2020]
5. Manjulatha VR, Anitha GS, Shivalingaiah N. Partogram: clinical study to assess the role of Partogram in primigravidae in labor. Int J Reprod Contracept Obstet Gynecol.. 2016;1014-25.
6. Lavender T, Hart A, Smyth RMD. Effect of partogram use on outcomes for women in spontaneous labour at term. Cochrane Database Syst Rev. 2013;7:CD005461.
7. Litwin LE, Maly C, Khamis AR, Hiner C, Zoungrana J, Mohamed K, et al. Use of an electronic partograph: feasibility and acceptability study in Zanzibar, Tanzania. BMC Preg Childbirth. 2018;18(1):147.
8. Zhang J, Landy HJ, Branch DW, Burkman R, Haberman S, Gregory KD, et al. Contemporary patterns of spontaneous labor with normal neonatal outcomes. Obstet Gynecol. 2010;116(6):1281-7.
9. Bernitz S, Dalbye R, Zhang J, Eggebø TM, Frøslie KF, Olsen IC, et al. The frequency of intrapartum caesarean section use with the WHO partograph versus Zhang's guideline in the Labour Progression Study (LaPS): a multicentre, cluster-randomised controlled trial. Lancet. 2019;393(10169):340-8.

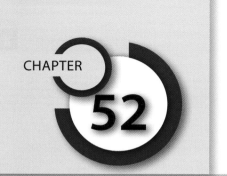

Nonstress Test

Prakash Mehta

◼ INTRODUCTION

The art of obstetrics is based on balancing of risks. By continuing a pregnancy, there might be a risk of death or damage in utero while termination could result in the risk of prematurity for the fetus and the risk of operative interventions for the mother. The primary objective of fetal surveillance is to prevent antenatal fetal deaths, which still account for greater than one-half of perinatal mortality. Antenatal fetal surveillance is a field of increasing importance in modern obstetrics, especially as results in perinatal care have made dramatic progress. It is an evolving field, and it is no longer acceptable just to wait and see when problems arise in pregnancy.

Several techniques for assessing fetal well-being are available to the obstetrician, including fetal movement counting, nonstress testing, contraction stress testing (CST), fetal biophysical assessment with real-time sonography, and Doppler ultrasonography for measuring umbilical and fetal blood flow. It is the obstetrician's reassurance that the fetal heart rate (FHR) pattern is normal and the nearly 100% certainty that the fetus is in a good condition which has made cardiotocography (CTG) so attractive and has induced its widespread use. However, as the father of CTG Hon has put it, "If you mess around with a process that works well 98% of times there is potential for harm."

◼ HISTORY[1]

The audibility of fetal heart tones was first described by Phillip Le Gaust in the 17th century. "The rate of the fetal heart is subject to considerable variations which affords us a fairly reliable means of judging as to the well-being of the child." This was excerpted from Dr J Whitridge Williams, in the second edition of Williams Obstetrics, in 1908.

As early as the mid-19th century, Kilian suggested that abnormalities of FHR, specifically tachycardia and bradycardia, indicated forceps delivery as soon as possible. The significance of interval changes in FHR began to be understood more fully in the 1950s and early 1960s after continuous fetal electrocardiogram monitoring was introduced by Hon. In 1969 Kubli et al. administered oxytocin to unmask uteroplacental insufficiency, and by 1972 Ray and colleagues introduced a formal technique for using oxytocin in this way, the oxytocin challenge test. In 1975, Freeman introduced the term "nonstressed antepartum monitoring" in the United States. That year, both Freeman and Lee and colleagues documented the association of FHR accelerations in response to spontaneous fetal movement with fetal well-being. They called this test the fetus acceleration determination test which was later christened as nonstress test (NST).[2]

◼ INSTRUMENT[3]

The cardiotocograph **(Fig. 1)**, more commonly known as an electronic fetal monitor or external fetal monitor (EFM) or NST, is used typically in the third trimester. A cardiotocograph measures simultaneously both the FHR and the uterine contractions, if any, using two separate disc-shaped transducers laid against the woman's abdomen. External measurement means taping or strapping the two sensors to the abdominal wall, with the heart ultrasonic sensor overlying the fetal heart and the contraction sensor measuring the tension of the maternal abdominal wall, an indirect measure of the intrauterine pressure. An ultrasound transducer similar to a Doppler fetal monitor measures the fetal heartbeat. A pressure-sensitive transducer,

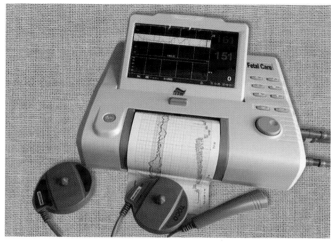

Fig. 1: Cardiotocograph.

called a tocodynamometer (toco), measures the strength and frequency of uterine contractions. Use of CTG and a computer network allows continual remote surveillance: a single nurse, midwife, or physician can watch the CTG traces of multiple patients simultaneously, via a computer station. The standard equipment consists of a multicrystal wide-beam transducer with a separate display for fetal heart sound and toco activity. A plain paper or high-resolution thermal array recorder is used for recording the trace. The Doppler transducer is with continuous autocorrelation processing with frequency –2.5 MHz and heart rate ranging from 30 to 240 bpm. The LED display, real-time FHR, and uterine activity (UA) value with a scaling of 30 bpm/cm settings on NST machines should be standardized so that paper speed is generally set to 1 centimeter (cm) per minute.

■ PHYSIOLOGY

The physiology behind the NST involves the fetal sympathetic and parasympathetic nervous systems and fetal baroreceptors. The sympathetic system is in the upper cardiothoracic nerves. These are the cardioaccelerator nerves and function from an earlier gestational age. The parasympathetic system matures later and works to slow the heart rate throughout pregnancy. This results in a decrease in baseline heart rate as the pregnancy matures. The aortic and carotid baroreceptors are responsible for moment-to-moment beating, and the chemoreceptors are stimulated by oxygen tension such that with acute hypoxia there will be increased variability, and with chronic hypoxia there will be decreased variability. Thus, the value of the NST is that in a nonacidotic, neurologically intact fetus, the heart rate should accelerate with fetal movements.

Technique

- The patient to be placed in a semi-Fowler's position or lateral tilt
- Blood pressure to be recorded
- Fluid volume assessment (hydrate patient when necessary)
- Avoid hypoglycemia (orange juice or coffee intake)
- Apply external monitors (Doppler as well as tocodynamometer)
- Instruct the mother to push button each time the fetus moves.
- Record a 20-minute window of heart rate monitoring regardless of the number of accelerations.
- If there are two accelerations of 15 bpm above baseline lasting for 15 seconds, NST is reactive.
- If the strip is nonreactive after 20 minutes, vibroacoustic stimulation may be used. An additional 20 minutes of examination is then required before the test is read as nonreactive.

Trace Analysis

The normal FHR pattern is characterized by a baseline frequency between 110 and 150 bpm, presence of periodic accelerations, a normal heart rate variability with a bandwidth between 5 and 25 bpm, and the absence of decelerations. The FHR pattern is abnormal when one or more of the following features are observed: a baseline frequency below 110 or above 150 bpm, absence of accelerations for >45 minutes, decreased or absent FHR variability, and existence of repeated variable or late decelerations. A baseline frequency between 100 and 110 bpm can be considered as normal when the duration of pregnancy has exceeded 41 weeks.[3] To identify the normal and abnormal FHR patterns,[4] the Rule of Four and Rule of Fifteen are applied. The four parameters are (1) the baseline heart rate, (2) variability and the periodic changes which include (3) acceleration, and (4) deceleration.

Baseline Heart Rate

Baseline heart rate is the mean level of the FHR when it is stable, excluding accelerations and decelerations. It is determined over a time period of 5 or 10 minutes and expressed in bpm. Preterm fetuses tend to have values toward the upper end of this range. A trend to a progressive rise in the baseline is important as well as the absolute values. The normal baseline FHR is 110–160 bpm, moderate bradycardia 100–109 bpm, moderate tachycardia 161–180 bpm, abnormal bradycardia <100 bpm, and abnormal tachycardia >180 bpm.

Fetal Tachycardia

Fetal tachycardia is defined as a baseline heart rate greater than 160 bpm and is considered a nonreassuring pattern. Tachycardia is considered mild when the heart rate is 160–180 bpm and severe when >180 bpm. Tachycardia >200 bpm is usually due to fetal tachyarrhythmia or congenital anomalies rather than hypoxia alone; persistent tachycardia > 180 bpm, especially when it occurs in conjunction with maternal fever, suggests chorioamnionitis. Fetal tachycardia may be a sign of increased fetal stress when it persists, but it is usually not associated with severe fetal distress unless decreased variability or another abnormality is present.

Causes of fetal tachycardia

- Hypoxia
- Maternal anxiety
- Maternal fever
- Maternal anemia
- Fetal anemia 4F
- Fetal state drugs
- Physiologic fetal
- Infections

- Tachyarrhythmia
- Thyrotoxicosis
- Doubling FHR

Fetal Bradycardia

Fetal bradycardia is defined as a baseline heart rate < 120 bpm. Bradycardia in the range of 100–120 bpm with normal variability is not associated with fetal acidosis. Bradycardia of this degree is common in postdate gestations and in fetuses with occiput posterior or transverse presentations. Bradycardia <100 bpm occurs in fetuses with congenital heart abnormalities or myocardial conduction defects, such as those occurring in conjunction with maternal collagen vascular disease. Moderate bradycardia of 80–100 bpm is a nonreassuring pattern. Severe prolonged bradycardia of < 80 bpm that lasts for 3 minutes or longer is an ominous finding indicating severe hypoxia and is often a terminal event.[1]

Causes of fetal bradycardia
- Hypoxia
- Idiopathic
- Hypopituitarism
- Hypotension
- Drugs
- Bradyarrhythmia
- Hypotension
- Halving of FHR

Baseline Variability[5]

Baseline variability is the minor fluctuations in baseline FHR occurring at three to five cycles per minute. It is measured by estimating the difference in beats per minute between the highest peak and the lowest trough of fluctuation in a 1-minute segment of the trace.
- *Normal baseline variability*: –5 bpm between contractions
- *Nonreassuring baseline variability*: <5 bpm for 40 minutes or more but <90 minutes
- *Abnormal baseline variability*: <5 bpm for 90 minutes or more. Loss of variability may be uncomplicated and may be the result of fetal quiescence (rest-activity cycle or behavior state), in which case the variability usually increases spontaneously within 30–40 minutes.

Causes of increased variability:
- Drugs (ephedrine)
- Increased fetal activity
- Cord compression
- Excessive uterine contraction
  - Meconium aspiration following variable deceleration

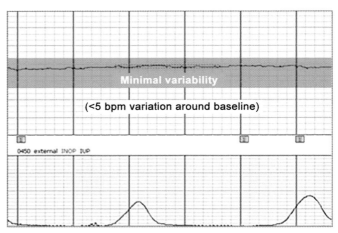

Fig. 2: Decreased FHR variability.

*Causes of decreased variability (**Fig. 2**):*
- Hypoxia
- Hypotension
- Fetal anomalies
- *Drugs*: CNS depressants: Diazepam/MgSO$_4$
  - *Parasympatholytics*: Atropine and hydroxyzine
- *Centrally acting adrenergic agents*: Methyldopa
- Physiological
- Arrhythmia

Saltatory Pattern[6]

Grossly increased variability of >25 bpm can be caused by acute hypoxia or mechanical compression of the umbilical cord. This pattern is most often seen during the second stage of labor. The presence of a saltatory pattern, especially when paired with decelerations, is a warning to look for and try to correct possible causes of acute hypoxia and to be alert for signs that the hypoxia is progressing to acidosis. Although it is a nonreassuring pattern, the saltatory pattern is usually not an indication for immediate delivery.

Periodic Fetal Heart Rate Changes

Accelerations (Figs. 3A and B)

Accelerations are transient increases in FHR of 15 bpm or more and lasting for 15 seconds or more. The significance of no accelerations on an otherwise normal CTG is unclear. They are usually associated with fetal movement, vaginal examinations, uterine contractions, umbilical vein compression, fetal scalp stimulation, or even external acoustic stimulation. The presence of accelerations is considered a reassuring sign of fetal well-being. An acceleration pattern preceding or following a variable deceleration (the "shoulders" of the deceleration) is seen only when the fetus is not hypoxic.[7] Accelerations are the basis for the NST.

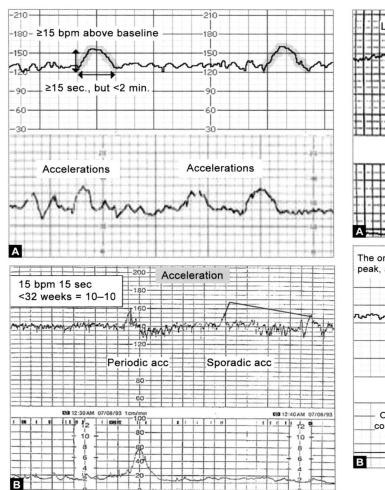

Figs. 3A and B: FHR acceleration.

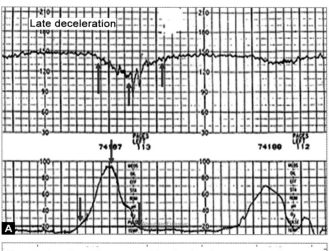

The onset, nadir, and recovery of the deceleration occur after the onset, peak, and recovery of the contraction respectively, in most cases

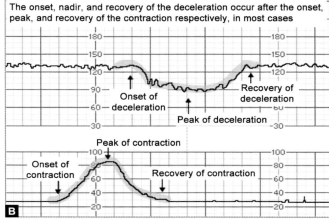

Figs. 4A and B: FHR deceleration.

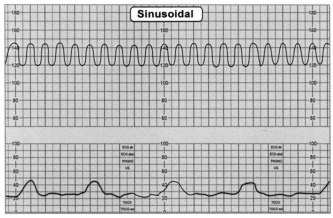

Fig. 5: Sinusoidal pattern.

Decelerations (Figs. 4A and B)

Decelerations are transient episodes of slowing of FHR below the baseline level of >15 bpm and lasting for 15 seconds or more.

Sinusoidal Pattern[8]

Sinusoidal pattern **(Fig. 5)** is a regular oscillation of the baseline long-term variability resembling a sine wave. This smooth, undulating pattern, lasting at least 10 minutes, has a relatively fixed period of 3–5 cycles per minute and an amplitude of 5–15 bpm above and below the baseline. It is also characterized by a stable baseline heart rate of 120–160 bpm and absent beat-to-beat variability. The true sinusoidal pattern is rare but ominous and is associated with high rates of fetal morbidity and mortality. It should be differentiated from the "pseudosinusoidal" pattern, which is a benign, uniform long-term variability pattern. A pseudosinusoidal pattern shows less regularity in the shape and amplitude of the variability waves and the presence of beat-to-beat variability, compared with the true sinusoidal pattern.

Causes of sinusoidal pattern

- Fetal anemia associated with Rh disease
- Acidosis
- Fetal anomalies

- Drugs
- Anencephaly following variable deceleration

Indication and Frequency

There are many indications for NST, and the frequency of testing also depends on the condition.

Condition GA Frequency

- Post-term pregnancy for 41 weeks
- Biweekly PROM at onset
- Daily bleeding for 26 weeks or at onset
- Biweekly oligohydramnios for 26 weeks or at onset
- Biweekly polyhydramnios for 32 weeks
- Weekly collagen disease/antiphospholipid antibodies (APLA) for 28 weeks
- Weekly diabetes class A1 (well-controlled) 36 weeks
- Weekly diabetes classes A2 and B (well-controlled) 32 weeks biweekly
- Chronic or pregnancy-induced hypertension 28 Weeks Weekly
- Biweekly severe anemia 32 weeks
- Weekly impaired renal function 28 weeks weekly
- Biweekly decreased fetal movements
- As per complaint once + Rpt SOS IUGR 28 weeks
- Biweekly previous intrauterine death
- Week before the event weekly

■ RESULT[3]

Reactive or Reassuring Nonstress Test (Fig. 6)

Reactive or reassuring nonstress test demonstrates two or more fetal movements accompanied by a FHR acceleration of 15 bpm or more lasting at least 15 seconds during a 20-minute period. Lack of fetal movement is nondiagnostic, and a repeat NST should be performed after a meal. Lack of movement for short periods of time may be attributable to fetal sleep. However, absence of movement for prolonged periods of time may be ominous.

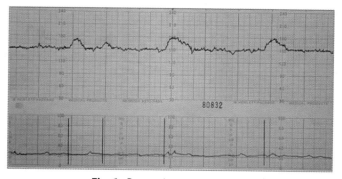

Fig. 6: Reassuring nonstress test.

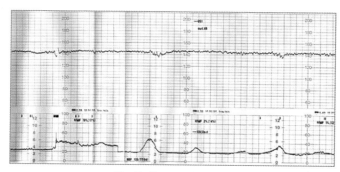

Fig. 7: Nonreactive CTG.

Nonreactive Nonstress Test (Fig. 7)

- No fetal movements or accelerations of heart beat (generally poor or no long-term variability)
- Baseline rate may be outside or within the normal range or decelerations are present.

Characteristics of Reassuring and Nonreassuring FHR Tracings

The reassuring FHR patterns include each of the following: (1) a baseline FHR of 110–160 bpm, (2) moderate variability, (3) gestational age-appropriate FHR accelerations, and (4) absence of FHR decelerations. The presence of all four of these criteria assures that no fetal acidemia is present. In the absence of accelerations, either spontaneous or elicited (i.e., by techniques such as scalp stimulation, vibroacoustic stimulation, or fetal scalp sampling), a combination of minimal or absent variability with late or variable decelerations typically constitutes a nonreassuring CTG and is predictive of acidemia.

Response

The dictum: Treat the patient, not the trace! Structured approach is a must.

Reactive Nonstress Test

With a high degree of certainty, a reassuring pattern indicates that there is no fetal acidemia at the time of testing. On the other hand, the nonreassuring pattern is suggestive of potential fetal acidemia and worsening fetal status, and the need for further measures to reassure the provider of the fetus's health. (1) The reactive NST should be performed each week if the medical problem appears to be persistent, i.e., chronic hypertension and renal disease. (2) The reactive NST may not need to be repeated in the potentially noncontinuous problem such as decreased fetal movement for which the fetus begins to move daily after this one episode.

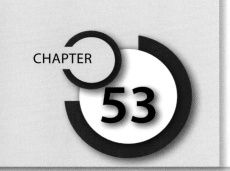

Sildenafil Citrate in Obstetrics and Gynecology

Suyajna Joshi D, Sanjana Kumar

INTRODUCTION

Sildenafil citrate, a phosphodiesterase type 5 (PDE5) inhibitor and the blockbuster erectile dysfunction drug, has been marketed across the globe since its approval by the Food and Drug Administration (FDA) in 1998. Its role in obstetrics has gained importance recently due to it's newer indications but still lacks adequate evidence through trials.

The drug has been used for improving the endometrial thickness for implantation, for improving uteroplacental circulation in FGR-oligoamnios. Many such indications have caught the attention of clinicians.

HISTORY

Sildenafil (compound UK-92,480) was synthesized by Pfizer scientists, Andrew Bell, David Brown, and Nicholas Terrett. The compound sildenafil was initially studied on an experimental basis for use in the treatment of hypertension and angina pectoris. The first clinical trials suggested that the drug had less effect on angina and could induce marked penile erections.[1] Pfizer thus started marketing it for erectile dysfunction, and this decision is often cited as an example of drug repositioning.[2,3] Informally called by the names *"blue pill,"* *"blue diamond"* (for it is marketed as a diamond-shaped blue pill by Pfizer), *"vitamin V"* and so on, sildenafil soon became a massively marketed drug.

Being the first to be named among the other PDE5 inhibitors such as Tadalafil, Vardenafil and Avanafil, sildenafil citrate has been commonly used orally followed by the intravenous route. However, recent trials have used the drug per vaginally for gynecological indications. The half-life of sildenafil citrate is 3–4 hours with an onset of action of 20 minutes. It is metabolized in the liver by CYP3A4.[4]

MECHANISM OF ACTION

Phosphodiesterase metabolizes cyclic guanosine monophosphate (cGMP) which brings about smooth muscle relaxation, and therefore inhibition of PDE5 by sildenafil causes increased cGMP with associated vasodilation independent of nitric oxide (NO) **(Fig. 1)**.

INDICATIONS

Due to its efficient vasodilatory effects, sildenafil citrate has been tried in all possible conditions requiring vasodilation, the most common of them being erectile dysfunction. Other common indications are pulmonary hypertension and peripheral vascular disease. The drug has recently been introduced to the world of obstetrics and gynecology, especially in assisted reproductive technology (ART), with its potential benefits to be addressed in the near future.

WELL-ESTABLISHED USES

The well-established uses of sildenafil citrate are given in **Box 1**.

INDICATIONS UNDER TRIAL

The indications that are under trial are given in **Box 2**.

COMMON ADVERSE EFFECTS[5]

The common adverse effects are given in **Box 3**.

CONTRAINDICATIONS[5]

- Patients on nitrates or nitrites
- Coronary heart disease
- Liver, kidney disease
- Peptic ulcer disease
- Leukemia
- Sickle cell anemia
- Myeloma
- History of allergy or hypersensitive reactions in the past

SILDENAFIL IN OBSTETRICS

Sildenafil: Pregnancy Category B Drug

Based on animal data, Sildenafil has shown no evidence of teratogenicity, embryotoxicity, and fetotoxicity even in maximum recommended human dose (MRHD). Due to its effectiveness and safety profile, it has made significant impact in its usage in obstetrics and also in ART.

Sildenafil potentiates the action of NO. With this effective action, it is used in the treatment of maternal

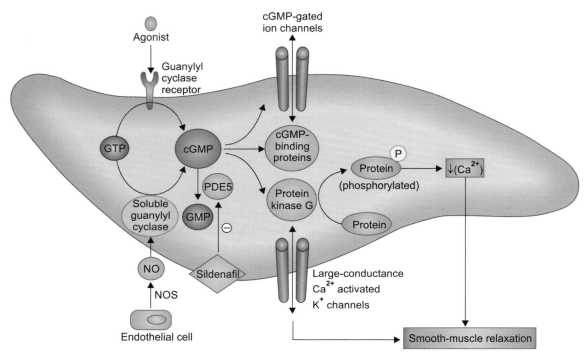

Fig. 1: Mechanism of action of sildenafil citrate. (cGMP: cyclic guanosine monophosphate; GTP: guanosine triphosphate; PDE5: phosphodiesterase type 5)

BOX 1: Well-established uses of sildenafil citrate.

- *Sexual dysfunction (males):*
  - Erectile dysfunction
  - Antidepressant-associated sexual dysfunction
- Pulmonary hypertension
- *Peripheral vascular disease:*
  - In Raynaud's phenomenon
  - To alleviate vasospasm, treat ischemic ulcers

BOX 2: Indications under trial

- High-altitude pulmonary edema
- In cardiac failure
- *Uses in obstetrics:*
  - Fetal growth restriction
  - Oligoamnios
  - Preeclampsia
  - Intrapartum fetal distress
  - Pulmonary artery hypertension in pregnancy
  - Threatened miscarriage in patients with recurrent pregnancy loss (RPL)
- *Uses in gynecology:*
  - Endometrial preparation before in vitro fertilization in cases with thin endometrium
  - For menstrual cramps and dysmenorrhea
  - To improve sexual arousal in women
- To improve exercise capacity in athletes

BOX 3: Common adverse effects.

- Headache (due to vasodilation)
- Flushing (due to vasodilation)
- Nasal congestion (due to vasodilation)
- Dyspepsia (due to relaxation of the gastroesophageal sphincter)
- Photophobia (week inhibition of PDE6 → interference with photoreceptor transduction in the retina)
- Blurred vision
- Cyanopsia
- Nonarteritic ischemic optic neuropathy
- Hypotension (due to PDE3 inhibition)

(PDE: phosphodiesterase)

---

which significant research and trials have been conducted to prove the beneficial impact of sildenafil are given in the following text.

Areas of Interests

Fetal Growth Restriction and Uteroplacental Insufficiency

Fetal growth restriction is defined as a pathological condition in which a fetus fails to achieve its growth completely and is often associated with variable degrees of uteroplacental insufficiency. It approximately affects 8% of all pregnancies contributing to perinatal morbidity and mortality due to many causes such as preterm births, fetal heart distress, asphyxia, neonatal encephalopathy, and altered immune function.[6] In the long term, growth-restricted babies have a risk of incidence of hypertension, diabetes mellitus, and coronary heart disease in adulthood.[7-9]

pulmonary arterial hypertension (PAH) for selective vasodilatation of the pulmonary vessels. It is also used in neonates (including those born preterm) for the treatment of persistent pulmonary hypertension. Other conditions in

Normal

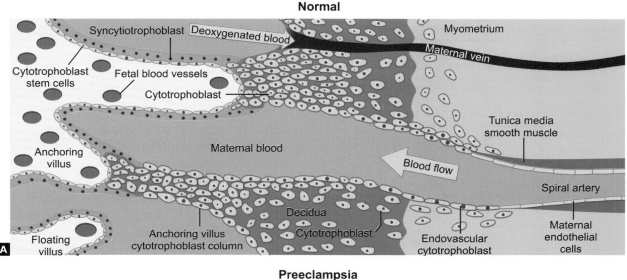

Preeclampsia

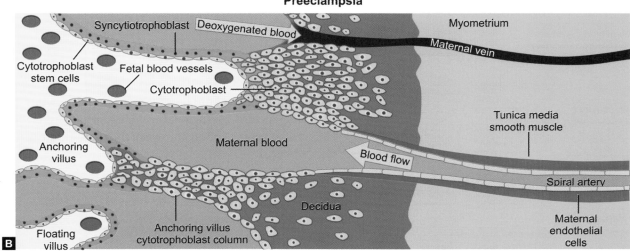

Figs. 2A and B: (A) Adequate trophoblastic invasion of spiral arteries converting them into low-resistance large caliber canals unresponsive to pressors; (B) Deficient trophoblastic invasion of spiral arteries leading to high-resistance vascular flow.

In a normal pregnancy with adequate trophoblast-driven modification of spiral arteries, blood flow through uterine vessels increases dramatically from approximately 50 mL/min at 10 weeks' gestational age to over 1,200 mL/min at term **(Figs. 2A and B)**.[10]

A poorly altered uteroplacental vasculature is the hallmark of the current pathogenic model of preeclampsia wherein aberrant spiral artery changes lead to a weakly perfused uteroplacental unit.[11,12]

Pathogenesis of preeclampsia and FGR: The pathogenesis of preeclampsia and FGR is shown in **Flowcharts 1 and 2**.

Fetal growth restriction is one condition in which the risk of expectant management and the hazards of preterm due to termination of pregnancy have to be delicately balanced. It has been approximated that for each extra day of prolongation of pregnancy between 24 and 32 weeks, there is a nonlinear gain of 1% in fetal viability.[13]

Currently, there are not many particular evidence-based therapies for severe early onset FGR. Nonspecific interventions mainly include lifestyle modifications, less work, rest at home, hospital admission for rest, and surveillance. Although these widely accepted methods of management are not based on conclusions from randomized controlled trials, they are used in the belief that rest will reduce the steal by the glutei and quadriceps from the uteroplacental circulation.

Therefore, there has been a constant search for an effective drug to treat uteroplacental insufficiency and give the benefit of expectant management to the baby. Based on studies conducted on guinea pigs and rats, sildenafil citrate is tried and is expected to cause a potential therapeutic strategy to improve uteroplacental blood flow in FGR pregnancies in humans.

Flowchart 1: Pathogenesis of preeclampsia and FGR-stage 1.

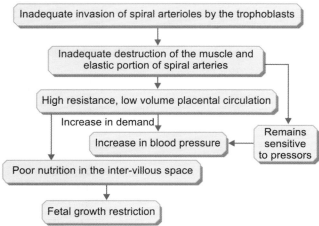

Flowchart 2: Pathogenesis of preeclampsia and fetal growth restriction-stage 2.

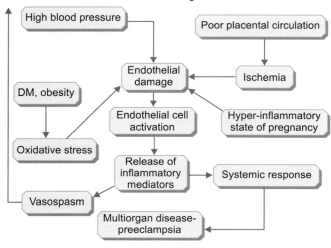

Role of sildenafil citrate in FGR:

- During pregnancy, NO is synthesized in the uteroplacental tissues and endothelial cells to maintain a low vascular resistance in the utero- and fetoplacental circulations.[14-16] Acting similar to NO, sildenafil can be considered to be an effective option for the management of FGR and uteroplacental insufficiency.
- The maternal side of the placenta has greater PDE5 than other sites, thus increasing the efficacy of sildenafil.[17] Also, it can obviously counterbalance the vascular dysfunction caused by augmented vasoconstrictors, i.e., the imbalance between the pressors and vasodilators in pregnancy.[18,19]

Because not many significant maternal and fetal side effects were observed in pregnant women using sildenafil for pulmonary artery hypertension, there was a change from preclinical to clinical studies for the use of sildenafil for FGR and preeclampsia.

Many single-center and multicenter clinical trials concluded that sildenafil significantly increases the placental blood flow and the perinatal outcome without any significant harm to the mother or baby.

However, the Dutch STRIDER (Sildenafil Therapy in Dismal prognosis Early-Onset Fetal Growth Restriction) trial conducted from 2015 to 2018 on 216 participants concluded with disappointing negative results that sildenafil does not improve severe FGR and it may increase the risk of neonatal pulmonary hypertension. The STRIDER trial was a placebo-controlled randomized controlled trial which included pregnant women between 20 weeks and 27 weeks 6 days gestational age with severe FGR **(Flowchart 3)**. The test group received sildenafil citrate 25 mg thrice a day, and the primary outcome was studied in terms of perinatal mortality and major neonatal morbidity until hospital discharge which did not differ significantly between the test and placebo groups.[20]

Similarly, the New Zealand and Australia STRIDER trial 2019 showed zero significant effect on fetal growth velocity in early onset FGR groups.

Multicenter studies on various population groups and different target gestational ages are warranted as evidence is still lacking regarding the use of sildenafil citrate in women with FGR.

Flowchart 3: Study design of STRIDER trial.

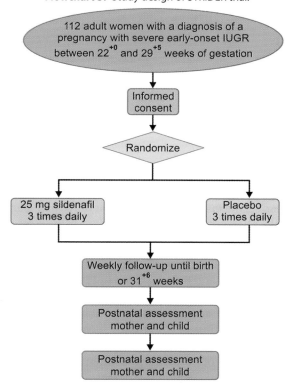

Preeclampsia

Preeclampsia accounts for 5–10% in pregnant population and is the leading cause of severe acute maternal morbidity and mortality. Early onset preeclampsia is most of the time associated with FGR and varying degrees of placental insufficiency as the two conditions share the common pathology of high-resistance uteroplacental circulation.

Therefore, the use of a drug like sildenafil that decreases the blood pressure and also improves the placental circulation would be of great value, especially in handling cases of early preterm with preeclampsia. Studies conducted have concluded that sildenafil citrate significantly lowers vasoconstriction and enhances the endothelial function of myometrial vessels in patients with preeclampsia and FGR.[21]

KEY POINTS

- Preeclampsia and FGR have a common pathogenesis of inadequate or defective trophoblastic invasion of spiral arteries causing high-resistance placental circulation in contrast to the low-resistance vascular channels not responsive to pressors seen in normal pregnancies.
- Poor placental blood flow decreases nutrition in the intervillous space→FGR.
- Sildenafil citrate, being a potent vasodilator, improves the placental blood flow and corrects the imbalances between pressors and vasodilators.
- Placenta is rich in PDE5 receptors.
- The dose most endorsed in most studies is 25 mg 8th hourly till delivery.
- The Dutch STRIDER study trial was abruptly stopped as it showed more risk of neonatal pulmonary hypertension.
- It warrants more studies and research trials to implement its use in routine practice.

Intrapartum Fetal Distress

In many pregnancies, placental function is sufficient to allow adequate growth of the fetus but not enough to meet the extra demands. Uterine contractions are accompanied with up to 60% decrease in uterine blood flow that could cause intrapartum hypoxia in these babies which clinically present as heart rate abnormalities and meconium-stained liquor.[22] Up to 63% of babies become compromised and suffer oxygen deprivation in labor and have no prior antenatal risk factors.[23] Events in labor account for as many as 20% cases of cerebral palsy in term infants, and almost 45% of stillbirths occurring during labor are usually due to hypoxia.[24]

Among the adequately grown fetuses at term, a part of them have evidence of cerebral redistribution similar to that seen in growth-restricted fetuses.[25,26] This cerebral redistribution is an adaptive response to suboptimal placental function and occurs before an obvious lag in growth velocity. So, there is always a possibility that suboptimal placental perfusion that has remained unrecognized presents itself for the first time during labor, and this calls for an active intervention so as to prevent adverse perinatal outcomes and unnecessary increase in caesarean section rates. Unfortunately, there are no interventions available for nonreassuring intrapartum fetal status but for delivery.

Role of sildenafil in intrapartum fetal distress **(Flowchart 4)**: Attributing to its vasodilator properties and mechanism of action similar to that in FGR and preeclampsia, sildenafil citrate has been tried in the management of intrapartum fetal compromise.

The RIDSTRESS (Reducing the risk of fetal distress with sildenafil study) was the first reported study evaluating the efficacy of sildenafil citrate on reducing the risk of intrapartum fetal compromise.

Methodology: RIDSTRESS was a phase 2 double-blind, randomized controlled trial wherein pregnant women with term pregnancy in latent labor or undergoing scheduled induction of labor were selected and randomly allocated into sildenafil citrate and control groups. The women in the sildenafil group received sildenafil citrate 50 mg orally every 8 hours (up to 150 mg) and those in the control group received a placebo.

Results: It was found that sildenafil citrate reduced the risk of emergency cesarean birth, meconium-stained liquor, and altered fetal heart rate patterns.[27]

However, larger phase 3 trials are necessary to recommend the clinical use of sildenafil citrate for intrapartum fetal compromise.

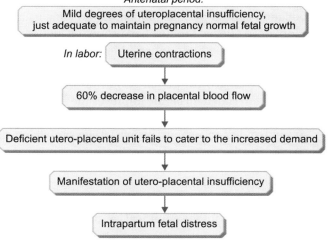

Flowchart 4: Pathophysiology of intrapartum fetal distress.

Antenatal period:

Mild degrees of uteroplacental insufficiency, just adequate to maintain pregnancy normal fetal growth

In labor: Uterine contractions

↓

60% decrease in placental blood flow

↓

Deficient utero-placental unit fails to cater to the increased demand

↓

Manifestation of utero-placental insufficiency

↓

Intrapartum fetal distress

KEY POINTS

- A small group among the adequately grown fetuses have mild degrees of uteroplacental insufficiency which manifests itself only during labor.
- Labor demands a 60% increase in blood flow which the already compromised placental circulation fails to provide → intrapartum fetal distress.
- Sildenafil citrate → vasodilation → improved placental circulation → decreases the incidence of intrapartum fetal compromise.
- The RIDSTRESS was the first reported study evaluating the efficacy of sildenafil citrate on reducing the risk of intrapartum fetal distress and it concluded that sildenafil citrate reduces the risk of emergency operative birth, meconium-stained liquor, and pathologic fetal heart rate patterns.

Recurrent Pregnancy Loss

Recurrent pregnancy loss is currently defined as three or more pregnancy losses prior to 20 weeks not necessarily consecutive of which more than half are unexplained. The routine workup done for RPL does not rule out the immunological and endometrial receptivity factors which could be the possible etiologies in a number of cases.

Role of sildenafil citrate in RPL:

- Decreased natural killer (NK) cell activity preventing implantation failure
- Vasodilation and increased uterine artery blood flow leading to improved endometrial width
- Uterine arterial blood flow indexes such as systolic/diastolic (S/D) ratio, resistive index (RI), and pulsatility index (PI) showed significant improved results.

While improving the uterine blood flow in the proliferative phase, NO may have ill effects on the endometrium during the implantation phase due to NO-facilitated release of cytokines from the NK cells—a possible cause of implantation failure. NO-independent vasodilation caused by sildenafil citrate explains its anti-inflammatory effects. Studies have shown a statistically significant decrease in peripheral blood NK cell activity after management with vaginal sildenafil.[29-31]

Endometrial growth depends on the uterine artery blood flow and sildenafil citrate improves the endometrial thickness by its vasodilatory effects.

Several studies have shown beneficial effects of sildenafil when used in prior menstrual cycles in achieving pregnancy by increasing the blood flow to endometrium and increasing the receptivity.[32,33]

However, according to consensus there are no recommendations for the empirical use of sildenafil citrate in women with RPL.

Pulmonary Hypertension in Pregnancy

Pulmonary hypertension is defined as an increase in the mean pulmonary pressure > 25 mm Hg at rest or >30 mm Hg with exercise.[34] Pregnancy in women with pulmonary hypertension is associated with a mortality rate as high as 30–56%.[35] The physiological changes associated with pregnancy allow a huge amount of fluid to collect in interstitial space. Following delivery, this fluid is shifted into maternal circulation, increasing preload and further increasing pulmonary hypertension.[36,37]

Sildenafil causes vasodilation of the pulmonary vascular bed and in systemic circulation. It also has a positive inotropic effect on the hypertrophic right ventricle.[38] Echocardiography is very useful in such situations to assess the severity. A multidisciplinary approach is must for tackling the situation. Being a category B medication, use of sildenafil in pregnant women with PAH has been tried and found to be safe.

KEY POINTS

- Sildenafil citrate has been found to have a role in improving the endometrial receptivity in cases of RPL.
- *Mechanisms*:
  - Decreased NK cell activity preventing implantation failure
  - Vasodilation and increased uterine artery blood flow leading to improved endometrial thickness
- Sildenafil has also been tried in the treatment of pulmonary hypertension in pregnancy. It makes vasodilation of the pulmonary vascular bed and in systemic circulation. It also causes a positive inotropic effect on the hypertrophic right ventricle.

Effect of Sildenafil on Maternal Hemodynamics in Pregnancies Complicated by Severe Early Onset Fetal Growth[39]

Unlike in normotensive pregnant women, impaired cardiac output has been reported in women who develop hypertensive disorders in the antenatal period. The same has been shown to be present in those with FGR. Arterial stiffness is a marker of vascular health and is a prognostic marker for cardiovascular disease in general population. Both pulse wave velocity (PWV), which is a direct measure of arterial stiffness, and augmentation index (AIx), which is a measure of arterial stiffness, can be measured noninvasively in pregnancy.

A multicenter cardiovascular substudy was conducted by Asma Khalil and colleagues in the UK on 135 women (70 women randomized to sildenafil and 65 to placebo) from 18 fetal medicine units in the UK between November 2014 and July 2016 with the aim to investigate the effect of

Flowchart 5: Mechanism of action of sildenafil on endometrial vasculature.

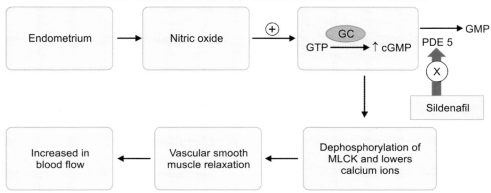

(cGMP: cyclic guanosine monophosphate; GTP: guanosine triphosphate; MLCK: myosin light-chain kinase)

sildenafil on maternal hemodynamics in pregnancies with severe early onset FGR.

The dose administered was 25 mg three times per day versus the placebo equivalent in pregnancies complicated by severe early onset FGR.

The results of this study showed the following:

- Sildenafil reduces maternal BP accompanied with a compensatory rise in heart rate.
- Even after adjusting for maternal BP and heart rate, sildenafil also reduces arterial stiffness in pregnant women with severe early onset FGR.
- However, these changes are less significant and have no short- or long-term clinical impact on the mother.

SILDENAFIL CITRATE IN GYNECOLOGY

For Endometrial Preparation in Assisted Reproductive Technology Cycles

Successful implantation of an embryo needs a receptive endometrium, a good-quality embryo, and synchronization between the two.[40] In spite of recent advances in ovarian stimulation protocols, an unresponsive and thin endometrium is still a challenge in assisted reproductive cycles.[41] The success of implantation is predicted by the thickness of the endometrium and the thickness by uterine blood flow.

Sildenafil citrate increases the blood flow to the uterine vessel **(Flowchart 5)** and in combination with estrogen, it leads to estrogen-mediated proliferation of endometrium.[42] As previously explained in this chapter, sildenafil also decreases the NK cell activity, inflammatory cytokines, and adds to the improvement in endometrial receptivity. Several studies have concluded that sildenafil citrate is effective in improving the outcome of fertility in women with recurrent implantation failure due to a thin endometrium. It can be used alone or in combination with estrogen considering the common causes for thin endometrium—poor uterine blood flow and deficiency of estrogen.

Outcomes of administration of Sildenafil citrate in ART-Salient studies:

- Sildenafil is effective in increasing the thickness of the endometrium and conception rates in infertility patients. Oral or vaginal preparations with dosage up to 100 mg/day from day 2 of cycle to day of human chorionic gonadotropin (HCG) trigger show promising results by increasing endometrial thickness up to 10–11 mm.[43]
- Use of sildenafil has shown significant improvements in Doppler indices in ART, especially in radial artery (RA-RI) and endometrial thickness.[44]
- Vaginally administered sildenafil has given better improvements in endometrial thickness as well as high implantation rates and good outcomes in ongoing pregnancy.[45]
- Addition of vaginal sildenafil as an adjuvant to oral estradiol valerate has significant concomitant effects in improving endometrium as well as pregnancy rates.[46]

Sexual Arousal in Women

For years, sildenafil citrate has been used for the treatment of sexual dysfunction in men. As there are similarities between male and female sexual responses, studies have assessed the effects of sildenafil citrate in women with a sexual arousal disorder.

The rationale behind the use of sildenafil citrate to improve sexual arousal in women is given in **Box 4**.

KEY POINTS

- Female sexual arousal disorder (FsAD) is more common than thought of.
- Conclusions from randomized controlled trials show that sildenafil citrate is moderately effective in treating FsAD.
- Sildenafil citrate is effective in patients with FsAD secondary to multiple sclerosis, diabetes, or

- antidepressant use; however, more trials in these patient populations are required to confirm hypothesis.
- Sildenafil citrate has a good safety profile in both sexes. However, limited data is available regarding this.

BOX 4: Rationale behind the use of sildenafil citrate to improve sexual arousal in women.

- PDE5 receptors are expressed in the vaginal, labial, and clitoral smooth muscles.[47]
- Sildenafil citrate → vasodilation → increased blood flow to the genitalia
- Engorgement of the clitoris and labia minora (modifications of the female analogue of penis in men) → improved sexual sensation and arousal
- Ultrafiltration of plasma by the capillary wall vessels contributes to lubrication of the vagina.[48]

(PDE5: phosphodiesterase type 5)

TABLE 1: Mechanisms of dysmenorrhea and the rationale of using sildenafil citrate for the same.

Mechanisms of dysmenorrhea	Mechanism of action of sildenafil citrate[43]
Poor uterine blood flow → ischemia → pain	Vasodilation → improved uterine artery blood flow → prevents ischemia
Increased myometrial contractions	Smooth muscle relaxation
Release of prostaglandins and mediators of pain	Increased blood flow → washout of prostaglandins and mediators of pain

Treatment of Primary Dysmenorrhea

Dysmenorrhea is a common gynecological problem for which newer treatment modalities have always been tried, but nonsteroidal anti-inflammatory drugs (NSAIDs) remain the mainstay of treatment. **Table 1** explains the mechanisms of dysmenorrhea and the rationale of using sildenafil citrate for the same.

Vaginal sildenafil citrate 100-mg single dose has been found to be effective in pain relief in primary dysmenorrhea.[49]

KEY POINTS

- The gynecological indications of sildenafil citrate under trial are: Recurrent implantation failure due to thin endometrium in ART, primary dysmenorrhea, and to improve sexual arousal in women.
- Sildenafil citrate increases the uterine blood flow and in combination with estrogen, it leads to estrogen-mediated proliferation of endometrium and also decreases the NK cell activity, inflammatory cytokines, and adds to improvement in endometrial receptivity.

- It has been found to improve sexual arousal in a small group of women, mainly due to increased blood supply to the genitalia and increased lubrication.
- Sildenafil has also been tried in the treatment of primary dysmenorrhea. It decreases pain due to smooth muscle relaxation and increase in uterine artery blood flow.

■ REFERENCES

1. ABM. (2008). Our clinicians regularly offer patients the opportunity to take part in trials of new drugs and treatments. Morriston Hospital in Swansea, was the first in the world to trial Viagra! [online] Available from https://web.archive.org/web/20080926034946/http://www.abm.university-trust.wales.nhs.uk/page.cfm?orgId=743&pid=29457 [Last accessed May, 2021]
2. Ashburn TT, Thor KB. Drug repositioning: identifying and developing new uses for existing drugs. Nature Rev Drug Discov. 2004;3(8):673-83.
3. Roundtable on Translating Genomic-Based Research for Health; Board on Health Sciences Policy; Institute of Medicine. Drug Repurposing and Repositioning: Workshop Summary. Washington (DC): National Academies Press; 2014.
4. Nichols DJ, Muirhead GJ, Harness JA. Pharmacokinetics of sildenafil after single oral doses in healthy male subjects: absolute bioavailability, food effects and dose proportionality. British J Clin Pharmacol. 2002;53(Suppl 1):5S-12S.
5. Tripathi KD. Essentials of Medical Pharmacology, 7th edition. New Delhi: Jaypee Brothers Medical Publishers; 2013. pp. 816–835.
6. Brar HS, Rutherford SE. Classification of intrauterine growth retardation. Semin Perinatol. 1988;12:2-10.
7. Barker DJ, Osmond C, Golding J, Kuh D, Wadsworth ME. Growth in utero, blood pressure in childhood and adult life, and mortality from cardiovascular disease. Br Med J. 1989;298:564-7.
8. Barker DJ, Gluckman PD, Godfrey KM, Harding JE, Owens JA, Robinson JS. Fetal nutrition and cardiovascular disease in adult life. Lancet. 1993;341(8850):938-41.
9. Barker DJ, Hales CN, Fall CH, Osmond C, Phipps K, Clark PM. Type 2 (non-insulin-dependent) diabetes mellitus, hypertension and hyperlipidaemia (syndrome X): relation to reduced fetal growth. Diabetologia. 1993;36:62-7.
10. Lang U, Baker RS, Braems G, Zygmunt M, Kunzel W, Clark KE. Uterine blood flow: a determinant of fetal growth. Eur J Obstet Gynecol Reprod Biol. 2003;110(Suppl 1):S55-61.
11. Lain KY, Roberts JM. Contemporary concepts of the pathogenesis and management of preeclampsia. JAMA. 2002;287:3183-6.
12. Roberts JM, Lain KY. Recent insights into the pathogenesis of pre-eclampsia. Placenta. 2002;23:359-72.
13. Manktelow B, Seaton S, Field D, Draper ES. Population based estimates of in-unit survival for very preterm infants. Pediatrics. 2013;131:e425-32.
14. Moncada S, Higgs A. The L-arginine-nitric oxide pathway. N Engl J Med; 1993;329:2002-12.
15. Learmont J, Poston L. Nitric oxide is involved in flow-induced dilation of isolated human small fetoplacental arteries. Am J Obstet Gynecol. 1996;174:583-8.
16. Lees C, Valensise H, Black R, Harrington K, Byiers S, Romanini S, et al. The efficacy and fetal–maternal cardiovascular effects of transdermal glyceryl trinitrate in the prophylaxis of preeclampsia

and its complications: a randomized double-blind placebo-controlled trial. Ultrasound Obstet Gynecol. 1998;12(5):334-8.

17. Ferreira RDdS, Negrini R, Bernardo WM, Simões R, Piato S. The effects of sildenafil in maternal and fetal outcomes in pregnancy: A systematic review and meta-analysis. PLOS One. 2019;14(7):e0219732.

18. Burke SD, Zsengellér ZK, Khankin EV, Lo AS, Rajakumar A, DuPont JJ, et al. Soluble fms-like tyrosine kinase 1 promotes angiotensin II sensitivity in preeclampsia. J Clin Invest. 2016;126:2561-74.

19. Ramesar SV, Mackraj I, Gathiram P, Moodley J. Sildenafil citrate decreases sFlt-1 and sEng in pregnant l- NAME treated Sprague-Dawley rats. Eur J Obstet Gynecol Reprod Biol. 2011;157:136-40.

20. Sharp A, Cornforth C, Jackson R, Harrold J, Turner MA, Kenny LC, et al; STRIDER group. Maternal sildenafil for severe fetal growth restriction (STRIDER): a multicentre, randomised, placebo-controlled, double-blind trial. Lancet Child Adolesc Health. 2018;2(2):93-102. [Erratum in: Lancet Child Adolesc Health. 2018;2(2):e2.]

21. Wareing M, O'Hara M, Myers JE, Philip PN. Sildenafil citrate (viagra) enhances vasodilatation in fetal growth restriction. J Clin Endocrinol Metab. 2005;90:2550-5.

22. Janbu T, Nesheim B. Uterine artery blood velocities during contractions in pregnancy and labour related to intrauterine pressure. Br J Obstet Gynaecol. 1987;94(12):1150-5.

23. Low JA, Pickersgill H, Killen H, Derrick E. The prediction and prevention of intrapartum fetal asphyxia in term pregnancies. Am J Obstet Gynecol. 2001;184(4):724-30.

24. McIntyre S, Taitz D, Keogh J, Goldsmith S, Badawi N, Blair E. A systematic review of risk factors for cerebral palsy in children born at term in developed countries. Dev Med Child Neurol. 2013;55(6):499-508.

25. Prior T, Mullins E, Bennett P, Kumar S. Prediction of intrapartum fetal compromise using the cerebroumbilical ratio: a prospective observational study. Am J Obstet Gynecol. 2013;208(2):124.e1-6.

26. Prior T, Mullins E, Bennett P, Kumar S. Umbilical venous flow rate in term fetuses: can variations in flow predict intrapartum compromise? Am J Obstet Gynecol. 2014;210(1):61.e1-8.

27. Dunn L, Flenady V, Sailesh K. Reducing the risk of fetal distress with sildenafil study (RIDSTRESS): A double-blind randomised control trial. J Transl Med. 2016;14:15.

28. Hosseini S, Zarnani AH, Asgarian-Omran H, Vahedian-Dargahi Z, Eshraghian MR, Akbarzadeh-Pasha Z, et al. Comparative analysis of NK cell subsets in menstrual and peripheral blood of patients with unexplained recurrent spontaneous abortion and fertile subjects. J Reprod Immunol. 2014;103:9-17.

29. Karami N, Boroujerdnia MG, Nikbakht R, Khodadadi A. Enhancement of peripheral blood CD56(dim) cell and NK cell cytotoxicity in women with recurrent spontaneous abortion or in vitro fertilization failure. J Reprod Immunol . 2012;95:87-92.

30. Park DW, Lee HJ, Park CW, Hong SR, Kwak-Kim J, Yang KM. Peripheral blood NK cells reflect changes in decidual NK cells in women with recurrent miscarriages. Am J Reprod Immunol. 2010;63(2):173-80.

31. Ramos-Medina R, García-Segovia A, Gil J, Carbone J, Aguarón de la Cruz A, Seyfferth A, et al. Experience in IVIg therapy for selected women with recurrent reproductive failure and NK cell expansion. Am J Reprod Immunol. 2014;71(5):458-66.

32. Makled AK, Sabaa HA, Esmail MA, Aboelmagd SATI. Effect of sildenafil citrate on peripheral natural killer cells in women with recurrent pregnancy loss. Nat Sci. 2019;17(9):147-52.

33. Webb DJ, Freestone S, Allen MJ, Muirhead GJ. Sildenafil citrate and blood-pressure-lowering drugs: results of drug interaction studies with an organic nitrate and a calcium antagonist. Am J Cardiol 1999;83:21C-8C.

34. Saleh SA, Sayed TM, Elkhouly NI, Elaidy ME. The use of sildenafil citrate versus nifedipine in women with recurrent miscarriages: a pilot study. Menoufia Med J. 2018;31:1238-43.

35. Galiè N, Hoeper MM, Humbert M, Torbicki A, Vachiery JL, Barbera JA, et al. Guidelines for the diagnosis and treatment of pulmonary hypertension: the Task Force for the Diagnosis and Treatment of Pulmonary Hypertension of the European Society of Cardiology (ESC) and the European Respiratory Society (ERS), endorsed by the International Society of Heart and Lung Transplantation (ISHLT). Eur Heart J. 2009;30:2493-537.

36. Weiss BM, Zemp L, Seifert B, Hess OM. Outcome of pulmonary vascular disease in pregnancy: a systematic overview from 1978 through 1996. J Am Coll Cardiol. 1998;31(7):1650-7.

37. Zamanian RT, Haddad F, Doyle RL, Weinacker AB. Management strategies for patients with pulmonary hypertension in the intensive care unit. Crit Care Med. 2007;35(9):2037-50.

38. Harsoor SS, Joshi Suyajna D. Anaesthetic management of parturient with primary pulmonary hypertension posted for caesarean section-a case report. Indian J. Anaesth. 2005;49:2235.

39. Goland S, Tsai F, Habib M, Janmohamed M, Goodwin TM, Elkayam U. Favorable outcome of pregnancy with an elective use of epoprostenol and sildenafil in women with severe pulmonary hypertension. Cardiology. 2010;115(3):205-8.

40. Khalil A, Sharp A, Cornforth C, Jackson R, Mousa H, Stock S, et al. Effect of sildenafil on maternal hemodynamics in pregnancies complicated by severe early-onset fetal growth restriction: planned subgroup analysis from a multicenter randomized placebo-controlled double-blind trial. Ultrasound Obstet Gynecol. 2020;55:198-209.

41. Maruyama T. Therapeutic strategies for implantation failure due to endometrial dysfunction. J Mammal Ova Res. 2009;26:129-33.

42. Ledee N, Chaouat G, Serazin V, Lombroso R, Dubanchet S, Oger P, et al. Endometrial vascularity by three-dimensional power Doppler ultrasound and cytokines: a complementary approach to assess uterine receptivity. J Reprod Immunol. 2008;77:57-62.

43. Sher G, Fisch JD. Effect of vaginal sildenafil citrate on the outcome of in vitro fertilization (IVF) after multiple IVF failures attributed to poor endometrial development. Fertil Steril. 2002;78:1073-6.

44. El-Maghrabi HA, El-Kasar YS, Elbaz ZM, Youssef L. Effect of sildenafil citrate on endometrial thickness and pregnancy rate in frozen-thawed embryo transfer cycles. Austin J Obstet Gynecol. 2020;7(1):1150.

45. Takasaki A, Tamura H, Miwa I, Taketani T, Shimamura K, Sugino N. Endometrial growth and uterine blood flow: a pilot study for improving endometrial thickness in the patients with a thin endometrium. Fertil Steril. 2010;93(6):1851.

46. Srilaxmi Y, Arun V, Reddy AS. Role of sildenafil on endometrial characters in ovulation induction cycle. J Med Sci Clin R es. 2020;8(5). https://dx.doi.org/10.18535/jmscr/v8i5.62

47. Uckert S, Ellinghaus P, Albrecht K, Jonas U, Oelke M. Expression of messenger ribonucleic acid encoding for phosphodiesterase isoenzymes in human female genital tissues. J Sex Med. 2007;4(6):1604-9.

48. Gragasin FS, Michelakis ED, Hogan A, Moudgil R, Hashimoto K, Wu X, et al. The neurovascular mechanism of clitoral erection: nitric oxide and cGMP-stimulated activation of BKCa channels. FASEB J. 2004;18(12):1382-91.

49. Dmitrovic R, Kunselman AR, Legro RS. Sildenafil citrate in the treatment of pain in primary dysmenorrhea: a randomized controlled trial. Hum Reprod. 2013;28(11):2958-65.

Index

Page numbers followed by *b* refer to box, *f* refer to figure, *fc* refer to flowchart, and *t* refer to table